Clinical Psychology, Research and Practice

Fourth Edition

Clinical Psychology, Research and Practice

AN INTRODUCTORY TEXTBOOK

Fourth Edition

Paul Bennett

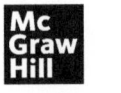
Open University Press

Open University Press
McGraw Hill
8th Floor, 338 Euston Road
London
England
NW1 3BH

email: enquiries@openup.co.uk
world wide web: www.openup.co.uk

First Edition published 2003
Second Edition published 2006
Third Edition Published 2011
First Published in this Fourth Edition 2021

A catalogue record of this book is available from the British Library

ISBN-13: 9780335248995
ISBN-10: 0335249000
eISBN: 9780335249008

Library of Congress Cataloging-in-Publication Data
CIP data applied for

Typeset by Transforma Pvt. Ltd., Chennai, India

Praise

"This book provides an excellent introduction to clinical psychology for undergraduate and postgraduate students. Written in an accessible style, the text effectively combines theory and research with practice examples and case studies. Chapter summary and discussion boxes offer a way to consolidate learning whilst the 'stop and think' boxes provide an opportunity to critically appraise and apply understanding to contemporary real world issues. Research boxes give the reader a detailed review of pertinent research studies whilst also modelling how research itself can be evaluated. This book is engaging, informative and offers incisive critique of key ideas throughout."
—Jason Davies, Professor of Forensic and
Clinical Psychology, Swansea University

"Comprehensive on key areas, theories and models, this book is well-suited to the undergraduate market. It would also be useful at postgraduate level, especially for conversion students as well as those starting to specialise in the more clinical aspects of psychology."
—Jessica Fielding, Lecturer in Psychology, University of Bristol

"This is an excellent, accessible introduction to clinical psychology that explores the key areas, controversies and debates in the field, while facilitating the development of students' critical appraisal skills. The book introduces various disorders from a psychological, social and biological perspective and different therapeutic interventions are thoroughly discussed. Particular strengths of this book include the use of comprehensive case formulations that bring to life the various disorders presented, and a scholarly discussion of developments in clinical practice including third wave cognitive behavioural therapies. I highly recommend this as a key text for practitioner psychology trainees and health care professionals working in medical settings."
—Christina Liossi, Chair in Paediatric Psychology,
University of Southampton and Honorary Consultant in
Paediatric Psychology, Great Ormond Street Hospital
for Children NHS Foundation Trust

Additional Resources

This fourth edition of *Clinical Psychology, Research and Practice* is supported by an Online Learning Centre, which can be accessed for free at: www.mheducation.co.uk/professionals/open-university-press/olc/bennett-clinical-psychology.

There you will find a range of additional resources for both students and instructors, to help bring the book's content to life.

Students can expect to find:

- Recommendations for popular films where themes of mental illness are explored, alongside analysis of how the portrayals in each film relate to the topics covered in this book
- Suggested resources for further study, including references for relevant fiction and non-fiction books, and links to YouTube videos and TEDX talks
- Sample essay questions, mapped to each section of the book, alongside suggested topics to cover in your response, and tips to avoid common mistakes

Instructors can expect to find:

- Lecture suggestions
- Proposed learning activities to run with students
- Suggested topics for lively classroom discussion and debate
- A ready-made PowerPoint for every chapter in the book, for use in your teaching
- Clearly articulated Learning Objectives and curriculum mapping

Brief Table of Contents

Detailed Table of Contents

Part 1

Background and methods

Part contents

1 Introduction

Chapter contents

This chapter introduces a number of issues relevant to mental health and clinical psychology, many of which are returned to in more detail later in the book. It starts by considering ways in which mental health problems have been conceptualized and treated over the years, before addressing modern concepts of mental health disorders from differing, and potentially challenging, perspectives. The chapter then examines a number of factors that contribute to the development and differing presentations of mental health disorders, focusing on genetic, biological, psychological, social, cultural, and familial explanations. Finally, it introduces the biopsychosocial approach, which attempts to integrate these various factors into one holistic model. By the end of the chapter, you should have an understanding of:

- Historical concepts and treatments of mental health problems
- Issues of diagnosis: the key diagnostic classification systems and their alternatives
- Models of the **aetiology** of mental health problems: genetic, biological, psychological, socio-cultural, developmental, and systemic or familial
- Psychotherapy versus **pharmacotherapy**.

1.1 Historical overview

Explanations of 'madness' have existed for much of history. Early Chinese, Hebrew, and Egyptian writings attributed bizarre behaviours to demonic possession. By the first century BCE, biological explanations were predominant. Hippocrates, for example, considered abnormal behaviour to result from an imbalance between four fluids, or humours, within the body: yellow and black bile, blood, and phlegm.

Excess yellow bile, for example, resulted in mania, while excess black bile led to melancholia. Treatment involved reducing levels of the relevant fluids through a variety of means. Levels of black bile, for example, could be reduced by a quiet life, a vegetarian diet, temperance, exercise, and celibacy. Although radical treatment approaches such as bleeding or restraint by mechanical devices were evident at this time, the first-line treatment of both the ancient Greeks and Romans was generally humane and included providing comfort and a supportive atmosphere.

By the Middle Ages, the dominance of religious thinking resulted in abnormal behaviour once more being considered the result of demonic possession. Treatment was provided by priests and included attempts to rid the individual of the demon through prayer, chanting, and administration of holy water. More radical approaches included insulting the devil, and starving, whipping or stretching the affected individual. Perhaps the most dramatic treatment of people supposedly possessed by demons was outlined in the Catholic Church's *Malleus Maleficarum* (witches' hammer), which provided a guide to the identification and treatment of witches – women who were blamed for any ills that occurred within society. The manual stated that a sudden loss of reason was the result of demonic possession, and that burning was the only way to expel the devil. Estimates of the number of women burned to death throughout Europe as a result of being considered a witch range from 1.7 to 9 million over a period of 250 years.

Towards the end of the Middle Ages, power again shifted to the secular authorities and biological theories of mental health problems became dominant. Institutions for the humane care of people with mental health problems were established. However, their initial success led to them become overcrowded. As a result, the quality of care they provided gradually deteriorated and became increasingly inhumane. One of the most famous of these institutions was Bethlem Hospital in London. Here, patients were bound by chains and, in certain phases of the moon, some were chained and whipped to prevent violence. Restraints were cruel and barbaric. The hospital became one of the most popular tourist attractions in London, with people paying to see the crazed inmates – hence the term 'bedlam'.

The care of mentally disturbed people changed once more in the eighteenth century. William Tuke in Britain and Phillipe Pinel in France re-established more humane treatments. Although asylums remained, their inmates were able to move around them freely. Treatments included working closely with inmates, reading and talking to them, and taking them on regular walks. Many were released from hospital as a result of their improved condition. This 'moral approach' was based on the assumption that if people with mental health problems were treated with care, they would improve sufficiently not to need further care. However, success rates did not reflect this optimism, and prejudice against people with mental health problems increased. Long-term incarceration once more became the norm.

Somatogenic and psychogenic perspectives

In the early twentieth century, theories and treatments of mental disorders diverged into two approaches: the somatogenic and psychogenic perspectives. The *somatogenic approach* considered mental abnormalities to result from biological disorders of the brain. A highly influential advocate of this approach, Emil Kraepelin, constructed the first modern typology of abnormal behaviour (Kraepelin [1883] 1981). He identified various clusters of symptoms, gave them diagnostic labels, and reported on their course. In addition, he measured the effects of various drugs on abnormal behaviour. Despite the rapid adoption of this approach, many of the interventions it led to, including remedies as diverse as tonsillectomy and **lobotomy**, proved ineffective. More recently, the somatogenic approach has led to the development of powerful drugs used in the treatment of conditions as varied as depression, **psychosis**, and panic attacks.

The *psychogenic approach* considered the primary causes of mental disorders to be psychological. It was initially led by an Austrian physician, Friedrich Mesmer. In 1778, he established a clinic in Paris to treat people with **hysterical disorders**. The treatment, called mesmerism, involved the patient sitting in a darkened room filled with music. Mesmer then appeared dressed in a flamboyant costume and touched the troubled area of the individual's body with a special rod, a treatment that proved effective in a number of cases. Despite these successes, he was considered a charlatan and eventually banned from holding his clinics in Paris. Other leading advocates of the psychogenic approach, Jean Charcot and then Sigmund Freud, used hypnotism in the treatment of hysterical disorders. Treatment typically involved hypnotizing the patient before encouraging them to identify the factors precipitating the onset of their symptoms and to re-experience their emotions at this time, a process known as **catharsis**. Freud later rejected this method in preference to free association and the use of **psychoanalysis**.

The latter part of the twentieth century saw a dramatic development in the psychological treatment of mental health problems. Humanistic therapies advocated by Rogers added to those of Freud and the analysts, as did the behavioural and cognitive behavioural approaches led by theorists such as Eysenck and Rachman in the UK, and Beck and Meichenbaum in the USA and Canada.

Care in the community

Modern treatments allow thousands of individuals with mental health problems to be treated in the community. In the UK, the movement of people from hospital to community began in the 1950s and reached its peak in the 1970s. Over this time, many people who had spent years, perhaps decades, in hospital were gradually moved back into the communities from which they came. This was not an easy process, as many had become totally institutionalized. Their behaviour was determined by the rules of the hospital, which were generally more accepting of deviance than the general population. They had limited self-care skills, as they had not been responsible for cooking, cleaning, and other elements of self-care for many years. Often the impact of living in an institution was more disabling than the condition for which they had originally been hospitalized, which could have been as non-problematic as vagrancy or being an unmarried mother. As a result, people discharged into the community had to be taught how to survive outside the hospital environment. Many found this very difficult, ending up as 'rotating door cases'; that is, as quickly as they were discharged into the community, they were readmitted to the hospital.

To avoid these difficulties, modern treatment seeks to minimize the use of hospital facilities and to maintain people within the community in which they live. In the UK, for example, people with relatively minor mental health problems, including most people with anxiety or mild-to-moderate depression, are treated by their general practitioner in a **primary care** setting or by easily accessible services such as the Increasing Access to Psychological Therapies (IAPT) network established in England. Established in 2008, this programme provides talking therapies to as many as one million people in a year (National Health Service [NHS], undated). It provides therapy for people experiencing a range of anxiety disorders, depression, or medically unexplained symptoms. It uses a stepped-care model in which participants are offered the 'least intrusive intervention' appropriate to their needs. This may vary from what are termed low-intensity interventions involving guided self-help, computerized cognitive behaviour therapy (CBT) or group-based programmes, to high-intensity interventions involving working with a specialist therapist. Interventions are evidence-based, and typically involve CBT, although a range of other approaches are available. Overall, around 60% of people across all conditions achieve what Clark et al. (2018) referred to as a 'reliable improvement', while 45% achieve a 'reliable recovery'.

More serious mental health problems are usually treated in the secondary care system. In the UK, this again focuses on 'care in the community' and usually involves outpatient appointments or visits to the individual's home by members of multidisciplinary teams of healthcare workers. Admission to hospital occurs only at times of crisis, with discharge back to the community as quickly as is reasonably possible. To facilitate this process, most healthcare providers have specialist teams that work with people in crisis (including feeling suicidal or experiencing acute psychosis) and their families to maintain them in the community. These teams provide psychological support (talking through problems, brief psychological interventions) and medication, as appropriate. Ideally, they are rapidly accessed with minimal bureaucratic processes. How well this service is provided varies across the country, with some teams working well and providing significant support, while others have been described as 'providing minimal risk management and medication delivery service' with limited access to some key professions (Lloyd-Evans and Johnson 2014).

Longer-term care is typically provided by multidisciplinary teams comprising a range of disciplines:

- Consultant psychiatrists who have medical responsibility for the care of their patients. They and more junior doctors are medical graduates who have specialized in the care of the 'mentally ill'. They are typically the prescribers of medication within the team, although many also engage in psychotherapy.
- Nurses within the team have a multifaceted role involving, among other things, monitoring an individual's progress, recommending or prescribing some changes in medication, providing basic psychological therapies, and acting as an advocate for the patient.
- Occupational therapists can help the individual develop or maintain life skills such as cooking or strategies for coping with stress.
- Clinical psychologists provide therapy for people with complex problems, and support others in their therapeutic work through **clinical supervision** and training in therapy skills.

- Social workers help the individual deal with social problems, including lack of money or employment that may contribute to their problems.

Historically, these teams have been 'led' by psychiatrists, but a more common model now is that any and all professionals within the team can act as coordinator of care of individuals referred to the team, with responsibility for ensuring all the relevant health and social care professionals are involved in the case and providing appropriate care.

1.2 Issues of diagnosis

The medical model

This book is organized around a set of diagnostic labels that can be ascribed to people with common mental experiences or who behave in similar ways, such as anxiety, depression, and so on. This approach is rooted in the 'medical model', which assumes that most mental health problems are the result of physiological abnormalities, generally involving brain systems. A disorder is considered as an illness, much as other medical problems are, and therefore can be treated with physical treatments, usually medication, that modify the underlying biological disorder. The type of treatment given is determined by a diagnosis.

Diagnosis involves identifying and labelling a condition through the presence of a number of pre-determined signs and symptoms. The historical roots of this approach lie in the work of Kraepelin in the late nineteenth century. He described a number of syndromes, each of which had a common set of symptoms differing from those of other syndromes, in a classification system which later formed the basis of the World Health Organization's (WHO) *International Classification of Diseases* (ICD: WHO 2018a). Indicating how such systems have struggled to accurately identify and classify mental health conditions, this is currently in its eleventh revision. The American Psychiatric Association (APA) devised its own classification system, known as the *Diagnostic and Statistical Manual* (**DSM**), which although having much in common with the ICD system, differs in a number of details. Like the ICD, it has changed over the years and, since its first publication in 1952, is now in its fifth full revision (DSM-5; APA 2013).

These classification systems provide clinicians with a dichotomous outcome that fits the medical model of treatment. Whether an individual is diagnosed with an 'illness' or not will determine whether or not they are treated, admitted to hospital, and so on. Proponents of the medical model have argued that a reliable diagnosis that is consistent both within and between countries ensures that:

- any individual presenting with a set of problems will receive the same diagnosis across the world
- they will therefore receive the same treatment wherever they are in the world
- research that informs treatment focuses on the same condition wherever it is conducted.

Diagnoses are particularly important in relation to drug therapies where a diagnosis will determine which class of drugs is used to treat the presenting problem: antidepressants for depression, antipsychotics for schizophrenia, and so on. An incorrect diagnosis will mean that incorrect medication is prescribed. In the case of research, an incorrect diagnosis will result in unreliable results from any treatment trial and will confuse rather than help the development of new treatments.

It is important to note that diagnoses assigned by DSM, which are used in this book, are social constructs. Indeed, they are the constructs of small but powerful committees of psychiatrists who over the generations of DSM have developed diagnostic criteria based on (at times very arbitrary) committee discussion and group consensus, generally in the absence of biological or any other sort of aetiological models of the disorders. As a consequence, many of the diagnoses – and the criteria on which they are based – have been strongly criticized. Davies (2013), for example, reported his interviews with the chair of the fourth DSM panel, who acknowledged that decisions to determine many diagnostic decisions on the basis of individuals having a number of symptoms from a larger pool (e.g. five symptoms out of a possible seven) were arbitrary and not based on any external criteria: six symptoms seemed too many, three too few! These unclear and subjective criteria have led to criticisms that two individuals may be given a diagnosis of an array of disorders, but to have no symptoms in common. The specificity required by a clear diagnosis is not always found or, indeed, possible. Interestingly, where the DSM committee has been unable to agree decisions, these may be opened to the wider membership of the APA. This approach was perhaps most blatant in 1973 when the membership of the APA was asked to vote on whether homosexuality should remain or be removed from the list of mental disorders: 5,854 psychiatrists voted for removal, while 3,810 voted to retain it. As a consequence, it was removed from DSM-IV as a mental disorder.

Revisions in the latest taxonomy, DSM-5, have been relatively minor, but not without controversy. Commentators have argued, for example, that by giving a number of problematic, but not necessarily pathological behaviours and experiences (e.g. temper tantrums in children, grief following a bereavement, and everyday forgetting in older adults) a diagnostic label, the DSM has pathologized normal behaviour and experiences. In addition, widening the criteria of established diagnoses, such as those for general anxiety disorder, have made them more akin to everyday experiences, allowing the possibility that many more people will be diagnosed with the condition. Some have even argued that such labelling is now serving pharmacological companies' interests by allowing the potential for pharmacological treatment of these new disorders or 'patients' (a claim which has robustly been refuted by the members of the DSM panel).

These philosophical assumptions underlying the medical model and its articulation through systems such as the DSM have been further challenged from a number of perspectives.

- The medical model implies that when an individual is ill, they behave or experience mental events that are in some way abnormal and different from those of 'normal' people – an argument rejected by the findings of cognitive psychology. There is increasing evidence that while the thought content and behaviour of people with and without mental health problems may differ from the norm, the cognitive processes underlying them are essentially the same.
- The approach fails to recognize the experience of the individual; they are assigned a diagnosis and the diagnosis is treated, not the individual. Two individuals may

be diagnosed with depression, but their experiences may be very different in terms of its cause, severity, and impact on their lives.

- The model implies that biological factors are primary in the development of mental health problems and that, therefore, biological treatments are also primary. This ignores findings that social and psychological factors appear to be critical in the development of mental health problems and that biological factors involved in mental health problems change as a result of changes in these factors. It also distracts from findings that pharmacological therapies may prove only partially effective in the treatment of a number of apparently biologically mediated conditions and that psychological therapies have proven more effective than pharmacological interventions in the treatment of many conditions (see subsequent chapters of this text).
- The medicalization of a number of behaviours has led to what many consider the inappropriate treatment of a number of 'disorders'. There is consistent evidence, for example, of significant labelling and medical treatment of children diagnosed with attention-deficit/hyperactivity disorder (ADHD) in the US when their behaviour may better be determined as 'naughty' (see Chapter 14).

A key criterion for the success of any diagnostic system is that it achieves reliable and valid diagnoses. That is, it achieves diagnoses that effectively discriminate between different conditions and which are consistently given when more than one clinician is making a blind diagnosis. A number of studies have shown problems in these areas. Vanheule et al. (2014), for example, subjected inter-rater reliability statistics of DSM-5 diagnoses to rigorous analysis and concluded that diagnostic reliability had not increased in accuracy since DSM-III. They summarized the reliability of a range of adult disorders considered in the DSM field trials, concluding that diagnosis of three conditions (post-traumatic stress disorder [PTSD], complex somatic disorder, and neurocognitive disorder) achieved very good reliability, seven diagnoses (including schizophrenia and alcohol use disorder) achieved good reliability, while four disorders achieved questionable levels of validity. The latter included major depressive disorder and generalized anxiety disorder, two of the most widely made diagnoses.

Reliability may be further influenced by a number of subtle, or not so subtle, factors. Barnes (2008) found systematic differences in diagnosis across ethnic groups in the US: African Americans were less likely to be diagnosed with bipolar and major depressive disorders, and more likely to be diagnosed with schizophrenia than white patients. By contrast, Mikton and Grounds (2007) found the ethnicity of the diagnosing physician impacts on diagnostic decisions. In this study, in which psychiatrists were asked to give a diagnosis based on a case vignette, Caucasian doctors were nearly three times more likely to assign a diagnosis of personality disorder than African Caribbean doctors.

One way to minimize these errors involves the use of a standardized diagnostic process. To this end, various authorities have developed standardized, structured or semi-structured, diagnostic interview protocols that systematically examine various aspects of the individual's functioning and symptoms, and according to the symptoms identified provide the clinician with a likely diagnosis. These are most commonly used in research studies, where accuracy and replicability of the diagnostic process are paramount. Schedules for adults include:

- *Structured Clinical Interview for DSM-5 Disorders* (SCID: First et al. 2016): available in a short and long form, with good reliability. The short SCID is relatively brief and applicable to most clinical disorders.
- *Clinical Diagnostic Interview* (CDI: DeFife et al. 2010): a 2–3-hour-long systematic and broad-based interview.

These instruments can also be used in day-to-day practice, although their length combined with the requirement for appropriate training and access to diagnostic and scoring protocols means that many psychiatrists do not use them. Instead, many adopt a less formalized, but nevertheless reasonably structured approach, known as the mental state examination. This systematically considers a variety of symptoms and background information that may contribute to a diagnosis, including physical appearance, behaviour, mood, attitude, orientation, attention and concentration, thought content and processes (to assess **delusions**), perception (to assess **hallucinations**), and insight and judgement. The final diagnosis is a subjective judgement based on this information rather than a score resulting from an interview.

Alternatives to the medical model

Any alternative to the medical/diagnostic model needs to differ from it on some important dimensions. In particular, it needs to do the following:

- make no dichotomy between abnormal and normal mental states
- consider the social and psychological processes that lead to and accompany any mental health problems
- make the affected individual (and not their diagnosis) the focus of assessment and treatment
- consider non-pharmacologically based interventions as (potentially) primary.

Two alternative approaches that address these issues are the dimensional approach and the psychological formulation.

Dimensional approach

While accepting the benefits of some form of diagnostic system, a number of commentators (e.g. Kim and Park 2019) have challenged the categorical approach adopted by the DSM. In DSM, diagnoses are based on the presence of a number of symptoms, such as poor sleep, feeling depressed, and so on. It provides a categorical classification: the individual either has the symptoms, and therefore a disorder, or does not. A dimensional approach rejects this all-or-nothing approach and the assumption that the mental states of people with a mental health problem are distinctly different from those of the 'normal' population. Proponents of the dimensional approach argue that categorical models of psychopathology are challenged by a number of problems, including:

- co-morbidity: an individual might satisfy the criteria for more than one diagnosis
- heterogeneity: two people with the same diagnosis can present with entirely different patterns of symptoms.

The dimensional approach suggests that some people who are now diagnosed as having a mental disorder may better be considered as being at the extreme end of a distribution of normality, not categorically different from others. Many of us have been anxious or depressed at one time or another, felt like not engaging with the world, or slept poorly. These experiences are not unique to people with a depressive disorder. Whether or not we consider them to be problematic depends on their frequency and the intensity with which they are experienced. The dimensional approach adopts this approach, believing it is the extent to which problems are experienced and their severity, not merely their presence or absence, that determines whether or not an individual has a mental health disorder. This approach is now developing a strong evidential base as being the preferred way of addressing these issues (e.g. Hankin et al. 2005). As a compromise with the diagnostic approach, some proponents of the dimensional system suggest that if a person scores above a threshold score, based on the severity and frequency of their experiences, they may be given some form of diagnosis.

The dimensional approach has a number of strengths. In particular it highlights which aspects of a person's life are problematic and for which they may require some form of help. It also avoids 'forcing' the presenting problems into a diagnostic category into which they do not easily fit. What it does not address is the processes causing or maintaining any problems. This level of assessment is provided by the psychological formulation.

Psychological formulation

Psychotherapists' understandings of mental health problems differ radically from the categorical and dimensional approaches. These approaches are both descriptive, albeit in differing ways. But psychotherapists require a deeper knowledge of individuals' experiences. They do not simply need to know that a person is depressed; they need to know the nature of the depression, the long- and short-term factors that led to or maintain this state, and so on. These then become the focus of any intervention. Psychological formulations attempt to identify the processes that led to and maintain the problems an individual is facing. These processes may be external (negative life events, rape, bereavement) or internal (distorted interpretations of the world, **hyperventilation** leading to panic disorder). They may also be short-term or longer-term sequelae to childhood events such as sexual abuse or poor parental relationships.

Although the content of a formulation will necessarily differ according to the orientation of the therapist, a typical cognitive behavioural formulation would consider:

- The presenting problem(s): what is troubling the individual?
- Predisposing factors: what factors have left them vulnerable to any problems they are experiencing?
- Precipitating factors: why have they developed problems now?
- Perpetuating cognitions and consequences: what thoughts are they experiencing and behaviours are they engaged in that are maintaining their problems?

A formulation is an explanatory hypothesis about the nature of the clinical problem. It has two main functions: to guide the therapist in their treatment plan and help establish criteria for evaluating its effectiveness. Formulations are not static and may change in the light of information emerging over time, as will the focus and form of any intervention. They are necessarily guided by the theoretical perspective of the therapist, which focuses the questions asked and the formulation established. These may be quite different for, say, a psychoanalyst and a cognitive behavioural therapist. This, of course, is both a strength and a weakness. A strength, because it allows the therapist to select, in a relatively parsimonious way from the myriad of potential contributors to a problem, those most likely to be relevant. A weakness, because these theoretical blinkers may focus the therapist too exclusively on what they consider to be important aspects of a **client's** experience, and too little on what may actually be important. On this basis, some have argued that good therapists are aware of several aetiological models and can either integrate them into a meaningful synthesis or identify which are relevant to particular clients. This approach assumes the theoretical stance taken by the therapist is coherent and scientifically valid. It also places significant emphasis on the skill of the therapist to identify salient processes and issues and place them within a coherent and accurate formulation. The risk is therefore that these assumptions may not always be met: a clear weakness of this approach. Nevertheless, so central is formulation to clinical psychology, and therapy in general, that each section in the final part of the book considers a formulation for one of the mental health problems described therein.

Finally, while psychotherapists may not comfortably assign a diagnostic label, they may use psychometric instruments as part of the assessment process and to measure changes over time. Frequently used measures include:

- *State-Trait Anxiety Inventory* (STAI; Spielberger et al. 1983). The STAI is a measure of anxiety, assessing both trait (general) and state (how you feel now) anxiety. Each scale comprises 20 items and has norms for clinical patients, working adults, and (the children's version) high school and college students.
- *Beck Depression Inventory* (BDI; Beck et al. 1996). The BDI comprises 21 questions relating to symptoms of depression such as hopelessness and irritability, cognitions such as guilt or feelings of being punished, and physical symptoms such as fatigue or lack of interest in sex. It can be used by people aged 13 years and upward, and provides cut-off scores indicating four levels of depression from minimal to severe.

Psychometric instruments may also measure processes such as beliefs or metacognitions (see Chapters 2 and 3) that contribute to distress or problematic behaviours, including:

- *The Meta-Cognitions Questionnaire* (MCQ; Cartwright-Hatton and Wells 1997). The MCQ taps into five relevant dimensions that include: positive beliefs about worry, negative beliefs about the controllability of thoughts, and negative beliefs about thoughts in general.
- *Paranoid, Persecutory and Delusional-Proneness Questionnaire* (McKay et al. 2005). This 54-item questionnaire comprises three subscales: persecutory paranoid ideation, non-persecutory paranoid ideation, and non-paranoid delusion-proneness. The questionnaire is suitable for use across both clinical and non-clinical populations.

1.3 The aetiology of mental health problems

There are diverse literatures focusing on factors that contribute to the development of mental health problems. The rest of this chapter provides an introduction to each type of explanation. The chapters in Part 2 of the book examine the issues in more detail in relation to specific disorders.

- *Genetic models* consider how genetic factors influence an individual's risk of developing a mental health disorder.
- *Biological models* focus on biochemical processes, usually involving chemicals known as **neurotransmitters**, which influence mood and behaviour. They also consider how damage to the brain can result in a number of mental health disorders.
- *Psychological models* focus on the internal mental processes that influence mood and behaviour. There are a number of psychological explanations of mental health disorders, the best known being psychoanalytic, humanistic, behavioural, and cognitive behavioural.
- *The socio-cultural approach* focuses on the role of social and cultural factors in mental health disorders.
- *Systemic models* focus on the role of social systems, frequently the family, in which the individual is situated. Disorders are considered to be the consequence of stressful or disordered interactions with families.
- *Developmental factors*, such as those that occur in childhood, influence vulnerability to a range of emotional difficulties, through processes such as attachment difficulties, inappropriate **cognitive schema**, and poor coping skills.

Genetic models

With the exception of egg, sperm, and red blood cells, each of the approximately 100 trillion cells of the body contain two complete sets of the human genome: one set from the individual's father, the other from their mother. Each genome comprises 23 pairs of **chromosomes**. Each set of chromosomes carries the 60,000–80,000 genes that contribute to both the physical and psychological characteristics of the individual.

Each gene in a set of matched genes affecting the same processes is known as an allele. The instructions in the sets of genes from each parent may be the same or quite different, for example blue versus brown eyes. Where the alleles are the same, the individual is described as homozygotic; where they differ, they are termed heterozygotic. The expression of these 'competing' genes is determined by whether the genes are dominant or recessive. Some genes, such as those determining the eye colour brown, are described as dominant and are expressed when linked to a gene with other instructions. Recessive genes are expressed only when matched with other recessive genes with the same instructions. The development of most mental health disorders is associated with recessive genes. If they were the result of dominant genes, their expression in each generation would be virtually guaranteed, resulting in continuing disadvantage and limited chances of reproduction.

Genetic studies of the aetiology of mental health problems have used several methods. Family studies measure whether those with genotypes that are more or less similar to the affected individual are at different risk for the disorder. If there is a genetic linkage in a disorder, one would expect someone with identical genetic make-up (a **monozygotic (MZ) twin**) to be more likely to develop the disorder than a non-identical or **dizygotic (DZ) twin**, who has roughly 50% of genes in common, who in turn would be more at risk than a cousin or aunt with even less genetic similarity. Many family studies focus on the degree to which both MZ and DZ twins develop the same disorder. Where more MZ than DZ twins are concordant for the disorder, this is taken to imply some level of genetic risk. This approach has a number of limitations. Critically, not only do closer family members share more genes, they also share a more common environment. MZ twins, for example, tend to be treated more similarly than DZ twins. Any concordance for a condition may therefore be attributable to a shared environment rather than shared genes.

In an attempt to separate out environment from genetic factors, many studies have examined concordance rates in twins brought up in differing environments, usually as a result of adoption. It is assumed that because the separated twins have a common genetic make-up and different environments, any concordance for the condition under examination is the result of genetic factors. However, there are a number of reasons why any **heritability coefficient** determined by this method may not prove totally accurate. First, even twins that are separated have factors other than their genes in common. If nothing else, they have shared the same prenatal experiences that may determine risk for various disorders. Another factor that can result in overestimation of genetic risk involves any genetic influence on the behaviour of a child, particularly where they are 'difficult' or 'problematic', instigating similar reactions from those caring for them. As a result, separated children may experience both a common genetic heritage and a common family background, despite their separation.

This kind of interpretive problem has resulted in new methodologies in this type of study. Rather than assume the nature of the environment in which the person lives, studies have now begun to measure genetic, environmental, social, and other life stresses. These data are then subject to statistical modelling techniques that allow the investigators to determine the degree to which genetic and environmental factors separately contribute to the development of the disorder under investigation.

Work on the human genome now also permits more fundamental research: the identification of specific genes responsible for specific disorders. In fact, most disorders are likely to result from a number of genes (that is, they are **polygenic**), and in some cases problems may arise from the absence of a gene, rather than its presence. There is evidence, for example, of a gene locus on chromosome 4 that may be protective against alcohol problems. Whatever the genetic linkages found, there is a general consensus that genes, at most, influence risk for a particular mental health disorder. Indeed, while risk for a particular disorder may be increased as a result of genetic factors, many if not most people with the disorder may not carry the relevant gene. Eighty-nine per cent of individuals diagnosed with schizophrenia, for example, have no known relative with the disorder. Not carrying the gene that increases risk for a disorder does not mean that you are immune to that disorder.

Biological models

Biochemical explanations of mental health problems focus on the biological processes underlying mood and behaviour. Both are regulated by brain systems, whose actions are mediated by neurotransmitters. These allow us to perceive information, integrate that information with past memories and other salient factors, and then respond emotionally and behaviourally. Disruption of these systems as a result of inappropriate neurotransmitter actions results in inappropriate perception, mood, and behaviour. The exact nature of the systems and the neurotransmitters involved in different mental health problems are considered in more detail in Chapter 4 and in each of the chapters in Part 2 of the book.

Other biochemical processes have been implicated in some conditions. Hormones such as melatonin appear to be involved in the aetiology of seasonal affective disorder, a type of depression considered in Chapter 7. Other disorders may be the result of problems in the architecture of the brain. Some of the symptoms of schizophrenia, for example, may arise from degeneration or failures of brain development that lead to fundamental errors in information processing, and disordered thoughts and behaviour. **Alzheimer's disease** results from progressive neuronal damage evident through the deterioration of cognitive functioning in later life.

Biochemical models are often considered to be in opposition to psychological explanations: mental health problems are seen as either psychological in nature *or* to have a biological cause. But this is a false dichotomy. A more appropriate way of thinking about the two approaches is that they provide different *levels* of explanation, somewhat analogous to the levels of explanation provided by physics and chemistry. Biochemical processes underpin all our behaviour at all times. The act of writing this sentence involves numerous sensory, motor, and neuronal processes, all of which are mediated by chemical transmissions. But understanding these fundamental processes explains only part of the behaviour: it does not easily account for the motivation for writing the sentence, the process of mental construction of the sentence or, indeed, my mood as it was written. To understand these, one needs to address the psychological processes driving the behaviour. In this way, both biochemical and psychological explanations of the behaviour are 'correct'.

Psychological models

In contrast to the biochemical and genetic models, wherein most scientists and practitioners believe in a common process through which mental health disorders arise, there are many psychological models. The very first of these psychological models was developed by Freud. His psychodynamic model focused on the competing unconscious battles between the **id**, **ego**, and **superego**, and how health functioning may be disrupted by developmental challenges in childhood.

Derivatives of Freud's original theory still form the theoretical basis of modern psychoanalytic therapy. However, mainstream psychology diverged markedly from this approach in the 1950s and 1960s. Behavioural theories (e.g. Wolpe 1982) rejected the notion of psychic processes influencing mood and behaviour and the unscientific nature of psychoanalysis. Its practitioners argued that behaviour is largely controlled by external events, and based their principles on the 'hard' science of **classical** and **operant conditioning**. At a similar time, humanistic theories (Rogers 1961) rejected psychoanalytic models, not because of their psychic nature, but because of the nature of their psychic phenomena. In contrast to psychodynamic models, which assume that behaviour and mood are influenced by past traumas, humanistic theories are based on the assumption that behaviour is driven by aspirations towards the future, with the potential of **self-actualization** available to all.

Behavioural explanations were, in turn, largely replaced by theories focusing on cognitive content; our beliefs or appraisals of the situations we face. Phobias were no longer seen as driven by conditioning but were explained by irrational beliefs and threat appraisals. In a more elaborate, developmental, model, Beck (2008) argued that fundamental beliefs about the self and the world (schema) are established in childhood. These beliefs then shape our responses to difficulties in adulthood. Depression is seen, for example, to be a consequence of negative schema developed in childhood (e.g. I am unloved and unlovable) as a result of childhood experiences subsequently being evoked as a consequence of low mood and adult experiences, such as difficulties in a relationship. These beliefs exacerbate low mood, evoke poor coping responses, and finally lead to depression.

This fundamental paradigm shift resulted in what has now become the dominant therapeutic approach within western psychology: cognitive behaviour therapy. However, even this approach is now changing and evolving. More modern cognitive theories focus not just on cognitive content but cognitive processes also. They consider processes such as the role of memory and attentional systems and poor coping strategies as central to our emotional problems. As an example of attentional bias, theorists such as Wells (2000) note that a spider phobic may have a range of beliefs about spiders when not in their presence, many of which may be benign. However, once in the presence of a spider, benign beliefs may be ignored, and attention given to high threat beliefs and memories of past fearful experiences. These, in turn, trigger a fear response and activation of a pre-programmed coping response usually involving avoidance of the threat.

By contrast, other theorists have placed behavioural explanations within a complex developmental framework. Strosahl et al. (2004), for example, argued that emotional responses occur as a consequence of learned associations between certain contexts and emotional states: their 'relational frame'. According to relational frames theorists, we are able to abstract elements from one set of frames and transfer them to other situations. A child who is trapped inside a wooden box and experiences great fear may later experience the same fear when trapped in other contexts, such as relationships. Although the contexts are very different, the responses are similar because the relational frame is the same. Because relational frames are verbally accessible (i.e. we are able to understand and describe them), they are also changeable. As a consequence, we may develop distorted concepts of relationships between elements within relational frames, and begin to respond to these distorted relational frames rather than the 'real' relational frames. As a result of this inappropriate relational framing, we may begin to avoid contexts in which negative emotions and behaviours are triggered. This avoidance results in a state of psychological rigidity, inappropriate coping attempts to minimize any distress we may experience, and a failure to learn that our fears are exaggerated and we can cope effectively with the feared situation. These various approaches are considered further in Chapters 2 and 3.

Socio-cultural models

All the models discussed so far assume that mental disorders arise as a result of problems within the individual, be they genetic, biochemical or psychological. By contrast, the socio-cultural approach assumes that external, social factors contribute to their development. Socio-cultural factors include a wide range of influences, from the family to wider socio-economic factors, some of which were identified in the British Adult Psychiatric Morbidity Survey (McManus et al. 2016). The survey revealed the highest rates of depression or anxiety to be among women, those living in urban settings, unemployed people, and those who were separated, divorced or widowed. Psychoses were more **prevalent** among urban than rural dwellers. Alcohol dependence was nearly twice as common among people who were unemployed than among those who were employed; drug dependence was five times higher among the unemployed than those in jobs. People who are members of ethnic minorities or in the lower socio-economic groups are also more likely to experience depression, non-specific distress, schizophrenia or substance abuse problems than those in other sectors of society (e.g. Veling et al. 2010). A number of – sometimes competing – theories to explain these differences have been proposed, each of which is discussed in more detail in Chapter 4.

Childhood adversity

- Although the root of all problems may not lie in childhood, many factors within our childhood do affect us later in life. Negative factors such as neglect and abuse may have an adverse impact, whereas strong and supportive families may be protective. The impact of these factors may be through a range of processes, including learning poor coping strategies to deal with adverse life events, negative self-beliefs, and poor emotional control.

Socio-economic status differences

- *Social drift*: this approach suggests that high levels of mental health problems among the lower socio-economic groups are the result of affected individuals developing a mental health problem, which renders them less economically viable. They may be unable to maintain a job or the levels of overtime required to maintain their standard of living, and drift down the socio-economic scale. That is, mental health problems precede a decline in socio-economic status.
- *Social stress*: this approach assumes that living in different socio-economic conditions results in differing levels of stress and resources to cope with that stress – the lower the socio-economic group, the higher the stress. That is, the stresses associated with social deprivation result in mental health problems, and an associated lack of resources (economic, social, psychological) fail to buffer these problems.

Gender differences

- *The experience of trauma*: women are more at risk of mental health problems as they are more likely to experience traumatic events including partner violence and sexual violation.
- *Role strain*: an alternative hypothesis suggests that women encounter more role strain and **spillover** between the demands of work and home than men. The resultant stress places them at increased risk for stress and mental health problems

Minority status

- *Confound with social class*: this model suggests that the apparent relationship between minority status and mental health problems is spurious. It suggests that people in ethnic minorities largely occupy the lower socio-economic groups. That they also have higher levels of mental health problems is a result of this association, not of being a member of an ethnic minority *per se*.
- *The effects of prejudice*: this suggests a more direct link between ethnic minority status and mental health. Mental health problems may result from the additional stresses, including overt and covert prejudice, experienced by the members of minority ethnic groups.
- *Cultural transitions*: a further source of stress may be the tension experienced as individuals adopt or reject some of the norms of their own or other cultures. Both may result in feelings of alienation, rejection by members of differing cultures, and consequent mental health problems.

Stop and think 1 ...

Most strategies for reducing the burden of mental health disorders have focused on treatment once they have developed. The importance of social and cultural factors points to another way of addressing the issue: to reduce the social, economic, and cultural factors that may contribute to poor mental health. This could be done in a number of ways – anti-bullying campaigns in schools, providing cheap or free crèches so that young, single mothers can access recreational facilities or have a break from child care, ensuring economic security for people in old age – that on the surface have little to do with mental health, but may actually have a significant impact on it.

So, if you had carte blanche, how would you change the society in which we live to maximize the mental health of the general population?

Social and cultural factors may also influence the type of problems people report, and how acceptable – or unacceptable – they are within a society. Some cultures positively affirm what might be considered hallucinations and signs of mental disturbance in others. People from different cultures may also report what we define as mental health problems in many different ways, and seek different treatments for them. Asian people, for example, often report mental distress framed as physical symptoms and their first line of treatment may involve herbs or other natural physical treatments. These issues are considered in more detail in Chapter 5.

Stop and think 2 ...

When I was writing the first draft of this text, the Stop and Think box above from the previous edition of the book seemed to encapsulate key issues for population mental health, and it is for that reason it is included here. But in the course of writing this edition, a much more acute clear and distinct danger to mental health established itself: Covid-19. In the UK, the number of clinical psychologists being trained is apparently increasing in anticipation of an 'avalanche' of mental health problems throughout the population over the next year and beyond. But who is most at risk for such problems and why? And how should we as a society respond to them?

Systemic models

A more enclosed system that impacts on mental health is the family. Family system theorists consider the individuals within a family to form an interacting system. Each has a reciprocal influence on those around them. The behaviour of individuals within these systems, and the communication between them, can lead to individual members behaving in ways that seem 'abnormal'. Perhaps the most extreme form of family dysfunction occurs when a member of a family sexually abuses a child within it. Levels of sexual abuse are very high among women who seek psychological therapy for conditions as varied as depression, anxiety, and anorexia (Jaffe et al. 2002).

One of the first models of family interactions in relation to mental health focused on people with schizophrenia. Brown and colleagues (e.g. Brown et al. 1972) were the first to identify a family characteristic, now termed high negative expressed emotion (NEE). They found that people diagnosed with schizophrenia living in families who were particularly critical, hostile or over-involved had a higher rate of relapse than those who did not experience such an environment. Reducing levels of NEE resulted in a dramatic reduction in relapse rates. A second, more complex, family system is thought by family therapists to contribute to the development of anorexia in young women (Minuchin et al. 1978). These and other family models of pathology are considered in more detail in Chapter 5 and other chapters in Part 2 of the book.

1.4 Psychotherapy versus pharmacotherapy

As a final word, despite the complex nature of mental health problems and their aetiology, the choice of therapies for people experiencing them boils down to a simple dichotomy: drug therapy versus talking therapy. It is possible to argue that, because biochemical processes underpin behaviour at a fundamental level, altering the levels of neurotransmitters that influence mood through pharmacological processes provides the most direct and effective form of treatment of mental health disorders. While there is some logic in this argument, it certainly does not hold for all cases and it implicitly assumes that psychological therapy does not influence the fundamental biological processes underpinning mental health disorders. This is not the case – there is a powerful reciprocity between the two forms of treatment. Psychological treatments cause changes at the biochemical level, otherwise they would not alter mood. Similarly, pharmacotherapy alters cognitions and behaviour (e.g. Mogg et al. 2004).

One argument favouring the use of psychological therapy is that many of the drugs prescribed are effective only while they are being taken. Once a course of drugs has finished, their action stops and the individual's biochemical status, and hence mood and behaviour, may revert to the state before the treatment was commenced. To prevent this, many people are now being prescribed drugs such as antidepressants for much longer than was initially considered to be necessary. The WHO, for example, recommends that antidepressant therapy should not be stopped earlier than 9–12 months 'after recovery' (WHO 2019). In contrast, some have argued that psychological therapy prepares the individual to cope with the stresses they face during therapy and in the future, making them at significantly less risk of relapse once therapy is terminated.

Both arguments may be overstating the case. There is good evidence that many people maintain good mental health following cessation of pharmacological treatments, although the reasons for this may be more psychological than pharmacological. A depressed individual who has withdrawn from family and social life, for example, may benefit from a drug treatment that helps them re-engage with people and enjoy life more. The pleasure gained from this may increase levels of the neurotransmitters that prevent depression (see Chapter 3) and maintain them in a healthy state once drug therapy is stopped. If they had not re-engaged so positively, the risk of relapse might have been much greater.

It is also true that some individuals do not benefit from psychological therapies, or they relapse following successful psychological treatments. They may find it difficult to adopt a psychological approach to reducing their problems. They may forget, be unable to use the new skills they have learned, or feel so overwhelmed by circumstances that they once more experience a deterioration in their mental health. For this reason, some advocates of psychological therapy suggest the need for 'booster' sessions some months after the completion of therapy to help maintain a positive mental state.

Both pharmacological and psychological therapies are reasonably effective in treating most mental health conditions. Psychological therapies seem to be more effective than drug treatments in treating conditions such as anorexia, panic disorder, mild-to-moderate depression, and some sexual problems. In contrast, although psychological treatments are increasingly being used in the treatment of psychosis, the mainstay of treatment remains drug therapy. The relative effectiveness of the two forms of treatment for some conditions such as severe depression is still hotly debated, as will be seen later in the book.

1.5 Chapter summary

1. Diagnosis of mental health conditions, such as those within DSM classifications, largely follows the biological or disease/medical model of mental health established by Kraepelin in the late nineteenth century.
2. According to this model, accurate diagnosis is important to ensure consistent treatment and research in relation to mental health disorders.
3. Diagnosis is typically based on the presence of a number of symptoms, including hallucinations, poor sleep, and so on. This categorical approach leads to a dichotomous diagnostic process in which the individual either has or does not have a disorder.
4. Dimensional approaches state that the experiences of individuals with mental health disorders differ in degree from those of the 'normal' population but are not categorically different.
5. Psychotherapists generally find diagnostic labels to be unhelpful. Instead, they focus on the nature of the factors that contribute to and maintain the individual's problems. These, usually in the form of a treatment formulation, become the focus of therapy.
6. A number of factors may contribute to the development of mental health disorders: genetic and biological factors, socio-cultural and family factors, and individual psychological factors. No one approach is able to explain the development of any one disorder, and most result from a combination of factors: the biopsychosocial approach.

1.6 For discussion

1. Should we limit the types of people with mental health disorders who are treated in the community? Should people such as psychopaths or so-called 'predatory' paedophiles thought to be at risk of reoffending be permitted to live or be treated outside hospital or prison?
2. What would you think if told an individual is 'schizophrenic'? How might this alter your interpretation of their behaviour or your responses to them?
3. Some severe psychiatric conditions such as Huntington's disease in which the individual develops increasing muscular spasticity and mental deterioration leading to death in middle age can be predicted by genetic testing. It cannot be prevented, but those who have the gene for the condition may choose not to have children and pass the gene on to them. Would you want to know as a young person whether you carry the gene?
4. If offered the choice of medication or psychological therapy for a mental health problem, which would you choose – and why?

1.7 Further reading

Ansari, A. and Osser, D. (2015) *Psychopharmacology: A Concise Overview for Students and Clinicians*, 2nd edition, North Charleston, SC: CreateSpace.

Bentall, R. (2004) *Madness Explained: Psychosis and Human Nature*, Harmondsworth: Penguin.

Fernando, S. (2010) *Mental Health, Race and Culture*, 3rd edition, London: Red Globe Press.

Frances, A. (2013) *Saving Normal: An Insider's Revolt Against Out-of-control Psychiatric Diagnosis, DSM 5, Big Pharma and the Medicalization of Ordinary Life*, New York: William Morrow.

Johnstone, L. and Dallos, R. (2014) *Formulation in Psychology and Psychotherapy*, London: Routledge.

Page, A. and Stritzke, W. (2015) *Clinical Psychology for Trainees: Foundations of Science-informed Practice*, Cambridge: Cambridge University Press.

2 The psychological perspective

Chapter contents

This chapter explores four major schools of psychological therapy developed since the late nineteenth century:

- *Psychoanalytic*: views childhood trauma and the unconscious as the causes of problems in adulthood
- *Behavioural*: considers psychopathology to arise from conditioning processes
- *Cognitive* or *cognitive behavioural*: assumes that the critical element of psychopathology is inappropriate, dysfunctional, cognitions
- *Humanistic*: considers psychopathology to be the consequence of deviation from the drive towards **self-actualization**.

To understand the rationale behind each therapy, it is necessary to understand the model of psychological disorder upon which it is based. The chapter therefore provides an overview of each approach's theory of psychological disorder as well as some of the strategies it uses to achieve change. Further developments in cognitive and behavioural theories and interventions are also considered in some detail in the next chapter. In addition, the effectiveness of various therapeutic approaches is considered in the context of specific conditions in Part 2 of the book. But for now, by the end of this chapter you should have an understanding of:

- key psychological models of the **aetiology** of mental health disorders: psychoanalytic, behavioural, cognitive behavioural and humanistic
- some of the widely used interventions based on these models.

2.1 The psychoanalytic approach

Freud

Sigmund Freud (e.g. Freud 1900) was one of the first clinicians to explore the role of childhood factors and the unconscious in explaining problems of adulthood. His work, conducted in the late nineteenth and early twentieth centuries, was highly innovative and based on his formulation of the unconscious, with insights largely derived from cases he saw in his practice in Vienna.

Freud considered personality to have three basic components: the **id**, **ego**, and **superego**:

- The *id* is driven by the basic instincts of sex and aggression, which Freud considered the basic motivating forces of human behaviour. It operates under the pleasure principle. That is, it seeks to maximize immediate gratification. It is greedy, demanding, and has no natural self-control.
- The *ego* is the realistic component of personality. It operates under what Freud termed the reality principle and also works to maximize gratification, but within the constraints of the real world.
- The *superego* contains the individual's morals and societal values. It acts as the conscience, creating feelings of guilt if social norms are violated.

These personality components are in a continuous struggle to control the individual. Sexual desire, for example, is rooted in the id. However, its immediate urge for sexual gratification is tempered by the superego's moralistic statements that such urges are a sin, and the ego's realistic consideration of the costs and benefits of various actions. The outcome of these competing processes is usually some form of socially acceptable sexual behaviour. However, should the id gain control, the likely outcome is rape or some other violent act.

Five stages of psychosexual development

According to Freud, the development of personality occurs through a five-stage sequence of psychosexual development. The first stage, known as the *oral stage*, is characterized by receiving gratification through oral means: sucking, crying or exploring objects with the mouth. The oral stage occurs between the ages of 18 and 24 months. At this time, children have only the id. Accordingly, the stage is characterized by an inability to delay gratification, together with selfish and demanding behaviour. Immediately following this is the *anal stage*, which continues until the child is between 42 and 48 months old. At this time, children achieve gratification through anal means. Freud argued that the process of toilet training is the first time the child becomes aware of their actions on other people, and learns to modify their behaviour to gain gratification from them. If the child satisfies parental demands, he or she receives praise and approval. If not, he or she experiences disapproval. Realistic expectation of these outcomes is the beginning of the ego development.

The third stage of psychosexual development is the *phallic stage*. This continues through to the age of 5 to 6 years. In this stage, the superego begins to develop as a result of the child's experiences of sexual conflicts and the means by which they are resolved. According to Freud, boys in the phallic stage develop sexual desires focusing on their mother, driven by the urges of the id. These desires are known as the Oedipus complex. By this stage, the ego is able to judge the realistic consequences of these actions and recognizes that they would meet the disapproval of their rival – their father. The boy also recognizes that if he were to enter into open rivalry with his father, he would be defeated. He begins to fear that his father will castrate him to prevent him from becoming a future rival for his mother, a phenomenon known as castration anxiety. The boy resolves this dilemma by identifying with his father. This permits him, at least symbolically, to make love to his mother as does his father. As part of this identification process, he begins to adopt the father's beliefs and values. He begins to develop a superego.

The young girl develops her superego in a similar way. Freud suggested that when a girl enters the phallic stage, she begins to recognize that she is different from boys. She experiences penis envy: she feels incomplete or inadequate as a result of her lack of a penis. She also believes that if she makes love with her father she will 'possess' her father's penis, at least temporarily. In addition, if she is made pregnant, she may bring a penis into the world by giving birth to a boy. In this way, the girl's basic sense of inferiority leads her to develop sexual desires focusing on her father. These feelings are resolved by the girl identifying with her mother, allowing her to symbolically make love to her father when her mother does so, and leading her to adopt her mother's moral values: her superego.

The fourth stage of development is the *latency stage*, which continues until puberty. During this stage, the individual channels their sexual and aggressive urges through age-appropriate interests and activities such as sports and hobbies. The final stage is the *genital stage*. This begins in puberty and continues throughout life. In it, the individual is driven by the two basic motivating forces: sex and aggression. Our bodies generate both sexual (libido) and aggressive energy. Healthy individuals discharge this energy through socially appropriate channels: sexual intercourse with age-appropriate adults, sports, career progression, and so on. Where people fail to find such outlets, energy builds until it can no longer be contained and is released in an uncontrolled fashion, guided by unconscious influences. To prevent the inappropriate discharge of these forces, the individual diverts or blocks them through a variety of unconscious mechanisms.

Defence mechanisms

According to Freud, mental health problems are the result of either ego anxieties or the **defence mechanisms** it establishes to prevent these anxieties becoming conscious. Ego anxieties frequently relate to troubling events experienced in early childhood. These can lead the individual to become fixated at a particular developmental stage, and to behave in ways appropriate to that stage during adulthood. Such behaviour forms an unconscious defence against anxiety caused by the experience and its memories. Its function is to prevent recognition of the hurt that was experienced at the time. Individuals may also regress to previous levels of psychosexual functioning through which they have successfully passed as a result of stresses in adulthood. The stage to which they regress is influenced by the severity of the stress, the similarity of the current stressor to problems experienced in previous stages, and the success with which each stage was passed through. Some of the repressed or fixated personality types in adulthood are summarized in Table 2.1.

A number of other defence mechanisms that do not involve regression may also be used to counter ego anxieties. The most basic Freudian defence mechanism is repression. In this, threatening material is unconsciously and actively blocked from awareness to prevent it from entering consciousness. Some other defence mechanisms are outlined in Table 2.2.

Table 2.1 Some adult personality characteristics associated with a failure to progress through Freud's development stages

Stage	Associated problems
Oral	Depression, narcissism, dependence
Anal	Obstinacy, obsessive-compulsive disorder, sadomasochism
Phallic	Gender identity problems, antisocial personality
Latent	Inadequate or excessive self-control
Genital	Identity diffusion

Table 2.2 Some Freudian defence mechanisms

Defence	Definition	Example
Repression	Blocking threatening material from consciousness	An adult unable to recall being abused as a child
Denial	Preventing threatening material from entering consciousness	A parent who cannot accept the death of their child
Projection	Attributing one's own unacceptable impulse or action to another	Someone who denies their homosexuality, and considers homosexuals to be constantly making sexual approaches
Displacement	Changing the target of an unacceptable impulse	'Kicking the cat' instead of whoever caused anger or upset
Reaction formation	Expressing the exact opposite of an unacceptable desire	A person who is considering ending a relationship, but continues to show strong affection for their partner
Sublimation	Expressing an unacceptable impulse in a symbolic manner	An individual with a strong drive for unattainable sexual relationships focuses their attention on achieving in their career or sport
Conversion	Expressing painful psychic material through symbolic physiological symptoms	A soldier who finds it unacceptable to shoot others develops paralysis in their hands
Undoing	A repetitive action that symbolically atones for an unacceptable impulse or behaviour	Repeated washing of hands following an extramarital affair

A classic case involving ego defence mechanisms was that of Little Hans. This young boy had an extreme fear of horses, which Freud suggested indicated a fear of his father – that is, castration anxiety. Hans's defence mechanism was to displace the fear of his father to more acceptable objects, horses, which were large and strong like his father, and acted as symbolic representations of him. Another condition which Freud identified as a defence mechanism was bed wetting, which he considered a symbolic form of masturbation. Its perpetrators expressed their underlying sexual urges by converting them to a more acceptable physical symptom.

Criticisms of Freudian theory

Freud broke new ground to develop a complex model of human development. His contribution to the development of theories of personality and psychopathology is without question. However, his theories have the weaknesses of any theory, particularly one so encompassing, developed before the present scientific method and its empirical process were established. Even though a number of researchers (e.g. Dollard and Miller 1950) have developed experimental studies to assess Freud's theory, it is beset with such fundamental interpretive problems that whatever the results of these studies, they provide little evidence to support or disprove Freud's theories. Because processes such as id drives, ego defences, and fixation are abstract and supposedly operate at an unconscious level, there is no way of knowing for certain whether or not they are occurring. In addition, the theory provides few, if any, testable hypotheses. If an individual engages in a set of behaviours predicted by Freud's theory, it may be considered supported. However, if they do not, the theory is not challenged or falsified, as it could be hypothesized this was a consequence of the individual's defence mechanisms.

Some other criticisms of Freudian theory include the following:

- Freud's theories were based on interpretation of information gleaned from a relatively small and specific group of patients, in particular, middle-class Viennese women. The ability to generalize from these cases to the wider population is questionable.
- Freud's views on women were misogynistic and based on cultural attitudes of his time, rather than a true scientific perspective.
- Freud's theory changed over time, sometimes without clear rejection of previous versions. It is therefore difficult to know which theory should be tested.

Freud's contemporaries and descendants

Jung

Carl Jung ([1912] 1956) was seen by Freud as the 'Crown Prince' of **psychoanalysis**. However, his beliefs became less and less congruent with those of Freud, and he broke away to develop his own analytical psychology. Jung considered Freud's emphasis on sex as the major motivator of human behaviour to be simplistic and reductionist. By contrast, Jung emphasized its psychological and spiritual influences. He also disagreed with Freud's notion that personality and adult neurosis are established in early childhood. He suggested that people are motivated by future goals rather than by past events. While Jung believed that our unconscious was developed through individual experiences, he also considered part of it reflected universal themes and ideas. He considered this 'collective unconscious' to be biologically based and evident through symbols and myths common to all races and times – a sort of race memory that influences our reactions to the present world. Jung considered that the goal of personal development is to expand conscious awareness through the ego making contact with the unconscious. The ultimate end of this process is union between the conscious and the unconscious, although this is rarely completely achieved. In this, Jung was close to the humanistic school, considered later in the chapter.

Klein

A generation later, Melanie Klein (1927) focused on the social drives that underpin our psychological development. Her work was based on object relations theory, which has the premise that human beings have an innate drive to form and maintain social relationships. Klein focused on the psychological processes involved in the relationship between mother and child in the first few months of life. She considered psychic structures to evolve from these interactions rather than the biologically derived tensions and conflicts, anxieties and sexual impulses proposed by Freud.

According to Klein, the infant goes through two key pre-oedipal developmental stages. The first, known as the paranoid-schizoid position, is dominant in children from birth to around 4 to 6 months old, although it is never completely outgrown and older children and adults can operate in this mode at times. This stage is characterized by paranoid anxiety. The child experiences this as fear of external objects, but it is actually driven by their death instinct. It is a fear of imminent annihilation, and is dealt with through a number of defence mechanisms, including one known as *splitting*. Through this, the child identifies objects as either completely good or completely bad. There is no integration of the two. In doing so, the child prevents the good being destroyed by the bad, and the child identifies him or herself with the good objects. According to Klein, the mother is initially represented by the child as 'part-object' of the breast, and is experienced as either a 'good object' or a 'bad object'. She is good when the child's needs are met through feeding; bad when these needs are not met. The baby responds to the bad object with feelings of terror, insecurity, and destructive rage.

The second developmental stage occurs roughly between 6 and 12 months. In this phase, known as the depressive position, the infant learns to bridge the gap between 'good' and 'bad' objects, and between his or her own experiences of love and hate, which created them. In doing so, the child is able to view the world in a more holistic manner, and objects can be accepted as having both good and bad elements. The child begins to see his or her mother as a more realistic 'whole object' rather than the part-object of the breast, and to understand that good and bad can co-exist in the same person. However, this revelation leads to a deep sense of disappointment and anger that a loved person can be bad as well as good. There is a primitive sense of loss and separation now the possibility of complete fusion with the 'good mother' is no longer possible. There may also be a sense of guilt, as the child feels he or she may be responsible for the end of this relationship.

In addition, fearing the loss of his or her object's love as a consequence of any destructive behaviour, the child attempts to inhibit such behaviours. In doing so, the child develops an increasing tolerance for ambivalence, and learns to mediate between the need for a loved object and his or her own instincts that threatened to destroy the object. This prepares the way for stable object relations, first with the mother and then with other social objects. However, the developing child and adult still carry the potential to revert to the paranoid-schizoid position, particularly at times of stress or distress, and the process of splitting (or other more Freudian defence mechanisms). This is more likely to occur if the individual has been traumatized as a child, and may adversely influence adult relationships.

The practice of psychoanalysis

Despite the differences between the various psychoanalytic theories, they all share a number of therapeutic goals, including gaining insight into the nature of the original trauma and bringing troubling material to consciousness so that the individual can cope with it without the use of ego defence mechanisms. By removing the need for the ego to engage its defence mechanisms, the symptoms may be 'cured'.

Freudian psychoanalysis

Freud experimented with a number of therapeutic techniques, including hypnosis and a form of suggestion in which he sat behind the patient, held their head in his hands, exerted mild pressure, and suggested that the troubling material would be 'released' when he released the physical pressure. He stopped using these methods as he came to believe that the patient–therapist relationship was critical to good psychotherapy. Instead, he used the process of free association. This involved the person speaking aloud whatever came to mind, with the therapist making no conscious effort to monitor or censor their speech. To facilitate the process, the person lay down so they were unable to see the therapist's face and could not be guided by any facial expressions resulting from their flow of thoughts.

Through free association, individuals may remember traumatic or problematic childhood events. However, given the ego's use of defence mechanisms, such revelations are unlikely. Instead, the therapist is guided more by what the person does *not* say than what they do. Absences, where the person is unable to think of a word or finish a sentence, or abrupt changes in topic may indicate the proximity of sensitive issues. Errors, in which a person may mean to say one thing and actually say something different (the so-called 'Freudian slip') may also be indicative of sensitive issues that the therapist would then explore more deeply.

Another technique used by Freud involved the interpretation of dreams, which he considered 'the Royal Road to the unconscious'. An example can be found in Freud's (1900) interpretation of the dream of one woman which included images of flowers as table decorations for a party. When asked to freely associate to the elements in her dream, she associated *violet* with *violate*, a word carrying both sexual and aggressive connotations. Freud interpreted the flowers as symbols of fertility and the birthday as a symbol of an impending birth or pregnancy. Accordingly, her dreams symbolized her desire to become impregnated by her fiancé.

A third source of information about childhood experiences can be found through examination of the person's relationship with their therapist. Freud suggested that a person may develop strong positive or negative feelings towards their therapist, a process known as **transference**. Positive transference may result in the person becoming dependent on the therapist or even falling in love with them. Negative transference includes resentment and anger. According to Freud, these feelings reflect those held for significant others earlier in the person's life. If they fall in love with their therapist, for example, this may mean they have failed to resolve an earlier oedipal conflict. Freud used the transference process in two ways: first, as a diagnostic process, and second, for resolving earlier conflicts by 'working through' the transference process. Freud contended that once having achieved insight, the individual may still need to work through the issues raised by an understanding of the trauma. In a process known as **catharsis**, the individual is encouraged to expresses the emotions previously damped down by the defence mechanisms.

Contemporary psychoanalysis

Classical psychoanalysis was extremely lengthy. Freud preferred to see persons six times a week, and even 'mild' cases were seen for three sessions a week. In addition, because psychoanalysis used free association to bring insight into the person's problems, and there may have been weeks or even months between sessions in which significant insights were attained, analysis took many months or even years. More recent versions of psychoanalysis tend to be shorter, typically lasting fewer than 25 sessions. They have three distinct phases: beginning, an active phase, and termination. Beginning involves assessment, developing a therapeutic alliance, and preparing the person for therapy. In the active phase, the therapist determines the direction of therapy and the issues addressed within it. Strategies may involve the use of interpretation of current feelings in terms of past experiences, and the elicitation of emotions experienced at the time of any trauma. Issues of transference are deliberately minimized, for example, by discouraging person dependence. The end of therapy is a negotiated process, in which issues of loss and separation are considered and dealt with.

Most people who take part in psychoanalysis in Britain do so by seeking private therapy. Not surprisingly, most find it a useful experience:

> I found the process remarkably useful. No one to judge you, no one to comment – you don't even have to talk to anyone. It provides a space for me without pressure to explore issues that are important to me that I cannot speak – quite literally – to anyone else about. I feel my unhappiness stems from my poor relationship with my parents – and this has provided me with a means to explore this, and disentangle some of the issues that confuse me about this time.

2.2 Behavioural approaches

The roots of **behaviour therapy** lie in the theories of classical and **operant conditioning** developed in the early to mid-twentieth century by Pavlov ([1927] 1960) and Skinner (1953). Although differing considerably in their explanations of behaviour, both theories held that:

- behaviour is determined by external events
- past learning experiences drive present behaviour
- behavioural change can be achieved through direct manipulation of external events – there is no need to explore or change the individual's 'psyche' or 'inner world'.

Classical conditioning

Classical conditioning was initially explored by Pavlov's work on the salivary response of dogs. Pavlov considered salivation to be a basic reflex to the presence of food that required no learning: an unconditioned response to an unconditioned stimulus. The novel element of Pavlov's work was that he noted that other salient stimuli present at the time of the elicitation of the unconditioned response subsequently come to elicit the same behaviours: in learning theory jargon, an initially neutral stimulus became a conditioned stimulus and elicited a conditioned response, identical to the unconditioned one. Repeated presentation of the conditioned stimulus in the absence of the unconditioned stimulus will result in a gradual fading of response to it, a process known as extinction.

The link between these processes and emotional disorders was made when it became clear that conditioning experiences may influence emotional as well as behavioural responses to stimuli. Behavioural explanations of phobias, for example, assumed that they result from a conditioning experience in which the inappropriately feared object or situation was associated with the experience of fear or anxiety at some time in the past. The conditioned stimulus subsequently evokes a conditioned fear response. The conditioning process can be so powerful when acute fear is experienced, that it may require only one conditioning experience to result in a long-term fear response (a phobia) that is difficult to extinguish. Being in a car crash, for example, may subsequently result in a phobic reaction to being in a car. This response has three components: a *behavioural element* involving avoidance or escape from the feared object, a high state of *physiological arousal* evident through a variety of symptoms including physical tension, increased startle response, tremor or sweating, and the *emotion* of anxiety and fear.

The most famous early example of the conditioning of a phobic response was Watson and Rayner's (1920) conditioning of 'Little Albert'. Eleven-month-old Albert was a hospitalized child who had a fear of furry animals induced through the experimental association of loud noises at the same time as being given a rabbit to play with. Over time, he developed a conditioned fear (phobic reaction) to the presence of furry animals, a fear which generalized to similar-looking stimuli including balls of cotton, white fur, and a Santa Claus mask. Sadly, although Albert was subsequently allowed to play with the toys in the absence of the loud noises, he was discharged from hospital with his phobia intact: an outcome now deemed ethically unacceptable.

Operant conditioning

In contrast to the reflexive behaviour associated with classical conditioning, operant conditioning attempts to explain behaviours that are voluntary and purposive. Skinner's basic premise was that behaviour that is rewarded (reinforced) will increase in frequency or be repeated; that which is not rewarded or is punished will decrease in frequency or not be repeated. His definition of a reinforcer was behavioural: that which is observed to increase the frequency or strength of a behaviour. He made no assumptions about internal mediating processes such as liking, pleasure or enjoyment.

Skinner distinguished between two types of reinforcer: *primary reinforcers*, such as food and water that have innate biological significance, and *conditioned reinforcers*, that have become associated with these primary reinforcers through a complex process of classical conditioning. In this way, reinforcers such as attention and social interaction, which are associated with the primary reinforcer of food and drink for young children, take on reinforcing properties in themselves.

Operant processes have been implicated in the development of a number of mental disorders. Lewinsohn et al. (1979), for example, considered depression to be the result of an individual being removed from a reward system they had previously occupied. Conversely, Seligman (1975) considered depression to arise from a failure to avoid punishment within the environment. His theory stemmed from a series of studies in which animals received electric shocks they were either able or unable to avoid. Animals that could avoid the shocks seemed to experience no ill-effects. Those that could not exhibited what Seligman termed **learned helplessness**. They were apathetic and, even when they were in conditions where they could avoid shocks, made no attempt to do so. This was seen as analogous to some elements of depression.

Combining classical and operant conditioning

The classical conditioning model of phobias so far considered is adequate in its description of the acquisition of anxiety and phobias. However, it is less able to explain why they are maintained over long periods, as repeated exposure to a feared object or situation in the absence of any negative consequences should lead to a reduction of anxiety through the process of extinction. Mowrer's (1947) two-factor theory combined both classical and operant processes to provide an explanation of this phenomenon. He noted that once a phobic response is established through classical conditioning processes, the affected individual tends to avoid the feared stimulus. This has two consequences. First, it prevents the classical conditioning process of extinction, as the individual does not experience the conditioned stimulus under conditions of safety. Second, because avoidance itself produces feelings of relief (it is reinforcing), the avoidance response is strengthened by operant conditioning processes. In this way, anxiety is potentially maintained over long periods.

Behaviour therapy

Behaviour therapy assumes behaviour and emotions to be governed by the laws of learning: disorders arise as a consequence of specific learning experiences and can be treated using the same principles. The type of therapy it engendered differed fundamentally from psychoanalysis, in that it focused directly on specific conditions such as phobias rather than attempting personality reconstruction, was relatively brief and actively directed by the therapist. Interventions were primarily developed for the treatment of anxiety disorders including phobias, with the goal of eliminating a conditioned fear response to previously feared stimuli.

Systematic desensitization

Systematic desensitization – or as a variant of it is frequently referred to now, exposure with response prevention (ERP) – involves repeatedly exposing the person to a series of stimuli, initially somewhat distant from, and then increasingly like, the feared stimulus, while in a state of relaxation. At the beginning of the intervention, the individual is taught to relax using standardized relaxation procedures (see below). At the same time, they construct a hierarchy of stimuli that progressively resemble the feared object or situation.

Therapy proceeds through a series of stages. In each stage, the person first relaxes and is then exposed to a stimulus within the hierarchy, starting with the most distant stimulus from the feared object or situation. On each exposure, they remain in the presence of the stimulus until they feel fully relaxed. This process is repeated several times until the stimulus no longer elicits an anxiety response. They then progress through the hierarchy of stimuli, repeating the same procedures until they are relaxed in the presence of their feared stimulus or situation (see Box 2.1). These procedures are thought to both extinguish the fear response to the stimulus and counter-condition a state of relaxation. It can be difficult to set up a graded exposure programme using real stimuli, as they may be difficult to obtain or control: snakes or driving in traffic, for example. In such circumstances, the 'traditional' approach was to establish and work through an imaginal hierarchy. Now, technology allows us to produce a much more immersive experience through the use of virtual reality, allowing the development of more closely controlled and constructed hierarchies than previously thought possible.

Flooding

The gradual approach of systematic desensitization is user-friendly, but relatively slow. Flooding involves a diametrically opposite approach. In it, individuals are exposed directly to their most feared stimulus and encouraged to remain with it until they no longer experience any fear, a process that may take an hour or more. It is based on the principles of *habituation*. We cannot sustain a fear response for prolonged periods of time: physical exhaustion results in a diminution of a fear response even under circumstances that initially provoke high levels of fear. Accordingly, even though initial levels of anxiety or fear may be extremely high, if the person remains in the feared situation sufficiently long, they will experience a reduction in anxiety to normal levels. This low level of fear is then associated with the previously feared stimulus. Repeated flooding is usually necessary to fully extinguish some fear responses. Flooding can be an effective form of therapy (see Chapter 6) and is now probably the favoured approach to the treatment of phobias. However, many therapists prefer to use desensitiza-

Box 2.1 Ruth's spider phobia: an example of systematic desensitization

The image of an individual with a spider phobia is a person who, when they see a spider, becomes anxious and jittery, and usually asks for someone to remove it from their presence. But for Ruth, the problem was much greater. From spring to autumn her fear of spiders was so strong that she would not enter a different room in her house without someone first checking there were no spiders in it. Similarly, she would not go into the hall or stairs of her house without a family member making checks. As a consequence, she remained restricted to one room in her house, unless there was someone in the house to check her 'safety'. If she saw a spider, she panicked, and would run as far away as possible from it.

Ruth entered a programme of systematic desensitization in the spring. She was taught to relax using deep muscle relaxation. At the same time, she developed a hierarchy of stimuli to be used in a desensitization programme. She also determined her desired end-point of the programme, which was to enter a room where there may be a spider without undue anxiety and be able to kill any spiders she noticed in the room. The initial hierarchy she and her therapist constructed included the following stimuli:

1. A pencil-drawn line, resembling the leg of a spider
2. A pencil oval, resembling the body of a spider
3. A pencil-drawn sketch of a spider
4. A picture of an actual spider
5. A dead spider in a jar
6. A dead spider on a nearby table
7. A live spider in a jar
8. A live spider constrained by the therapist
9. A live, unconstrained spider.

Ruth worked through this hierarchy over a period of weekly meetings. On each occasion, she used the relaxation techniques and was exposed to the relevant stimulus within the hierarchy on several occasions. Each time, she remained in the presence of the stimulus until she was fully relaxed and calm. The stimulus was removed and then re-presented, and the procedure repeated, until there was good evidence that she was fully relaxed at that stage in the hierarchy and she felt confident to move to the next stage.

Once she was able to be relaxed in the presence of a live spider, Ruth began a second hierarchy:

1. Walking into a room with a constrained spider in it
2. Walking into a room with the possibility of an unconstrained spider in it, remaining by the door
3. Walking into a room in which she knew there was a spider and killing it with a heavy object

4. Walking into a room with the possibility of an unconstrained spider in it, and sitting down in the room for several minutes.

Most people with a phobia of spiders would not require such a gradual or extended treatment programme. Nevertheless, this programme provides a good example of the process of systematic desensitization.

tion methods, as they do not provoke the high levels of **client** distress associated with flooding. Nor do they run the risk of the recipient leaving before extinction of the fear is achieved, something that may actually add to their problems as avoidance of the feared stimulus is once more reinforced.

Relaxation techniques

Relaxation is a key element of both systematic desensitization and flooding. It reduces the high sympathetic nervous system activity (the flight–fight response) activated during fear (see Chapter 4). However, it does not come naturally at such times, and most people have to be taught how to relax. The relaxation process most commonly taught is a derivative of Jacobson's deep muscle relaxation technique. This involves alternately tensing and relaxing muscle groups throughout the body in an ordered sequence. The order in which the muscles are relaxed varies, but a typical exercise may involve the following stages (the tensing procedure is described in parentheses): hands and forearms (making a fist), upper arms (touching fingers to shoulder), shoulders and lower neck (pulling up shoulders), back of neck (touching chin to chest), lips (pushing them together), forehead (frowning), abdomen/chest (holding deep breath), abdomen (tensing stomach muscles), legs and feet (push heel away, pull toes to point at head: not lifting leg). With practice the individual can learn to relax without the prior tensing, using this process immediately before exposure to feared stimuli, whether in the clinic or 'real world'.

2.3 Cognitive approaches

While behavioural therapies achieved (and still do achieve) some notable successes, particularly as treatments for anxiety disorders, the 1970s saw a shift towards a more cognitive approach to our understanding of both anxiety and mood disorders. By this time, conditioning theories were finding it increasingly difficult to account for emerging experimental and clinical findings:

- Many phobics were unable to identify any traumatic conditioning incident
- Many common phobias were to relatively benign stimuli, such as spiders, or rarely encountered stimuli, such as snakes
- By contrast, rates of phobias to many frequently encountered and potentially frightening stimuli (such as traffic) were relatively low
- Phobias tend to 'run' in families

Seligman (1971) provided one explanation for some of these findings. He suggested that some basic anxieties may be biologically 'hardwired'. This has survival advantages, in that avoidance of small, quick, and possibly dangerous animals is likely to be of significant survival benefit to individuals who live in dangerous and wild environments. These instinctual reactions become problematic when we no longer live in such surroundings, but because they are hardwired, we find it difficult to stop responding in this basic way (see Chapter 6 for further discussion of this issue).

While Seligman's theory gave some support to the behavioural model, other findings made it increasingly difficult to maintain purely behavioural models of fear acquisition. One of the more interesting challenges stemmed from cases such as the individual whose initial fear of beetles generalized to several other stimuli including Volkswagen cars and the Beatles pop group (Carr 1974). While behavioural theory acknowledged the potential for the generalization of a fear response to similar stimuli, this was based on the physical characteristics of the related stimuli. In this case, the associations between feared stimuli were of a semantic nature – that is, they were mediated by cognitive processes.

At the same time as these problems emerged, other theorists were beginning to explore the role of cognitive processes in directing behaviour. Social learning theory (Bandura 1977), for example, identified that we can learn fear responses without having direct experience of the feared object. Instead, fear can be acquired from observation of other people's responses, through a process known as **vicarious learning**. A fear of flying, for example, may develop as a result of seeing air crashes on the television or hearing the accounts of those involved. Social learning theory can also provide a cognitive explanation of why phobias run in families: children may acquire fears from observation of their parents' fearful behaviour or stories. Finally, Bandura also provided a cognitive explanation of the therapeutic mechanisms of systematic desensitization and flooding: reductions in anxiety were the result of the individual's increasing confidence, or self-efficacy as Bandura termed it, in their ability to cope with the presence of the feared object.

Emerging clinical models

Further pressure to shift from purely behavioural interventions stemmed from the emerging cognitive therapies of Aaron Beck (e.g. Beck 1976) and Albert Ellis (1977) used in the treatment of mood disorders such as depression. Both clinicians assumed that our cognitive response to events, not the events themselves, determine our mood, and that mental health problems are a consequence of 'faulty' or 'irrational' thinking: misinterpretations of environmental events. These thoughts impact on our mood, our behaviour, and our physiological state. Ellis referred to this process as the *A-B-C theory* of personality functioning, where:

- A is an activating event: something that triggers an emotional response
- C is the emotional or behavioural reaction to that event
- B is the intervening cognitive processing, the individual's beliefs about the event.

Beck referred to the immediate thoughts that drive negative emotions as automatic negative thoughts (ANTs). They come to mind automatically as the individual's first response to a particular situation and are without logic or grounding in reality. Despite this, their very automaticity means they are unchallenged and taken as true. He also identified a more fundamental set of beliefs known as a *cognitive schema* (plural *schemata*): unconscious beliefs about the self and the world that influence our surface cognitions.

Beck hypothesized that our cognitive schemata develop in childhood. Some may exert a consistent influence throughout life. People with avoidant personalities, for example, may hold the fundamental belief that 'If people get close to me, they will discover the "real" me and reject me'. As a consequence, they continually avoid others to prevent this catastrophe occurring. Other schemata, such as those underlying depression, may impact only at certain times. According to Beck, many vulnerable individuals are able to override negative schemata for much of the time. However, when they encounter situations as adults that echo previous negative childhood experiences (divorce or separation, for example, reflecting earlier experiences of parental rejection) and there is an initial lowering of mood, underlying negative schemata are activated, influencing surface cognitions and triggering an episode of depression.

Cognitive behavioural therapy

Acceptance of the role of cognitions in mood disorders did not lead to the wholesale rejection of behavioural techniques. There was a therapeutic evolution rather than revolution, and cognitive behavioural therapy (CBT) uses both behavioural and cognitive strategies to achieve change. That said, the primary goal of CBT is to change distorted cognitions, albeit through the use of both cognitive and behavioural techniques.

Cognitive techniques

The simplest method of directly changing cognitions involves the use **self-instruction training** (Meichenbaum 1985). This involves interrupting the flow of negative 'stressogenic' thoughts by replacing them with pre-prepared realistic or 'coping' ones. These typically fall into one of two categories: reminders to use any stress-coping techniques the person has practised, and reminders that the individual can cope effectively with the situation ('You can cope with this … you have before … remember to relax …').

A more complex approach, known as **cognitive challenge**, involves identifying and challenging the reality of the negative assumptions an individual is making. In this, the person is taught to 'catch' their thoughts and identify the association between thoughts, emotions, and behaviour. They then learn to treat their negative cognitive responses to particular situations as hypotheses or guesses, not reality, to challenge their veracity, and to replace them with more appropriate and less emotionally disturbing thoughts ('I'm feeling faint. I'm going to pass out and make a fool of myself' versus 'Well, I've felt this way before and nothing bad happened – It won't happen this time …). This skill can be practised within the therapy session, before being used in the 'real world'.

Ways of identifying and changing negative assumptions can be taught through what Beck (Beck et al. 1979) called *Socratic dialogue* or *guided discovery*. This involves the therapist helping the person to identify distorted patterns of thinking and encouraging them to consider different ways of thinking or evidence that may challenge them. Within this process a strategy known as the *downward arrow technique* (Beck et al. 1979) can be implemented. Key questions include:

- What is your concern about …?
- What would the implications be …?
- What would the consequences be …?
- What would the ultimate consequences be …?

One example of their use is provided by this extract from a session with a problem drinker:

Therapist: You feel quite strongly that you need to be 'relaxed' by alcohol when you go to a party. What is your concern about being sober?
Person: I wouldn't enjoy myself and I wouldn't be much fun to be with.
T: What would be the implications of that?
P: Well, people wouldn't talk to me.
T: And what would be the consequence of that?
P: I need to have people like me. My job depends on it. If I can't entertain people at a party, I'm no good at my job …
T: So, what happens if that is the case?
P: Well, I guess I lose my job!
T: So, you lose your job because you didn't get drunk at a party?
P: Well, put like that, I think I may have not had it in the right perspective.

Here, the downward arrow technique has been used both to identify some of the individual's core beliefs and to help him to reconsider their accuracy by showing how disproportionate they were.

Behavioural strategies

Behavioural strategies may also be used to facilitate cognitive change. This typically involves setting up behavioural experiments within a therapy session or as homework that directly test the cognitive beliefs that people may hold, in the expectation that negative beliefs are disconfirmed – and more positive ones affirmed. This may be the most fundamental process of emotional change. Cognitive challenge allows the possibility that the individual *may* be thinking inappropriately, behavioural hypothesis-testing establishes it to be the case. In the case of the problem drinker above, for example, the individual may be encouraged to challenge his thoughts in relation to the outcome of a party if he does not drink, but actually finding out he can socialize and entertain at a party without getting drunk provides definitive proof, and is likely to engender longer-term change.

One interesting behavioural challenge used by a colleague in the treatment of two people with schizophrenia involved simultaneously testing their assumptions about their unusual abilities. One felt that their thoughts were being 'broadcast' and heard by other people; the other believed that they could hear what other people were thinking. As a test of both their beliefs, the two of them were put in a room. One was asked to look at cards often used to test extrasensory perception (ESP), and asked to broadcast an image of each of the cards he looked at. The other was asked to write down the images that he was 'receiving'. Of course, the received images bore no relationship to the images that were actually being 'broadcast', so both sets of beliefs were challenged by this particular behavioural experiment.

The flow of therapy

Much of cognitive behaviour therapy actually takes place outside the therapy sessions. The flow of therapy usually involves exploration of a particular issue within a therapy session, perhaps using Socratic dialogue to identify and challenge cognitive distortions. Based on this process, a homework assignment may be made in which the individual monitors a key therapy indicator such as mood or anxiety, or engages in some form of behavioural challenge. At the next session, this homework is reviewed, a new issue is considered, and further homework is set in an iterative progressive process. The homework assignments are as important, if not more important, as the therapy 'hour'.

Experiencing cognitive behavioural therapy

Here are some views about the experience of CBT:

> I found it really helpful – but it was difficult. The therapist asked me to, like, question my thoughts. I found that really difficult. I couldn't really work out what I was thinking … let alone try to question them! But I remember one appointment when we talked through how I felt when I went on holiday, and I felt really sad at the beginning of the session. By the end I felt really good about myself! And I began to see how thinking about things differently could help me feel better. In the end I found this part of therapy really useful.

> I found the relaxation really good … I really enjoyed it. Yeah, it worked well – the rest wasn't easy. But I really valued the support of my therapist. I actually think that that was the most important thing I got out of therapy.

> I found it good to take a gradual approach to dealing with my panics. The therapist was very good as they listened to my concerns, and gave me advice about what to do to stop me panicking. I don't think I would have liked just talking – and telling her about my childhood, and so on – I can't see the point in that.

These comments reflect some of the problems that people face in CBT and the importance of the relationship between person and therapist, even in the relatively structured use of cognitive behavioural techniques.

Research box 1

Leuzinger-Bohleber, M., Hautzinger, M., Fiedler, G. et al. (2019) Outcome of psychoanalytic and cognitive behavioural long-term therapy with chronically depressed patients: a controlled trial with preferential and randomized allocation, *Canadian Journal of Psychiatry*, 64: 47–58.

This research paper is interesting firstly because it challenges the dominance of cognitive behaviour therapy (CBT) as a treatment approach, and secondly because of its relatively novel design. Cognitive behaviour therapy has become the dominant therapeutic approach across many healthcare systems partly because of the weight of evidence of its effectiveness, which other approaches lack. For other approaches to be adopted requires them to achieve a substantial research base. Psychoanalytic approaches have struggled to achieve evidence of effectiveness in the past, and have therefore been excluded as a therapeutic approach in many healthcare systems. Accordingly, a study directly comparing CBT and psychoanalysis is an important contribution to the psychotherapeutic literature. The study is also interesting because rather than being a randomized controlled trial, in which participants are randomly assigned to a therapeutic approach they may or may not be sympathetic to, it adopted a 'preference trial' approach. In this, participants were given a choice over the treatment they received, potentially facilitating adherence to, and the effectiveness of, each therapeutic approach.

Method

Participants

Participants were aged 21–60 years with chronic depression or low mood (dysthymia) lasting at least one year. Level of depression was confirmed by meeting the criteria for these diagnoses using the Structured Clinical Interview (SCID; see Chapter 1), and having a score of 17 or above on the Beck Depression Inventory (BDI) and a clinician rating of more than 9 points on the Quick Inventory of Depressive Symptomatology (QIDS; Rush et al. 2003). Participants with stable dosage of antidepressants were included in the trial.

Interventions

Psychoanalysis considered depression in the context of developmental processes, particularly pathological processes involving unconscious fantasies and conflicts. It focused on: (i) developing a differentiated, integrated, and realistic basic feeling of self and identity; (ii) facilitating the ability to engage in satisfying reciprocal interpersonal relationships; and (iii) the ability to unfold creativity in work, developmental tasks matching the individual's life-cycle, and satisfying management of everyday life situations. It involved discovering unconscious determining factors due to failures in development (e.g. archaic unconscious fantasies stimulated by traumatizations, pathological relationships), and working through idiosyncratic unconscious fantasies and conflicts due to developmental deficits and traumatizations in the 'here and now' of the therapeutic relationship.

Cognitive behavioural therapy followed the model of Beck and involved: (i) problem analysis, goals, **psychoeducation**, rationale for treatment, explanation of intervention steps; (ii) behaviour-oriented interventions, including activation, increasing pleasant activities, balance of negative and positive activities, structuring day and week; (iii) cognitive interventions, including focus on automatic thoughts and alternatives, influence of basic assumptions and schemata; (iv) skill training, including social and problem-solving skills using role-play and homework; and (v) maintenance and relapse prevention.

Adherence to the required protocols was checked through assessment of randomly selected audiotapes by three independent raters.

Outcome measures

Key outcome measures were a questionnaire-based assessment of depression (Beck Depression Inventory; BDI) and a clinician-based assessment, the Quick Inventory of Depressive Symptomatology (QIDS). All assessments were by trained clinicians blind to treatment condition. QIDS scores were recorded and independently rated, with high ($r = 0.95$) inter-rater reliability.

Group allocation

At entry into the study participants were given a choice of intervention, and assigned to their treatment of choice. Those with no preference were randomly assigned to one or other condition. Accordingly, there were four 'arms' to the trial and analysis: (i) preferred CBT (P-CBT), (ii) preferred psychoanalysis (P-PA), (iii) allocated CBT (A-CBT), and (iv) allocated PA (A-PA)

Trial flow

Of 554 people interviewed, 252 fitted the **DSM** criteria for entry into the study. Measures were taken at entry, and 1-, 2-, and 3-year follow-up.

Results

Data was analysed in two ways: linear changes in scores on the BDI and QIDS, and categorical shifts from scores above the diagnostic criterion (case) to below this criterion (non-case). These are outlined in the table below.

	P-CBT (N = 63)	P-PA (N = 101)	A-CBT (N = 41)	A-PA (N = 47)	Sig. time change	Sig. between condition
BDI score						
Baseline	32.0 (7.8)	31.2 (7.8)	32.6 (7.0)	33.9 (9.2)		NS
Change						
Year 1	14.4 (12.1)	10.7 (11.1)	12.6 (13.3)	12.0 (12.7)	<0.001	NS
Year 2	15.2 (9.7)	13.9 (12.7)	11.9 (12.2)	15.2 (12.7)	<0.001	NS
Year 3	17.2 (10.7)	15.8 (10.9)	17.5 (12.4)	20.1 (11.9)	<0.001	NS
QIDS						
Baseline	14.1 (3.0)	14.3 (3.0)	13.3 (2.6)	15.2 (3.4)		
Change						
Year 1	7.1 (4.0)	5.7 (4.4)	6.6 (4.8)	6.8 (4.9)	<0.001	NS
Year 2	7.8 (4.5)	8.0 (4.4)	6.9 (5.9)	8.6 (4.9)	<0.001	NS
Year 3	7.0 (5.5)	8.0 (5.1)	9.7 (3.7)	10.4 (5.9)	<0.001	NS
BDI non-case						
Year 1	38%	28%	47%	32%	<0.001	NS
Year 2	45%	38%	47%	32%	<0.001	NS
Year 3	43%	44%	50%	44%	<0.001	NS
QIDS non-case						
Year 1	54%	33%	41%	33%	<0.001	NS
Year 2	57%	44%	46%	44%	<0.001	NS
Year 3	52%	55%	79%	68%	<0.001	NS

Discussion

A number of interesting points are raised by the data. First, the apparent preference for psychoanalysis. The study was conducted in French-speaking Canada. Psychoanalysis is still very popular in France, and although CBT is increasingly used, there may be a cultural preference for this approach. Accordingly, this preference may be culturally specific and not found in other populations. Second, all the interventions appear to be equally effective, even when allocated and not the choice of the individual. Third, the success rates are relatively high for both interventions for this 'difficult to treat' group of individuals, who have typically not responded to other treatment approaches. From a methodological perspective, the study struggled to keep participants engaged in the research, and at times the response rates were less than ideal. Nevertheless, it appears that CBT and psychoanalysis are equally effective. A success story for psychoanalysis? Well, not quite actually. The somewhat hidden information here that becomes evident at the end of the results section was the shear length of the interventions. Participants in the PA intervention received an average of 234 sessions over the entire period of the trial, while the CBT participants received an average of 57 sessions, lasting up to 15 months. Accordingly, from a methodological perspective, the interventions were not comparable, with the potential for an effect simply of seeing a therapist being more sustained in the PA condition. From a healthcare provider perspective, neither approach is realistic. Modern CBT interventions provided by formal healthcare systems are now likely to last between eight and ten sessions. The requirement and costs of continued therapy for this sustained period of time are simply not tenable.

2.4 Humanistic approaches

The humanistic school of psychology was founded in the 1950s in the USA. Its therapeutic approach was developed by Carl Rogers (1961). Humanism formed as a 'Third Force' as a reaction against both psychoanalysis and behaviourism. Humanists considered psychoanalysis to be too pessimistic, as it emphasized the pathological, irrational, unconscious fragmentation of personality. Behaviourism was rejected because of its mechanistic approach to understanding the human condition. By contrast, humanistic psychologists wanted a psychology that focused on healthy, rational, higher motivations.

The approach has two key foundations:

- Behaviour is understood in terms of the subjective experience of the individual: the *phenomenological* perspective. This accepts the subjective experience of the individual as a valid source of information about their values, motives, and the meaning of their behaviour.
- Behaviour is not constrained by either past experiences or current circumstances. The individual has 'free will' and makes behavioural choices independent of past learning history or the unconscious influence of innate drives.

Carl Rogers's (1961) theory of the individual has been termed a *self-theory*, in that it focused on the individual's self-concept and their subjective experience of the world. Rogers's basic premise was that all individuals have an innate drive to grow, develop, and enhance their abilities in ways they choose: a process he called self-actualization. This 'actualizing tendency' stimulates creativity and leads us to seek new challenges and skills that motivate healthy growth. When the individual is in touch with their actualizing tendency, their behaviour is directed in ways that foster positive growth and happiness. When they are not, the result is sadness, anxiety or depression.

Rogers also noted that we live in subjective worlds of our own creation: the *phenomenal field*. In many ways, this maps onto reality, but it may also be distorted and inaccurate. Nevertheless, our reaction to events, be they emotional or behavioural, is based on our perception of the world, not 'objective' reality. Within this framework, the most significant element is the sense of self, our understanding of 'who we are'. Rogers considered the self to be constantly in a process of forming and re-forming. We experience it as unchanging only as a result of biases and selectivity in attending to those elements of our phenomenal field that are consistent with our prior experience. Our sense of self is influenced by past experiences, our present situation, and expectations of the future. However, unlike the psychoanalysts, he argued that the past is only as important as the individual chooses to make it, through conscious choice. Free will allows us to break away from the past, and for our behaviour and emotions to be related more to the present, and perhaps the future.

Although as individuals we acknowledge our *actual self*, our actualizing tendency drives us towards another version of the self: the *ideal self*. This reflects who we would like to be: the goals and aspirations of our lives. Like the self, this is a changing and evolving concept. The degree to which the actual and ideal selves match each other has a profound effect on our emotions and behaviour. When the two are relatively similar (what Rogers termed congruent), we experience positive emotions; when the two are incongruent, we experience sadness and other negative emotions, and the actualizing process is inhibited.

For many, the beginnings of incongruence lie in childhood. Rogers argued that the way parental love and approval are given has a strong impact on the developing person. Subtle elements of parent–child interactions contribute to the development of pathology. One important process, known as *conditional positive regard*, occurs when parents simultaneously show their disapproval both of bad behaviour and of the child ('Your behaviour is bad, and I don't love you when you behave in this way'). Love and approval are granted only if the child behaves in a way that his or her parents want them to. As a result, children adopt their parents' 'conditions of worth'. That is, the child comes to associate their self-worth with their behaviour and begins to adopt behaviours that are valued by their parents. The child begins to internalize the goals of his or her parents into its ideal self, and work towards achieving them rather than his or her own goals and aspirations. As a result, the child fails to progress towards self-actualization.

According to Rogers, three elements of the individual's interactions with others can facilitate their move towards self-actualization:

- *Unconditional positive regard*: acceptance and love that are not contingent upon the individual behaving in the required manner: 'I do not approve of your behaviour ... but I love you nonetheless'.
- *Genuineness*: an environment in which the individual is able to freely express their own sense of self, rather than playing a role or hiding behind a façade.
- *Empathy*: an environment in which the individual is involved with people who can understand the world from their viewpoint – who share their phenomenal field.

Humanistic therapy

There are several schools of humanistic therapy, with the *person-centred therapy* of Rogers being pre-eminent. Rogers considered pathology to be the result of a deviation from the self-actualizing process, usually as a consequence of experiencing conditional positive regard. Therapy involves the individual realigning with their own actualizing tendency.

Early in the history of Rogers's therapy, he described his approach as non-directive. The role of the therapist was to help the individual explore issues relevant to them and their development, with an equal relationship between therapist and person giving the person control over the issues explored. However, careful analysis of therapy transcripts by Truax (1966) indicated that rather than act as a neutral facilitator, the therapist (in this case Rogers himself) unconsciously reinforced statements that indicated progress on the person's part, and ignored those that were less positive. Acknowledging the impossibility of total neutrality by the therapist, Rogers abandoned the term non-directive, but still emphasized that therapy should focus on the development of the individual, not the interpretations or actions of the therapist. The name 'client-centred therapy' (later changed to person-centred) was deliberately chosen by Rogers to contrast with the medicalization and power structure implied by use of the term 'patient' by the psychoanalysts.

The goal of person-centred therapy is to provide an environment in which the individual can identify their own life goals and how they wish to determine them: to place them on the pathway to self-actualization. Rogers stated that therapy does not rely on techniques or doing things *to* the person. Rather, the quality of the interpersonal encounter is the most significant element in determining effectiveness. The goal of the therapist is to provide a setting in which the individual is not judged but is free to explore new ways of being. That is, therapy provides the conditions necessary for growth identified earlier. To achieve this, the therapist must have three characteristics:

- they are integrated and genuine in their relationship with the person
- they gain an empathic understanding of the person's perspective and communicate this to them
- they provide unconditional positive regard.

Being genuine means that the therapist shares feeling or gives feedback about how they feel as a consequence of what the person is telling them. Such feedback may be positive or negative, and shows that the therapist is human with human feelings. It may involve expressions of sadness or even anger in response to the individual's stories. Empathy involves the therapist gaining an understanding of the individual's situation, problems, feelings, and concerns, from *their* perspective, and showing the person that they have achieved this level of understanding. The most frequent method by which this is achieved is through a process of reflecting back the therapist's understanding of the person's perspective. The final component of the therapeutic relationship is that the therapist is not judgemental, and does not repeat the past experiences of conditional positive regard.

Rogers suggested that these three therapist characteristics can facilitate a shift from the externally imposed standards of others to the identification and shift to the pathway towards self-actualization. This is thought to be achieved through a series of seven stages, in which the individual:

1. fails to acknowledge feelings, and considers personal relationships to be dangerous
2. is able to describe their behaviour, but rarely their feelings, which are not 'owned'

3. can begin to describe their emotional reactions to past events, and recognize contradictions in their experience
4. develops an awareness of their current feelings, but finds it difficult to cope with them
5. begins to explore their inner life in a more meaningful and emotional way
6. is able to fully experience feelings while talking of past events
7. develops a basic trust in their own inner processes: feelings experienced with immediacy and intensity.

The therapist's actions facilitate each of these processes. Empathic feedback encourages and validates the exploration and expression of personal feelings and meanings of statements made in therapy. Acceptance and genuineness encourage the growth of trust in the self and increased risk-taking in the expression of previously withheld thoughts or emotions.

Experiencing person-centred therapy

Here are some reactions to this type of approach:

> I found it really quite disconcerting. All my therapist seemed to do was to repeat back to me things that I'd said to him. I wanted someone to suggest things and advise me what to do to help me cope with my problems. But all he seemed to do was to avoid this and say it was up to me!

> I really liked the space to sit and think – without someone on my back or things to deal with. Just thinking things through can help you change your perspective or think how to do things different. Just unloading some of the shit I'd had during the week really helped.

> I found it really useful – it gave me time to think and develop my plans for the future. Sometimes you need this sort of space, with someone you can trust and who does not sit in judgement on you – even if some of the things you say may not always put you in the best light.

These comments reflect some of the benefits that many people get from humanistic therapy. They also hint that different people may benefit from different types of therapeutic approach. The first person here, for example, may have benefited from a more structured form of therapy. Finally, they also draw attention to the non-specific benefits of therapy, which may just involve expressing negative emotions that cannot be expressed elsewhere.

2.5 How effective are the different therapies?

The therapeutic approaches outlined in this chapter developed from different historical roots and at different times. Nevertheless, they are all still practised in one form or other, although the dominant method is now the cognitive behavioural approach. The reasons for this can be attributed to a number of factors, including the dominance of cognitive psychology within the broader discipline of psychology and the accessibility of the approach to both practitioner and recipient.

As the number of studies of interventions in specific conditions proliferate, comparisons between the various approaches have increasingly become condition- or therapy-specific. However, several early **meta-analyses** drew together evidence of the relative effectiveness of each of the therapeutic approaches over a broad spectrum of disorders. These consistently showed cognitive behavioural approaches to be superior to both psychoanalytic and humanistic approaches. One of the most stringent of these early meta-analyses was reported by Shapiro and Shapiro (1983), who identified 143 studies that compared different therapies both to one another and to a control condition. They found the following **effect sizes**: psychoanalytic therapy, 0.40; behavioural therapy, 1.06; CBT, 1.42. These compared with an effect size for **placebo** interventions of 0.71. These data both emphasized the relative strength of cognitive behavioural interventions and showed the analytic therapies to be marginally less effective than placebo.

Since then, the dominance of CBT has become more questionable. Barth et al. (2013), for example, conducted a meta-analysis on the effect of seven therapeutic approaches for the treatment of depression. Interventions included short-term psychodynamic therapy, supportive counselling, and cognitive behavioural therapy. All were more effective than a **waiting list control**, but there were few differences in effectiveness between them. In a theoretical commentary on the findings of a range of similar findings, Cuijpers et al. (2019) admitted that the relative effectiveness of differing intervention approaches is proving difficult to determine, with a number of meta-analyses finding no differences between the various types of intervention; although those that do find differences tend to favour cognitive behavioural interventions. So frequent are these findings of 'no differences' across the therapies, that some (e.g. Gelso 2014) have argued for a common factors model of therapeutic gain through which processes common to all therapeutic approaches may be significant drivers of change. These include:

- The personal relationship between therapist and recipient, and 'the extent to which each is genuine … and experiences the other in ways that befit the other' (Gelso 2014). That is, the core elements of the humanistic therapies. This provision of care may be particularly beneficial for those people who lack caring relationships elsewhere.
- Therapy provides an explanation or rationale for why the person is experiencing their difficulties.
- Therapy provides expectations and support of actions to remedy their problems, using the strategies appropriate to the form of therapy they are engaged in. It indicates change can be achieved and supports individuals while they attempt to make changes.

More succinctly, Lambert and Ogles (2014) suggested that therapy provides support, learning, and facilitates action. Accordingly, although therapists may have allegiances and skills in particular therapeutic approaches, many factors common to a range of therapies are also key to therapeutic benefit. In addition, soft-therapist skills are also essential to the outcome of therapy. According to Wampold (2015), these include:

- a sophisticated set of interpersonal skills, including verbal fluency, interpersonal perception, affective modulation and expressiveness, warmth and acceptance, and empathy
- ensuring that the person feels understood, trusts the therapist, and believes the therapist can help him or her
- building a working alliance with a broad range of persons – the working alliance involves the therapeutic bond, but also importantly agreement about the task of goals of therapy
- adjusting therapy if resistance to the treatment is apparent or the person is not making adequate progress
- providing an acceptable and adaptive explanation for the person's distress
- developing a treatment plan that is consistent with the explanation provided to the person
- being influential, persuasive, and convincing.

Stop and think ...

Some years ago, when I was head of a clinical psychology service, I read two simultaneous government guidelines on the provision of psychological therapy. The first stated quite clearly that the use of any intervention needs to 'evidence-based' – that is, there should be a significant amount of evidence supporting its use. The second stated that the choice of intervention should be that of the recipient. These were clearly contradictory statements, and were clearly problematic. What if a service user requested a form of intervention I believed to be unhelpful? What if they asked for a treatment approach for which no one had the training? How would anyone naïve to therapy have any real idea what may benefit them most? By contrast, many potentially useful interventions may not have a strong empirical support. They may be new, or as in the case of psychoanalysis rarely effectively evaluated. So, how should we determine the therapies provided by the NHS, and how should we train our clinical psychologists? Is the continued focus on cognitive behaviour therapy as a primary form of intervention justified? Or should we teach a wider range of therapeutic approaches?

2.6 Chapter summary

1. Different psychoanalytic models of psychopathology place differing emphases on sexual and developmental issues. They are central to Freud's theory, but not those of Jung and Klein. All, however, place childhood experiences and trauma at the centre of later psychopathology.
2. Psychoanalytic therapy is aimed at gaining insight into the traumas that lay the foundations for future emotional problems. Insight may lead to catharsis, the

expression of emotions previously withheld from consciousness by ego defence mechanisms.

3. Behavioural models of psychopathology have focused mainly on various types of anxiety. Phobias, for example, are considered a conditioned response to a particular stimulus, with fear maintained through operant conditioning processes.

4. Behavioural therapies are based on classical and operant conditioning paradigms. Key approaches involve flooding and systematic desensitization. These are thought to result in counter-conditioning or habituation of the fear response.

5. Cognitive understandings of psychopathology place cognitions as central to psychopathology. Therapists such as Beck have provided insight into the thought content associated with a variety of disorders.

6. Cognitive behavioural interventions involve changing inappropriate cognitions, which leads to changes in mood and behaviour.

7. Humanistic therapies aim to provide the individual with the emotional space to reorient them towards the path to self-actualization.

8. The key factor within humanistic therapy is the relationship between therapist and person, which removes conditions of worth imposed by parents and others, and allows the individual to move towards self-actualization.

9. Cognitive behavioural therapy has long been considered the most effective psychotherapy. However, evidence is now emerging of equality of effectiveness of a range of psychotherapies and an increasing focus on common therapeutic factors.

2.7 For discussion

1. Some clinical psychology training courses encourage their trainees to undertake a course of psychotherapy during their training. How might this be useful to their practice as clinicians? Should all clinicians receive some form of psychotherapy while practising?

2. One of the claims of the early behaviour therapists was that therapy could be delivered without the need of a therapist. Written and now computer-driven programmes could provide the skills and structure to treat mental health problems. Was this a realistic claim?

3. Consider the contention that Freud's theory has been under-rated over the years, and still has much to contribute to our understanding of mental health problems.

4. How accessible are the thoughts that influence mood, and how easy is it to change them?

5. What commonalities and differences are there between the various schools of therapy?

6. 'It's not who you are, but what you do as a therapist ...' Discuss this statement in the context of the treatment of mental health disorders.

2.8 Further reading

Corrie, S., Townsend, M. and Cockx, A. (2015) *Assessment and Case Formulation in Cognitive Behavioural Therapy*, London: Sage.

Lemma, A. (2015) *Introduction to the Practice of Psychodynamic Psychotherapy*, Chichester: Wiley.

Mearns, D., Thorne, B. and McLeod, J. (2013) *Person-centred Counselling in Action*, London: Sage.

Wampold, B.E. (2019) *The Basics of Psychotherapy: An Introduction to Theory and Practice*, Washington, DC: American Psychological Association.

Westbrook, D., Kennerly, H. and Kirk, J. (2016) *An Introduction to Cognitive Behaviour Therapy: Skills and Applications*, London: Sage.

3 Beyond cognitive behavioural therapy

Cognitive behavioural therapy (CBT) is the dominant therapeutic approach within professional healthcare settings. It is attractive to healthcare providers as there is a wealth of research showing its effectiveness across a wide range of problems, and the relatively short time-frames in which such changes can be achieved. At its most fundamental, CBT skills are also relatively easy to teach and implement; although skilled use of CBT remains a complex process, and therapist skill is a key determinant of the success or failure of therapy (Keijsers et al. 2000). In addition, national bodies that establish treatment guidelines (in the UK, the National Institute for Health and Care Excellence, or NICE) identify CBT as the psychological treatment of choice for most mental health problems.

Despite its ubiquity CBT has also undergone a number of fundamental changes and challenges to its underpinning theory, and the therapeutic approaches and methods used by its adherents. Since the pioneering work of Beck and Ellis considered in the previous chapter, a number of theorists and clinicians have taken the basic tenets of cognitive therapy and developed them in various ways. Some cognitive models of psychopathology (e.g. Wells 2000) have developed more dynamic models, combining cognitive content (as considered by Beck and Ellis) with processes such as attention, long-term memory retrieval, and other processes within more general information processing models. Others (e.g. Hayes et al. 2006) have adopted a more radical behaviourist stance and questioned both the central role of cognitions in psychopathology and developed interventions that do not attempt cognitive change. We consider both approaches in this chapter. By the end of the chapter, you should have an understanding of factors influencing these new developments and some key therapeutic advances:

- The transdiagnostic model
- The S-REF model and metacognitive therapy
- Relational frames theory and acceptance and commitment therapy.

3.1 Beyond CBT

Behavioural therapy was first established in the mid-1950s. It and its derivates have their own history, often described in terms of 'waves' of theory and practice. The first wave, **behaviour therapy**, focused on identifying and changing contingencies between external contextual cues, emotions, and behaviour. The second wave, led by Beck and Ellis, shifted the focus of therapy to internal events: cognitions. The central tenet of this generation of therapies was that if we can identify aberrant cognitions and then challenge and change them through logic, we can reduce the emotional distress associated with them. Hayes et al. (2006) described this as a common-sense model of psychopathology, but that it had its limitations. With this in mind, a number of theorists and clinicians have argued that the second-wave theories have critical limitations, including an exclusive focus on the *content* of cognitions to the exclusion of other cognitive *processes* and the development of condition-specific theories. A third generation of theories and interventions has attempted to shift from these foci, sometimes in quite opposing ways, but also with a significant degree of commonality. These newer theories are often referred to as 'third-wave' theories and therapies.

The third wave: an introduction

The first theory to be addressed in this chapter, the transdiagnostic theory (Harvey et al. 2004), takes its name from its originators' contention that the degree of co-morbidity between mental health problems is so great that psychological theories need to focus on factors common to differing disorders rather than those that differentiate between them. They noted that while any cognitive content may be specific to each disorder (as suggested by Beck), a number of psychological processes, including those related to biases in attention and memory, will be the same. These underlying processes became the focus of their theoretical model. They stopped short, however, of developing a specific intervention based on their theoretical framework.

Other models have focused on both understanding the causes of mental health disorders *and* treating them. The first to be considered in this chapter, the Self-Regulatory Executive Function (S-REF) model, was developed in the UK by Wells (2000). It is avowedly cognitive and has much in common with the transdiagnostic approach. Like the transdiagnostic approach, it focuses on processes such as attentional bias and memory retrieval, but also focuses on factors (including cognitive content) specific to different conditions. Indeed, Wells has developed a number of condition-specific theories (some of which are considered later in the book), each of which can be interpreted in the light of the S-REF model. He has also developed an intervention approach, known as metacognitive therapy, which can be applied to a number of conditions.

The third approach to be considered in the chapter is markedly different from either of the first two models. Like the transdiagnostic model, it provides a model of psychopathology that is relevant to a number of conditions. However, it adopts a radical behaviourist approach, and challenges the basic assumption that cognitive change is central or even relevant to therapeutic change. In an early critique of CBT, Beidel and Turner (1986) argued that there was little need for the 'cognitive' in cognitive behavioural therapy. They argued that rather than changes in cognitions being necessary to facilitate behavioural and emotional change, behavioural change may itself change cognitions and emotions: an anxious individual may feel more confident and less anxious after successfully confronting a fear, a depressed person may benefit emotionally from engaging in a pleasant activity, and so on. This being the case, they argued, the most direct therapeutic route is behavioural: cognitive change is an additional, and unnecessary, step within therapy.

This view gained support from a British cognitive therapist, Teasdale (e.g. Teasdale 1993), who argued that changes in cognitions made within the therapy session were only short-term in nature. They lead the individual to engage in behaviours that test the old and new assumptions developed within the therapy session: the person with a phobia may approach their feared object with less expectation of being harmed; the depressed person may try out a new, more active, way of dealing with their problems with greater expectations of success. However, longer-term cognitive, emotional or behavioural change occurs only after these new assumptions are tested and confirmed. This model suggests that the role of cognitive interventions is essentially one of encouraging the individual to engage in some form of behavioural change. The logical outcome both for Beidel and Turner and for Teasdale is that a behavioural intervention in which the **client** is directly encouraged to test their assumptions without any cognitive preparation should prove effective in engendering emotional change. Strongly linked to this theoretical perspective is the therapeutic model of acceptance and commitment therapy (Hayes et al. 2006).

3.2 The transdiagnostic model

In one of the largest surveys of psychiatric co-morbidity so far conducted, Kessler et al. (1994) estimated that the average individual diagnosed with a mental health disorder would not have just one disorder: their symptoms would lead them to be diagnosed with an average of 2.1 disorders. Of course, just like the family with 2.4 children, such an individual would never actually exist; but the key issue here is that many people could be diagnosed with a number of co-existing disorders. The extent of this co-morbidity is emphasized by the findings of Jacobi et al. (2004) highlighted in Table 3.1, which shows the percentage of people with various diagnoses found to have up to three or more additional diagnosable disorders. Of note also is that in the few intervention trials that have examined this issue (e.g. Tsao et al. 2002), improvements in one disorder seem to be matched by improvements in others that are not the focus of the intervention.

Together, these data led Harvey and colleagues (2004) to argue that these co-morbid conditions must be driven by similar processes, amenable to the same therapeutic interventions, and that psychological models should attempt to

Table 3.1 The percentage of individuals diagnosed with various DSM disorders that would be co-morbid for at least one additional disorder

Disorder	Pure disorder	One additional diagnosis	Two additional diagnoses	Three or more additional diagnoses
Eating disorders	35	21	31	13
Generalized anxiety disorder	6	15	25	53
Obsessive-compulsive disorder	15	12	10	63
Bipolar disorder	25	25	15	35
Possible psychotic disorder	27	20	13	40

Source: Adapted from Jacobi et al. (2004).

determine factors common to them all, not those specific to each condition. This is not to say there are no differences in the factors that contribute to differing conditions. Indeed, Harvey at al. identified a number of cognitions (or concerns as they refer to them) that delineate *between* conditions: panic disorder is associated with concerns about bodily sensations, obsessive-compulsive behaviour involves intrusive thoughts about responsibility of harm to others, and so on. However, their focus is on factors common to the various conditions. They drew on clinical and experimental cognitive studies to determine the key drivers of a range of disorders:

- *Errors of attention* may maintain a disorder when an individual selectively attends to information that is consistent with their concerns or fails to attend to information that is *inconsistent* with their concerns and which would change their understanding of the situation or help them cope better with it. In addition, focusing on their own thoughts, feelings, and actions may make the individual more likely to make self-attributions and take the blame for failure rather than looking for external factors. Finally, the automatic nature of attentional memories may lead some people to feel that their mind is not under their own control, leading to fears of 'madness'.

- *Errors of memory* may occur in the encoding or retrieval stages of memory. Encoding errors may occur as a result of our attentional bias. We tend to preferentially attend to stimuli pertinent to our survival. For this reason, people who experience severe life-threatening trauma tend to remember the threatening aspects of the situation. Our memory is also affected by our schema of the world. This guides our attention and thus the encoding process to certain aspects of our environment, resulting in the encoding of significantly biased information. One frequent bias in retrieval of memories occurs as a result of a phenomenon known as mood-dependent memory. This process results in recalling memories from the past that are consistent with our present mood. If, for example, we are feeling depressed or anxious, we are more likely to recall memories consistent with that mood, which may in turn exacerbate any depression or anxiety.

- A number of *reasoning errors* may also result in mood disorders. These errors map on to those identified by Beck and other second-wave theorists, and include errors of interpretive reasoning, expectancy reasoning, and a failure of hypothesis-testing (biasing such tests to support rather than challenge negative beliefs).

- *Thought processes* involved in mood disorders include intrusive thoughts, worry, and rumination. Worry is a chain of difficult-to-control thoughts and images that trigger negative mood states. Rumination is dysfunctional, redundant, repetitive, and stereotypical thinking. It may repetitively focus an individual's attention on his or her negative feelings, and the nature and implications of those feelings. The higher the frequency of negative thoughts, the more impact such thoughts are likely to have on mood.

- A number of behaviours are also implicated in the initiation and continuation of emotional disorders. As noted in the previous chapter, escape from, or avoidance of, feared situations may serve to maintain long-term anxiety. Such avoidance may involve behavioural avoidance; it may also involve the use of cognitive avoidance strategies such as distraction from distressing thoughts. Although these actions may reduce distress in the short term, in the longer term they may maintain anxiety, as the individual fails to habituate to worrying thoughts. Both cognitive and behavioural avoidance prevents the individual learning their fears are exaggerated, and they will not actually experience the harm they assume will occur.

3.3 The Self-Regulatory Executive Function (S-REF) model

In an argument consistent with that of Harvey and her colleagues, Wells (2000) noted that second-wave theories focused on the *content* of dysfunctional thoughts and ignored the mechanisms that gave such thoughts their power. His S-REF model was developed to remedy this deficiency. The model focuses on both the content of cognitions and the processes associated with them across a range of mental health problems. In psychological jargon, the theory links schema theory (focusing on the content of thought) with information processing and self-regulation theory.

The model assumes three interacting levels of cognition:

- A stimulus-driven network of processing units that guide routine responses to routine events around us
- 'On-line' processing, involving the conscious focusing of attention, appraisals of events, and control of actions and thoughts
- Information about the individual stored in long-term memory.

According to Wells, low-level processing is largely automatic, and requires little active attention. By contrast, on-line processing requires attention and conscious awareness. In addition, the content and outcomes of this processing are influenced by self-knowledge derived from long-term memory. Wells identified two key 'modes' in which these various elements operate:

1. *Object mode*: thoughts and perceptions are unevaluated and form an accurate perception of events. They are not subject to analysis and interpretation. Wells considers this to be our 'default setting'.

2. *Metacognitive mode*: in this context, the individual is distanced from their thoughts and perceptions and actively evaluates them. They think about their thoughts, feelings, and perceptions and in doing so may arrive at accurate, or frequently inaccurate, analyses of them. Some people, for example, may believe that they *have* to worry about issues that concern them ('Worrying helps me cope with my problems; if I don't worry, things will get out of control ...') and as a result may spend significant amounts of time worrying about even quite irrelevant things despite the discomfort they experience while doing so.

Wells refers to patterns of activation of the system as differing 'configurations' and refers to the configuration most closely linked to psychopathology as the S-REF configuration. This involves both an appraisal of a disjunction between an actual state and a desired state, and the development of plans to reduce or obviate this discrepancy. This may be a simple, short-term, process. Feeling hungry (and thus differing from the desired state of feeling comfortably full), for example, may trigger the plan and then action of eating a meal. Once the meal is eaten, the S-REF configuration ceases to exist, and the individual moves on to other issues. By contrast, many mental health conditions result from repeated unchanged, and unsuccessful, attempts to reduce this discrepancy. Phobic anxiety, for example, may be maintained over long periods of time as a result of the individual repeatedly following plans to avoid a feared situation. Here, the coping effort is successful in reducing the immediate discrepancy between feeling fearful and the desired state of not being fearful, but maintains fear in the long run as it prevents the individual from learning that any fears they have are exaggerated. This explanation is not dissimilar to that of Mowrer (1947), discussed in the previous chapter.

According to Wells, S-REF processing is initiated either by some form of external threat or internally generated threat-related thoughts. In response, we develop plans to reduce the discrepancy between the actual and desired self (see Figure 3.1). These coping plans are guided by a series of beliefs – or metacognitive knowledge as Wells refers to it. Plans are often unconscious and relatively automatic, although individuals may be able to verbalize them. Thus, an individual with generalized anxiety disorder may unconsciously scan their environment for threats and be able to verbalize this as, 'I must be vigilant so I won't be taken by surprise'; someone with depression may verbalize their plans as, 'I must be pessimistic, so I can avoid disappointment', and so on. A second type of belief is also relevant: declarative beliefs about ourselves: 'I am worthless, vulnerable', and so on.

Part of any plan may be to attend to these beliefs, making them salient at times of stress or distress, even if the individual may hold a number of differing beliefs. A spider phobic, for example, may pay attention to catastrophizing cognitions when faced with a spider and in S-REF configuration, but be more rational about the threat (or lack of threat) associated with spiders when not faced with a spider, and therefore not in S-REF configuration. In this example, there is a clear time point at which the S-REF configuration becomes redundant, and the individual can shift into another, less stressful, configuration. But what maintains individuals in the S-REF configuration or allows an individual to shift away from the S-REF configuration in less clearly defined situations? In cases where there is no external evidence of safety (for example, obsessional washing to prevent contamination by

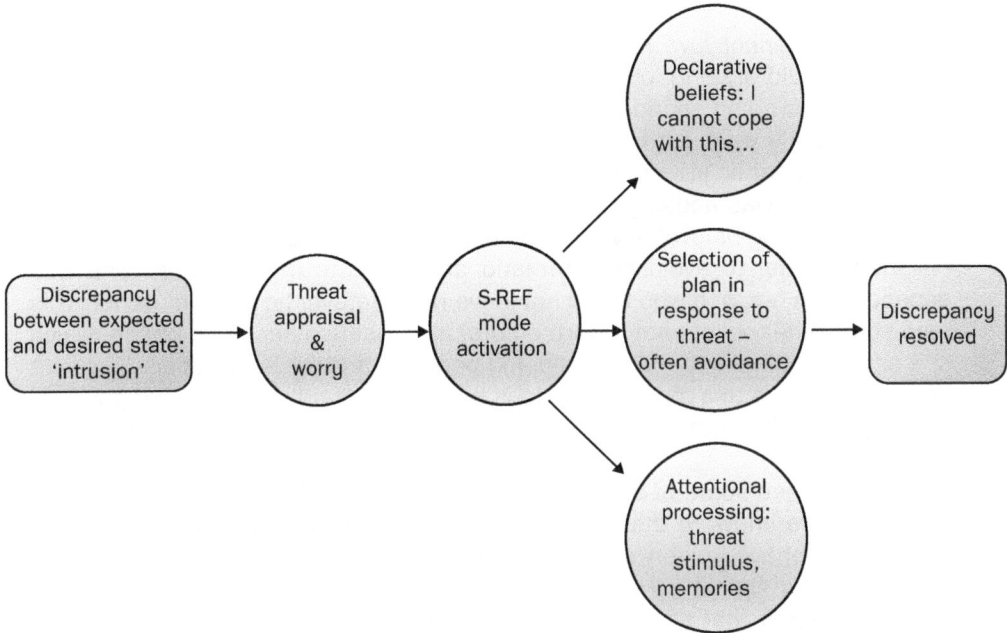

Figure 3.1 Simplified version of Wells' S-REF mode

germs), the individual may continue in S-REF configuration until it 'feels right' or they 'know' they can stop (i.e. after five washing rituals). The problem with such criteria is that they require high levels of perceived security before the S-REF configuration can be left. Accordingly, the obsessive individual may check a situation or engage in safety rituals on many occasions – sometimes a disabling number of occasions – before they feel safe to stop doing so.

Box 3.1 When do you believe beliefs?

Mrs Jones was a chronically depressed, severely obese, woman. She had married a man with long-term health problems who had since died. She had limited contact with a small group of friends, all of whom also had long-term mental health problems, and she rarely saw her family. This situation stemmed from her childhood, during which she was sexually abused by a family friend on several occasions. As a consequence of her abuse, she developed a number of beliefs as a child that continued into adulthood:

- '*I am a bad person*': she believed this because she felt that of all the people that her abuser could have chosen, he had chosen her. She believed this indicated that he knew she was bad and had therefore selected her from a number of other potential victims.

- *'My parents cannot love me'*: this stemmed from a number of perspectives. First, how could anyone love such a bad person as she was? In addition, she had been allowed so spend the night and weekends in the home of her abuser, while her family went out for the night or on weekend trips. This must indicate that they thought so little of her that they allowed her to spend time with someone they knew was abusing her.
- *'I am undeserving of love'*: a variant on her belief of being bad and unloved, and one that led her to avoid social relationships and to marry a man who was dependent on her, and who could not leave her whatever he thought of her. This (and some other beliefs not reported here) also justified her being obese, which she saw as a barrier to men developing personal and sexual relationships with her. Her marriage to a man with serious health problems also gave her power in their relationship, both in general and in particular in sexual relationships.

Therapy challenged some of these fundamental beliefs. She came to believe that her parents were unaware that she was being abused. She described, for example, how she behaved when she stayed with her abuser. She would smile and look happy when she was with her parents as she did not want them to know about the abuse or that she dreaded spending time in his house. She was also able to determine that the abuser's choice of her was based on convenience and the ability to manipulate her, rather than because she was inherently bad. As a result of this, Mrs Jones was able to argue coherently that she did not believe she was a bad person, that her parents did love her, and that she both deserved friendship and could establish friendships. But her mood did not improve despite making quite fundamental changes to her cognitive set, and neither did her feelings about herself. Why should this be the case?

One key phenomenon that can be explained by this process is the frequently reported lack of association between intellectual and emotional beliefs. In this, the individual may state that he or she logically knows the belief is false but that they still 'feel' as if it is correct. A feeling of this kind may be metacognitive in nature.

Metacognitive therapy

A key goal of Wells' metacognitive therapy is to make the individual aware of their unhelpful avoidance plans, to change them to ones that involve confronting previously feared situations, and to tolerate the distress that may result from such a confrontation. More broadly, metacognitive therapy aims to:

- teach individuals to develop more flexible coping strategies to use in stressful situations – to 'unlock' themselves from previous patterns of inappropriate coping responses
- help participants to gain new experiences of mastery and control over previously emotionally difficult circumstances
- change long-term memory, and beliefs about the self

- teach participants 'a higher metacognitive mode', which allows them to process information in ways that do not trigger high levels of S-REF activity.

In order to achieve these goals, therapy focuses on changing the plans that lead to inappropriate coping responses and/or the individual's responses to any metacognitions or declaratory cognitions they experience. In direct opposition to second-wave therapies, the latter goal involves teaching the individual to tolerate or become emotionally detached from any distressing cognitions rather than directly trying to change them. Accordingly, key processes within metacognitive therapy include:

- changing the metacognitive beliefs (plans) that drive inappropriate coping responses and learning to adopt more realistic goals
- learning skills such as mindfulness that allow individuals to access potentially distressing thoughts without triggering high levels of S-REF activity and distress.
- reducing attention to worries and other unwanted cognitive content – through the use of attentional control skills.

The next sections focus on two of these strategies (mindfulness and attention control skills) in more detail.

Mindfulness

Mindfulness has a central role in the teaching of the Buddha. According to Buddhist learning, mindfulness is necessary on the road to enlightenment and is achieved through the meditative process of focusing one's awareness on the present – not memories of the past or possible creations of the future. Through meditation, we can learn that 'thoughts are just thoughts' that may or may not be true; as, of course, do the cognitive therapists. However, we can also learn to be aware of potentially distressing thoughts without them evoking an emotional reaction. Bishop et al. (2004) proposed a two-component model of mindfulness:

- *Self-regulation of attention.* Mindfulness involves being fully aware of our current experience – observing and attending to our changing thoughts, feelings, and sensations as they occur. This allows us to be aware of these phenomena as they arise, but not to elaborate on them. Rather than getting caught up in ruminative thoughts, mindfulness involves a direct non-judgemental experience of events in the mind and body. This leads to a feeling of being very alert and 'alive'
- *An orientation toward one's experiences in the present moment characterized by curiosity, openness, and acceptance.* The lack of cognitive effort given to the elaboration on the meanings and associations of our various experiences allows us to focus more on our present experience. Rather than observing experience through the filter of our beliefs and assumptions, mindfulness involves a direct, unfiltered awareness of our experiences.

Clearly, mindfulness is not simple, and requires significant effort to learn. Most programmes that teach mindfulness involve some form of meditation, often taught over sessions spread over many weeks or months. During meditation, participants learn to focus on a particular physical stimulus such as a picture, or a sensory stimulus such as the sound of a repeated mantra, and to be aware of – but not focused on – unwanted intrusive sensations, thoughts or emotions. Participants also practise mindfulness during ordinary activities like walking, standing, and eating. Wells argued that mindfulness can be used to help people be aware of and change their cognitions and metacognitions without being overwhelmed by them. It can also be used at times when potentially distressing thoughts come to mind. Rather than challenge such thoughts, practitioners of mindfulness are aware of them, but they only form a small, unattended part of their perceptual awareness. Other factors provide a stronger focus of their attention.

As well as a component of therapy, mindfulness can form a primary intervention in itself. The most frequently cited method of mindfulness training is the mindfulness-based stress reduction (MBSR) programme of Kabat-Zinn (e.g. Kabat-Zinn 1990). The programme is conducted as an 8- to 10-week course for groups of up to 30 participants who meet weekly for around 2 hours for instruction and practice in mindfulness meditation skills, together with discussion of stress and coping, and homework assignments. An all-day (7–8-hour) intensive mindfulness session usually is held around the sixth week. Several mindfulness meditation skills are taught. For example, the 'body scan' is a 45-minute exercise in which attention is directed sequentially to numerous areas of the body while the participant is lying down with eyes closed. Sensations in each area are carefully observed. In sitting meditation, participants are instructed to sit in a relaxed and wakeful posture with eyes closed and to direct attention to the sensations of breathing. Hatha yoga postures are used to teach mindfulness of bodily sensations during gentle movements and stretching. Participants also practise mindfulness during ordinary activities like walking, standing, and eating.

Participants in MBSR are instructed to practise these skills outside group meetings for at least 45 minutes a day, 6 days a week. Audiotapes are used early in treatment, but participants are encouraged to practise without tapes after a few weeks. For all mindfulness exercises, participants are instructed to focus attention on the target of observation (e.g. breathing or walking), and to be aware of it in each moment. When emotions, sensations or cognitions arise, they are observed non-judgementally. When the participant notices that their mind has wandered into thoughts, memories or fantasies, the nature or content of them is briefly noted, if possible, and then attention is returned to the present moment. Thus, participants are instructed to notice their thoughts and feelings but not to become absorbed in their content. Even judgemental thoughts (e.g. 'This is a waste of time') are to be observed non-judgementally. Upon noticing such a thought, the participant might label it as a judgemental thought, or simply as 'thinking', and then return attention to the present moment. An important consequence of mindfulness practice is the realization that most sensations, thoughts, and emotions fluctuate, or are transient, passing by 'like waves in the sea'.

Attentional control skills

Attentional training is somewhat easier to master than mindfulness. Unlike mindfulness, attentional training does not help participants to tolerate the experience of distressing thoughts. Rather, it gives the individual 'time out' from them. Wells argues that because avoidance of worrisome thoughts is a core contributor to continued distress, distraction is not to be used at times of high distress – at such times, mindfulness should be used to help the individual learn to tolerate their distressing thoughts. Rather, it can be used to 'reset maladaptive thought processes' at times when the individual is not experiencing particularly high levels of distress. The process is first taught in a therapy session, and then used as homework. It involves initially fixating on a visual stimulus such as a mark on the wall and then focusing attention for several moments on each of a series of different sounds, such as the therapist's voice, tapping, the ticking of a clock. The individual is instructed to focus exclusively on only the sound. They then shift their attention rapidly between the set of sounds, before listening simultaneously to all the sounds, trying to be aware of as many of them as possible. The whole sequence takes between 10 and 15 minutes to enact.

Metacognitive formulation and treatment approaches

Although Wells uses a number of strategies to help people cope with emotion-laden cognitions through the use of mindfulness and attentional control, his approach also includes a degree of **cognitive challenge**, albeit in a more elaborate manner than the traditional second-wave therapies. This moves the therapist from exploring the A-B-C pattern of antecedents, cognitions, and emotional and behavioural responses outlined in the previous chapter (see Figure 3.2) to what Wells calls the A-M-C unit of analysis. Here, antecedents (A) lead to metacognitions (M), which direct attention to declarative beliefs, which drive both emotional and behavioural consequences (C) (see Figure 3.3).

In the example shown (see Figures 3.2 and 3.3), a Beckian analysis of a depressed person's response to an argument with a friend may involve negative thoughts such as 'I can never keep friends', which maintains or increases feelings of depression and behavioural avoidance. The additional step added by Wells involves metacognitions. In this, the individual makes a conscious decision to access memories of previous failures and problems, as well as to ruminate about

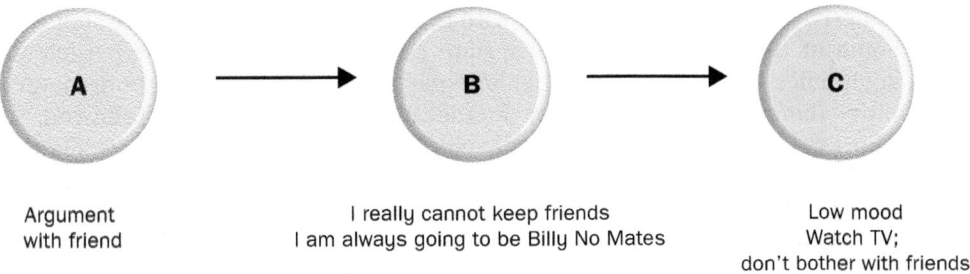

Figure 3.2 The Beckian analysis of depression, linking antecedents to cognitions, and cognitions to their emotional and behavioural consequences

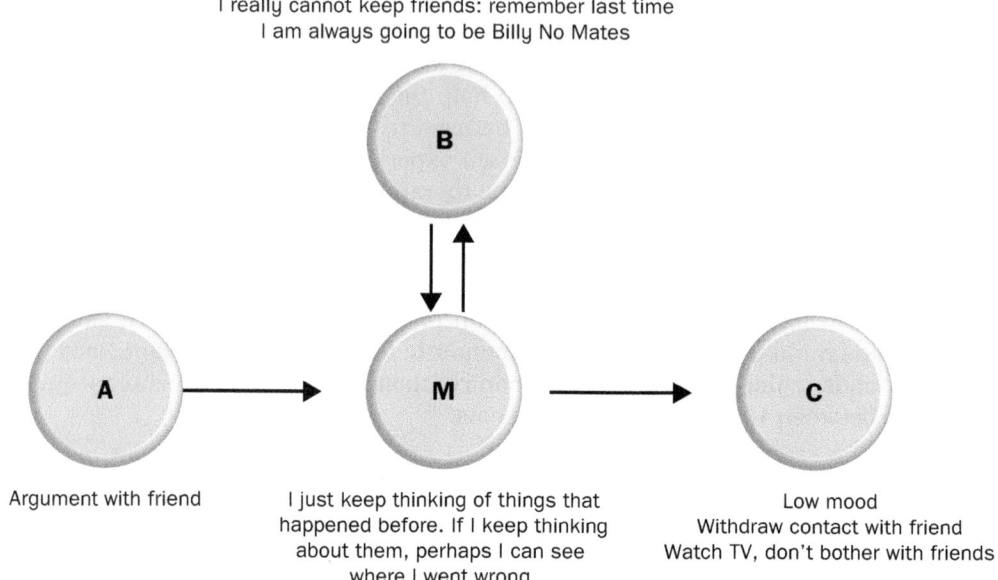

I really cannot keep friends: remember last time
I am always going to be Billy No Mates

Argument with friend

I just keep thinking of things that
happened before. If I keep thinking
about them, perhaps I can see
where I went wrong

Low mood
Withdraw contact with friend
Watch TV, don't bother with friends

Figure 3.3 The MAC complex of Wells, in which antecedents trigger meta-cognitions and related beliefs, which link to emotional and behavioural consequences

the situation in an attempt to try and sort it out. As a response to these metacognitions (or plans), the individual deliberately both retrieves negative memories that reinforce their negative beliefs, and chooses to dwell on them, significantly adding to their depressed feelings.

Changing inappropriate beliefs, behaviours, and emotions involves what Wells calls the P-E-T-S protocol. Here, the individual **P**repares for change, is **E**xposed to the feared situation and **T**ests new responses to it, and then **S**ummarizes their responses to the situation as part of gaining an understanding of the factors contributing to the problem and developing further interventions.

- The *prepare stage* involves identifying problematic situations and the maladaptive responses used to cope with them, exploring the evidence supporting some of the potentially inappropriate cognitions the person experiences at such times (in a classic Socratic dialogue), and teaching them about metacognitive therapy as a rationale for the therapeutic approach to be followed.
- The *expose/test* stages involve developing and implementing new plans for coping with difficult situations. These involve both adopting new behaviours and developing strategies for managing any fears the individual may experience while engaging in new behaviours. These will include mindfulness, avoiding attending to memories of previous problems, and so on. In contrast to second-wave therapy that would encourage the individual to evoke and challenge worrisome thoughts as they occur in such situations, mindfulness strategies allow the individual to experience such thoughts but not make them the focus of their attention

- The *summarize* stage involves reflecting back on the previous stage, to determine its effectiveness and to develop further interventions designed to challenge previous inappropriate fears and coping strategies.

Research box 2

Arch, J., Eifert, G.H., Davies, C. et al. (2012) Randomized clinical trial of cognitive behavioral therapy (CBT) versus acceptance and commitment therapy (ACT) for mixed anxiety disorders, *Journal of Consulting and Clinical Psychology*, 80: 750–65.

Cognitive behavioural therapy (CBT) is the most widely accepted treatment for most emotional disorders, and is the key intervention approach recommended by most treatment guidelines. However, there are good theoretical reasons to assume that other approaches may be equally or more effective. Research is needed to compare the effectiveness of these emerging approaches to allow reconsideration of the treatment of choice for a number of disorders. The study by Arch et al. provides one such analysis, directly comparing CBT with acceptance and commitment therapy (ACT) in the treatment of a range of anxiety disorders.

Method

Participants

The participants ($N = 143$) were recruited through adverts placed in local flyers, local newspaper adverts, and Craig's List. They all met the **DSM** criteria for a diagnosis of a range of anxiety disorders (social anxiety, panic disorder, specific phobia, obsessive-compulsive disorder, and generalized anxiety disorder) and were blind to the treatment they were to receive (15 dropped out before receiving treatment). Participants were either medication-free or on a stable dose and had not received psychotherapy for their anxiety in the 6 months prior to the study. Exclusion criteria included severe depression, suicidal ideation, or a history or **psychosis** or bipolar disorder.

Design

Participants were assessed before treatment, at the end of treatment, and at 5 and 12 months follow-up.

Participants were randomly allocated to either CBT or ACT. In each condition, they received 12, weekly, one-hour sessions following manuals to ensure adherence to the required intervention approach and intervention strategies. These were followed by six, monthly, phone calls lasting 20 to 35 minutes to enhance long-term outcomes. The 39 therapists were all doctoral students on the UCLA clinical psychology training programme.

Cognitive behavioural therapy: Session 1, assessment, self-monitoring, and **psychoeducation**; Sessions 2–4, cognitive restructuring with hypothesis-testing, self-monitoring, and breathing retraining; Sessions 5–11: exposure with response prevention, including interoceptive (for panic), in-vivo, and imaginal contexts; Session 12, relapse prevention.

Acceptance and commitment therapy: Sessions 1–3, psychoeducation, experiential exercises, and discussion aimed at accepting and learning that efforts to control anxiety were ineffective and interfered with achieving life goals; Sessions 4–5, mindfulness, acceptance, and cognitive defusion; Sessions 6–11, continued use of acceptance, mindfulness, and defusion, as well as exploration of, and encouragement to pursue, valued life activities. Behavioural exposure used to provide opportunities to practise making room for, mindfully observing, and accepting anxiety, and engaging in valued activities while experiencing anxiety; Session 12, review and future planning.

Measures

- *Diagnostic Interview* using the Anxiety Disorders Interview Schedule-IV. This provided 'clinical severity ratings' (CSR) on a 0–8 scale for each condition. Interviews were recorded and blindly rated by a second rater. Inter-rater reliability of the diagnosis was 100%. The correlation between severity ratings was 0.65.
- *Anxiety Sensitivity Index (ASI)*: assesses fear of anxiety-related sensations such as shortness of breath and the belief that such sensations are harmful.
- *Penn State Worry Questionnaire (PSWQ)*: measures the presence of clinically significant worry.
- *Fear Questionnaire (Fear Q)*: single-item scale rating degree of avoidance of primary phobic object.
- *Quality of Life Index (QLI)*: measures values and life satisfaction.
- *Acceptance and Action Questionnaire (AAQ)*: measures psychological flexibility.

Results

No differences emerged between the characteristics of participants in the two conditions except that there were more people with panic disorder (49%) in the CBT group than the ACT group (32%). Participant ratings of 'treatment credibility', taken immediately before the second therapy session, were significantly higher for CBT than for ACT. Ratings of therapist competence did not differ between the conditions, and measures of treatment protocol adherence indicated that the therapists adhered to the treatment protocols. Completion of therapy also did not differ between conditions (CBT, 68%; ACT, 65%).

Changes over time

Two types of analysis were conducted. The first, an 'intention to treat' analysis, included data from all participants in the study, based on the assumption that participants who dropped out of the study did not change on any variable. A second analysis examined outcomes of those who completed all measures at each assessment point (see Table 1).

Table 1 Mean and standard deviation of scores on each outcome measure

Measure	Pre-treatment	Post-treatment	6 months	12 months
CSR				
ACT	5.70 (0.89)	3.11 (2.21)	2.77 (2.39)	2.33 (1.98)
CBT	5.55 (0.94)	2.90 (2.12)	2.67 (2.24)	2.94 (2.52)
ASI				
ACT	31.81 (11.25)	18.65 (11.89)	14.56 (10.14)	17.05 (12.62)
CBT	27.60 (11.81)	18.68 (11.16)	20.47 (12.90)	15.64 (8.04)
PSWQ				
ACT	46.52 (11.93)	39.89 (11.01)	37.79 (10.87)	39.32 (12.26)
CBT	45.00 (12.82)	37.63 (15.22)	37.72 (13.04)	37.14 (12.72)
Fear Q				
ACT	5.84 (2.34)	4.13 (2.37)	4.00 (2.66)	4.28 (2.72)
CBT	5.34 (2.95)	4.06 (2.96)	4.22 (3.12)	3.82 (2.70)
QLI				
ACT	0.19 (1.85)	1.42 (1.88)	0.50 (1.43)	1.17 (1.51)
CBT	0.55 (2.10)	1.78 (1.35)	1.45 (1.52)	1.86 (1.88)
AAQ				
ACT	59.01 (12.35)	70.82 (13.14)	72.14 (10.86)	71.71 (11.42)
CBT	58.49 (11.84)	69.43 (14.75)	68.38 (13.76)	68.43 (11.65)

Intention to treat analysis

Measures of anxiety

After controlling for demographic and clinical covariates, multiple linear modelling showed that both conditions showed equal and significant reductions in CSR-measured anxiety between pre- and post-treatment measures. However, the ACT group continued to make improvements up to 12 months follow-up, while CBT maintained but did not improve (B = 0.58, SE = 0.28, $t(126) = 2.03$, $p = 0.04$). All other measures showed significant improvements in all groups over time ($p < 0.01$), with no differences between the groups at any time.

Wider measures

Both the AAQ and QLI showed significant improvements over time ($p < 0.001$) with no differences. between conditions.

Completers analysis

ACT achieved lower CSR ratings that CBT (B = 1.01, SE = 0.49, $t(83)$ = 2.04, p = 0.04), with all other measures of anxiety showing no difference in outcome between the conditions and significant change over time. ACT also achieved higher ratings on the AAQ, while those in the CBT condition reported higher levels of quality of life on the QLI. Participants in the ACT condition were also more likely to have received additional psychotherapy beyond that provided in the trial, although regression analysis found this was not predictive of any outcome.

Discussion

This was an impressively controlled, conducted, and analysed study. Both CBT and ACT achieved substantial improvements over time on all measures of anxiety and quality of life. Gains made immediately after therapy were maintained over time. Key differences between the two interventions emerged following treatment, with ACT achieving steeper improvement rates and better outcomes on the key measure of anxiety at one-year follow-up. By contrast, and to the surprise of the authors, those in the CBT group had higher measures of quality of life at follow-up, despite the focus on valued life experiences being a key focus of ACT. The study had a number of strengths and weaknesses. The focus on a mixed range of anxiety disorders prevents assessment of the specificity of the intervention effect, but reflects the 'real life' case mix of most therapists. The use of trainee **psychotherapists** may also have reduced the impact of the interventions, although any effect is likely to be equal across the conditions. Indeed, as ACT is more complex than CBT, any impact may have been more on the ACT condition than CBT. Overall, therefore, the study provides clear evidence that ACT is a viable alternative to CBT. Finally, the authors note that the very similar outcomes of two very different interventions suggests there are many common therapeutic factors that may have contributed to these findings, as discussed in the chapter.

3.4 Relational frames theory

In contrast to Wells, who considers pathology to be the outcome of cognitive processes, relational frames theory considers cognitions to be relatively unimportant in the development of pathology. Interestingly though, despite its philosophical differences from the S-REF and its radical behavioural roots, relational frames theory also concludes that the key to psychopathology is the continued engagement in inappropriate behavioural responses to contextual cues within our environment. Relational frame theory (e.g. Hayes et al. 2006) assumes that we naturally attend to, and respond to, relationships between various elements of our environment. These relationships can be defined in three key ways:

- *Relational context*: we can identify the direct relationship between two elements within our environment – the brighter of two colours, the larger of two people, and so on.
- *Combinatorial entailment*: this involves logically combining relations. For example, if we learned that Stephen is larger than John, and John is larger than Mary, we also know that Stephen is larger than Mary.
- *Functional context*: this involves relating to *functions* of elements within our environment, not simply their physical relationships. For instance, using the above example, we may also consider that Stephen is better at carrying heavy objects than Mary.

Together, these three features of any context are referred to as its 'relational frame'. Hayes et al. (2006) argue we are able to abstract elements from one set of frames and can transfer them from one situation to another. They note, for example, that a child who is trapped inside a wooden box and experiences great fear may later experience the same fear when trapped in other contexts, such as relationships. Although the contexts are very different, the responses are similar because the relational frame is the same. According to Hayes et al., the developing child develops more and increasingly complex frames over time. These relational frames are brought to bear on new situations through analogies, stories, metaphors, and rules. Recognition of a situation in terms of its relational frame triggers operantly conditioned responses to that context. According to Hayes, these relational frames are the dominant determinants of our behaviour and experience.

Critical to the development of psychopathology is Hayes's argument that because relational frames are verbally accessible (i.e. we are able to understand and describe them), they are also changeable. Accordingly, over time we may develop distorted concepts of relationships between elements within relational frames, and begin to respond to these distorted relational frames rather than the 'real' relational frames, at the same time as becoming less sensitive to the real outcomes of our behaviour. Hayes et al. refer to the process by which we interact with events on the basis of our 'verbally ascribed functions' rather than their 'direct functions' as involving cognitive fusion. We take our cognitively distorted view as being an accurate representation of a relational frame. In this way, worry about the future becomes worry about an *actual* future, rather than a *constructed* future. Similarly, the thought 'life is not worth living' is a conclusion about life and its quality, rather than a transitory, verbal evaluative process of the here and now.

One consequence of inappropriate relational framing is that individuals may begin to avoid contexts in which negative emotions and behaviours are triggered. This prevents us experiencing distress, but also prevents us having more positive experiences in these contexts. The individual with agoraphobia stays at home to avoid the anxiety attack that is sure to occur if they go to the supermarket. The depressed person avoids a family reunion in response to the idea that people will avoid her. These contingencies can be considered in terms of rules: 'If I don't go out of the house, then I won't feel panicky – which is good', 'I can avoid feeling miserable and bad about myself if I don't go to the party where people will avoid me', and so on. Hayes et al. contend that the consequence of cognitive fusion and experiential avoidance results in a state of psychological rigidity. In this, we engage in inappropriate coping attempts to minimize any distress we may experience. We may persevere doing things that are best stopped, and stop doing things when perseverance is the best option. These failed coping attempts become problems in themselves. So, by a different route, the S-REF and relational frames theory arrive at the same explanatory conclusion.

Acceptance and commitment therapy

Based on relational frames theory, acceptance and commitment therapy (ACT; pronounced, 'act') is a therapy approach *that uses acceptance and mindfulness processes as well as commitment and behaviour change processes to produce a greater psychological flexibility* (Hayes et al. 2006). ACT is rooted in radical behaviourism, as it assumes that psychological events (thoughts, emotions, behaviour) are the result of an interaction between the individual and the context in which they are in, that is both historically (e.g. prior learning histories) and situationally (current antecedents and consequences, verbal rules) defined. That is, they are the outcomes of both **classical** and **operant conditioning** processes. In addition, ACT does not consider thoughts or feelings to necessarily direct behaviour. Change can be achieved through changing contextual variables rather than attempts to change internal processes such as cognitions, emotions, sensations, and so on. Accordingly, ACT encourages clients to focus on living according to their own values rather than challenging any misconceptions about their situation.

The goals of ACT

In common with the S-REF model, ACT teaches the individual to be aware of ongoing private events (thoughts), but not to be driven by them: to be in touch with the present moment as fully as possible, and to either change or persist in behaviours in order to achieve valued goals. All ACT interventions aim to increase the individual's flexibility in responding to situations they face. This flexibility is established through a focus on five, related, core processes: acceptance, defusion, contact with the present moment, values, and committed action.

- *Acceptance* involves being aware of thoughts, feelings, and bodily sensations as they occur, but not to be driven by them. Instead, the aim is to experience non-judgemental awareness of these events and actively embrace them. Therapy emphasizes that attempts at inappropriate control are stressful and paradoxically serve to maintain the distress the individual is trying to control: 'control is the problem, not the solution'. Acceptance is taught through a variety of techniques, including mindfulness, and the use of graded exercises showing it is possible to feel intense feelings or notice intense and bodily sensations without harm.
- *Cognitive defusion* involves the experience of thoughts as simply 'thoughts', feelings as feelings, memories as memories, and physical sensations as physical sensations. None of these experiences are inherently damaging. Indeed, harm occurs when they are seen as harmful experiences that need to be controlled and eliminated. Thoughts form just one interpretation of events, and

there are many others that may be equally appropriate to any situation. In contrast to second-wave interventions, however, individuals are encouraged to accept their presence, and not try to change or control them.

- *Contact with the present moment* involves effective, open, and undefended contact with the present moment. There are two features to this process: first, observing what is present in the environment and in private experience (i.e. thoughts and emotions); and second, labelling and describing what is present, without excessive judgement or evaluation. Together these establish a sense of 'self as a process of ongoing awareness' of events and experiences. Mindfulness is one technique through which this can be achieved.
- *Values* relates to the motivation for change. In order for an individual to face feared obstacles, they need a purpose for doing so. ACT aims not simply to rid the person of their problems, but to help them build a more vital, purposeful life; to enable progress towards valued life goals without the hindrance of worries, emotions, and other private events.
- *Committed action* relates to individuals developing strategies for achieving desired goals. Once they have begun to understand how fusion and avoidance are preventing them from moving towards such goals, they are encouraged to define goals in specific areas and to progress towards them. Progress towards these goals becomes a key part of therapy.

In summary, the key goal of ACT is not to change what its originators describe as 'private events', such as emotions, thoughts, and physiological reactions, although these may be secondary outcomes of any intervention. Rather, it involves enabling the individual to work towards valued goals, which they define, and to prevent historically developed patterns of thoughts and emotions preventing such progress. It aims to do so by teaching participants to distance themselves from negative thoughts and emotions, to be able to note their presence but not be responsive to them, while actively engaging in positive behavioural change. ACT is not a condition-specific intervention. Rather, it is applicable to a wide range of conditions, from generalized anxiety disorder, through depression, to psychosis; and, incidentally, it has the same goals, if not therapeutic techniques, as Wells' metacognitive therapy.

The process of therapy

ACT is a complex intervention and is not conducted in a standardized manner. Interventions involve the use of metaphors, experiential exercises, and behavioural tasks. Strosahl et al. (2004) identified a number of broad strategies to help people make changes in each of the domains identified above.

- *Developing acceptance*: communicating that the individual is not 'broken', but is using unworkable strategies; helping them make direct contact with the paradoxical effect of emotional control strategies; encouraging them to experiment with stopping struggling for emotional control and suggesting acceptance as an alternative; using a graded and structured approach to acceptance in which they learn acceptance of painful emotions in gradually more demanding situations.

- *Undermining cognitive fusion*: helping the person to identify emotional, cognitive, behavioural or physical barriers to change and the impact these have on their willingness to engage in new or previously avoided behaviours; learning through experience that unwanted private experiences are not 'toxic' and can be accepted without judgement; distancing themselves from thoughts, learning that they are *experiences*, not the individual themselves.
- *Contact with the present moment*: modelling by the therapist of contact with and the expression of feelings, thoughts or sensations as they occur within the therapeutic relationship; using exercises to expand awareness of experience as an ongoing process; showing how to pull away from worries or ruminations and come back to the present moment
- *Defining valued directions*: clarifying valued life directions and distinguishing between values and goals.
- *Building patterns of committed action*: identifying value-based goals and building a concrete action plan; identifying and working through perceived and potential future barriers to change; appreciating the qualities of committed action, including vitality and sense of growth.

As you can see, ACT is a complex therapy involving the use of a variety of behavioural methods as well as stories, metaphors, and mental exercises to encourage change. As such, the approach cannot be fully considered within the present chapter. However, the key aim of their approach is that the primary process of change is to engage in previously avoided behaviours or refrain from previous ineffective and problematic coping behaviours, to learn to cope or reduce the distress involved in doing this through the use, for example, of mindfulness, and thereby learn that the feared consequences will not occur. As such, despite many differences in philosophy and approach, both the cognitive approach of Wells and the behavioural approach of the ACT therapists have much in common.

Stop and think ...

The theoretical models considered in this chapter provide a more complex understanding of the processes underpinning a range of mental health problems than those of the second-wave theories and therapeutic interventions. But as we will see in subsequent chapters, this additional modelling has not resulted in substantial gains in the effectiveness of our therapeutic endeavours – the outcome of second- and third-wave interventions appears remarkably similar. Why might this be the case? Have we failed to identify new processes that influence mood or behaviour or fundamentally change the process of therapy? In the end, are the fine-grain elements of therapy irrelevant, and (as discussed in the previous chapter) are the human elements of therapy more important determinants of outcome – and should this be where future research is focused? How do we further improve the outcomes of psychological therapy?

3.5 Chapter summary

1. The transdiagnostic model of Harvey et al. notes that many mental health problems co-occur, and that explanations for this should explore common processes across conditions rather than cognitive differences between conditions. These processes involve attention, memory, errors of reasoning, thought and behavioural processes. This approach has been explicitly adopted by a number of therapeutic approaches, including that of Wells.

2. Wells' Self-Regulatory Executive Function model notes three interacting levels of cognition: unconscious processing, processing that occurs at the time of emotional distress involving focusing attention, appraisal of events, and planning and executing behavioural responses, and information stored in memory.

3. According to Wells, emotional and behavioural problems occur as a result of a failure to adapt to stressful circumstances, and repeating ineffective plans (often involving avoidance and guided by metacognitive processes) which prevent the individual learning that a feared consequence will not occur should they confront the issue directly.

4. Therapy involves adopting new plans that directly confront feared contexts, and using strategies such as mindfulness to help individuals cope with the emotional consequences of these revised plans.

5. In common with the second wave of therapists, clients may also be encouraged to challenge inappropriate declarative beliefs. However, this is not central to the process of therapy.

6. Acceptance and commitment therapy comes from a radical behavioural perspective, and is based on relational frames theory. According to Hayes, people with mental health problems develop distorted 'relational frames', with inaccurate expectations of the outcomes of behaviour and the relationship between our behaviour and its outcomes. In turn, these distorted relational frames lead to inappropriate behaviour and emotional responses to events.

7. Hayes uses the term cognitive fusion to express the failure of people to treat their thoughts as interpretations of events or future possibilities – instead, thoughts are taken as truths, which leads to experiential avoidance and a state of psychological rigidity.

8. As with Wells, the therapeutic approach to reducing avoidance and psychological rigidity is to engage in previously avoided responses to difficult situations, and learn to cope with the emotions this process may arouse.

9. The core aspects of ACT are: acceptance, cognitive defusion, contact with the present moment, developing values supporting change, and committed action. Although its aims are similar to Wells' metacognitive therapy, ACT involves a more complex use of metaphor, stories, and mental exercises to encourage change. However, at its core, it involves engaging in previously difficult behaviours, and learning that doing so will not result in the feared outcomes.

3.6 For discussion

1. Consider the relationship between the behavioural therapies, the second-wave cognitive behavioural therapies, and the third-wave therapies described in this chapter. What do they have in common, and how do they differ?
2. The second-wave cognitive therapies of Beck et al. consider changing cognitive content to be the primary agent of emotional change. In the light of the shift from this theoretical stance in the third-wave therapies, how important do you consider this process to be?
3. Is it realistic to expect to develop a single model for the development of mental health problems that cuts across all diagnoses?
4. Should therapists trained and competent in second-wave therapies train to be third-wave therapists?

3.7 Further reading

Bennett, R. and Oliver, J. (2019) *Acceptance and Commitment Therapy (100 Key Points)*, London: Routledge.

Harvey, A., Watkins, E., Mansell, W. et al. (2005) *Cognitive Behavioural Processes Across Psychological Disorders: A Transdiagnostic Approach to Research and Treatment*, Oxford: Oxford University Press.

Hofmann, S.G. and Asmundson, G.J.G. (2008) Acceptance and mindfulness-based therapy: new wave or old hat?, *Clinical Psychology Review*, 28: 1–16.

Kabat-Zinn, J. (2013) *Full Catastrophe Living: How to Cope with Stress, Pain and Illness Using Mindfulness Meditation*, New York: Delacorte.

Wells, A. (2011) *Metacognitive Therapy for Anxiety and Depression*, New York: Guilford Press.

Wells, A. and Fisher, P. (2015) *Treating Depression: MCT, CBT and Third Wave Therapies*, Chichester: Wiley.

4 Biological explanations and treatments

The basis of biological explanations and treatments of mental disorders is that behaviour and mood are regulated by brain systems. These allow us to perceive information, integrate that information with past memories and other salient factors, and then respond emotionally and behaviourally. Their disruption results in inappropriate perception, mood, and behaviour. This may occur as a result of structural damage, or disruption of chemicals, known as **neurotransmitters**, responsible for activating different areas of the brain. By the end of the chapter, you should have an understanding of:

- Basic neuroanatomy as it relates to mental health disorders
- The neurotransmitter systems and the key neurotransmitters that influence mood and behaviour
- The drug treatments that are used to alter neurotransmitter levels and, hence, mood and behaviour
- Three physical interventions used to treat mental health problems: **electroconvulsive therapy (ECT)**, transcranial magnetic stimulation (TMS), and psychosurgery
- Some of the controversies and issues raised by each treatment method.

4.1 The behavioural anatomy of the brain

The brain is an intricately patterned complex of nerve cell bodies. It is divided into four anatomical areas: the hindbrain, midbrain, forebrain, and cerebrum.

Hindbrain, midbrain, and forebrain

The hindbrain contains the parts of the brain necessary for life: the *medulla oblongata*, which controls respiration, blood pressure, and heartbeat; the *reticular formation*, which controls wakefulness and alertness; and the *pons* and *cerebellum*, which correlate muscular and positional information.

Above these lies the midbrain, which also contains part of the reticular system together with the sensory and motor correlation centres, which integrate reflex and automatic responses involving the visual and auditory systems and are involved in the integration of muscle movements.

Many of the key structures that influence mood and behaviour are situated in the forebrain. These include the following:

- *Thalamus*: links the basic functions of the hindbrain and midbrain with the higher centres of processing, the cerebral cortex. Regulates attention and contributes to memory functions. The portion that enters the limbic system is involved in the experience of emotions.
- *Hypothalamus*: regulates appetite, sexual arousal, and thirst. Also appears to have some control over emotions.
- *Limbic system*: a series of structures including a linked group of brain areas known as the Papez circuit: hippocampus – fornix – mammillary bodies – thalamus – cingulated cortex – hippocampus. The hippocampus – fornix – mammillary bodies circuit is also involved in memory. The hippocampus is one site of interaction between the perceptual and memory systems. A further part of the system, known as the amygdala, links sensory information to emotionally relevant behaviours, particularly responses to fear and anger. It has been called the 'emotional computer' because of its role in coordinating the process that begins with the evaluation of sensory information for significance (such as threat) and then controls the resulting behavioural and autonomic responses.
- The *ventral tegmental area* (VTA): an important nerve tract within the limbic system. Activation of the VTA sends messages to clusters of nerve cells in the nucleus accumbens and the frontal cortex. This linkage, known as the mesolimbic dopamine system, forms the brain's primary reward pathway.

Cerebrum

Above these three sets of structures lies the cerebrum, the most recently evolved part of the brain. It contains a number of structures:

- *Basal ganglia*: a dense mass of neurons at its core. It includes the corpus striatum responsible for complex motor coordination.
- *Cortex*: the convoluted outer layer of grey matter comprising nerve cell bodies and their synaptic connections. It is the most highly organized centre of the brain. Most cortical areas are involved to some degree in the mediation of any complex behaviour, although there are centres of functional control within it. It is divided into two functional hemispheres, linked by the *corpus callosum*, a series of interconnecting neural fibres, at its base. It is divided into four lobes: frontal, temporal, occipital, and parietal (see Figures 4.1 and 4.2). As these are

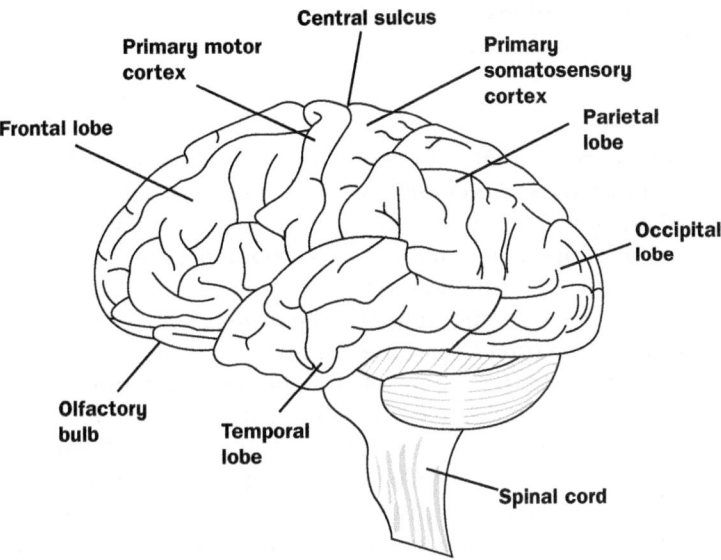

Figure 4.1 The gross anatomy of the brain

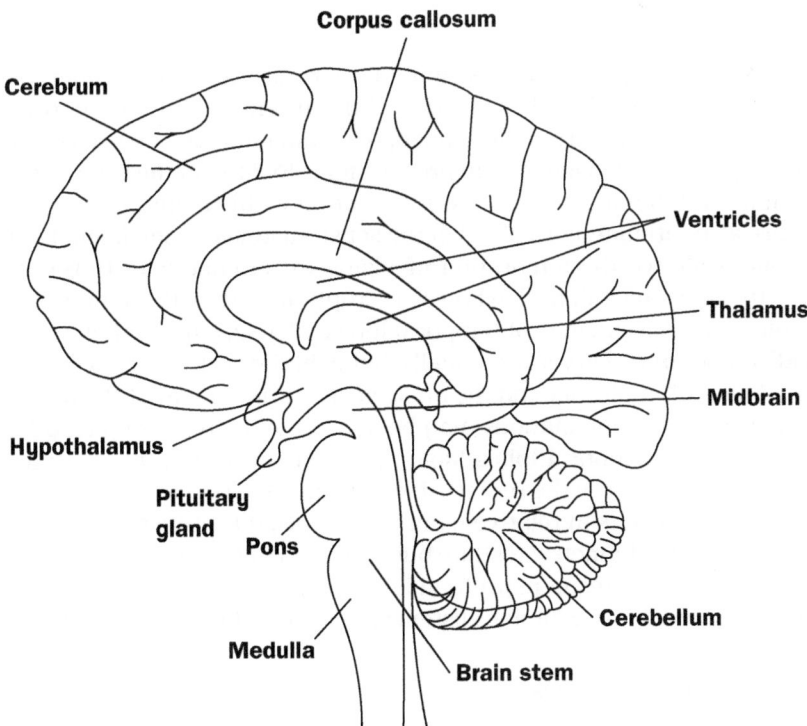

Figure 4.2 Cross-section of the brain showing key brain structures

involved in the **aetiology** of a number of mental health and neurological disorders, the function of each will now be considered in more detail.

Frontal lobes

The frontal lobes make up about one-third of the mass of the brain. The frontal cortex has an **executive function**, as it coordinates a number of complex processes, including speech, motor coordination, and behavioural planning. Loss of this executive function, as a consequence of damage, can result in a number of outcomes, including diminished anxiety and concern for the future, impulsiveness, lack of initiative and spontaneity, impairments in recent memory, loss of capacity to think in abstract terms, and an inability to plan and follow through a course of action or to take account of the outcome of actions. Individuals with frontal damage become inflexible and rigid. An individual may have difficulty shifting from one concept or task to another and changing from one established habit or behaviour to another. This can result in **perseveration**, where a particular behaviour is continued even in the face of clear instructions to change. The frontal lobes also seem to influence motivation levels. Damage to them can lead to a condition known as adynamia, evident through a complete or relative lack of verbal or overt behaviour. The prefrontal lobes are connected to the limbic system via the thalamus and motor system within the cortex. Links between the prefrontal cortex and the limbic system are activated during rewarding behaviours.

Temporal lobes

Although their functions are distributed, there are also clear functional centres within the temporal lobes. The location of these centres differs according to handedness. In people who are right-handed, the main language centre is located in the left hemisphere, and visuo-spatial processing is located in the right hemisphere. In left-handed individuals, there is less localization within hemispheres. The temporal lobes are also intimately involved in the sense systems of smell and hearing. They are responsible for the integration of visual experience with those of the other senses to make meaningful wholes. Disruption within the temporal lobes, for example, as a consequence of temporal lobe epilepsy, can result in visual illusions or **hallucinations**. Olfactory (smell) hallucinations have also been reported, although less often. Reflecting the multifaceted functioning of the temporal lobes, these illusions or hallucinations may be accompanied by strong emotions, in particular fear. The temporal lobes have an important role in memory and contain systems which preserve the record of conscious experience. Damage to one of the temporal lobes results in relatively minor memory difficulties, some of which may be evident on psychometric testing, but may not cause problems to the individual. Damage to both can result in profound memory deficits. Finally, they have an intimate connection with the limbic system and link emotions to events and memories.

Occipital and parietal lobes

These lobes are primarily involved in the integration of sensory information. Their functions are distributed and there are no clear functional centres. The occipital lobe is primarily involved in visual perception. Links to the cortex permit interpretation of visual stimuli.

Synapses

Each of the millions of interconnecting nerves within the brain is known as a neuron. Activation of systems within the brain is the result of small electrical currents progressing along many different neurons. Critical to the flow of this current are the small gaps between neurons, known as synapses. Here, chemicals known as neurotransmitters are responsible for activation of the system.

Each neuron has a number of fine branches known as axons at its terminal. At the end of these is an area known as the presynaptic terminal, which, in turn, is in close proximity to the postsynaptic terminal within the axon of another neuron. Between them is an enclosed area known as the synaptic cleft (see Figure 4.3). Neurotransmitter chemicals are stored within the axon in small pockets known as synaptic vesicles. Electrical stimulation of the nerve results in release of the vesicles' contents into the synaptic cleft. Once the transmitter has been released into the synaptic cleft, it moves across the gap between the two axons, where it is taken up by specialist cells within the postsynaptic membrane – the receptor cells. Once in the receiving neuron, chemicals known as second messengers are released and trigger firing of the neuron, continuing the activity of the activated neurological system. If all the transmitter is not taken up by the postsynaptic receptor, further activation may be inhibited either by re-uptake of the unused molecules back into vesicles in the initiating neuron or by degradation by other chemicals, such as monoamine oxidase released into the synaptic cleft.

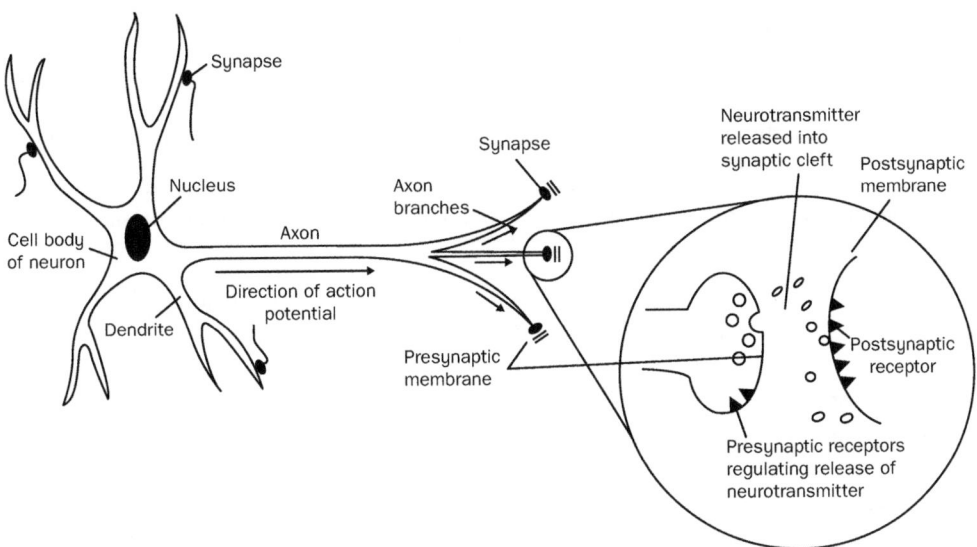

Figure 4.3 A neuron and close-up of the synaptic cleft

Neuronal activity itself is mediated by small electrical impulses that travel down the nerve axon towards the nerve ending. When a neuron is at rest, the outside of the cell wall is lined with sodium ions, and the inside wall is lined with potassium ions. When the neuron is stimulated by an incoming message at its receptor site, the sodium ions move from the outer side of the cell membrane to its inside. This starts a wave of electrochemical activity that continues down the length of the axon and results in it 'firing'. Immediately following this, the potassium ions shift from the inside to the outside of the neuron, returning it to its original resting state.

Neurotransmitters

A relatively small number of neurotransmitters have been implicated in the aetiology of the most common mental disorders. The effects of those considered in this chapter are summarized in Table 4.1 and are considered in more detail in the relevant chapters later in the book.

Serotonin

First identified in the 1950s, serotonin is an amino acid, and is synthesized from its precursor l-tryptophan. It is found in the striatum, mesolimbic system, forebrain, cortex, hippocampus, thalamus, and hypothalamus. It is thought to be involved in moderating mood, with low levels associated with conditions such as depression and obsessive-compulsive disorder.

Norepinephrine

Norepinephrine is a second neurotransmitter involved in depression as well as a number of anxiety disorders. Among other areas, it is found in the hypothalamus, cerebellum, and hippocampus. It belongs to a family of chemicals known as catecholamines.

Table 4.1 The key neurotransmitters, some of the drugs that affect them, and their role in key mental health disorders

Neurotransmitter	Primary disorder	Treatment	Mode of action
Monoamines			
Serotonin	↓in depression	Tricyclics, SSRIs	Prevent re-uptake
Dopamine	↓in schizophrenia	Phenothiazines	Block receptor sites
		Reserpine	Block vesicular storage
Catecholamines			
Norepinephrine	↓in depression	MAOIs	Prevent degradation
		Tricyclics	Prevent re-uptake
Amino acids			
GABA	↓in anxiety	Benzodiazepines	Enhance GABA

Dopamine

Neurons mediated by dopamine are found in the mesolimbic system, in a brain area known as A10, with links to the thalamus, hippocampus, frontal cortex, and the substantia nigra. Dopaminergic dysregulation has been associated with conditions as varied as schizophrenia, autism, and attentional deficit/hyperactivity disorders.

GABA

A group of drugs known as benzodiazepines were found to be an effective treatment for anxiety before their mode of action was understood. It is now known that they enhance the action of a neurotransmitter known as gamma-aminobutyric acid (GABA). This carries inhibitory messages: when it is received at the postsynaptic receptor site, it prevents the neuron from firing. Sites of GABA include the brain stem, cerebellum, and limbic system.

4.2 The autonomic nervous system

Although most explanations of mental health problems focus on neurotransmitters and neurological processes, another system, known as the autonomic nervous system, is also involved in some conditions, particularly those involving stress or anxiety. The autonomic nervous system links the brain to many of the body organs, including the heart, gut, and smooth muscles. Its job is to control the activity of these organs in response to the various demands being placed on them, for example by increasing heart rate, blood pressure, and breathing rate during exercise. Overall control of the autonomic nervous system is provided by the hypothalamus. It receives blood-borne and nervous system inputs concerning the state of the body, such as oxygenation and acidity of the blood. In addition, it receives inputs from the cortex and limbic system regarding behavioural and emotional factors. Based on these various inputs, the hypothalamus either increases or decreases activity within the autonomic nervous system and the various organs it controls.

Autonomic processes

The autonomic nervous system comprises two subsystems, known as the sympathetic and parasympathetic nervous systems. These arise in the medulla oblongata in the brain stem and travel down the spinal cord. At various points along the spinal cord, they link with other nerves connected to target organs such as the heart, arteries, skeletal muscles, and colon. The *sympathetic system* is involved in arousal, and its activity within the brain and spinal cord is controlled by norepinephrine. High levels of norepinephrine result in increased arousal and activation of the target organs. The *parasympathetic system* is involved in calming or reducing arousal, and its activity is controlled by levels of the neurotransmitter acetylcholine. The two systems tend to work antagonistically and the level of physical activation of the individual at any one time is a function of the relative dominance of each system.

Endocrine responses

Neurotransmitters act quickly, but are unable to maintain activation for long. To enable a sustained response to stress, a second system is activated by the sympathetic nervous system. High levels of sympathetic nervous system activity cause part of the adrenal glands, known as the adrenal medulla, situated above the kidneys, to release hormonal counterparts of the neurotransmitter norepinephrine (and to a lesser extent epinephrine) into the bloodstream. These travel to the target organs, are taken up by receptors, and sustain the action initiated by the neurotransmitters.

When the emotion of stress is experienced, the sympathetic nervous system gains dominance, activates the body, and prepares it to deal with physical damage. At its most dramatic, this response is known as the *fight–flight response*. At such times, sympathetic activity is clearly dominant, the heart beats more quickly and more powerfully, blood is shunted to the muscles and away from the gut (hence the experience of 'butterflies'), skeletal muscles tense in preparation for action, and so on. The individual may shake, pace or want to engage in some form of physical activity. This ancient response is clearly advantageous at times when the causes of stress are acute and life-threatening: chronic activation in response to long-term stress or short-term activation at inappropriate times, such as while in a supermarket or bus queue, is more problematic.

4.3 Drug therapies

Activation of brain systems is dependent on the activity of individual neurons, which, in turn, are influenced by the amount of neurotransmitter available at the postsynaptic receptor site: too much and the system is overactive; too little and it is underactive. The goal of drug therapies is to ensure appropriate levels of key neurotransmitters. They do this by one of two actions:

- *Increasing the availability* of the neurotransmitter by preventing re-uptake at the synapse, preventing degradation within the synaptic cleft, or replacing low levels of a particular neurotransmitter with its pharmacological equivalent. Drugs that increase the action of a neurotransmitter are known as **agonists**.
- *Decreasing availability* of the neurotransmitter by depleting levels of the available transmitter or replacing the active transmitters with an inert chemical. Drugs that inhibit the action of a neurotransmitter are known as **antagonists**.

Drugs are usually administered by mouth or injection into muscles, and then enter the bloodstream. They enter the brain by permeation from the small blood vessels that pass through it. Designing drugs to influence brain activity has not proven easy. The brain is protected from infection and other blood-borne insults by the blood–brain barrier. In the rest of the body, drugs pass from the blood vessels to target sites through pores in the walls of the blood vessels. The blood vessels in the brain lack these pores, and drugs have to pass directly through the cells of the blood vessel wall. This mechanism means that only drugs using relatively small molecules can pass this barrier, and even then their perfusion will be less than in the rest of the body.

Treating depression

Drugs that increase norepinephrine: MAOIs

The first potent antidepressants to be developed were known as **monoamine oxidase inhibitors** (**MAOIs**). These prevent degradation of norepinephrine (and to a lesser extent, serotonin) by monoamine oxidase within the synaptic cleft and help sustain its action. As was the case of a number of early psychiatric treatments, the discovery of the antidepressant qualities of MAOIs was accidental. Their first use was in the treatment of tuberculosis, where they were found to improve mood in those treated and became a standard treatment for depression, with a success rate of about 50%.

Despite this therapeutic benefit, MAOIs are now rarely used. As well as working in the brain, they prevent the production of monoamine oxidase in the liver and intestines, where it breaks down tyramine, a chemical that can result in potentially fatal and sudden increases in blood pressure if allowed to accumulate within the body. In order to prevent this, people who take MAOIs have to avoid foods such as cheeses, red wines, Marmite, bananas, and some fish that contain tyramine. Eating these foodstuffs may trigger a sudden and potentially fatal rise in blood pressure. Some newer MAOIs, known as reversible selective MAOIs, have been developed that avoid these problems. However, as more recent research has suggested that serotonin is more important than norepinephrine in the aetiology of depression, treatment has mostly changed to drugs that affect serotonin levels.

Drugs that increase serotonin: tricyclic antidepressants, SSRIs, and SNRIs

Three drug groups increase serotonin levels by inhibiting its re-uptake into the presynaptic terminal: the **tricyclics** (e.g. imipramine, amitriptyline), **selective serotonin re-uptake inhibitors** (**SSRIs**; e.g. fluoxetine, sertraline), and **serotonin and norepinephrine re-uptake inhibitors** (**SRNIs**; e.g. venlafaxine, milnacipran, duloxetine). Both tricyclics and SNRIs (clearly!) also increase levels of norepinephrine.

The first tricyclic, imipramine, was used initially as a treatment for schizophrenia. It was unsuccessful in this, but did reduce levels of depression in many people. Between 60% and 65% of those who take tricyclics experience some improvement of symptoms (Hirschfeld 1999). Their effects, and those of other drugs that increase serotonin levels, can take 10 days or more to become evident, probably due to an initial reduction in the amount of serotonin produced at the presynaptic terminal in response to more being available within the synaptic cleft. Improvements in mood occur as the system adapts to the drug and begins to release normal amounts of serotonin again, with re-uptake prevention finally resulting in an increase in available serotonin. It is important to maintain a therapeutic regime for some months after changes in mood have been achieved: about 50% of users will relapse within a year if tricyclic use is stopped prematurely (Montgomery et al. 1993).

Selective serotonin re-uptake inhibitors are a more recent pharmacological treatment. They increase serotonin without affecting norepinephrine levels. Although they are no more effective than tricyclics (Anderson 1998), this selectivity means they have fewer side-effects such as constipation, blurred vision, increased appetite and weight gain, and an uncomfortably dry mouth. They are also less dangerous in overdose. They are not without side-effects, however, which include fatigue, insomnia, nausea, headache, and tremor. Of concern also is evidence of a characteristic SSRI discontinuation syndrome (Haddad and Anderson 2007). It is usually mild, commences within one week of stopping treatment, resolves spontaneously within 3 weeks, and comprises a number of physical and psychological symptoms, of which the most frequent are dizziness, nausea, lethargy, and headache. Restarting use of an SSRI leads to resolution within 48 hours. To minimize this risk, SSRIs, like other antidepressants, need to be withdrawn gradually. Because SNRIs work on both serotonin and norepinephrine levels, they are generally considered more effective in the treatment of severe depression than SSRIs. However, the gains from their use are modest, and they may be less tolerated by patients than SSRIs due to the greater likelihood of side-effects (e.g. Lam et al. 2010).

Side-effects such as a dry mouth may appear somewhat trivial, but they can have a significant impact on those taking these drugs, as one user pointed out:

> The worst thing about the drug was the dry mouth I got with it. And when I say 'dry mouth', I really mean it. My mouth and lips were dry all the time. I wanted to drink all the time, so I could refresh my mouth. But that didn't help much – so I ended up chewing gum all the time – and I hate gum! It may not sound much, but when you are already feeling down, it just adds to the bad feeling.

Another woman, who benefited from taking SSRIs, commented on a perhaps less obvious side-effect.

> Taking these drugs was great – I felt so much better on them. But one problem did arise. When I was depressed, the last thing I wanted to do was to have sex with my husband. Now, I can't wait … but the most frustrating thing is I can't climax! We have great fun, but it is so frustrating!

The problem with Prozac

The introduction of SSRIs was not without problems. Perhaps the most widely known controversy involved one of the first of this type of drug to be widely available – Prozac (otherwise known as fluoxetine). This was described by its makers as the first of a new generation of side-effect-free antidepressants. In addition, it rapidly gained a reputation as the only antidepressant that could not only help people who were depressed, but also improve the quality of life of people who were not. It seemed to increase confidence and sociability and to reduce shyness and social anxiety. As a result, it became widely prescribed in the USA, among both those who were depressed and those who needed the emotional lift that it provided.

This initial success was soon mitigated by a series of claims alleging that Prozac had far more side-effects than was initially reported by its makers, the most dramatic of which involved significant behavioural disinhibition that could result in either self-harm or violence towards others. Perhaps the most notorious association between Prozac and violence was the case of Joseph Wesbecker, who shot 20 people in his former workplace, eight of them fatally, before killing himself while he was taking Prozac.

Of course, small case studies and sensationalist stories cannot be considered convincing evidence of a link between Prozac and dangerous behaviour, but they did increase the publicity surrounding prescription of the drug. More empirical studies have now put this controversy to rest. Fergusson et al. (2005), for example, found no evidence of any greater risk of suicide associated with SSRIs than with tricyclics in a **meta-analysis** of the relevant trials. In addition, Yerevanian et al. (2004) found that suicide rates did not differ across SSRIs and tricyclics, and that suicide rates were higher following discontinuation of both SSRIs and tricylics than during active treatment. Perhaps this latter finding is the most disappointing aspect of SSRIs, which were hoped to be an effective and relatively short-term treatment. Instead, they can have a high incidence of relapse following discontinuation, with rates varying between 13% and 90% depending on the duration of treatment and history of depression (Raynsford 2019).

Treating anxiety

Drugs that enhance the action of GABA: the benzodiazepines

A group of drugs known as benzodiazepines was found in the 1960s to be an effective treatment of anxiety. This class of drugs replaced the use of low doses of barbiturates, which made people drowsy, could prove fatal as they led to respiratory failure, and were highly addictive.

Benzodiazepines appear to enhance the action of GABA, but do not bind to the same postsynaptic receptor sites. As well as impacting on sites within the brain such as the limbic system, they provide a relaxant effect as a result of their effect on GABA within the spinal cord. The first benzodiazepine was known as chlordiazepoxide (Librium). The best known, Valium, was marketed several years later. By the mid-1980s, benzodiazepines were the most widely prescribed **psychotropic medication**. However, their prescription has not been without cost. When their use is stopped, levels of anxiety frequently return to pre-morbid levels or above (Chouinard 2004). Sudden withdrawal of these drugs typically results in the rapid recurrence of previous symptoms combined with withdrawal symptoms, including sweating, shaking, nausea, and vomiting. As a consequence, up to 80% of people who stop taking benzodiazepines after a long period of use relapse and require further treatment. Many people have to be gradually withdrawn from the drugs over extended periods of time, often many months. Benzodiazepine use has also been associated with a number of undesirable side-effects, including drowsiness, memory loss, and depression. Around 1% of people taking benzodiazepines may have paradoxical responses, including aggressive or suicidal behaviour as a consequence of disinhibition (Dodds 2017). Despite these concerns, benzodiazepines are still regularly prescribed, but now on a more short-term basis than previously.

Drugs that increase serotonin (and norepinephrine)

There is increasing evidence that a number of anxiety conditions, including generalized anxiety and obsessive-compulsive disorder, are mediated, at least in part, by serotonin. For these conditions, treatment with antidepressants, in particular

SSRIs (e.g. Bighelli et al. 2018) but to a lesser extent SNRIs, has proven more effective than traditional anxiolytics and have become the treatment of choice.

Treating schizophrenia

Biological theorists have implicated dopamine in the aetiology of the **positive symptoms** of schizophrenia (see Chapter 13). Individuals with these symptoms do not show raised levels of dopamine but appear instead to have an excessive number of dopamine receptor sites on the postsynaptic terminal, making them over-reactive to normal levels of dopamine. The goal of therapy is usually therefore to reduce the number of receptor sites accessible to the dopamine by filling them with inert drugs that mimic dopamine's chemical composition. A less frequent intervention involves reducing the amount of available dopamine.

Drugs that reduce dopamine

The origin of the present pharmacological treatment of schizophrenia lies in the observations made in the 1940s by a French surgeon, Henri Laborit, that one of the drugs he used as an antihistamine had a profound calming effect on his patients prior to surgery. The drug was called chlorpromazine. In the early 1950s, this was used experimentally with patients with **psychotic** symptoms, and rapidly became established as the primary treatment of schizophrenia.

Chlorpromazine belongs to a class of drugs variously known as **phenothiazines**, **neuroleptics** or **major tranquillizers**. They work by blocking the dopamine receptors in the postsynaptic receptor sites. Unfortunately, while successful in the short term, their use results in a proliferation of dopamine receptor sites (Strange 1992), adding further to the sensitivity of the postsynaptic receptors and resulting in the need for long-term treatment. They also have a number of significant side-effects. For these reasons, clinicians maintain people with schizophrenia on the lowest effective dose or gradually reduce and stop medication after a period of time in which the individual is functioning normally (see Chapter 13).

The phenothiazines' main side-effects occur as a result of their impact on the extrapyramidal areas of the brain, including the substantia nigra. These areas are involved in the control of motor activity and coordination. The most common **extrapyramidal symptoms** are Parkinsonian symptoms. These include stiffness in the arms and legs, facial expressions that are flat and dull, and tremors, particularly in the hands. These symptoms can usually be relieved by drugs that reverse the effects of phenothiazines or a reduction in the amount of drug prescribed. About 20% of those who take phenothiazines for an extended time develop a second condition, known as tardive dyskinesia. Its primary symptoms include involuntary writhing or tic-like movements of the face or whole body. Facial movements include involuntary chewing, sucking and writhing of the tongue in and out of the mouth. Body movements include jerky, purposeless movements of the arms, legs, and torso. Its severity varies between a single symptom and a severe whole-body problem. These symptoms are difficult to treat and can be irreversible. If detected early, and treatment is stopped immediately, most symptoms will remit. However, many symptoms are similar to those found in schizophrenia and may not be observed or even result in increased phenothiazine being prescribed. The longer an individual has taken phenothiazines, the less likely their symptoms are to remit, even after the cessation of therapy.

A second approach to the treatment of schizophrenia involves reducing the amount of dopamine available to be released into the synaptic cleft. The action of a drug known as reserpine is to inhibit the synthesis of dopamine. Once existing stores have been utilized, it can take up to 2 weeks for them to return to normal levels during treatment with reserpine.

Drugs that reduce NMDA levels

One additional form of drug has proven effective in the treatment of schizophrenia. Atypical neuroleptics achieve their benefits through their impact on NMDA receptors. Drugs such as phencyclidine (PCP, 'angel-dust') and ketamine are thought to increase activity in these receptors and cause symptoms similar to those of schizophrenia. Their activity seems to be blocked by the drugs clozapine and risperidone (Morimoto et al. 2002). These drugs may also reduce dopamine activity, possibly indirectly through their influence on serotonin levels, which control dopamine release at times of stress (Pehek et al. 2006).

These atypical neuroleptics are now the first-line treatment of schizophrenia, as they are generally more effective than phenothiazines and consistently cause significantly fewer extrapyramidal symptoms (Huhn et al. 2019). Success rates with phenothiazines of about 65% are typical; for the new drugs the success rate is about 85% (Awad and Vorungati 1999). Unfortunately, the medication still carries some costs, and these can be severe. Between 1% and 2% of those who take the drug go on to develop **agranulocytosis**, a potentially fatal reduction in white blood cells, resulting in a need for all those prescribed these drugs to have regular blood tests so they can be withdrawn before this disorder becomes problematic.

Adherence to drug treatments

Any drug can achieve its potential only if it is taken regularly and at therapeutic levels. This is not always the case: up to 50% of people prescribed psychotropic medication either do not take the recommended dose or do not take the drug at all. Bulloch and Patten (2010), for example, reported non-adherence rates in their survey of over 6,000 people taking psychotropic medication of 34.6% for antipsychotics, 34.7% for sedative-hypnotics, 38.1% for mood stabilizers (in the treatment of bipolar disorder), and 45.9% for antidepressants.

The most frequent reason for non-adherence is forgetting. More conscious decisions whether or not to take tablets are often based on a form of cost–benefit analysis, in which the benefits of taking medication, usually in terms of relief from symptoms, are weighed against the costs of taking it – usually the side-effects of the drug. The more side-effects a drug has, the lower the rates of adherence, particularly where there are no immediate changes in symptoms when doses of a drug are taken or missed, as is the case for many psychiatric drugs. An example of this can be found in the findings of Demyttenaere et al. (1998), who found that 36% of people prescribed the tricyclic amitriptyline failed to take their medication, compared to 6% of those prescribed the SSRI fluoxetine. Level of depression was not predictive of drop-out. However, younger men who experienced severe side-effects were least likely to take the medication.

Not surprisingly, some side-effects are more problematic than others, although these may not be immediately obvious. Achtyes et al. (2018), for example, found potential weight gain was the most important determinant of medication choice among people with a diagnosis of schizophrenia. Other factors may also be involved. Day et al. (2005) found that a poor relationship with the prescriber, experience of coercion during admission, and low insight predicted a negative attitude towards treatment. Niolu et al. (2015) found that low adherence in people prescribed antipsychotics was associated with the absence of a caregiver, poor insight, a negative attitude towards medication, and a high degree of perceived self-control over their problems. Sirey et al. (2001) found high adherence to medication to be associated with lower perceived stigma of taking drugs, higher self-rated severity of illness, being aged 60 or over, and absence of 'personality pathology'. Finally, simply considering the medication you are taking to be 'necessary' is a powerful factor in adherence (Jónsdóttir et al. 2008).

Research box 3

Schulze, L.N., Stenzel, U., Leipert, J. et al. (2019) Improving medication adherence with telemedicine for adults with severe mental illness, *Psychiatric Services*, 70: 225–28.

Even before lockdown for Covid-19, telemedicine, or remote engagement between healthcare professionals and their patients, had become increasingly popular. It allows easy, regular, and cost-effective contact between health worker and those they are working with. This paper combines this approach with the important role of maintaining adherence to antipsychotic medication, which can typically drop to below 50%. It assessed the effectiveness of standardized telephone calls and text messages, an approach previously found to be of value in people with anxiety and mood disorders.

Method

Participants

Participants were people with a confirmed diagnosis of either schizophrenia or bipolar disorder, aged 18 years or over, who had been discharged from three German psychiatric hospitals, and who had no scheduled out-patient consultations within the time-frame of the study. Participants who were actively suicidal were excluded from the study at any point this was detected.

Conditions

Active intervention: standardized, regular telephone calls every second week delivered by trained nurses. The calls always used the same overall structure:

- Opening the conversation: check mood, what happened since last call?
- Individual topics: personal content, e.g. chat about hobby, family, etc.
- Medication: any changes, side-effects, problems with adherence
- Suicidal tendencies: questionnaire addressing suicidal thoughts, planning, etc.
- Ending: take home message, topic for next call.

Participants were also asked whether they wished to receive weekly reminder texts. If they opted to do so, these were sent on a weekly basis.

Usual care: basic 'medical care' involving 'occasional' visits to physician to evaluate convalescence. No measure of frequency of contact was made.

Measures

- A standardized measure of adherence, the Medication Adherence Report Scale – Deutsch (MARS-D) is a psychometrically strong measure of adherence to medication. It comprises five items measuring adherence to medical regimens. Items include: 'Do you every forget to take your medication?', 'When you feel better, do you sometimes stop taking your medication?'
- Social desirability was measured using a brief Social Desirability Scale. This was used as a covariate in analyses of change in medication adherence in an attempt to reduce the biases in reporting adherence that may reflect participants' desire to 'please' the researcher.

After discharge from hospital, participants were randomly allocated to the active intervention or usual care control condition. Assessments of adherence were conducted by telephone at 3- and 6-month follow-up.

Results

Baseline measures were taken on 120 participants who conformed to the study requirements. By 6 months, 88 remained in the study (42 in the active intervention, 46 in the control). Drop-out rates did not differ significantly across the conditions. The mean age at baseline was 42 years. Half the study population was female and half male. Eighty per cent were diagnosed with schizophrenia, 20% with bipolar disorder.

Adherence was measured using logistic regression, which provides an odds ratio (OR) of the likelihood of adherence in the active intervention compared to that in the control condition. The OR for reported adherence at 6-month follow-up was 4.11 (95% confidence interval [95% CI] = 1.47–11.45, $p = 0.007$), indicating that those in the active intervention were over four times more likely to report being adherent than those in usual care. This (OR) was found after controlling for age, gender, and baseline adherence scores. Adding the social desirability score did not negatively impact on this finding. Indeed, the OR between the conditions rose to 6.79 (95% CI = 1.98–23.28, $p = 0.002$) when this was added to the regression equation.

Discussion

Measuring adherence to medication is difficult, as invasive measures such as diary-keeping tend to increase adherence, almost forming an intervention in themselves. The optimal approach is to provide medication in containers that unobtrusively record the number of times they are opened and which either transmit this data to a remote recorder or are returned by the user and the data is then extracted. This approach is clearly expensive and difficult to establish in the 'real-world' setting in which this study was conducted. Accordingly, while the self-report measure used on this study is clearly not without problems (being in a study in which you are clearly being exhorted to maintain adherence to your medication is likely to have the demand characteristic of over-reporting adherence), the researchers attempted to at least reduce this bias by partialling out the effects of social desirability. A stronger study, with more participants may usefully have also considered factors such as relapse rates and use of healthcare support services, which may have added value and strengthened any conclusions that could be drawn from the data. Finally, the intervention could have proven quite expensive, and at a time when healthcare resources are scarce, some consideration could usefully have been given to the cost-effectiveness of the intervention.

Stop and think ...

Taking medication has both benefits and costs. It is relatively simple and does not require the effort required to engage in psychotherapy. We may experience a relief from symptoms. However, we may also experience a number of side-effects. Most of these are relatively innocuous – although they may have a significant impact on the individual. The dry mouth associated with some antidepressant medications, for example, sounds relatively trivial but, in reality, is a significant and uncomfortable consequence. The side-effects of some other types of medication may have a longer-term and more significant impact on health. Of note in this context is that these side-effects are frequently experienced immediately an individual starts taking medication – the benefits may take some time, often weeks, before becoming evident.

So, what would influence your willingness to take and adhere to a medication regimen? Would you accept significant side-effects in the hope of future gain – and, if so, for how long? Many people have an 'against medication' bias. If you do, how severe would any mental health problem have to be before you decided to take medication? Perhaps even more pertinent given the high levels of relapse following cessation of medication, how long would you be willing to continue taking medication? Months, years? What factors would influence your decisions in this regard? And finally, how much would the knowledge of alternative intervention approaches such as psychotherapy influence your decisions?

4.4 Electroconvulsive therapy

Electroconvulsive therapy (ECT) is the brief discharge of an electric current through the brain with the aim of inducing a controlled epileptic convulsion to achieve an improvement in an abnormal mental state. Its origins lie in observations made in the 1930s that stunned pigs appeared particularly sedated and quiet in abattoirs, and justified by anecdotal evidence that people who had epilepsy rarely evidenced any form of **psychosis** and that their mood following epileptic seizures often improved.

Extrapolating from these observations, physicians attempted to induce epileptic fits in an attempt to treat mood disorders, initially using injections of camphor – a process that proved fatal in a number of cases. An alternative approach was pioneered by two Italian psychiatrists, Ugo Cerletti and Lucio Bini, who found that they could induce seizures by applying electrical currents to patients' heads, and improve the symptoms of schizophrenia. Cerletti later abandoned ECT and sought alternative treatments as a result of his concerns over the physical damage, including jaw dislocation and broken bones, and neurological effects such as memory loss that resulted from the seizures provoked by his treatment.

Until the 1950s, ECT involved placing electrodes on each temple and passing an electric current of between 65 and 140 volts through these 'paddles' for half a second or less. This provoked an epileptic fit lasting from half to several minutes. Initially, this was given 'straight'; that is, with the patient fully conscious. Vigorous convulsive muscle activity frequently led to bone fractures until the introduction of the muscle relaxants given prior to ECT. As awareness of this paralysis led to high levels of anxiety on the part of the recipient, this was soon accompanied by administration of an intravenous barbiturate to render them unconscious during the procedure, a process known as modified ECT. More recently, the electrodes have been placed over the non-dominant hemisphere only, a process known as unilateral ECT. This is thought to result in fewer side-effects. ECT is typically administered two or three times a week in courses ranging from 4 to 12 treatments. Less commonly, it is given fortnightly or monthly for 6 months or longer to prevent relapse, a process known as continuation or maintenance ECT. Even now, how ECT achieves any benefits is not fully understood (Oltedal et al. 2017), although Fosse and Read (2013) speculated it may increase activity in the dopamine system and reduce activation of the frontal and temporal lobes.

The use of ECT peaked and then began to decline substantially in the 1950s following the introduction of a range of psychotropic drug treatments. Nevertheless, its use is still recommended by many psychiatric authorities, including NICE (2009a), who recommended its use in the treatment of depression, but only when this has proven resistant to multiple drug and psychological treatments. NICE did not recommend its use with a second patient group for whom ECT has been frequently prescribed, those with a diagnosis of schizophrenia (NICE 2009b), unless they are experiencing potentially life-threatening catatonia or severe or a prolonged manic episode. How effectively these guidelines have been followed is difficult to assess. Following a freedom of information request to 56 UK mental healthcare providers (NHS Trusts), Read et al. (2018) found some Trusts were using ECT 12 times more frequently than others, indicating significant variability in its use by differing psychiatrists. Of concern was that only ten Trusts were able to provide data on how many people received psychological therapy prior to ECT (as recommended by NICE). Among these, the figures varied from zero to 100% – again indicating a wide variation in practice, and failures to adhere to guidelines.

The ECT controversy

The use of ECT has not been without controversy. Those against its use oppose it on moral grounds as well as question its effectiveness. Even the psychiatric authorities that endorse its use have acknowledged the controversy. The US National Institutes of Health (NIH) Consensus Statement (1985) observed that ECT had been used inappropriately to treat disorders where there was no evidence of effectiveness and that many of these efforts proved harmful. It also noted that the use of ECT as a means of managing unruly patients, exemplified in the film *One Flew over the Cuckoo's Nest,* contributed to its perception as an abusive instrument of behavioural control for patients in mental institutions.

The controversy around ECT revolves around the potential harm that may result from its treatment. The short-term effects are associated with being given an anaesthetic and fitting. Adverse events are rare, but do occur. The NIH Consensus Statement suggested a rate of up to 4.5 deaths per 100,000 treatments, a risk comparable to the use of short-acting barbiturate anaesthetics in other conditions. They also noted that the risk of physical injury was low but still evident, with a complication rate of 1 per 1,300 to 1,400 treatments. Problems included tooth damage, vertebral compression fractures, uncontrollable fitting, peripheral nerve palsy, and skin burns. Some people also find ECT a terrifying experience, an abusive invasion of personal autonomy, or even experience a sense of shame because of the social stigma they associate with it (Johnstone 2003).

Effect on memory

Perhaps the most problematic outcome of ECT is its effect on memory. People who have had ECT typically experience an acute phase of confusion following treatment: it can take them 5 or 10 minutes to remember who they are, where they are or what day it is. It also impairs the ability to learn and retain new information for a period of time following administration and may impact adversely on memories of events that occurred months or even years before treatment. Feliu et al. (2008), for example, found that nearly a month after receiving ECT, patients performed less well than before their treatment on objective measures of recognition memory, and short-term memory of both verbal and visual memory, despite improvements in mood. Similar findings have been found in tests of autobiographical memory. Lisanby et al. (2000) followed 55 people with major depression, randomly allocated to either unilateral or bilateral ECT. Prior to treatment, they obtained detailed autobiographical and impersonal memories and then tested recall of these memories immediately following the course of ECT and at 2-month follow-up. A control group who did not have depression or ECT underwent the same testing procedures. All those who received ECT recalled fewer personal and impersonal memories, and in less detail, than controls on both testing occasions. By the second assessment, differences between the two groups who received

ECT also emerged: those given bilateral ECT recalled less than those who had unilateral ECT. The degree of memory impairment can also be linked to the amount of electrical stimulation during ECT. Kronsell et al. (2019), for instance, followed a cohort of people treated with ECT for depression and found that 44% of those with a high 'dosage' experienced significant subjective memory loss. Of those receiving a 'low dosage', the equivalent figure was 25%.

Alternatives to ECT

Given the problems associated with ECT, a number of researchers have attempted to find alternative methods to achieve the same clinical results, without the unwanted side-effects. Transcranial magnetic stimulation (TMS) is one such approach. It involves passing a series of electrical pulses close to the brain. The coil is held on the scalp and the magnetic field passes through the skull and into the brain. Small induced currents can then make brain areas below the coil more or less active, depending on the settings used. TMS can influence many brain functions, including movement, visual perception, memory, reaction time, speech, and mood. Its most obvious effects last for relatively brief periods following stimulation. However, there is some evidence that the procedure may prove an alternative approach to the use of ECT, and its use in depression has recently been endorsed by a European Expert Group (Lefaucheur et al. 2020). In one relevant study, Schulze-Rauschenbach et al. (2005) compared TMS with unilateral ECT in the treatment of major depression. Treatment response was comparable: 46% of people treated with ECT and 44% of those treated with TMS showed significant clinical improvements. More encouragingly, while patients treated with ECT showed evidence of memory deficits, those treated with TMS showed no decrement and even improvements in memory. Quite how TMS impacts on mood is not clear. However, animal studies suggest it may result in increases in serotonin and a number of other neurotransmitters including dopamine (Kanno et al. 2003). Although there has been some interest in the use of TMS in other conditions such as anxiety and obsessive-compulsive disorder, it has yet to be shown to be effective (Pigot et al. 2008).

4.5 Psychosurgery

The modern practice of psychosurgery began in the 1930s, when two Portuguese neurologists, Egas Moniz and Almeida Lima, began severing connections to and from the frontal lobes in people with 'psychoneuroses'. By 1936, the procedure developed into what was termed a prefrontal leucotomy (sometimes referred to as a **lobotomy**). This operation was initially fairly crude, as the surgeon had to estimate where to lesion the brain without any form of neuroimaging and did so freehand. However, it gradually became more precise in its anatomical location and procedures. Between 1936 and 1961, over 10,000 people received this type of treatment in the UK. Of these, an estimated 20% of those diagnosed with schizophrenia and about 50% of those with depression gained some degree of benefit (Malizia 2000). However, 4% died as a result of surgery, 4% developed a severe loss of motivation, 15% developed epilepsy, while up to 60% developed 'troublesome' personality changes. Despite these problems, the approach had many advocates, probably because there were no viable alternatives to this treatment for much of this time.

Rates of psychosurgery have fallen dramatically since effective pharmacological alternatives became available. Now, only about 20 operations are conducted in the UK each year, and only for conditions that have proven unresponsive to a variety of alternative treatments. New, more specific, surgical procedures have also been developed, including the stereotactic subcaudate tractotomy and stereotactic cingulotomy. Stereotactic interventions involve a device called a stereotactic frame, which is placed over the brain during operations and, in combination with neuroimaging, allows highly accurate lesions to be conducted. Neurosurgeons use a 'conservative' approach, creating small initial lesions, which can be added to with later operations should this be required.

Most lesions are created with heated electrodes, with the exception of the subcaudate tractotomy, which involves placing radioactive rods in the target area, destroying parts of the subcaudate brain area through a brief burst of radioactivity before becoming inert. It is usually used for the treatment of severe, intractable depression. Stereotactic cingulotomy is the most commonly used procedure for the anxiety disorders, including obsessive-compulsive disorder (see Chapter 6). The operation is conducted under general anaesthetic and involves placing electrodes into the cingulate bundle in each hemisphere. The tips of the electrodes are then heated to 85°C for about 100 seconds.

How psychosurgery achieves any therapeutic gains is not fully understood. In obsessive-compulsive disorder, for example, it may sever the brain systems driving the behaviours (see Chapter 6). However, preliminary evidence suggests that people with obsessive-compulsive disorder do not improve immediately following surgery; it may take several weeks or months before any benefits are observed. Jenike (1998) speculated that secondary nerve regeneration or metabolic alterations in brain areas other than those actually lesioned may be involved in any changes. This lack of understanding of what surgeons are actually doing provides critics of this approach with strong concerns about the nature and use of psychosurgery.

Post-operative effects

Rates of psychosurgery have fallen dramatically over the past decade, partly as a consequence of the findings reported by Malizia above. More dramatically, perhaps, a number of people have taken their own lives following surgery. Whether this is a result of the surgical procedure or would have happened without this intervention is difficult to judge. It is possible that some people who viewed the operation as the treatment of last resort may have died by suicide after disappointing results or simply did not benefit from the treatment. Jenike et al. (1991), for example, found that 4 of a series of 33 individuals who underwent cingulotomy for the treatment of obsessive-compulsive disorder took their own lives in the 13 years following the operation. All four had experienced severe depression with prominent suicidal ruminations prior to surgery. Perhaps the most scathing summary of the outcomes of surgery comes from one person, Henry Marsh (then a nurse, now an eminent neurosurgeon) intimately involved in the care of these patients: 'It reflected … bad medicine, bad science, because it was clear … patients who were subjected to this procedure were never followed up … If you saw the patient after the operation they'd seem alright, they'd walk and talk and say thank you doctor … The fact they were totally ruined as social human beings probably didn't count' (Levinson 2011).

Availability of psychosurgery

Given the issues raised above, it is perhaps not surprising that psychosurgery is banned by law in some countries, including Germany, Spain, and some US states, and treatment guidelines in the UK do not recommend it as a form of treatment for obsessive-compulsive disorder, depression or anxiety. While it remains possible to have psychosurgery in the UK in extreme cases, this is very rare. One of two hospitals in the UK to perform this type of surgery, Ninewells Hospital in Scotland, performed only four operations between 2015 and 2016 (MIND 2018). The criteria for the operation are stringent. The individual has to be resistant to all other attempts to treat the condition. In treating depression, for example, a candidate for surgery would typically have made more than two serious suicide attempts, have had an initial onset at least 18 years previously, and their present episode would have lasted 7 years without a period of remission of at least 6 months. They would have received over 30 ECT treatments, 'unusually large' doses of antidepressants, and been severely depressed on psychometric testing. The law in relation to psychosurgery differs across the mainland countries of the UK. However, in all of them, a panel of representatives has to be appointed by an appropriate governmental body overseeing health provision to assess that the person is providing full consent to the operation and that they are likely to benefit from it. No patient can be given psychosurgery without their consent.

4.6 Chapter summary

1. The brain is divided into a number of anatomical areas, most of which are in some way related to functions that influence mood or behaviour.
2. Damage to most brain areas will result in deficits that may be evident as emotional or mental health problems.
3. Activity within the brain is mediated by neurotransmitters, which act at the neuronal synapse.
4. Neurotransmitters mediate the activity within brain systems that are responsible for mood and behaviour. The most important to mental health are serotonin, dopamine, GABA, and norepinephrine.
5. Drug therapies affect the activity within brain systems by increasing or decreasing levels of neurotransmitters. Antidepressants increase the availability of serotonin (and to a lesser extent norepinephrine), anxiolytics increase levels of GABA, and neuroleptics decrease levels of dopamine.
6. ECT involves passing an electrical current through the temporal lobes of the brain to induce a seizure.

7. Treatment with ECT remains controversial; although it is now much safer than previously, it still evokes strong emotional arguments, among both those who support its use and those who oppose it. A number of medical authorities recommend its use in cases of depression that resist treatment using other methods.

8. ECT is linked to significant measurable memory problems that last a significant period of time. A new alternative, transcranial magnetic stimulation, may prove effective and has fewer such side-effects.

9. Psychosurgery is now used only in extreme cases of obsessive-compulsive disorder or depression.

10. Psychosurgery achieves a moderate degree of clinical benefit in a population where previous, more conservative treatments have failed, but carries with it a small but significant risk of subtle cognitive deficits.

11. How psychosurgery acts to relieve symptoms is not clear. It may interfere with activity within brain systems that mediate obsessive-compulsive disorder or depression. However, the time-frame in which changes occur following surgery indicates the possibility of other, as yet unknown, mechanisms.

4.7 For discussion

1. Drug treatment for schizophrenia carries both risks and benefits. What considerations should a doctor have when prescribing phenothiazine medication?

2. What contextual, social, and psychological factors are likely to influence adherence to a medication regimen?

3. Under what conditions, if any, would you consider having ECT or psychosurgery if others thought you might benefit from either treatment?

4. If offered a choice, would you opt for a medical or psychological treatment for a mental health condition that could be treated equally effectively with either approach?

4.8 Further reading

Bentall, R. (2010) *Doctoring the Mind*, London: Allen Lane.

Gibb, B. (2012) *A Rough Guide to the Brain*, London: Rough Guides.

Harrington, A. (2019) *Mind Fixers: Psychiatry's Troubled Search for the Biology of Mental Illness*, New York: Norton.

Healy, D. (2016) *Psychiatric Drugs Explained*, Edinburgh: Churchill Livingstone.

National Institute for Health and Care Excellence (NICE) (2009) *Guidance on the Use of Electroconvulsive Therapy*, London: NICE.

5 The individual and beyond

Very few of us live isolated lives that do not involve interacting with other people or wider society. And these interactions impact on our mental well-being. Good relationships, for example, appear to be protective against mental health problems; poor relationships or living in a stressful environment increase our risk. The first part of the chapter considers how the nature of relationships close to us, within the family, may contribute to mental health problems, and how these may be addressed in family therapy. It then considers more distal psychosocial influences and how these may be addressed through individual, public health or economic initiatives. Finally, the chapter considers how differing cultural factors may result in people from different cultures expressing distress in different ways, and how these need to be addressed within therapy. By the end of the chapter, you should have an understanding of:

- Theories of family functioning and interventions that involve the whole family
- The impact of factors such as socio-economic status (SES), gender, and ethnicity on mental health
- How health promotion and public health programmes may improve the mental well-being of individuals and populations
- How mental health problems may present and be treated across different cultures.

5.1 A systems approach

Family models of mental health disorders and their treatment are based on systems theory, and their related therapies are known as 'systemic therapies'. These view the family or other social groups as an interrelated set of individuals. The behaviour of each person within the system does not occur in isolation. Instead, behaviour follows a principle of circularity in which no one behaviour is seen as starting or being the outcome of events. The behaviour of X affects Y, whose behaviour reciprocally affects X, whose response to this affects Y, and so on. They form a continuous causal loop, with no beginning or end. Change in this continuous system can therefore be achieved by intervening at any point within it.

The chapter considers two systemic therapies that have emerged from very different theoretical perspectives: structural family therapy and strategic family therapy. Other forms of family therapy are described in the following chapters as appropriate. Whichever systemic therapy a family engages in may appear complex and confusing. It may involve whole families and even extended families. There are frequently two or more therapists involved, one or more of whom may not be obvious to the family, but they will know of their presence. Often a team of therapists sits behind a one-way mirror and tracks the progress of therapy. They may discuss issues raised within the session, identify the nature of the interactions among family members, and develop intervention strategies. They provide support to the therapist in the room with the family, who may be too involved in managing the process of therapy to notice all the complex interrelationships that occur. These observers may take an active role. They may communicate with the therapist in the room, either by telephone or by the therapist stepping out of the room for consultations with them, and share developing formulations about the nature of the problem. They may even tell the therapist to take a particular action or ask a specific question. The experience of family therapy is therefore very different from that of individual therapy, as is reflected in these participants' negative and positive responses to an initial therapy session:

> I I found it unpleasant and uncomfortable. We didn't all want to be there, and when we did get there, it was not at all clear what was going on. I didn't feel it right that we were watched by people through a mirror. You can't see their reaction to what's going on … that is really uncomfortable. didn't like it at all. I don't think we'll come back.

> It was weird, and not what I expected. The therapist was moving about talking to us all. He even got some of us to move around! Not what you expect. I thought they would be quiet and make us take it in turns to talk to them … not move around and interrupt and things … It was unnerving to know that people were watching through the mirror. But you couldn't see them, and I began to forget about them, especially when we were dealing with difficult things in the therapy session.

Structural family therapy

The structural school of family therapy was initially developed by Salvador Minuchin (e.g. Minuchin et al. 1978) and is now a widely practised approach to the treatment of family dysfunction and affected individuals. The core premise of this approach is that well-functioning families have a clear structure. When a family lacks such a structure, it fails to deal with any problems it faces from either internal or outside sources. This lack of structure may not be apparent to the family: they may not present complaining of family problems. More typically, one person from the family is seen as having mental health or behavioural problems. This 'identified patient' is a symptom of a dysfunctional family, and the family as a whole would benefit from change.

According to Minuchin, families develop structures in order to carry out roles. One important family structure involves the rules that govern the way in which family members relate to each other. The father, for example, will relate to different people in different ways at different times: partner, father, disciplinarian, friend, and so on. The rules that regulate these various relationships differ. However, each is governed by overt and covert rules.

Minuchin also identified a series of elements that combine to determine each family's organization and style of interaction. Subsystems are small units within the family that share a common element: generation, gender, interest, and so on. One individual may be a member of several subsystems, but boundaries exist between each subsystem and between the family and the outside world. According to Minuchin, clear boundaries are required to allow subsystems to carry out their specific functions and to develop autonomy and a sense of belonging. Problems arise when these boundaries are incorrectly established within families. Diffuse boundaries are highly permeable, and information flows readily between subsystems. In such cases, family members are extremely close. Indeed, they may become too close, leading to a state of enmeshment in which individual members do not experience a state of autonomy or independence. Conversely, boundaries that are too rigid and which prevent information flow between subsystems result in a process of disengagement and emotional detachment between family members.

Subsystems are organized hierarchically. The parental subsystem is generally considered to be superordinate to others, such as sibling subsystems, and to have an **executive function**. It makes key family decisions. There may also be disruptions or temporary subsystems established, in the form of alliances. Here, members of different subsystems cooperate, typically on a short-term basis. Father and son may combine forces to influence the mother, and so on. These alliances, particularly if they are long term, are thought to disturb the family hierarchy and to be an indication of dysfunction.

Minuchin identified the characteristics of functional families as having clear boundaries, appropriate hierarchies, and sufficiently flexible alignments to adjust, change, and foster individuals within them. Dysfunctional families have the opposite constellation of characteristics. According to Minuchin, when an individual presents with problems seen as requiring therapy, these 'symptoms' actually represent systemic problems. Minuchin's group associated particular diagnoses with specific types of family dynamics. The characteristic of 'anorexic families', for example, is being enmeshed, overprotective, rigid, and conflict-avoidant, with unexpressed parental conflict (Minuchin et al. 1978; see Case formulation box, p. 101). According to Minuchin, the stresses associated with an adolescent's push for independence within such a family increase the risk of the parental conflict becoming overt. To avoid this, the adolescent develops anorexic behaviours to prevent total dissension within the family. These behaviours may hold the family together as it unites around the 'identified patient' and deflect attention away from parental conflict.

The goal of therapy is to identify where these dysfunctions lie and to change them: to establish a 'normal' family structure in which the parental subsystem has executive powers, the boundaries between and around generations are clear, and long-term alliances do not exist. Each family member should have age-appropriate independence while still feeling part of the family.

Structural family therapy is behavioural, directive, and dynamic. The therapist is active within therapy sessions. They may move about, change the positions of family members to develop or disrupt alliances, interrupt particular allegiance patterns, and align with different members of the family. Treatment of the family involves three elements:

- challenging the family's perception of reality
- providing alternative possibilities that make sense to them
- once the family has tried out new patterns of transactions, developing new relationships and structures that are self-sustaining.

The therapeutic process involves a series of stages:

1. *Joining with the family*: the therapist enters the system, joining or establishing rapport by accommodating to the family's culture, mood, style, and language. The therapist may physically sit within the family and engage with them
2. *Evaluating the family structure*: the therapist examines boundaries, hierarchies, and alliances. This may be a very dynamic process. Individuals or subsystems are observed interacting using role play. The therapist may even set up conditions for these to be real interactions. Minuchin et al. (1978), for example, frequently held therapy sessions with the families of children with anorexia at lunchtime, when the family would be invited to have a meal together. These sessions could demonstrate, for example, the inability of parents to work together to encourage their child to eat, or a shifting pattern of coalitions between each parent and the child. This may lead to discussion among family members about the reasons for these various behaviours.
3. *Unbalancing the system*: during this phase, the therapist deliberately unbalances existing, dysfunctional, behavioural patterns in order to put the family into a state of disequilibrium. This process is highly directive and may involve the therapist aligning him or herself with different subsystems or alliances. An example of this process can be found in the case of a depressed woman who was pessimistic and hopeless at the start of a therapy session, but whose mood improved as she vented her feelings of frustration with her husband and her husband's family, who were critical and demanding of her. Rather than remain neutral, as would be the case in most one-to-one therapies, the therapist began to take sides with her husband, sympathizing with the problems he was having trying to keep everyone in the family happy, but also suggested that the two of

them sit down and attempt to establish limits on the intrusiveness of his family on their relationship.

4. *Restructuring operations*: once the system has been unbalanced, attempts follow to establish a normative family structure. This may involve a series of strategies, including:

   a) *actualizing family transactional patterns*: developing more appropriate transactional patterns through strategies including role play, guided practice, and physical manipulation of individuals into appropriate subsystems (by, for example, sitting mother and father together and jointly interacting with members of other systems);

   b) *escalating stress*: blocking recurrent inappropriate transactional patterns and developing conflict in order to encourage new alliances within more appropriate subsystems.

It is assumed that any changes are mutually reinforcing and that families will continue to develop without the need for further intervention. Therapy may nevertheless continue at weekly intervals for several months. One advantage of this approach is that it presents a clear model of therapy. Targets and goals are clearly stated, and the process of change and the strategies through which they can be achieved are well delineated. However, its simplicity may also be a disadvantage, and many new therapists attempt to restructure the family before they have sufficient grasp of family rules. The application of too rigid a blueprint of family functioning can have the effect of imposing the therapist's solution on the family, which may, of course, be incorrect.

Strategic family therapy

In contrast to the rigid structural model of the effective family developed by Minuchin, the approach adopted by Watzlawick et al. (1974) was less formal and more flexible. The focus of this approach was on the problem-solving strategies families used in response to pressures from within or without. They noted that when a family faces a problem, its members typically interact in repetitive ways and adopt previously used strategies to deal with the problem. If this is successful, the problem is resolved. When these strategies are unsuccessful, some families will adopt novel approaches in their attempts to resolve the problem. Others may continue to apply the same unsuccessful strategy to try to achieve change. Where this occurs, the attempts at problem resolution may themselves become the problem. An example of this process can be found in the man who responds to his wife's lack of engagement with him with upset and anger. In his anger, he attempts to persuade his wife to be more forthcoming in their relationship. However, in response to his anger, she becomes more withdrawn and avoidant, which results in him becoming more angry, her becoming more avoidant, and so on. Here, his anger, used in an attempt to change the original problem, has become part of the problem, not the solution – as has the woman's withdrawal. It is important to note that *both* repetitive responses exacerbate the problem – not just his anger or her lack of communication, which is what individual therapy may focus on.

The goal of therapy is to identify and change these repetitive and, ultimately, destructive attempts at problem resolution. The family's tendency to look for a cause of the problems and to attribute them to one individual is minimized, as this is seen as contributing to, rather than helping, the problem. The strategic school placed significant emphasis on both verbal and non-verbal communication between family members. All behaviour was thought to act as a form of communication. One cannot fail to communicate: inaction provides a message just as much as action.

The goal of strategic therapy is to disrupt behavioural cycles that maintain the problem, and to introduce the conditions for more appropriate transactional patterns. Therapy follows discrete stages:

1. Detailed exploration and definition of the difficulties to be resolved
2. Developing a strategic plan of action to break up the sequences of interactions that are maintaining the problem
3. Delivery of the strategic interventions, often involving homework between therapy sessions, the goal of which is to disrupt the problematic sequences
4. Feedback on the outcome of these interventions
5. Reappraisal of the therapeutic plan, including revision of homework or other interventions employed.

The style of the therapist is one of emotional distance from the family. To avoid confrontation, they may adopt a one-down approach rather than expert position. They also do not insist that the whole family attends therapy sessions: they will work with whoever attends. Therapy focuses on two key strategies of change: positive reframing and paradoxical interventions.

- *Positive reframing* involves placing a positive interpretation on the behaviours that are contributing to the problem. That is not as difficult as it may sound because, according to the strategic therapists, these behaviours are erroneous but genuine attempts at resolving a problem. In this way, a couple who are constantly antagonistic towards each other may be told that the good thing about their arguing is that it shows they both have sufficient commitment to the relationship to continue fighting in an attempt to make it work. The reframing challenges the family's perception of the presenting problem and encourages its members to redefine and give a new meaning to it. Having redefined the problem, the family can no longer apply the same solutions, and new solutions and patterns of interaction become possible.
- *Paradoxical intervention* involves family members being asked to engage in tasks that are paradoxical or contrary to common sense. The arguing couple, for example, may be asked to *continue* arguing – perhaps linked to the positive reframe of 'because this shows your continuing care for each other'. By the use of paradox, the therapist creates a therapeutic bind by suggesting that there are good reasons why it is advisable *not* to change – while hoping to have the opposite effect. The paradox is intended to give the problem a new meaning so that those involved will be forced to decide on change or no change – itself a change within the system.

A number of paradoxical strategies have been identified. The above example is known as *symptom prescription*. A similar technique, known as *pretending*, involves a family member deliberately and consciously pretending to have a particular problem, with the family enacting their usual pattern around the presenting 'symptom'. Again, this is meant to disrupt the normal family interactions and facilitate behavioural change. The approach has a number of strengths, and the strategic group reported some impressive therapeutic gains (Watzlawick et al. 1974). However, the ethics of the approach have been challenged, as the power lies with the therapist and the method of treatment is not clear to its recipient. The formulation box illustrates two differing formulations of one problem from the structural and strategic perspectives.

Case formulation

Jane's anorexia: an example of structural versus strategic therapy

Strategic and structural approaches view the problems that people have quite differently. Here are two formulations of the problems associated with anorexia. Jane is an adolescent girl diagnosed with anorexia: the 'identified patient' indicative of structural problems within a family. The therapist has heard how the mother and father try to encourage her to eat, but have so far failed to do so.

A structural approach

A structural view of this situation would be that the family is enmeshed: they are overly concerned about their daughter's behaviour and so close to her that they deprive her of her independence and decision-making autonomy. The power invested in the girl to control the family has inverted the power hierarchy within the family, and the parental system is weak: they cannot get her to eat. The goal of therapy is to remedy these deficiencies, in particular, to strengthen the parental subsystem and restore the appropriate power hierarchy. One way in which this may be achieved is for the therapist to actively change the structure and to support the parents in their attempts to control the behaviour of their daughter.

A strategic approach

A different formulation of the problem may be gained by a strategic approach. One possible formulation is that as Jane entered adolescence she tried to gain more autonomy and independence. However, her parents were overprotective and controlling and did not accommodate to these changes. She therefore started to diet as an expression of control and autonomy. However, her dieting and loss of weight simply increased her parents' concern over her health and increased their desire to control her and ensure she ate 'properly'. Accordingly, they increased their attempts at controlling her eating. As a direct consequence, she rebelled and escalated her diet, which, in turn, increased her parents' concern and protective behaviour, which ... and the cycle continues. The pattern of interaction that is established is the main concern of the strategic therapist – not the initiating problem.

This chapter has described two very different approaches to working with families. However, there are many other approaches, some of which will be described in subsequent chapters. Evaluation of the effectiveness of systemic interventions is therefore not a simple matter. Nevertheless, it is clear that family therapy of one sort or another is an effective intervention for a number of problems. Family interventions targeted at young people, for example, have been found to be more effective than usual treatment for problems as diverse as anorexia (e.g. Fisher et al. 2019), perinatal depression (Cluxton-Keller and Bruce 2018), and adolescent behavioural disorders and drug misuse (e.g. Hartnett et al. 2017). However, it has also been acknowledged that much of the research is of a relatively low quality, and studies with stronger methodologies and comparisons with individual therapies may be of benefit in this context.

5.2 Psychosocial explanations of mental health problems

Risk for mental health problems has been linked to a number of social and economic factors. The results of the British Psychiatric Morbidity Survey (McManus et al. 2016), for example, provided evidence typical of the wider findings. The survey found mental disorders were more common in people living alone, those in poor physical health, and the unemployed. A higher proportion of women than men, and particularly younger women, were diagnosed with common mental health problems such as anxiety and depression. There were significant differences in access to mental health services across ethnic groups with black males having particularly low treatment rates. Around a quarter of men drank alcohol at hazardous levels, while around 13% of women did the same. Earlier iterations of this survey had shown that unemployed people were twice as likely to abuse alcohol as employed people and five times more likely to be dependent on other types of drugs. **Psychoses** were more prevalent among urban than rural dwellers. The **prevalence** of neurotic disorders among hostel residents was 38%, among night shelter residents 60%, and among those sleeping rough 57%. Rates of **psychoses** and alcohol and drug dependence were similarly high. Accordingly, explanations of mental health problems need to include the wider environment in which we have lived and continue to live.

Developmental processes

Events and relationships within childhood can have lasting impacts on later mental health, both for good and bad. Many children experience challenging circumstances yet go on to have a healthy adulthood. These factors increase risk but are by no means sole determinants of later problems. Pirkola et al. (2005), for example, found that 60% of participants in a large Finnish cohort study retrospectively reported at least one childhood adversity, including maternal problems with alcohol, paternal mental health problems, family discord or being bullied at school. Of these, 17% were given a psychiatric diagnosis while an adult. By contrast, 10% of adults who did not experience adversity received a similar diagnosis. Some gender-specific effects were also found. Men whose father experienced mental health problems were over four times more likely to develop depression than those without this experience. Women whose mother experienced mental health problems were three times more likely to develop depression. Authoritarian, intrusive, over-protective or controlling parenting increases risk for anxiety disorders both in children and the adults they become (e.g. Varela and Hensley-Maloney 2009). By contrast, parental acceptance, warmth, sensitivity, and responsiveness are associated with lower levels of anxiety.

Of note also is that while sexual abuse may be a headline issue, empirical studies do not support this prioritization. Cecil et al. (2017), for example, conducted one of many studies that have found various forms of maltreatment to frequently co-occur, and that emotional abuse may be the most important predictor of subsequent mental health problems in both men and women. Similarly, Swannell et al. (2012) found adults who reported being physically abused or neglected as a child were around two and half times more likely to report self-harming than those without these experiences. Sexual abuse was not associated with self-harm.

Childhood factors go on to interact with subsequent events to influence risk for adult disorders. McLaughlin et al. (2010), for example, found the more adverse childhood circumstances an individual experienced, the more likely they were to experience later problems. In addition, they found an interaction between childhood and adult adversity, with a doubling of risk for disorders, including depression, post-traumatic stress, and anxiety if both factors were present. Similarly, Bromberger et al. (2017) found the best predictors of women's depressive symptoms over a 15-year period were a history of childhood maltreatment combined with ongoing financial difficulties, stressful life events, low social support, low role functioning, and poor health.

Of course, childhood risk factors include more than family dynamics. Negative factors may also occur outside the home. Wolke et al. (2012), for example, found that children who experienced long-term physical bullying were around five times more likely to develop symptoms of borderline personality disorder than their peers. The risk for those who experienced both physical and social bullying, such as exclusion from social groups, was seven times greater. Cyber-bullying is now emerging as a significant problem, with both recipients and bullies appearing to be at greater risk of depression and suicide than those not involved (Bonanno and Hymel 2013).

It is important to consider not just that these risk factors exist, but *how* they influence risk. Identifying the mediating processes between such abuse and later psychopathology is critical to our understanding of them. Abuse can establish a range of negative beliefs about the self: beliefs that the person is bad, deserving of ill-treatment or abuse, unloved and unlovable. These beliefs can then influence future relationships in negative ways. The individual may avoid close relationships, or lose faith in parents or potential friends, leading to loneliness, depression, self-harming behaviours, and so on. In this way, the abuse is the first part in a series of negative psychological and social processes that ultimately lead to long-term distress (see Salokangas et al. 2018). From a different theoretical perspective, Widom et al. (2018) found that adults who had experienced neglect and/or physical abuse as a child were likely to develop anxious or avoidant attachment styles in adulthood, which in turn were associated with high levels of anxiety and depression, and poor self-esteem.

Socio-economic status

There is consistent evidence (e.g. WHO/CGF 2014) that mental health problems are more prevalent among lower socio-economic groups. Socio-economic status (SES) may provide an omnibus concept subsuming a range of specific challenges to mental health. People in lower socio-economic groups are likely to have a range of life experiences including financial insecurity, poor housing, and high numbers of negative life events and hassles that place them at particular risk for stress in general and mental health problems in particular. Poor housing, for example, if experienced for significant periods, increases risk for mental health problems (Pevalin et al. 2017). Any financial strain is likely to be exacerbated at times of economic pressure. Living under constrained economic circumstances can be challenging while in a job (Mental Health Foundation 2016). Losing a job or being in a precarious job can be equally if not more difficult. Among young people, being in precarious work can increase risk for mental health problems by around 50% (Canivet et al. 2016). Myles et al. (2017) found increased levels of subclinical psychological distress as Australia's economy experienced a downturn and unemployment increased, although clinically diagnosable levels of distress were less influenced by the recession. The peak levels of distress were some months after being laid off, presumably as money ran out and future job prospects became worryingly reduced. By contrast, moving from unstable to stable employment is associated with improved mental health (Reine et al. 2008), as does living in accommodation when the rent or mortgage is not associated with significant financial pressure (Mason et al. 2013).

Social causation versus social drift

Two opposing hypotheses have been proposed to explain higher rates of mental health disorders among people in lower socio-economic groups. *Social causation models* suggest they result from higher levels of stress experienced by the less well-off – that is, low SES 'causes' mental health problems. The *social drift model* opposes this view. It suggests that mental health problems lead to a decline in SES. According to this model, when an individual develops a mental health disorder, they become less economically viable. They may be unable to maintain a job, or the levels of overtime required to maintain their standard of living. They therefore drift down the socio-economic scale – that is, mental health problems 'cause' low SES.

Of course, both processes may be involved. Ritsher et al. (2001), for example, followed a cohort of people whose parents had either experienced an episode of major depression or were depression-free. They hypothesized that if the social causation model held, the children of blue-collar parents were at increased risk of developing depression. If the social drift model held, having depressed parents placed participants at risk of a low SES. Their data supported the social causation hypotheses. The children of blue-collar workers were more than three times as likely to develop a major depressive disorder as those of white-collar workers. Parental depression did not predict the SES of their offspring. Nor was there any evidence of drift following the onset of depression. By contrast, O'Donoghue et al. (2014) found that 43% of their Irish cohort presenting with first-time psychosis were likely to drift down the socio-economic scale over a 6-year period, an outcome exacerbated by the use of self-medication through drugs such as cannabis. Finally, Lund and Cois (2018) found evidence of both social causation and drift in a 2-year-long cohort study of South Africans presenting with depression.

Differential vulnerability

As well as more economic resources, people in higher socio-economic groups also appear to have more social and psychological resources known to be protective against mental health problems than the less well-off. Examples of this can be found in the research of Grzywacz et al. (2004), who found that high levels of education formed a buffer against stress and moderated, at least in part, the association between SES and mental health. Matthews et al. (2008) found an association between low levels of what they called 'reserve capacity' (a combination of optimism, self-esteem, and social support), negative emotions, and low SES. In addition, social support, which is highly protective against a number of mental health problems, is frequently less available to those in the lower socio-economic groups (Chaix et al. 2007).

The role of social capital

While social stress and lack of resources appear to be direct contributors to many mental health problems, Wilkinson and Pickett (2018) argued that *relative* lack of income may also contribute. They argued that wide disparities in wealth across society result in low levels of *social capital*, which is associated with both individual distrust and dissatisfaction, and social factors such as high levels of crime. This, Wilkinson and Pickett contended, is inherently stressful and results in high levels of mental health problems among those individuals who experience it.

The impact of social capital on health is now well established, to the extent that Ehsan et al. (2019) were able to conduct a systematic review of 20 previous systematic reviews exploring the role of social capital in both physical and mental health. Within it, they identified several types of social cohesion, including: (i) *cognitive*, referring to the perception of trust, reciprocity, norms, and values within a community; (ii) *structural*, relating to the quantity of relationships and membership in institutions that can bring individuals and groups together; and (iii) *bonding*, involving the social resources available to individuals through close networks or groups with similar socio-demographic characteristics. Of the reviews they considered, 9 found strong evidence of a relationship between social capital and health, while 16 provided weak to moderate evidence, with cognitive social capital providing the strongest overall association.

Research box 4

Fitzsimons, E., Goodman, A. and Smith, J.P. (2017) Poverty dynamics and parental mental health: determinants of childhood mental health in the UK, *Social Science and Medicine*, 175: 43–51.

Mental health problems can be inter-generational due to a range of proximal factors, such as parental behaviour and attitudes. But wider factors may also affect children's mental health, including their experiences of school, peers, and the socio-economic context in which they live. And this is the focus of this study. It reports on the social and economic factors, as well as the mental health of parents, that impacted on the mental health of a large cohort of British children born in the early years of the twenty-first century.

Method

Participants

The Millennium Cohort Study is a longitudinal cohort study following the outcomes of 18,827 children born into 18,552 families throughout the UK in 2000 and 2001. Following baseline measures at birth, six 'sweeps' have been conducted to identify their outcomes, at ages 3, 5, 7, 11, and 14 years. The present report focused on data taken in sweep 3, when the children involved were aged 5 years, and sweep 5, when they were aged 11 years.

At age 5, data were gathered in relation to 14,792 children from a 'main' parent (14,792, natural mother; 394, natural father) or alternative close relative (most frequently a grandmother), the partner of the main respondent (11,145, natural father; 303, natural mother) or alternative, the majority of which were step-parents (560 respondents). At age 11, data were recorded in relation to 13,588 cases with a similar distribution of participants

Measures

A range of measures were taken at each time point. The key measures in relation to the present paper were:

- *Strengths and Difficulties Questionnaire (SDQ)*: a behavioural screening questionnaire for 3–16-year-olds, to identify behavioural and emotional problems. It identifies: (i) 'internalizing problems', involving emotional distress and difficulties with peers, and (ii) 'externalizing problems', involving conduct problems and hyperactivity.
- *Family background*: this focused on family structure (number of siblings, parent's relationship status), child gender, and ethnicity. Socio-economic status (SES), and in particular poverty, was indicated by family income being less than 60% of the national 'median equalized income'.

- *Early childhood environment*: a range of adverse measures including low birth weight, bedwetting, and concerns about child speech at age 3 years.
- *Parental mental health*: measured using the Malaise Inventory, which measures levels of psychological distress or depression. It provides a cut-off score to determine 'moderate' distress (>4) and 'severe mental illness' (>13).
- *Parental physical health*: this included any chronic physical health problems, and whether either parent smoked prior to pregnancy.

Results

The paper focused on the relationships between the predictor variables and SDQ outcomes of internalizing and externalizing problems. Table 1 shows the percentage of children with problematic SDQ scores on each measure of mental health problems in five quintiles of family income (from lowest to highest bands of income within the study). There is a clear and statistically significant gradient of problems across each level of income. Logistic regression found all differences between SES groups to be significantly different ($p < 0.001$) after controlling for a number of potential confounding variables.

Table 1 Percentage of children in each quintile of income to experience mental health problems

Income quintile	Emotional difficulties	Problems with peers	Conduct disorder	Hyperactivity
Age 11 years				
Lowest	15.6	17.2	18.8	16.3
Second	13.2	14.0	13.8	14.5
Third	10.1	9.4	7.9	8.6
Fourth	9.1	7.8	5.1	7.2
Highest	6.5	7.1	3.3	5.8
Age 5 years				
Lowest	8.8	11.5	17.7	16.7
Second	7.1	10.0	13.5	13.0
Third	4.0	6.0	7.5	6.1
Fourth	4.0	4.3	5.5	6.1
Highest	2.4	3.8	4.6	5.3

A second set of data showed the percentage of children who developed mental health problems in each of a number of changing financial contexts between the ages of 5 and 11 years (see Table 2). Rates of all mental health problems differed significantly ($p < 0.001$) across contexts, with higher rates in all poverty conditions, even among those whose parents moved out of poverty compared to those individuals who did not experience poverty. Again, significant differences between rates of disorders in children who did and did not have experience of poverty were consistently statistically significant ($p < 0.001$) after controlling for potential confounding variables.

Table 2 Percentage of children in each poverty context to experience mental health problems

	Emotional difficulties		Peer difficulties	
Change 5–11 years	**Present**	**Absent**	**Present**	**Absent**
Moving into poverty	6.3	2.3	4.8	2.4
Moved out of poverty	5.6	1.6	4.7	1.7
Stayed in poverty	6.5	2.0	4.7	2.0
	Conduct disorders		Hyperactivity	
Moving into poverty	8.2	2.3	12.6	4.9
Moved out of poverty	6.4	2.0	6.2	1.1
Stayed in poverty	8.0	1.8	7.6	0.09

Finally, the risk for mental health problems for children whose mother and/or father had mental health problems was evaluated, this time with transitions between the ages of 5 and 7 years.

Table 3 Percentage of children in each parental mental health context to experience mental health problems

Change 5–11 years	**Emotional difficulties**	**Peer difficulties**	**Conduct disorders**	**Hyperactivity**
Mother moved into poor mental health	6.7***	4.5***	3.5***	5.2***
Mother moved out of poor mental health	3.5***	0.7	0.6	2.1*
Mother stayed in poor mental health	9.9***	5.9***	7.0***	5.4***
Father moved into poor mental health	1.3	0.8	1.8	2.5*
Father moved out of poor mental health	0.3	0.6	0.04	0.1
Father stayed in poor mental health	3.8*	0.7	2.1	1.3

*** $p < 0.001$, * $p < 0.05$.

Table 3 reports the percentage of children in each parental mental health context to experience mental health problems. The significance is based on comparisons of the same disorders in children with no such experiences. As can be seen, the influence of parental health is largely driven by maternal mental health, with risk for child mental health problems primarily among those whose mothers moved into, or maintained, poor mental health. Transitions to better health reduced the risk for child mental health problems. By contrast, the influence of fathers' mental health is much lower and inconsistent.

Discussion

Childhood poverty had a consistent impact on child mental health across all the conditions measured. However, parental, and in particular maternal mental health, was the most powerful predictor of poor child mental health. This is not surprising given that typical parenting patterns still involve a greater involvement of the mother in childcare. The processes through which these conditions impact on child mental health is not explored, but are likely to involve processes such as child neglect, inappropriate responses to child behaviours, and so on. They are also likely to be cross-generational. Previous studies have indicated that poor mental health as a child can lead to a reduced income as a future parent due to reduced chances of a good education, likelihood of employment, and being married.

Gender differences

According to the WHO (e.g. de Jonge 2018), although overall lifetime rates of mental health problems differ little between men and women, there are 'striking differences' between the prevalence of key common disorders across the sexes. Women are more likely to experience depression, anxiety, and somatic complaints, for example. Once established these disorders may also be more persistent in women. By contrast, men are more likely to be diagnosed with alcohol dependence and antisocial personality disorder. There are no marked gender differences in the prevalence of **psychotic** disorders, although the prognosis for women who develop them may be worse than that for men. The WHO identified a number of gender-specific factors that particularly influence risk for women, including gender-based violence, socio-economic disadvantage, low income and income inequality, and 'unremitting responsibility for the care of others'.

What evidence there is suggests that women experience more hardship in their work and family roles than men. Even when working full time, women tend to do more in the home than their partners. This process, known as work–home **spillover**, is now well recognized as contributing to high levels of stress in those who experience it and has been shown to treble risk for depression in women, particularly when this is combined with other risks such as low income (e.g. Okechukwu et al. 2012). A second type of additional home demand involves engaging in a caring role beyond the normal family responsibilities. The care of a person with dementia, for example, is highly stressful, and associated with issues such as difficult behaviours, accidents, as well as the sheer grind of day-to-day care. This role appears to disproportionately affect women and those who rely on income and social support (e.g. Byeon 2019). From a different perspective, Ketcher et al. (2020) identified the stresses involved in caring for a spouse with advanced cancer. Female caregivers reported significantly higher levels of perceived stress, depression, anxiety, and social strain compared with their male counterparts.

Women are also more subject to physical assault within the family, rape, and other traumatizing events than men, and these can have a devastating effect. Rees et al. (2014), for example, reported a retrospective case–control study comparing mental health outcomes in women with no prior history of mental health problems who subsequently did or did not experience partner violence. Among those who experienced violence, 37% experienced their first mental health problems in the year following the incident, of whom over half were diagnosed with post-traumatic stress disorder. Among those who did not experience such problems, only 1% experienced mental health problems in the comparative year. A diverging approach has been to suggest that women may be particularly dependent on coping resources such as social support, and vulnerable to disruptions within them. However, it now seems that men may be equally dependent on these networks, and equally susceptible to their disruption (e.g. Lee and Dik 2017).

Minority status

Minority status can be conferred by a number of factors: ethnicity, sexual orientation, appearance, and so on. However, it is usually taken to mean obvious differences as a result of ethnicity. Considering issues of ethnicity is not without its dangers. It encompasses a variety of issues: language, religion, experience of races and migration, culture, ancestry, and forms of identity. Each of these may individually or together contribute to differences between the mental and physical health of different ethnic groups. It is dangerous to reify 'ethnicity' as a single factor which alone impacts on mental health. Any brief review of the relevant literature can therefore only scratch the surface of a complex subject and suggest only some issues that may explain some differences in some mental health problems across some minority groups.

Differential exposure

One explanation for higher levels of mental health problems among social minorities is that they are exposed to more stress than the majority groups. One general stress to which many people in ethnic minorities are exposed is that associated with low SES. In the UK, for example, rates of unemployment, poverty, and homelessness are highest among minority groups, and even when employed, people from minority groups may receive less salary than the majority (Mental Health Foundation 2019). With this in mind, some commentators have suggested that any distress resulting from being a member of an ethnic minority is the result of being part of a lower socio-economic group, not being part of an ethnic minority *per se*. Sachs-Ericsson et al. (2005), for example, found in their large US sample that more African Americans reported high levels of depression than white people. However, this relationship was mediated by a number of indices of SES. In an interesting study of the impact of a single traumatic event experienced by a whole population, Ali et al. (2017) explored the mental health impact of Hurricane Katrina, which devastated New Orleans in 2005. Following this event, the odds of developing depression were much higher among African Americans than Caucasians. However, after partialling out factors such as social support, SES, and trauma-specific factors, the relationship between race and risk for depression was no longer significant. Accordingly, it appears that much if not all of the relationship between ethnicity and mental health is linked to the social context in which individuals find themselves.

There are, however, social stressors to which minority social groups are uniquely exposed. One obvious stressor is that of racial prejudice, and there are a number of research papers showing evidence of its negative emotional impact. In one such study, Noh et al. (2007) identified what they termed 'overt' and 'subtle' discrimination, and found that overt discrimination was particularly associated with low positive affect, while the experience of subtle discrimination was associated with high levels of depressive symptoms. In an interesting study of immigrants to Sweden, Lecerof et al. (2016) found that key determinants of poor mental health were discrimination (people who experienced discrimination were nearly three times more likely to experience poor health), financial difficulties, and housing problems. These effects were reduced if individuals had a high level of trust in those around them, and thus participated socially, reflecting on the power of social capital. Prejudice, or fear of prejudice, may also impact on other minorities.

Discrimination at a group level can also impact on mental health. The term 'neighbourhood racial discrimination' has come to mean discrimination at multiple levels, including limited access to valued resources, such as jobs and education, and being targeted by the police. Above these functional issues is the higher-level perception that one's racial group is devalued in society. These processes and beliefs have been shown consistently to predict mental health problems such as depression (e.g. English et al. 2014) and lie at the heart of the Black Lives Matter movement (https://blacklivesmatter.com).

Stop and think …

At the time of writing this book, there are protests across America, the UK, and many other countries as a response to institutional racism, frequently focusing on the way ethnic minorities have been treated by the police. Sparked by the death of George Floyd, the US protests have become a bitter (literal) battleground between races and people of differing socio-political views. The response of the US president has been to send in the National Guard and others to, firstly, attempt to quell the protests, and then to arrest people through the use of unnamed and unidentified agents of various governmental bodies, despite their only 'offence' being the pursuit of lawful protestation. Is this the best way to handle the situation? How *should* local and national government respond to what may be considered decades of discriminative practices against whole communities in both the short term and the long term?

A third source of stress experienced by ethnic minorities may be a consequence of tensions as individuals adopt or consciously reject some of the customs and values of other cultures, including those of the host culture. Both may result in feelings of alienation and rejection by members of the larger or one's own culture. In one study of this phenomenon, Lai (2004) studied Chinese immigrants to Canada, and found that the highest levels of depression were among those who established more cultural barriers against the new culture, and who identified more with traditional Chinese cultural values.

5.3 Mental health promotion

Given the powerful role of social and economic factors in determining mental health, it may be beneficial to address these factors directly. The WHO (2004) acknowledged this need, noting the influence of culture and social capital on mental health as well as noting the importance of interventions at differing 'levels', aimed not just at preventing ill-health, but also at promoting positive health. This perspective involves:

- having a holistic approach to health
- respecting diverse cultures and beliefs
- promoting positive health as well as preventing ill-health
- working at a structural (societal) not just individual level
- using participatory methods.

Removing the jargon, this means that public health services should work not just with individuals, but also at a societal level to bring about improvements in health. They should involve communities and attempt to improve health and quality of life, not just prevent disease. They can work at a legislative level, with communities, and with groups and individuals within them. Initiatives can be conducted by a variety of people, some of whom would label themselves as workers in health promotion, and others who would not. Some examples of the range of public health activities that can be conducted, in this case to minimize levels of alcohol-related problems, are outlined in Table 5.1. Here, interventions are aimed at the whole population of drinkers as well as those who drink to excess.

Individual interventions

Despite the wide variety of potential interventions, most mental health initiatives have involved improving access to psychiatric and psychological care for individuals who develop mental health problems and who have poor access to healthcare: the economically deprived, people without housing, and so on. Other interventions have been aimed at preventing relapse (Neto et al. 2008).

An approach of more relevance to *preventing* mental health problems involves providing relatively simple psychological interventions that are open to all. One such programme (Galla et al. 2015) provided mindfulness classes (see Chapter 3) in urban Los Angeles. Given that mindfulness training is a highly successful intervention for people experiencing mental health problems, it should not be surpris-

Table 5.1 Examples of differing levels of public health initiatives aimed at minimizing alcohol related harm

Level of approach	Examples of practice
Whole population	
Central government	Establishing drink-drive laws
	Higher taxation on high-percentage alcoholic drinks
	Government guidelines on consumption limits
Local government	Local police policies on public houses and drink-driving
	Licensing of new pubs and drinking time limits
Media	Drink-drive campaigns
	Television programmes on the harmful effects of alcohol and promoting sensible drinking
Supermarkets/shops	Giving priority to visibility and pricing of low-alcohol drinks on the shelves
Population of drinkers	
Individual pubs/ brewers	Establishing local minibus services to prevent drink-driving
	Provision of low-alcohol beers
	Discouraging the obviously intoxicated from drinking alcohol (in the USA, a bartender can be sued for an incident – e.g. car accident – involving a drunk individual if they served them alcohol while visibly drunk)
Supermarkets/shops	Policing of drinking-age requirements for purchase of alcohol
Individual drinkers	
Healthcare/social services	Provision of detoxification services
	Therapy to prevent excess alcohol consumption
	Therapy to prevent relapse in people who have successfully stopped or reduced their excess drinking

ing that it was equally effective as a preventive intervention, achieving significant gains on measures of mindfulness, self-compassion, and stress. More widely, a systematic review and **meta-analysis** conducted by Joyce et al. (2018) examined data from 11 controlled trials and concluded that both cognitive behaviour therapy and mindfulness 'had a positive impact on individual resilience'.

The workplace can also provide a setting for learning **stress management skills**. In a meta-analysis of over 2,500 participants in 17 studies of occupational stress management interventions, Routsalainen et al. (2008) found that they resulted in 'small but probably relevant' (and statistically significant) reductions in stress, emotional exhaustion, anxiety, and burnout compared to no intervention. Despite these various successes, some caution should be given to interpretation of the data, as these types of programme typically attract only between 10% and 40% of the workforce, and many of those who attend have little to gain, while many anxious individuals do not attend them. As a consequence, a number of studies have begun to evaluate more innovative ways of providing these types of intervention. Mistretta et al. (2018), for example, compared live training in the workplace of a mindfulness-based stress management programme with the same programme delivered via smartphone. Unfortunately, from the perspective of widest access, the live programme came out on top, achieving gains on measures of stress and emotional burnout not found in the smartphone programme.

Another place in which preventive interventions can be conducted is schools. Interventions here can focus on developing life skills as well as specific ways of handling stress, and provide a potentially life-long benefit. An example of this approach is provided by the Promoting Alternative THinking Strategies (PATHS) programme (www.pathstraining.com/main). This approach teaches pupils a number of cognitive strategies, social competencies, and social problem-solving skills to help them regulate their social relationships and emotions. It is intended to be taught at least twice weekly for between 20 and 30 minutes through the academic year, with different packages for different school grades. Kam et al. (2004) found the intervention to be effective in improving social problem-solving, emotional understanding, self-report of conduct problems, teacher ratings of adaptive behaviour, and cognitive abilities related to social planning and impulsivity for up to 5 years following the intervention. More recently, a number of studies have shown mindfulness programmes also to be of benefit in both early years education (e.g. Flook et al. 2015) and older children (e.g. Schonert-Reichl et al. 2015) on measures as wide ranging as pro-social behaviour and peer acceptance, empathy, perspective-taking, and mindfulness.

Not all interventions need to be provided by 'experts'. Indeed, over the past decade there has been considerable development of programmes led by peers, whether they be workmates, people facing the same issues or problems, or fellow school students. Some of the best work in this context has come from interventions in school settings. One of the more established suicide prevention programmes in the US, for example, is known as the Sources of Strength programme. One evaluation (e.g. Pickering et al. 2018) explored its roll-out in 20 schools, in which over 500 peer educators were trained and nearly 4,000 school pupils were targeted. In each school, individual students were identified as being influential among their peers. These students were then taught a number of strategies for developing healthy relationships, building social bonds, as well as learning about suicide and suicide prevention. They then became a resource for, and influence on, their peers. A key additional role was to identify and report peers with suicidal ideation to appropriate adults. The intervention achieved a four-fold difference in the likelihood of trained peer leaders referring potentially suicidal individuals to trusted adults compared to untrained individuals.

Based on the success of the Sources of Strength programme, Pisani et al. (2018) explored the effect of an automated text-based intervention for young people attending schools in rural US communities. The Text4Strength programme took advantage of the now almost obligatory use of texting in young people, to provide students with 28 interactive messages on their mobile phone over a period of 9 weeks, focusing on being a positive friend, mentoring, the use of family support, engaging in healthy activities, medical access, emotion regulation strategies, and the values of generosity and spirituality. More than 70% of participants found the texts useful, including many who did not actively respond to them, while between 35% and 100% of participants engaged with differing elements within the programme.

This second approach involves a now increasingly used strategy for influencing individual mental health – the use of apps, which can provide relevant information and graded skills such as mindfulness or wider strategies for improving mental health. In one outcome study of a mindfulness app, Bostock et al. (2019) compared outcomes in participants randomized to use an app providing 45 pre-recorded mindful meditations for a period of 8 weeks and a **waiting list control**. During this period, participants in the mindfulness condition completed an average of 17 meditation sessions, and reported significant gains on measures of well-being, distress, work stress, and perceived social support within the workplace. These gains were broadly maintained 2 months later and are typical of similar studies in a range of populations.

Systemic interventions

Large-scale societal changes such as those outlined in Table 5.1 are clearly constrained by political factors. However, there are some enclosed communities such as the workplace or school where interventions designed to change the entire working or learning environment are more possible and may impact on the mental health of all those within them.

One of the few worksite interventions to report a systemic approach to reducing stress was reported by Maes et al. (1998). Their intervention drew upon studies that identified working conditions that can enhance both the well-being of workers and productivity. These included individuals working within their capabilities, avoiding short and repetitive performance tasks, having some control over the organization of work, and having adequate social contact. With these factors in mind, they attempted, within the constraints of production, to change the nature of each worker's job in a number of large factories to bring it closer to the ideal. Although measures of 'stress' were not taken as part of the research programme, these changes resulted in an increase in the quality of work and lower absenteeism rates – both indicative of an increase in well-being at work.

In another context, the School Transitional Environment Project (STEP) (e.g. Felner et al. 1993) changed the school environment to make it less threatening to students during transitions from lower to higher schools. It aimed to reduce the complexity of the new school environment, to make teachers more supportive, and to create a 'stable support mechanism' through a consistent set of peers and classmates. This resulted in significantly lower levels of stress and anxiety, depression and delinquent behaviour than in schools where these changes were not instituted. It also proved more effective than a teaching programme focusing on coping and problem-solving skills. A similar programme known as Friendly Schools (Cross et al. 2018) developed a complex intervention addressing the content of teaching, school policies and procedures, as well as the social and physical environment, pastoral care provided, and school–home–community links. The intervention achieved gains across a range of outcomes, including the frequency of bullying, depression, anxiety, stress, and loneliness in the first year of school. These effects faded by the end of the second year. A much simpler (at least in theory) approach was suggested by the findings of a systematic review by McCormick (2017), who found that simply providing green spaces within and beyond the school and encouraging young children to play in them may also benefit their mental health.

Even broader approaches have been taken to reduce the stress linked with one aspect associated with low SES: poor living conditions. Aubry et al. (2019) measured the effects of providing stable housing to people with significant mental health problems in a small Canadian city. This simple act resulted in significant improvements in quality of life and recovery. At an even wider level of intervention, White et al. (2017) explored the mental health impact of the regeneration of entire neighbourhoods in Wales. They distributed questionnaires to over 10,000 residents in Wales asking whether the area in which they were living had been regenerated under a Welsh Government programme and linked the results to a wider dataset providing longitudinal data on mental health in these areas. The measure of mental health was somewhat crude (a 5-point scale) and differences on this measure between areas were small. Nevertheless, at a population level they were significant, with the population in areas of regeneration experiencing significant gains in mental health.

5.4 Cross-cultural issues

This chapter has already noted that people from minority cultures tend to experience more mental health problems than the majority population. But there are other, perhaps more fundamental differences in the experience of mental health and mental health problems across cultures. The next section considers two facets of this phenomenon.

Presentation of problems

Not surprisingly, perhaps, many common conditions present in ways that reflect the culture in which they are experienced. Members of the Inuit population, for example, may develop a condition known as *kayak angst* – a feeling of panic associated with being alone in a kayak in the Arctic wastes. This may be termed 'agoraphobia with panic disorder' in societies where there are lots of houses and busy streets, and no kayaks. Mental distress may also result from exaggeration of culturally specific normative behaviours or concerns. In Japan, where ritual and politeness are extremely important, a condition known as *taijin kyofusho* is an incapacitating fear of offending or harming others through one's own awkward social behaviour, glancing at their genital areas or imagined physical defect.

Similar problems may also present quite differently in various parts of the world. One of the key differences across cultures is the greater or lesser emphasis placed on physical symptoms as either a metaphor for, or means of expressing, emotional distress. It is generally acknowledged that people from Eastern cultures tend to 'somatize' their distress, talking about it in terms of physical symptoms, while people from Western cultures talk more about psychological symptoms.

In South and East Asia, presentation of mental health problems through physical complaints is common. In an early report of this phenomenon, Kleinman (1977) reported the experiences of a group of Taiwanese people with 'depressive syndrome'. Eighty-eight per cent of them initially complained only of physical symptoms, and did not report any emotional or psychological problems when directly asked about them. Twenty-eight per cent rejected the idea that they were depressed even when they had experienced symptom relief following antidepressant medication. In a similar group of American patients, only 4% presented complaining of physical symptoms. Similarly, Hoge et al. (2006) compared presentation of what the **DSM** would term generalized anxiety disorder in people in Nepal and the USA, and found that the Nepalese people were more likely to report high levels of somatic symptoms such as dizziness and indigestion, while the Americans were more likely to report psychological symptoms including being scared or nervous.

Kleinman (1977) suggested that differing presentations reflect differing social beliefs, norms, and attitudes towards mental health problems. He argued that people from cultures that stigmatize mental health problems, or where treatments for such problems are usually somatic, are more likely to report physical rather than mental problems. An example of this was provided by Kirmayer et al. (2004), who reported a study of Vietnamese people who had emigrated to Canada. Many of them expressed emotional distress in terms of a condition they termed *uat u'c*. This was described in terms of having bodily aches, being cold, and depleted of energy. However, further discussion with these individuals revealed that their symptoms resulted from a predicament that involved indignation over a social injustice that could not be denounced because of their status within the social hierarchy and a need to maintain social harmony. Similarly, Karasz (2005) examined conceptual models of depressive symptoms in South Asian and European immigrants to the USA. Participants were presented with a vignette describing depressive symptoms and then asked about their understanding of the symptoms presented. The Asian people identified the problem in the vignette in social and moral terms, and suggested treatment should involve self-help and non-professional help. The Europeans typically held one of two models. The first was similar to that of the Asians; the other emphasized biological explanations including 'hormonal imbalance' and 'neurological problems'.

More radical differences in beliefs about the nature of mental health problems have been found in a variety of non-Western countries, including some in Africa and Asia. In Malaysia, Razali (1995) found that 53% of people with mental health problems attributed them to supernatural agents, such as witchcraft or possession by evil spirits. Interestingly, belief in supernatural causes of mental illness was not significantly associated with age, gender, level of education or occupation. A second example can be found in research from Zimbabwe, reported by Patel et al. (1995), who found that angered ancestral spirits, evil spirits, and witchcraft were potent causes of mental health problems. Similar levels of belief in supernatural causes of mental health problems were found in Nigeria by Adebowale and Ogunlesi (1999), although they also found that 17% of people attributed their mental health disorder to biological factors, and 23% believed their condition was the result of psychosocial factors. The latter beliefs were more common among urban than among rural dwellers, suggesting that beliefs about the cause of mental health disorders may change as people become aware of alternative causal explanations. This change from traditional models of mental health problems to more Western understandings has been tracked over time in Kerala, southern India, where Halliburton (2005) reported a transition from explanations of mental health problems in terms of spirit possession to more Western understandings of 'depression' and 'tension' over time. Nevertheless, there are still strong academic and lay beliefs in non-Western causal models. Liao et al. (2017) from the China Medical University Hospital, for example, attributed depression in haemodialysis patients to deficiencies in Yang ('the harmony of all the opposite elements and forces that make up existence') and Qi ('vital energy'). Furthermore, Grupp et al. (2018) found that asylum-seekers from Eritrea and Somalia, while acknowledging the role of trauma as one cause for their symptoms of post-traumatic stress, were also likely to acknowledge religious and supernatural causes. They were also more likely to seek help from religious authorities than from more psychologically oriented practitioners.

Seeking help

Not surprisingly, the beliefs individuals hold about the cause of any problem will influence the type of help they seek. Razali and Najib (2000), for example, found that 69% of Malay patients in their sample had sought help from a traditional healer called a *Bomoh* before consulting a psychiatrist. Treatment by a *Bomoh* differs according to their diagnosis of the problem. If the condition appears to be caused by a spell, the *Bomoh* identifies the ingredients of the spell and removes or neutralizes them. If the problem is caused by ghosts or evil spirits, they try to drive out or defeat them. This involves going into a trance, carrying out an exorcism, communicating with spirits, and reciting special prayers or verses from the Koran. Similar patterns of help-seeking also occur in a number of African countries. Abiodun (1995) found the first point of contact for about one-third of patients attending a mental health service in Nigeria had been a traditional or religious healer. By contrast, Appiah-Poku et al. (2004) found that only 6% of Ghanaian people using their local psychiatric services had seen a faith healer before coming to the service. Again, these data allow the possibility of shifting cultural understandings of the causes of mental health problems and the type of help that is sought. To put these data in some context, Elkins et al. (2005) found that 44% of their sample of US psychiatric in-patients had tried to treat their condition with herbal therapies before seeking professional help; 30% had used spiritual healing.

Care should be taken not to adopt a too Western-centric approach to consideration of the effectiveness of these varying interventions. While the benefits of ritual healing and such approaches have yet to be shown to be effective in empirical trials, there *is* clear evidence of the effectiveness of a number of non-Western approaches. A number of herbal treatments, including the use of saffron (Lopresti and Drummond 2014) for example, have been shown to be effective in the treatment of depression, while acupuncture has been shown to add to the benefits of **serotonin re-uptake inhibitors** (**SSRIs**; see Chapter 4), and also in the treatment of depression (Chan et al. 2015).

The potential clash between Western and other cultural approaches was highlighted in an article by Sax (2014), who noted that ritual healing was widespread in parts of India, and was the most common form of treatment sought by people with serious mental health problems. So incompatible was this approach with Western psychiatric models, Sax argued, the two could not work together, and it was best that the formal healthcare services (which provided a more Western-based service) turn a blind eye to this alternative approach, and neither attempt to challenge it directly or work with its practitioners. Van der Watt et al. (2017) also noted the challenges associated with the introduction of Western biomedical approaches into cultures with strong alternative beliefs in Central Africa. Their work involved interviews with healthcare practitioners who adopted a biomedical approach, as well as faith and traditional healers. They identified significant distrust and negative attitudes between these groups. Like Sax, they considered the likelihood of collaboration between them as 'remote'.

Stop and think ...

Imagine waking up feeling miserable, sad, and finding it difficult to face the day. How serious do these feelings need to be before you seek help? Do they have to last a week, a month? And who do you tell about your problems? Your doctor? Your friends? And how much do you confide and how do you describe your problems? Admitting both to yourself and others that you have a mental health problem is not always easy. But what factors influence when and how an individual decides to tell others about any emotional distress they are experiencing – and how much they tell? Decisions to seek help for mental health problems are likely to be influenced by a range of factors, including: (i) the duration and severity of symptoms, (ii) the family and social support available, (iii) the accessibility and perceived benefits of **pharmacotherapy** or psychotherapy, (iv) perceived stigma towards mental health problems, and (v) attitudes towards help-seeking. So, should we be encouraging people to seek support for mental health problems early in their history? If so, how can we as a society facilitate this outcome among all groups within society?

5.5 Chapter summary

1. Both small and large social groups and other social factors impact on levels of mental health conditions.
2. Family models of mental health note the reciprocity between family members, and that mental health problems arise as a consequence of interactions between family members.
3. Structural family therapy adopts a model of a well-functioning family, based on the boundaries between units within the family. It uses behavioural strategies to shift dysfunctional families towards this model.
4. Strategic family therapy has no model of appropriate functioning. It uses two strategies of change: positive reframing and paradoxical manipulations.

5. Three major social variables impact on levels of mental health within the population: socio-economic position, gender, and minority status.
6. Explanations for these differences include differences in levels of stress and coping resources and, perhaps, processes of social comparison.
7. Cultural factors may influence the causal explanations for mental health problems and the treatment individuals from differing cultures seek.
8. Proponents of radical health promotion suggest that health inequalities can best be addressed through economic and political changes.
9. Those involved in promoting mental health have typically done so using more circumscribed interventions, including using the media and open-access classes to teach stress coping skills. Some projects have also addressed working and school environments to make them less stressful.

5.6 For discussion

1. Virtually all conditions treated with family therapy can also be treated by one-to-one therapy. What are the advantages and disadvantages of each approach?
2. How effective is a white middle-class therapist likely to be when providing therapy for someone from a different social class and culture? How can they alter the approach they take with such an individual?
3. Consider how you could promote mental health within the wider population or specific groups, such as people from ethnic minorities or single mothers.
4. If mental health disorders result at least in part from social conditions, should psychologists be actively involved in attempts to influence public health policy and relevant government decisions?

5.7 Further reading

Dallos, R. and Draper, R. (2015) *An Introduction to Family Therapy: Systemic Theory and Practice*, Maidenhead: Open University Press.

Fernando, S. (2014) *Mental Health Worldwide: Culture, Globalization and Development*, Basingstoke: Palgrave Macmillan.

Walker, R. (2020) *The Unapologetic Guide to Black Mental Health: Navigate an Unequal System, Learn Tools for Emotional Wellness, and Get the Help you Deserve*, Oakland, CA: New Harbinger.

Wilkinson, R. and Pickett, K. (2018) *The Inner Level: How More Equal Societies Reduce Stress, Restore Sanity and Improve Everyone's Well-being*, London: Allen Lane.

World Health Organization (WHO) (undated) *Gender Disparities in Mental Health*, Geneva: WHO [https://www.who.int/mental_health/media/en/242.pdf].

Part 2
Specific issues

Part contents

6 Anxiety disorders

Anxiety is a useful emotion. Without it, we are likely to be reckless, and engage in activities that could lead to harm or danger. However, when levels of anxiety become inappropriately high, they stop being a proportionate response to the threats within the environment and become problematic to the individual experiencing them. **DSM**-5 includes three of the four disorders considered here within its category of anxiety disorders: simple phobia, panic disorder, and generalized anxiety disorder (GAD). Obsessive-compulsive disorder (OCD) has historically been situated within this category, but now has been given its own. Nevertheless, because the experiences of people with OCD and relevant theories have much in common with those associated with anxiety, it is also considered here. Accordingly, by the end of the chapter, you should have an understanding of:

- The nature and **aetiology** of each condition from a number of theoretical perspectives
- The types of interventions used to treat each disorder
- The relative effectiveness of each of these interventions.

6.1 A common biological pathway

Although the exact aetiology of the different anxiety disorders does vary, there appear to be some fundamental neurophysiological mechanisms influencing risk for anxiety, with the 'type' of anxiety the person experiences resulting from an interaction between their neurophysiological predisposition and life experiences. Anxiety is associated with overactivation of a brain system involving the sep-to-hippocampal system (linking the septum, amygdala, hippocampus, and fornix) and the Papez circuit (otherwise known as the circuit of emotion: linking the mammillary bodies, thalamus, cingulate gyrus and hippocampus, prefrontal cortex, amygdala, and septum). Gray (1983) called this the behavioural inhibition system (BIS), because activation of these brain circuits is thought to interrupt ongoing behaviour, and redirect attention to signs of threat or danger. According to Gray, the BIS receives information about the environment from the sensory cortex. It then checks this against predictions it makes about future changes. When a mismatch occurs, the system is activated and the individual experiences the emotion of anxiety. In anxiety the criteria for such discrepancies may be 'set' too low, resulting in the individual constantly responding to perceived mismatches and the system being chronically activated.

Central to the development and maintenance of fear are the amygdala and hypothalamus. The amygdala modulates our experience of anxiety, aggression, fear conditioning, and emotional memory. It has links to the hypothalamus, which regulates the autonomic nervous system's response to these experiences. Activation of the sympathetic arm of this system results in high levels of physiological arousal: the so-called fight–flight response. Activity within the amygdala is modulated through both serotonin and GABA. Low levels of serotonin within the amygdala are associated with high levels of fear, an effect which is obviated by treatment with **SSRIs** (e.g. Adamec et al. 2004). Importantly, though, the influence of serotonin may actually be indirect, and mediated by its influence over levels of GABA (see Chapter 4). Low levels of serotonin may lead to low levels of GABA (Celada et al. 2013), and low levels of GABA within the amygdala result in a low threshold to the perception of threat. In turn, threat perception leads to activation of the sympathetic nervous system by the hypothalamus modulated by the two **neurotransmitters** and hormones, norepinephrine and epinephrine.

6.2 Specific phobias

A specific phobia is an unrealistic fear of a clearly identified object or situation. This fear will have cognitive, physiological, and behavioural components; the latter usually involving movement away from, or avoidance of, the source of the fear. DSM-5 identifies the following criteria for this diagnosis to be met:

- Marked fear or anxiety in relation to a specific object or situation
- The phobic stimulus almost always provokes immediate fear or anxiety
- The fear or anxiety is disproportionate to the actual danger posed by the phobic stimulus and its socio-cultural context
- The phobic stimulus is actively avoided or endured with intense fear or anxiety
- The symptoms typically last for 6 months or more.

The DSM further notes that phobic responses can occur in response to a variety of types of stimuli, including animals, natural environmental factors (heights, water), blood–injection–injury, specific situations (aeroplanes, lifts), and 'other' fears, including fear of vomiting, contracting an illness, and so on. More complex disorders, such as a phobic fear of social situations and agoraphobia, receive separate diagnoses.

Studies across different cultures and times estimate an overall **prevalence** of around 5.5%, with females having higher rates than males (Wardenaar et al. 2017). Age of onset tends to follow a particular pattern, with phobias relating to animals, blood-injury, dentists, and natural environments beginning in childhood, while others such as claustrophobia and agoraphobia typically start in adolescence and early adulthood. Once established, phobias tend to be long-lasting and may persist for decades. They are also strongly associated with, and may predate, other anxiety, mood, and substance use disorders (see Eaton et al. 2018).

Some common and not so common phobias are as follows:

Mysophobia	Fear of germs or contamination
Claustrophobia	Fear of enclosed spaces
Trypanophobia	Fear of injections
Monophobia	Fear of being alone
Helminthophobia	Fear of (parasitic) worms
Taphephobia	Fear of being buried alive
Triskaidekaphobia	Fear of the number 13
Ailurophobia	Fear of cats
Aviophobia	Fear of flying
Arachnophobia	Fear of spiders

Phobias such as a fear of snakes or spiders appear to be universal. The nature and prevalence of other phobias, however, appear to be influenced by cultural factors. A very specific social phobia common in Japan but almost non-existent in the West is known as *taijin kyofusho*. This involves an incapacitating fear of offending or harming others through one's own awkward social behaviour, glancing at their genital areas or imagined physical defect. The focus of this phobia is on the harm to others, not on embarrassment to self as in social phobias in the West. As such, it appears to be a pathological exaggeration of the modesty and sensitive regard for others that, at lower levels, are considered proper in Japan.

Aetiology of phobias

Psychoanalytic models

According to Freud (1906), phobias act as a defence against the anxiety experienced when impulses formed by the **id** are repressed, resulting in a displacement of the repressed feelings onto the object or situation with which it is symbolically associated. These become phobic stimuli and the individual is able to avoid dealing with their repressed conflicts by avoiding them. These conflicts often involve childhood trauma or conflict. The most famous case of a phobia discussed by Freud is that of Little Hans. Hans was a 5-year-old boy who was afraid of horses, and avoided leaving the house for fear of being bitten by one. He also developed a specific fear of the blinkers and muzzles on horses' faces. Freud considered his fears to relate to the Oedipus complex (see Chapter 2), and that he was having sexual fantasies about his mother and feared his father's retaliation. He therefore displaced the fear of his father onto horses who reminded him of his father. A more prosaic explanation for these fears may have been his witnessing an incident in which a horse fell down in the street in front of him. Another psychodynamic interpretation, in which the feared object or behaviour is seen as symbolic of other fears or issues (agoraphobia as a response to feeling trapped within a marriage), may be less sexually charged than Freud's interpretation but of relevance to more modern psychodynamic therapies.

Behavioural models

Early behavioural models of phobias considered them to result from conditioning experiences, in which the inappropriately feared object or situation was associated with the experience of fear at some time in the past. The conditioning process can be so powerful when acute fear is experienced, this association need happen only once to result in a long-term fear response that is difficult to extinguish. Being in a car crash, for example, may result in a phobic reaction to being in a car, and subsequent avoidance of cars or driving. This response has three components:

- a *behavioural* element involving avoidance or escape from the feared object
- high levels of *physiological arousal* evident through a variety of symptoms, including physical tension, increased startle response, tremor or sweating, and driven by the sympathetic nervous system
- the *emotion* of anxiety and fear.

The most famous early example of conditioning a phobic response was Watson and Rayner's (1920) **classical conditioning** of 'Little Albert', discussed in Chapter 2. The classical conditioning model of the acquisition of phobias is clearly consistent with examples such as this, but is less able to explain why phobias persist over long periods. Learning theory suggests that repeated exposures in the absence of any negative consequences should lead to a reduction of anxiety through the process of extinction. In response to this weakness, Mowrer (1947) added a second factor to the conditioning model. His two-factor theory combined both classical and operant processes. He noted that once a phobic response is established through classical conditioning, the affected individual tends to avoid the feared stimulus. This has two consequences. First, it prevents the classical conditioning process of extinction, as the individual does not experience the conditioned stimulus under conditions of safety. Second, because avoidance itself produces feelings of relief (i.e. it is reinforcing), the avoidance response is strengthened by **operant conditioning** processes. In this way, phobic anxiety is potentially maintained over long periods.

Despite this addition, by the 1970s conditioning theories of the acquisition of fear and other emotional responses were finding it increasingly difficult to account for emerging experimental and clinical findings (e.g. Davey 1997):

- Many people with a phobia were unable to identify any traumatic conditioning incident. This seemed particularly true of some animal phobias and fears of heights and water. Less than 10% of snake phobics had been attacked or bitten by a snake. By contrast, over 90% of people reporting a dental phobia had at least one painful episode at a dentist (Davey 1997).

- Many people exposed to trauma do not develop a phobia. Only about 16% of people who attend hospital following a serious road traffic accident, for example, develop a phobia or fear of travelling by car (Mayou et al. 2001).
- Many common phobias are to relatively benign stimuli (e.g. spiders).
- Many common phobias are to stimuli rarely if ever directly encountered by most individuals (e.g. snakes).
- By contrast, rates of phobias to many frequently encountered and potentially frightening stimuli (e.g. traffic, knives, guns) are relatively low.
- Phobias tend to 'run' in families.

A cognitive behavioural model

In response to these concerns, more recent models of the aetiology of phobias have retained the conditioning processes of the early models but added a number of other processes. The most important of these is the addition of cognitive variables as mediators of both the acquisition of a phobias and their potential time course (Hofmann 2008).

Factors that may influence the *acquisition* of phobias include:

- The degree of familiarity with the feared stimulus. The more trauma-free associations an individual has had with a particular stimulus, the less likely they are to develop a phobia if that stimulus subsequently becomes associated with high levels of fear: a process known as latent inhibition. Conversely, the more negative emotions are associated with a particular stimulus prior to a traumatic event, the more likely an individual is to develop a phobia.
- Information from other people or observation of someone else expressing high levels of fear in the context of a particular stimulus. The latter process is known as **vicarious learning** and provides one explanation for the high prevalence of the same phobias in some families (Bandura 1982).

Factors that influence the *maintenance* of phobias, include:

- Socially or verbally transmitted information about the feared stimulus. Unfortunately, it seems easier to increase fear by telling people that a trigger event was more horrific than it appeared at the time than to reduce fear through reassurance that it was less horrific.
- Rehearsal and overestimation of the possible adverse outcomes that may occur should the individual encounter the feared stimulus. The more this occurs, the stronger the fear reaction during 'live' encounters with the feared stimulus.

Biological/evolutionary model

A second influential theory used to account for the non-random distribution of phobias is known as preparedness theory. Seligman (1971) proposed that some phobias or fears are more easily acquired as a result of their evolutionary usefulness than others. He contended that at some time in our evolutionary history it was beneficial to have a fear of potentially dangerous stimuli such as snakes, small animals, and so on – stimuli he termed 'phylogenetically relevant cues'. As a result, we may be hardwired, or biologically prepared, to react fearfully to stimuli that were once threatening to prehistoric man. Note that Seligman did not suggest we have an inborn fear of snakes, spiders, and so on. Rather, he suggested that we acquire fear to such stimuli more easily following some form of conditioning experience than we do to others. The theory has four key predictions (Merckelbach and de Jong 1999):

- The most prevalent phobias should be to stimuli that were potentially dangerous in a pre-technological age: this does seem to be the case (Merckelbach and de Jong 1999).
- Fear of these stimuli is easily acquired (and more easily than other phobias): again, this may the case. Marks (1977), for example, gave an example of a woman who was looking at a picture of a snake at the time she was involved in a car accident. She became phobic to snakes, but not to cars.
- Because of their biological significance, they are non-cognitive.
- They resist extinction: experimental work by Öhman and colleagues (see Öhman and Mineka 2001) found that once a conditioned response to phylogenetically relevant stimuli was established in the laboratory, it took longer to extinguish than other conditioned phobias.

Accordingly, although not all the evidence is strongly supportive of the model (see Merckelbach and de Jong 1999), the consensus seems to be that some evolutionary/genetic processes may be involved in the acquisition of phobias. Confirmation of this preparedness hypothesis requires evidence of some genetic involvement in the disorder. In one exploration of this issue, Skre et al. (2000) found measures of agoraphobia, social phobia, and animal phobias were more strongly correlated in **monozygotic (MZ)** than **dizygotic (DZ) twins**. They calculated a genetic heritability of 0.47 for common phobic fear of small animals and of 0.30 for agoraphobic fear. However, there was no evidence of heritability for the fear of 'nature phenomena' and situational fear. These findings support a modest genetic contribution to at least some phobias and a predisposition to a fear of small animals in particular. The exact location of any genetic loci has yet to be established (Meier and Deckert 2019).

Biological mechanisms

The most obvious biological response to a phobic object is a high degree of physiological arousal. This is known as the fight–flight response and is driven by the sympathetic arm of the autonomic nervous system. At such times, the heart beats quickly and powerfully, blood is shunted to the muscles and away from the gut (hence the experience of 'butterflies'), the skeletal muscles tense, and blood pressure rises. These and other processes prepare the body for rapid and dramatic action. This may be apparent through running away from a feared situation, or shaking, breathlessness, sweating, and dizziness. These experiences can be so extreme they can lead to fear of having a heart attack. The one exception to this occurs in people who have a phobia concerning blood-injury or injection. When they encounter these stimuli, they typically experience an initial acceleration followed by a reduction in heart rate and blood pressure – a parasympathetic response. As a consequence, they experience nausea, dizziness, and may faint. Up to 70% of blood-phobic individuals report having fainted at some time (Öst and Hellström 1997).

Less obvious, but equally important, may be more central neural processes that serve to maintain phobias in the longer term. These link back to the role of the amygdala, serotonin, and GABA, considered earlier in the chapter. In this extended model, phobias may be established by some form of conditioning event, which results in high levels of sympathetic arousal driven by the hypothalamus. Over time, low levels of GABA within the amygdala, and therefore high activation of the hypothalamus in response to previously conditioned events, may contribute to a failure to habituate to any conditioned stimulus (Garcia 2017).

Treatment of phobias

Cognitive/behavioural treatments

The premise underpinning behavioural treatments of phobias was outlined in Chapter 2. They involve exposure to the feared stimulus either directly (flooding) or in a series of hierarchical stages (systematic desensitization). These approaches may be augmented by teaching people skills such as relaxation or cognitive strategies to counter negative expectations and fear of catastrophic outcomes. However, the effects of these additions have been mixed, with both treatment gains and losses, indicating that the core of any treatment involves direct exposure to the feared stimulus and staying with it until any fear is extinguished (Wolitzky-Taylor et al. 2008).

Given the well-established success of behavioural interventions, recent research has involved attempts at fine-tuning them and making them cost-effective. One important strand of research has focused on the effects of single-session exposure to the feared stimulus. These sessions may be fairly lengthy, sometimes over 3 hours. In one study of its effectiveness, Hellström et al. (1996) reported outcomes of a group treatment of people with a spider phobia. They were randomly assigned into one of two conditions: small groups of three to four people and larger groups of seven to eight people. All groups received one 3-hour session in which the principles of the treatment (flooding) were explained to participants. They watched as the therapist was exposed to the spiders and coped with their fear. They were then encouraged to handle four spiders and shown how to cope with this experience. Immediately after treatment, 82% of people in the small groups had made clinically significant improvements, compared to 70% of those in the large groups. By one-year follow-up, the equivalent percentages were 95% and 75%, respectively. These and other data have led reviewers such as Davis et al. (2019) to conclude that this single-session exposure approach is of significant benefit across a range of ages, including young adults and children.

A second approach to making treatment both more available and cost-effective has been through the use of the internet. In a trial of an intervention for which live exposure is necessarily limited, Campos et al. (2019) explored the impact of NO-FEAR airlines, an intervention involving exposure to experiences related to flying that used images and sounds associated with each phase of flying from take-off to landing (and even plane crashes). Participants were randomly allocated to one of three conditions: self-applied exposure, exposure with therapist guidance involving a weekly phone call with guidance adapted to the individual treatment phase and pace, and a **waiting list control** condition. Although the number of flights made after the interventions did not differ across the groups, those in both active interventions travelled with lower levels of anxiety and less 'safety behaviours'. Around 80% of those in the active interventions were considered 'recovered' on one measure of fear of flying, compared to 9% of those in the waiting list.

A third strand of therapy has involved the use of virtual reality, which may be particularly beneficial when the hierarchical progression may be difficult to control, such as a phobia of driving. In one study of this approach, Walshe et al. (2003) treated car phobics using a virtual reality exposure programme involving up to 12 one-hour sessions. The participants improved significantly on measures of travel distress, avoidance, and maladaptive driving strategies. This approach is clearly more expensive and complex than the treatment for spider phobia described above. However, where exposure to a controlled or safe 'live' exposure may be difficult to establish, it can be of benefit and is no less effective than live exposure in most cases (Wechsler et al. 2019).

Pharmacological treatments

Despite the potential role of serotonin/GABA in the maintenance of phobias, evidence of significant benefit from SSRIs, while promising, has yet to be fully established. Alamy et al. (2008), for example, found benefits favouring an SSRI over **placebo** on a measure of global impairment for people with a range of specific phobias, but their sample was very small (12 participants) and so their results should be viewed with caution. As a consequence, even **pharmacotherapy** advisory sources (e.g. Swinson and McCabe 2019) indicate the first line of treatment for specific phobias should be cognitive behavioural therapy (CBT).

6.3 Panic disorder

A panic attack is a period of intense fear or discomfort that reaches a peak within 10 minutes, and is associated with at least five symptoms, including breathlessness, palpitations, dizziness or trembling, nausea, and tingling sensations in the arms and fingers. People who have specific phobias may experience high levels of arousal or even panic in the presence of their feared object. However, they will not be diagnosed with panic disorder. Critical to this diagnosis is that panic attacks, at least initially, are unexpected and not associated with a specific stimulus; although links between feelings of panic and specific contexts may become evident over time. According to DSM-5, to be given this diagnosis the individual will report recurrent unexpected panic attacks, at least one of which has been followed by either or both of:

- a month or more of persistent concern or worry about additional panic attacks or their consequences

- a month or more of significant maladaptive change in behaviour related to the attacks, including behaviours designed to avoid having panic attacks, such as avoidance of unfamiliar situations.

Charles Darwin provided one of the first descriptions of a panic attack when he described one of his own, although his condition at the time was tentatively diagnosed as 'dyspepsia with an aggravated character', 'catarrhal dyspepsia', and 'suppressed gout' (Barloon and Noyes 1997). He was not unusual, and the prevalence of panic attacks may be increasing. The prevalence of US citizens to report having had at least one panic attack rose from 5.3% to 12.7% between 1980 and 1995 (Goodwin 2003). However, the number of people achieving the diagnostic criteria for panic disorder is much lower. Olaya et al. (2018), for example, synthesized data from three large Spanish studies and found an overall population prevalence of around 4–5%. The prevalence of the disorder was lower in older adults (3.2 %), and much higher in those aged 30–39 years (9.5%). The condition is universal and consistent across geographical and cultural boundaries, although triggers to panic may vary across cultures. In the Arctic, a fear of being alone known as *kayak angst*, and a Chinese anxiety syndrome involving the fear of penile retraction into the body resulting in death known as *koro*, show striking similarities to panic disorder.

Aetiology of panic disorder

Biological mechanisms

Panic, or physiological arousal close to panic, can be experienced by individuals with specific phobias. It should be no surprise, therefore, that the central and peripheral neurological processes are the same in both conditions. In addition to these neurological processes, a defining feature of a panic attack is known as **hyperventilation**. This involves disruption of breathing, which becomes rapid, with short inhalations and exhalations. As a consequence, carbon dioxide is rapidly exhaled and not absorbed into the bloodstream, while oxygen is over-absorbed, leading to the many physical sensations associated with panic. As the normal breathing response is triggered by high levels of carbon dioxide within the circulation, the physiological trigger to breathe does not occur, resulting in feelings of shortness of breath, which encourage further over-breathing. It is at times such as this that the eponymous 'brown bag' can come in useful. Placing one over the mouth and nose ensures that the person re-breathes the carbon dioxide they are exhaling, increasing its absorption from the lungs into the blood, stabilizing the breathing pattern and stopping the symptoms.

Evidence that panic disorder has a genetic component can be found in studies such as that by Kendler et al. (1993), who found concordance rates of 24% between MZ twins and 11% between DZ twins. These and other data included in a **meta-analysis** by Hettema et al. (2001a) indicated that panic disorder has a **heritability coefficient** of 0.40. Specific genes related to panic disorder are now being identified, although these are likely to be associated with a broad tendency towards anxiety rather than panic disorder *per se* and may involve those that influence serotonin, norepinephrine, and also dopaminergic responses to stress (e.g. Jacob et al. 2010).

Social factors

High levels of social stress increase risk for panic disorder. The highest rates of panic disorder are among those who are widowed, divorced or separated, live in cities, or have limited education. More specifically, Scocco et al. (2007) found that of their sample of individuals with panic disorder, 93% had experienced a role transition in the previous year, 86% reported 'interpersonal deficits', 75% a role dispute, and 38% had suffered the loss of a relative or significant other. Compared to non-panic comparison groups, Batinić et al. (2009) found much higher levels of physical health problems and conflict with or separation from important others among people with panic disorder. They may also have experienced early parental loss and physical or sexual abuse. Bandelow et al. (2002), for example, compared the experiences of people with and without panic disorder and found that those with the disorder found their parents to be more restrictive and less loving than controls. They were also more likely to report negative childhood events such as the death of a father, sexual abuse or violence within the family. By comparison, a careful study by De Venter et al. (2017) following a cohort of individuals with a range of anxiety disorders, including over 500 with panic disorder, found that while over 50% reported experiences of childhood trauma and neglect, these factors were more strongly associated with measures of severity and chronicity in people with social phobias than those with panic disorder. Not surprisingly, childhood anxiety, which may be related to poor attachment with parents, also predicts panic disorder in adulthood (Biederman et al. 2005).

Psychological explanations

Most psychological theories have focused more on immediate factors associated with the condition than historical ones. Given the apparent link between panic and phobias, Mowrer's (1947) conditioning model of fear acquisition and maintenance would appear to be relevant to this condition. However, the theory assumes high levels of conditioned anxiety to be triggered by the presence of a feared stimulus. It has difficulties in explaining high levels of anxiety in the absence of an obvious stimulus – a defining characteristic of panic disorder.

The most influential alternative model is that of Clark (1986). A key element of panic disorder is that the individual experiencing panic can see no obvious link between the feelings of panic they experience and the context in which they occur – in other words, they come 'out of the blue'. According to Clark, this is because the initiating event may be the experience of 'normal' high levels of arousal as a consequence of such things as a high caffeine intake, rushing or anger. Because this high arousal 'makes sense' in this context, it may not even be noticed by the individual. However, it may become classically conditioned to the context in which it occurs, such that the next time the individual finds themselves in this context, they experience a similar physiological state, for which they now have no immediate explanation. Instead, they identify it as being anomalous: a sign of potential or imminent physical harm.

These thoughts lead to activation of the fight–flight response, resulting in an increase in physiological arousal, which is further interpreted in a catastrophic

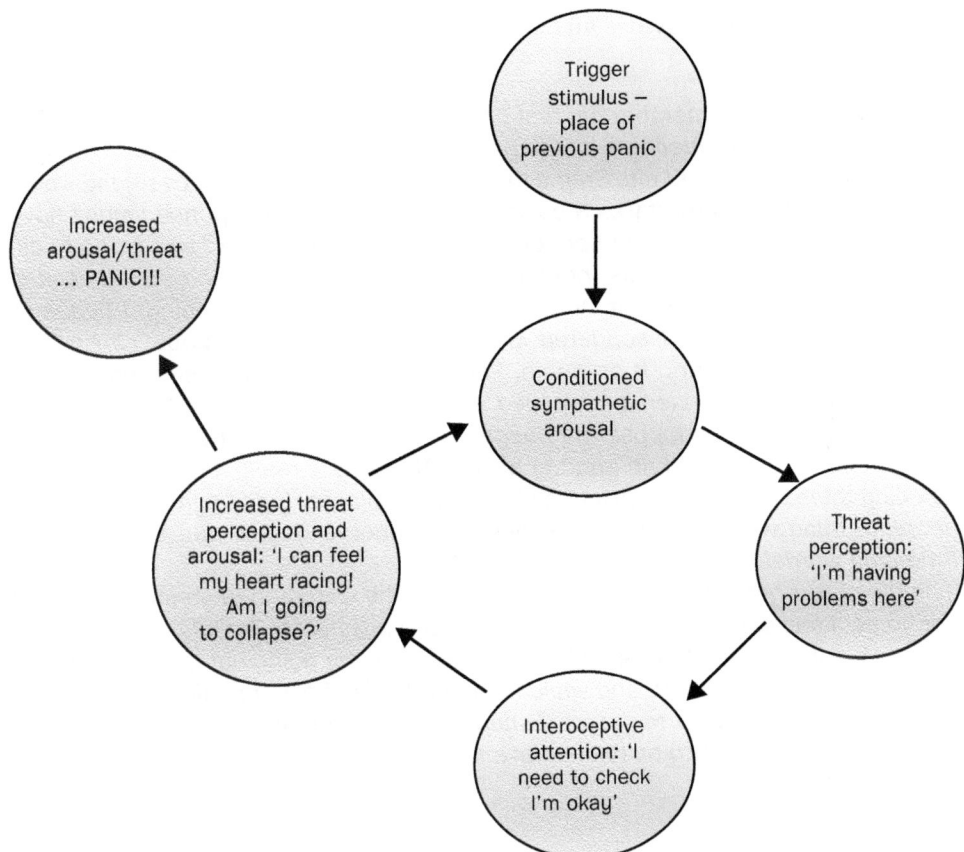

Figure 6.1 The panic cycle

fashion ('Yes, my heart really is pounding; I really am heading for a heart attack'). These anxiety-laden cognitions further increase arousal and its associated bodily sensations, which lead to further levels of arousal: a vicious circle which culminates in a panic attack (see Figure 6.1).

Once an individual has developed a tendency to interpret bodily sensations catastrophically, two further processes contribute to the maintenance of panic disorder. First, because they are frightened of certain sensations, they become hypervigilant and repeatedly scan their body checking for them. Any sensations then identified are taken as further evidence of the presence of a serious physical or mental disorder. Second, safety behaviours, usually involving not entering a feared situation, or leaving it at the onset of symptoms, tend to maintain the individual's negative interpretations. Such avoidance prevents the individual from learning that the symptoms they have experienced are not as dangerous as they think, and serves to maintain their anxiety (Wells 2000).

The case of Sue provides an example of these processes:

When did it begin? I remember my first panic – who wouldn't? It was in the car park in Tesco's. I remember feeling a bit faint. I thought I was going to pass out. I thought I would look such a fool if I did. Stupid to pass out in a car park. And everyone would look at me ... Now I know it was a panic attack. But when it happened I didn't have a clue what was going on. I felt bad for no reason ... I didn't think I was going to die or anything like that, but I was frightened I would collapse and end up in hospital. I think I could have got over it OK, but the next time I went shopping, I began to think about things again. I wondered whether there was anything about Tesco's or shopping that might bring it on again. Perhaps I had pushed myself too hard ... I was in a bit of a rush when it happened – I don't know. They weren't very sensible thoughts, really. But I suppose they began to wind me up. Anyway, the next time I went shopping ... yes, I had another attack. That was it really, I just thought, 'I'm not going there again'. So I started to shop in other places, but I began to worry that the same thing would happen, and then I had another panic, and that just confirmed my worries.

In the end, it got easier to stay at home out of the way than to go out. I quite like it at home. I feel safe, and I watch TV without any hassle. My friends come and see me, so it's not as if I don't have a life. I was never one for going out much. If I go out, then I worry before I set off, and while I am out. I often have a panic, so it's just not worth going out. I can get to the local shop if I go with my husband. And I can go in the car with him – as long as I don't have to get out. But I don't like to go far ...

The example of Sue fits Clark's (1986) model of the development of panic disorder. She also hinted at a further factor that can contribute to the development of the disorder or its associated problems: a process known as secondary gain. Being restricted to the house was quite pleasant for Sue. She gained sympathy from her husband and quite enjoyed being at home. These secondary rewards contributed to the maintenance of her avoidant behaviour once it had been initiated.

Clark's model has been experimentally tested in a number of ways. These have examined key elements of the theory, including:

1. Cognitions can trigger panic in vulnerable individuals
2. People with panic disorder are more likely to panic if they experience unusual physical symptoms than people without the disorder
3. If people with panic disorder experience unusual symptoms and are given an appropriate explanation, they will experience less panic than those not given such an explanation.

Perhaps the most dramatic evidence of the first premise comes from what is now a rather old but insightful study reported by Clark et al. (1988). They asked a group of individuals with panic disorder and 'typical' controls to read out loud a series of word pairs. Some of these pairings included combinations of body sensations and catastrophic feelings or thoughts typically made by individuals while panicking, for example 'breathless – suffocate'. Each group was asked to rate their anxiety before and after reading the cards and to rate any changes in any panic symptoms. The manipulation proved unexpectedly powerful. Ten out of the 12 people with panic disorder, but no controls, had a panic attack while reading the cards.

Investigation of the second and third elements of the theory has frequently involved use of an experimental paradigm known as respiratory challenge. In this, participants take a breath of air with higher than usual levels of carbon dioxide (various studies use between a 5% and 50% carbon dioxide mixture). This induces feelings similar to those that occur during hyperventilation: shortness of breath, light-headedness, tingling in the arms and legs, and so on. There is consistent evidence that following this procedure, people with panic disorder are significantly more likely to panic than are people with obsessive-compulsive disorder, GAD or depression (e.g. Vickers et al. 2012).

This panic may be moderated if individuals are given a non-catastrophic explanation for any symptoms they experience. In one study of this effect, Rapee et al. (1986) gave different information about the sensations likely to be experienced as a result of a single inhalation of 50% carbon dioxide and 50% oxygen to people with panic disorder. Half their participants were given a detailed explanation of all the possible sensations they could experience, and told they resulted from inhalation of the gas. The others were given no explanation of what to expect. As expected, participants in the detailed explanation group reported less catastrophic cognitions and less anxiety than those in the naïve condition. Of note also is that if people with panic disorder are simply told (incorrectly) that their heart rate is increasing in response to a psychological task, they experience more panic symptoms than do individuals who do not have panic disorder (Story and Craske 2008).

Stop and think ...

We often talk about risk factors for various disorders, but rarely if ever think about protective factors. We know some: men benefit from being married (the advantage is less for women), and women benefit from having a wider support system. But what factors may be protective, in both the long and the short term, against the anxiety disorders discussed in this chapter? Given the high levels of mental health problems within society (and the frighteningly high impact of Covid-19 on mental health), should society work to reduce risk for them? If so, how, how much resource should be devoted to such efforts, and how widespread and contextual should they be? Should mental health skills be taught in schools? Should work practices be established that minimize stress and support individuals who may be struggling with their mental health? We can intervene from a range of levels (e.g. individual, institution, society) and with a range of methods (e.g. provision of therapy, education to reduce stigma, occupational policy to reduce occupational stress). So, how far is it reasonable to go, and where should any efforts be directed?

Treatment of panic disorder

Cognitive behavioural interventions

Some of the most successful treatment programmes for panic disorder have been based on Clark's aetiological model. Clark et al. (1994), for example, developed a two-phase treatment approach. The first phase involved teaching participants the cognitive model of panic. The second involved three elements:

- relaxation to reduce physiological arousal at the time of stress
- cognitive procedures to change panicogenic cognitions
- behavioural procedures to control panic symptoms.

Relaxation involves learning to physically relax and to slow and control breathing. These techniques can be applied before potential panic attacks, for example, when approaching a situation where a panic attack has occurred previously, and during them. Cognitive procedures include **self-instruction training** and **cognitive challenge** (see Chapter 3). The goal of the behavioural procedures is to teach the individual, through direct experience, that the outcome they fear at times of panic will not actually happen.

Increasingly, therapists instigate the symptoms of panic within the therapy session and practise its control through the use of cognitive and relaxation techniques. Symptoms may be generated by a variety of procedures, including reading words linking bodily sensations and catastrophic outcomes, and hyperventilating, a process known as interoceptive exposure. These behavioural experiments can show how thoughts and behaviours influence symptoms previously considered the result of unknown factors and allow rehearsal of cognitive and relaxation panic control strategies. Once control over symptoms has been achieved within the therapy sessions, these skills can be used in real-life situations. This may be done gradually, starting with relatively easy circumstances and moving on to more difficult ones in a process of graded exposure.

Overall, CBT is an effective intervention for panic disorder. Summarizing the data, Ham et al. (2005) calculated an overall success rate of 73% for CBT (i.e. participants considered panic-free), compared with 27% for those who did not receive treatment. Forty-six per cent of participants remained panic-free at one-year follow-up. Given these various components to the therapy, it is of interest which are most effective – an issue explored by Pompoli et al. (2018). They examined the outcomes of 72 studies of CBT for panic disorder, identifying the elements that were more or less useful in these interventions, and concluded that interoceptive exposure and face-to-face therapy settings were critical both to outcomes and acceptability to recipients. Muscle relaxation and the use of virtual reality were of less value, while graded *in vivo* exposure, usually seen as central to any behavioural intervention, improved acceptability but had only small effects on efficacy. Even within the CBT paradigm, they identified a seven-fold difference in outcome between those interventions that used the optimum combination of strategies and those that used the least effective. These differences in strategy and outcome may have contributed to Carpenter and colleagues' (2018) conclusion that the overall effectiveness of therapy for panic disorder was less than that associated with CBT interventions for phobias and GAD.

Pharmacological treatments

The standard pharmacological treatment for panic disorder now involves the use of SSRIs (Batelaan et al. 2012), which have been shown to reduce the frequency of panic attacks in 36–86% of people treated using them (Kasper and Resinger 2001). In a direct comparison of SSRIs with a psychological intervention, van Apeldoorn et al. (2010) followed a cohort of people with a primary diagnosis of panic disorder who were treated with CBT, an SSRI combined with regular meetings with the prescribing clinician, or a combination of the two for a period of one year. Nine months into treatment, the pharmacological intervention proved superior, with the SSRI alone and in combination with CBT proving more effective than CBT alone. However, 3 months later, the CBT group had continued to improve, while those in the SSRI condition were more likely to relapse, with CBT then proving superior to the SSRI (remission rates of 44% in the CBT group, 25% in the SSRI condition, and 52% in the combined intervention). By one-year follow-up, remission rates in each of the conditions were as follows: CBT 31%, SSRI 25%, and combined therapy 48%.

6.4 Generalized anxiety disorder

DSM-5 defines generalized anxiety disorder (GAD) as excessive or ongoing anxiety and worry, occurring on more days than not, over a period of at least 6 months. In addition:

- the individual finds it difficult to control their worry
- anxiety and worry are associated with three or more of the following:
  o restlessness, feeling 'keyed up' or 'on edge'
  o being easily fatigued
  o difficulty concentrating
  o irritability
  o muscle tension
  o sleep disturbance.

The worries reported by people with GAD usually involve relatively minor, everyday matters. Nevertheless, they find both their worries difficult to control and the extent to which they have them distressing. The prevalence of GAD within the UK is 4.4% (McManus et al. 2016), and usually begins in childhood or adolescence. Once established, it tends to be a chronic disorder: up to 80% of people diagnosed with GAD report having been worried or anxious much of their lives, and its **incidence** appears to increase in older adults (Krasucki et al. 1998). It has high levels of co-morbidity with mood and somatoform disorders (Conway et al. 2006). Rates are highest among women, middle-aged people, people living alone, and those of low income. As GAD can almost be trait-like in its nature, given its chronicity, its prevalence may not be subject to acute stresses. Nevertheless, a 35% prevalence of symptoms potentially diagnosable as GAD recently found in a large representative Chinese sample (Huang and Zhao 2020) indicates the emotional cost of the Covid-19 pandemic in that country. Rates of 20–22% may be more typical of European populations (e.g. González-Sanguino et al. 2020), levels which are not markedly different from those found among healthcare workers, where rates averaging 23% have been found (Pappa et al. 2020).

Aetiology of GAD

Biological mechanisms

The biological mechanisms underpinning GAD have already been considered, and involve the behavioural inhibition system (BIS), amygdala, and to a lesser extent the hypothalamus and sympathetic nervous system. It is noteworthy that this chronic activation of the BIS leads people with GAD to experience less *acute* anxiety than on average, probably a consequence of chronically high levels of norepinephrine resulting in the receptivity of that neurotransmitter at the postsynaptic site becoming less sensitive over time (Spiegel and Barlow 2000). The influence of genetic factors on the risk of developing GAD appears to be modest. Hettema et al. (2001b), for example, obtained a lifetime history of GAD through interviews with 3,100 pairs of twins. Concordance rates between the pairs were relatively low, leading the authors to estimate the heritability of GAD to be about 15–20% across both sexes. Links have been made between GAD and polymorphisms of the *RGS2* gene, which may also be implicated in bipolar disorder (Koenen et al. 2009), and a unique risk through the *ITM2B* gene (Davies et al. 2015).

Psychoanalytic explanations

Freud distinguished two routes to general anxiety in adulthood, both of which have their roots in childhood: too rigorous punishment and over-protection. He suggested that both 'neurotic' and 'moral' anxiety begin when the child is repeatedly punished for, or prevented from, expressing their id impulses. This leads them to believe that such impulses are dangerous and have to be controlled. In adulthood, when parental control is no longer operating, the individual fears that their id impulses will be uncontrollable, and they may take actions they do not want to. By contrast, a child protected from threats and frustrations will not develop **defence mechanisms** adequate to deal with the demands of adult life. As a consequence, relatively small threats result in feelings of high levels of anxiety. Chorpita and Barlow (1998), for example, found over-protectiveness, excessive punishment, and critical comments as a child to be associated with high levels of anxiety in adulthood.

Humanistic explanations

A further explanation of any link between parental control and the development of GAD is provided by the humanists. Humanists consider GAD to occur when individuals fail to accept themselves for who they are. As a consequence, they experience extreme anxiety and are unable to fulfil their potential as a human being. According to Rogers (1961), this negation of self stems from childhood experiences of excessive discipline. If the individual is subject to criticism and harsh standards as a child, they adopt the standards of those around them, in order to receive conditional positive regard for doing so. They subjugate their own beliefs and desires and try to meet these externally imposed standards by repeatedly denying or distorting their true thoughts and experiences. Despite such efforts, threatening self-judgements can break through and cause intense anxiety. While theoretically elegant, this theory has not been subject to empirical testing, and the importance of these processes is largely unknown.

Socio-cultural factors

Social stress influences the prevalence of GAD. Its prevalence is relatively high among people in low socio-economic groups, ethnic minorities, urban populations, people living in countries subject to war and political oppression, and those experiencing chronic work stress (e.g. Melchior et al. 2007). As the demands of everyday living become more complex, the proportion of the population experiencing GAD has increased. Prevalence in the USA, for example, rose from 2.5% in 1975 to 4% by the early 1990s (Regier et al. 1998).

Surprisingly, few studies have considered longer-term antecedents to GAD – and these have found little evidence of a particular role of childhood trauma. Bulik et al. (2001), for example, investigated retrospective reports of child sexual abuse in women who had experienced major depression, GAD, bulimia nervosa, panic disorder, or alcohol or drug dependence. Although many of the women reported experiencing childhood sexual abuse, this was not uniquely predictive of any diagnosis. Similarly, as noted above, the role of parental style presents mixed evidence. More important may be the transmission of anxiety across the generations in combination with individual characteristics. Murray et al. (2008), for example, followed a group of young children of socially anxious and less anxious mothers over time, and found that only children identified as having both high levels of behavioural inhibition (see earlier in this chapter) and a socially anxious mother became more anxious and avoidant over time, suggesting an interaction between biological vulnerability and environmental processes. Children appear to learn fear from their parents as a consequence of observational learning of both the signs of anxiety and poor coping strategies associated with anxiety, such as avoidance (Murray et al. 2009).

Cognitive explanations

Beck provided a more cognitive account of this process, consistent with the childhood learning model. According to Beck (1997), people who experience high levels of generalized anxiety initially interpret a relatively small number of situations as dangerous and threatening. Over time, they apply these assumptions to more and more situations and develop an increasingly generalized anxiety. Beck identified a number of **cognitive schemata** that underpin this anxiety, including 'a situation or a person is unsafe until proven safe', and 'it is always best to assume the worst'. As a consequence of such thoughts, the individual becomes alert to the possibilities of danger and threat throughout their everyday life, and responds with the emotion of anxiety. The process may also work in reverse. Beck noted a form of reasoning he called emotional reasoning, which suggests that if we feel an emotion such as anxiety in certain situations, this leads us to have cognitions that support this anxiety: 'If I am feeling anxious, there must be something to be anxious about here'. Thus, the individual may enter a cycle of negative emotions driving negative cognitions, which in turn drive negative emotions, and so on.

An alternative cognitive model of GAD was developed by Wells (1995), who proposed that the core feature of GAD was excess worry. He identified two types of worry experienced by people with GAD:

- Type 1 worries are the typical worries that most of us experience, albeit at an amplified level: worries related to work, social, health, and other issues
- Type 2 worry, or 'meta-worry', involves the negative appraisal of one's own worries: 'Worrying will drive me mad ...', 'I worry about my worries taking me over ...'.

Type 1 worries are relatively common in population samples. Type 2 worries are common in samples of people with GAD. Wells therefore suggested that individuals with GAD are defined by high levels of Type 2 worries. These worries, while unpleasant, also form a coping response to reduce distress: 'Worrying helps me cope with my problems ...' (see discussion of the S-REF in Chapter 3). As a result, the individual may be motivated to continue worrying, despite their discomfort doing so. At the same time, they may hold increasingly negative views about their worrying. They may believe it is uncontrollable and that it has negative effects on their psychological, social, and physical functioning. However, these beliefs co-exist with the more positive beliefs about worry, and the individual may vacillate between trying to avoid worrying and active worry. This combination of processes led Dugas et al. (2005) to suggest that the central elements of GAD are an intolerance of uncertainty, positive beliefs about worry, poor problem orientation, and cognitive avoidance. The latter strategy may prove ineffective, as attempts to suppress intrusive thoughts typically make them more frequent and salient (e.g. Muris et al. 1998).

Claire provides an example of the worries and meta-worries that people with GAD experience:

It's a family joke, but it's true ... one day we set of from home to shop in Nottingham – a journey of about an hour and a half ... and from the minute we got in the car I was worried about where we were going to park, what the traffic would be like when we got there, and so on. I just worried the whole trip and drove my family mad. It sounds funny, but it's true!

I worry about everything and nothing. I worry if the kids are late back at night. They know I worry, so they really try to be back on time. I've given them a mobile phone so they can ring me if there are any problems or if they are going to be late ... and they do because they know I'll be in a right state when they get home if they don't. I worry about the food – I won't eat it if it's over the recommended date even though my husband assures me that that's OK and we're not going to get any disease. You name it, I'm sure I've worried about it. It does get me down ... I can see me worrying myself into an early grave ... But I can't stop worrying. My husband says 'Just get on with things, try not to worry'. But I can't. I sit and knit or watch the television in the evening trying not to worry about things, but once something's on my mind it's really difficult to stop – however hard I tell myself to. I worry about my health – the slightest thing, and I'm off to the doctor. I know I'm going to worry about things when we have stopped talking. Sometimes it really feels as if I'm going mad. It does get me down, because every day I cannot relax and just get on with things like most people. Mind you, I think many people worry too little … just cruise through life without a care in the world … that can't be right either …

What sounds even more mad is that I worry about NOT worrying. What if the worrying I do does stop bad things happening? I know it doesn't really, but I could never forgive myself if something happened to the children and I had just been getting on with things and didn't have their safety in mind. I could never forgive myself. What sort of a person would that make me – not caring for them when they were in danger?

Treatment of GAD

Cognitive behavioural treatment

Early behavioural interventions in the treatment of GAD involved exposure to feared situations combined with response prevention, much as in the treatment of phobias. Unfortunately, while effective in the treatment of some other anxiety disorders, these methods have proved of little value in the treatment of GAD as the situations that threaten people with GAD are so diffuse. Cognitive behavioural interventions did not prove effective in the treatment of GAD until they incorporated three key strategies:

- worry exposure assignments
- cognitive restructuring of anxiety-provoking thoughts
- relaxation training.

Many people with GAD attempt to mentally block or distract from negative or catastrophic thoughts. As a result, they fail to extinguish the associated anxiety and continue to be worried by their thoughts. Worry exposure involves the individual focusing on these frightening or catastrophic thoughts or images for increasing periods of time, eventually up to between 25 and 50 minutes. Anxiety typically rises and then falls, as the images are held and the individual habituates to them. This process may be augmented through the addition of coping skills, including relaxation or cognitive strategies such as cognitive challenge. Exposure may initially be conducted in the imagination and then shift to real situations the person encounters, either in a planned progression or more naturalistic way. This approach has proven relatively effective. One **meta-analysis** of 41 studies comparing CBT with placebo in the treatment of a range of anxiety disorders (Carpenter et al. 2018) found those engaging with CBT were three times more likely to make significant improvements than those receiving placebo across all disorders. GAD had some of the most positive outcomes, with those receiving CBT five times more likely to make significant treatment gains than those in the placebo interventions.

An alternative cognitive approach involves the use of metacognitive therapy (MCT; see Chapter 3), which challenges the core beliefs driving worry. Nordahl et al. (2018) explored the impact of such a programme, incorporating five components: (i) education about the MCT approach and development of case formulation; (ii) modification of beliefs about the uncontrollability and danger of worry; (iii) challenging positive beliefs about the utility and advantages of worry; (iv) implementation of alternative coping strategies; and (v) relapse prevention. This approach was compared with a more conventional CBT approach and a waiting list control. The MCT was superior, with recovery rates of 65% in the MCT condition and 38% in the CBT condition immediately following therapy, and 57% and 31% respectively at 2-year follow-up. A second alternative to the 'standard' CBT approach involves the application of mindfulness (see Chapter 3). In perhaps the best test of this approach, Wong et al. (2016) compared the effectiveness of an 8-week course of mindfulness-based cognitive therapy (Kabat-Zinn 1990), CBT-based **psychoeducation**, and usual care (essentially, no treatment). The two active interventions proved equally effective, and more effective than usual care immediately following treatment and up to one-year follow-up.

Psychoanalytic therapy

One study has examined the effectiveness of psychoanalytical therapy in the treatment of GAD, comparing it with a cognitive intervention (Durham et al. 1994). Psychoanalytical therapy involved the exploration and understanding of the individual's problems within the context of their current relationship, their developmental context, and in terms of the **transference** and resistance within the therapeutic relationship. Cognitive behavioural therapy proved significantly more effective than psychoanalytical therapy, both immediately following therapy and at 6-month follow-up. By this time, 76% of those receiving CBT were 'better' or 'very considerably' improved; 42% of those in psychoanalytic therapy achieved the same levels of success. Using a more conservative criterion of 'return to normal functioning', the results were less supportive of analytic therapy: 20% of those receiving psychoanalytic therapy achieved this criterion versus 66% of those in the cognitive therapy condition. Drop-out from therapy was much lower in the cognitive therapy group than in the analytic therapy condition: 10% versus 24% respectively.

Pharmacological therapy

Given the role of serotonin and GABA in GAD, it should be no surprise that both **tricyclics** and SSRIs appear effective in the treatment of GAD, although the fewer side-effects associated with SSRIs, and the greater levels of adherence to them, make them the pharmacological treatment of choice (see Mitte et al. 2005). Combining psychological and drug therapy may be of limited benefit. Crits-Christoph et al. (2011), for example, found no additional benefit of allocating people already on an SSRI to CBT.

6.5 Obsessive-compulsive disorder

Obsessive-compulsive disorder (OCD) is a chronic and disabling condition. It typically involves intrusive thoughts that some form of harm will occur if the individual does not perform certain acts or rituals. This results in high levels of anxiety which can usually be reduced by performing the required acts or rituals, known as safety behaviours. According to DSM-5, a diagnosis of OCD requires the following criteria to be met:

- Recurrent and persistent thoughts, impulses or images that are intrusive, inappropriate, and cause significant anxiety or distress (the obsession).
- The individual attempts to ignore or suppress these thoughts, urges or images, or to neutralize them with some thought or action (the compulsion). The characteristics of these are:
  - Repetitive behaviours (for example, hand washing, checking) or mental acts (such as praying, repeating words silently) that the person feels driven to perform, according to rules that must be applied rigidly.
  - Compulsions are used to prevent or reduce distress, or prevent some dreaded event or situation. They are not connected in a realistic way with what they are designed to neutralize or prevent, or are clearly excessive.

The obsessions or compulsions must cause marked distress, last at least one hour a day, or cause clinically significant distress or impairment in social, occupational or other important areas of functioning.

Rachman (2003) identified some of the more common obsessions as concerning:

- *aggressive actions*: thoughts of harming or harm being inflicted on family or children
- *sexual acts*: a fear of inappropriate acts or gestures ('I will molest a young child'), images of sex with inappropriate partners
- *blasphemous acts*: a fear of making sacrilegious gestures in a holy place, pollution of prayers with impure thoughts.

Rachman also identified some frequent compulsions in which people with OCD engage to counter particular concerns, some of which are summarized in Table 6.1.

Table 6.1 Frequent obsessions and compulsions reported by people with obsessive-compulsive disorder

Obsession	Compulsion
Concern with cleanliness (dirt, germs, contamination)	Excessive and ritualized washing, cleaning or bathing
Concern about body secretions (e.g. saliva, urine)	Rituals to remove or avoid contact with body secretions
Sexual obsessions (fear of forbidden urges or aggressive sexual actions)	Ritualized and rigid sexual relationships
Obsessive fears of harming self or others	Repeated checking of doors, cookers, alarms or locks; when driving, retracing route for fear of having run over someone
Concern with exactness (symmetry, order)	Ritualized arranging and rearranging
Obsessions with health (or fear of ill-health)	Checking and rechecking vital signs, rigid dietary intake, constantly checking for new information about health, death, and dying

An example of the nature of OCD and its associated problems is provided by Stephen. He was a factory worker frightened of catching AIDS from 'contamination' in his work area as a consequence of someone he believed to be HIV-positive having touched a nearby workbench some months previously. To avoid this, he engaged in a number of protective behaviours, including turning on taps using his elbows, waiting by doors so that someone else would open them, and using disposable towels to avoid the possibility of contamination. He washed his hands frequently through the day to make sure no stray contamination affected him. On each occasion he washed his hands until his skin was raw and bleeding. If he touched an area he feared was contaminated, he became extremely anxious and had to wash his hands repeatedly until he could reassure himself that he was not contaminated and reduce his anxiety. He described his situation as follows:

I am frightened to touch anything M has been in contact with – well I won't touch it. I know he had venereal disease and he could have AIDS, and you know how it can spread ... and you cannot, like, avoid it. It's invisible – and I can't take the risk of coming into contact with it. I was really angry when he came into where I work. It's one thing avoiding things when I could kick doors open, but when I knew he had touched my workbench, I was horrified ... because I didn't want me and my family to get the disease, and I didn't know how to avoid it. I washed and scrubbed it down with disinfectant and rubbed my hands raw – but you can never guarantee that things are entirely clean. So, I start each day by cleaning my work area, hands, and arms for security ... to protect me and my family from the dirt that this man has spread ... Once that's done, I can relax ... I've got eczema on my hands because of the washing and they get really sore but it's worth it. It stops me worrying about things – and that's a lot worse. If I worry I think about getting AIDS and dying and my family dying. I just can't stop until I've got things sorted.

From the minute I come into work, I get really anxious. I get anxious on the way to work, because I have to face the risk of catching venereal disease ... it feels such a relief when I have finished washing, even though my hands are sore. I wash before I go home, and I take my clothes off before going into the house when I get back from work. I put them in the washer and wash them straight away – my wife can't touch them ... I have a shower before I do anything else and wash myself thoroughly. I would never forgive myself if I brought the disease into the house ... I leave my shoes outside.

I don't care if other people use my workbench – unless they work with M. I don't worry for them – that's for them to look out for. But if they don't get a disease it doesn't reassure me, because I know that these things are hidden ... just because they don't seem to have the disease doesn't mean they don't have it. If they know M, then I have to redo the washing, because I worry that they may be contaminated.

Aetiology of OCD

Biological mechanisms

Biological theorists (e.g. Maia et al. 2008) have identified two interconnected brain systems that are implicated in OCD. The first is a loop connecting the orbitofrontal area, where sexual, violent, and other primitive impulses normally arise, to the thalamic region, where the individual engages in more cognitive and perhaps behavioural responses as a result of this activation. A second loop connects the orbito-frontal region to the thalamic region, but via the corpus striatum. The striatal region is thought to control the degree of activity within the systems. It tends to filter out high levels of activity within the orbitofrontal area so that the thalamus does not over-respond to these initial impulses. In OCD, it may fail to correct overactivity in the orbitofrontal-thalamic loop, so the individual over-responds to environmental stimuli, and is unable to prevent their cognitive and behavioural responses to them. The first system appears to be mediated by the excitatory neurotransmitter glutamic acid. The second system appears to be mediated by a number of neurotransmitters including serotonin, dopamine, and GABA.

Evidence of a genetic risk for OCD is mixed. Andrews et al. (1990) found no evidence of higher concordance in MZ than in DZ twins. Similarly, Black et al. (1992) found 2.5% of their large sample of relatives of people with OCD had the disorder, a figure not dissimilar to the 2.3% prevalence among their control group and population norms. More recent studies, however, measuring dimensions of OCD symptoms rather than the presence or absence of a diagnosis of OCD have identified a genetic influence ranging from 45% to 65% (see van Grootheest et al. 2005). In addition, Noh et al. (2017) were able to identify four gene variants (*NRXN1*, *HTR2A*, *CTTNBP2*, and *REEP3*) that disrupt synapse development and interfere with neural pathways in the cortico-striatal loop, affecting serotonin and glutamate regulation, increasing the risk for OCD.

Psychoanalytic explanations

Freud (1922) considered OCD to result from the individual's fear of their id impulses and their use of **ego** defence mechanisms to reduce this anxiety. This 'battle' between the two opposing forces is not played out in the unconscious. Instead, it involves explicit and dramatic thoughts and actions. The id impulses are typically evident through obsessive thoughts, while the compulsions are the result of ego defences. Two ego defence mechanisms are particularly common in OCD: undoing and reaction formation. *Undoing* involves overt behaviours designed to counter the feared outcome, such as washing to avoid contamination. *Reaction formation* involves the adoption of behaviours diametrically opposed to the unacceptable impulses. The compulsively clean individual, for example, may experience strong 'inappropriate' sexual compulsions that are countered by their cleanliness and orderliness.

The origins of OCD lie in difficulties associated with the anal phase of development. Freud suggested that children in this stage gain gratification through their bowel movements. If their parents prohibit or curb this pleasure through, for example, over-zealous potty training, this may result in a state of anger and aggressive id impulses expressed through soiling or other destructive behaviour. If the parents respond to this with further pressure, and if they embarrass the child in attempts to encourage toilet training, the child may feel shame and guilt as a consequence of their behaviour. So, the pleasure of the id begins to compete with the control of the ego. If this continues, the child may become fixated in this stage and develop an obsessive personality. Traumas experienced in adulthood may result in a regression to this stage if the passage through it is incomplete.

Not all psychodynamic theories are in agreement with Freud, although all agree that OCD involves competition between aggressive impulses and attempts at controlling them. Kleinian analysts suggest that as a consequence of stress some individuals may lose the ability to see both good and bad in the same object. Rather, they consider it to be either good *or* bad: there is a *splitting* of good and bad with no shades of feelings in between. Obsessive-compulsive disorders arise where the individual protects themselves against these 'bad' thoughts that would make them a 'bad' person through the use of obsessional behaviours.

Behavioural explanations

The behavioural model of OCD is based on the two-process model of Mowrer (1947): fear of specific stimuli is acquired through classical conditioning and maintained by operant processes. What differentiates OCD from phobic or panic disorders is that anxiety arises in conditions from which the individual cannot easily escape. As a result, reductions of distress are achieved by engaging in covert or overt ritual or obsessive behaviours the individual believes will counteract the obsession. These form escape or avoidant behaviours, and reduce anxiety in the short term. However, they maintain longer-term anxiety and avoidant behaviour, as the affected individual fails to learn that no harm will occur in their absence. The individual also attempts to prevent initial contact with a feared stimulus.

Cognitive explanations

Salkovskis's cognitive model (Salkovskis and Kirk 1997) identifies obsessions as intrusive cognitions which the individual interprets as indicating they may be responsible for harm to themselves or others unless they take some form of preventive action. This belief leads to a state of fear or distress which the individual tries to reduce by: (i) trying to suppress these thoughts, and (ii) taking actions intended to reduce their responsibility for any negative outcomes – so-called safety behaviours. Typically, these beliefs place significant responsibility on the individual, more so than on others: 'I know that if I don't wash my hands, I will spread contamination – if *you* don't wash your hands, this is less likely (and I don't care)'.

Unfortunately, attempts at suppression of intrusive thoughts can, paradoxically, make them more frequent and salient. Salkovskis and Kirk (1997), for example, reported a series of single case studies in which people with OCD used a diary to record the frequency of intrusive thoughts on alternate days in which they either attempted to suppress their thoughts or not. They found a clear difference in the number of intrusive thoughts during each phase of the study: during 'suppression' days, levels of intrusive thoughts were about double the rate reported on non-suppression days. The failure to suppress obsessive thoughts can lead to other safety behaviours, including:

- *Compulsive behaviour*: such as excessive washing to remove the threat of contamination, ritual or repeated checking.
- *Neutralization*: a cognitive equivalent of compulsive behaviour. This can involve thinking a thought to counter the original thought. Thoughts related to evil or harm may be countered by repeating phrases such as 'Jesus cares for me' several times.
- *Avoiding situations*: related to the obsessional thoughts.
- *Seeking reassurance*: repeatedly asking for reassurance that the feared outcome will not happen.
- *Diluting or sharing responsibility*: asking others to take some responsibility for an action, or provide reassurance that the individual is not fully responsible for potential harm to others.

Engaging in these strategies may reduce anxiety in the short term, as the individual feels relief once they have occurred. Unfortunately, they maintain long-term anxiety, because the individual never experiences the lack of harm in their absence. They therefore cannot learn or gain confidence that not using them will not result in harm,

In his metacognitive, S-REF model (see Chapter 3), Wells (2000) argued that OCD is driven by the individual's beliefs about the nature of their beliefs – their metacognitive beliefs. According to Wells, people with OCD often blur the boundaries between thoughts and reality. They may believe, for example, that having a thought about an event will make that event happen ('If I think of the devil, the devil will appear') or that thinking about an event in the past must mean that it actually happened ('If I think I have abused her, I probably have'). The metacognitive model identified three types of fusion beliefs:

- *Thought–event fusion*: the belief that having a thought means an event has happened, will happen, or will make an event happen
- *Thought–action fusion*: the belief that thoughts will lead to uncontrollable engagement in unwanted actions
- *Thought–object fusion*: the belief that thoughts, feelings, and memories can be transferred into objects and/or 'caught' from objects.

These types of beliefs, combined with the meta-belief that behavioural or cognitive rituals may prevent harm arising from any potentially damaging thought fusion, lead to OCD. In a study comparing the Wells and Salkovskis models, Myers and Wells (2005) examined the relationship between responsibility, metacognitions, thought fusion, and various measures of OCD in a non-clinical sample. Their results indicated a clear association between levels of obsessive-compulsive symptoms and cognitions related to perceived responsibility (Salkovskis model). However, in their multivariate analysis, after controlling for metacognitive beliefs, the relationship between responsibility and obsessive-compulsive traits was no longer statistically significant. From these data they argued that the metacognitive model was a better explanation of obsessive-compulsive symptoms than the responsibility model.

Treatment of OCD

Behavioural and cognitive behavioural approaches

Behavioural treatment of OCD typically involves exposure and response prevention. In this, the individual is exposed to their feared stimulus, frequently in a graded manner, and then helped to prevent avoidance through their use of escape rituals: 'contaminating' hands and not washing them, and so on. This is thought to extinguish the fear response as the individual learns the lack of association between the occurrence of harm-related thoughts and any of the expected negative consequences. Relaxation may also be taught to help people cope with the high levels of physiological arousal associated with the fear response.

Many clinical studies using this approach achieved moderate success, although complete remission was achieved by less than half of those who engaged in such programmes (Salkovskis and Kirk 1997). Behavioural treatments were also difficult to apply to people who ruminated or who had no ritualistic behaviour, and treatment refusal and dropping out were relatively common. Accordingly, as models of the disorder have evolved, so have the treatment programmes, which now focus increasingly on the cognitive factors that maintain the disorder.

The cognitive approach still involves exposure to a feared stimulus and response prevention, which is seen as a central element to any intervention. However, these procedures are augmented by a number of cognitive strategies, including:

- challenging inappropriate thoughts
- mind experiments
- behavioural hypothesis-testing.

Mind experiments allow the individual to test the validity of their expectations, particularly focusing on the threat associated with their thoughts. Someone who is frightened that their thoughts may kill someone, for example, may be encouraged to test the reality of this assumption by a mind experiment in which the therapist and then **client** test out this assumption by thinking the feared thoughts – hopefully with no negative effects!

Unfortunately, although cognitive behavioural interventions are consistently better than no intervention or treatment as usual (Gava et al. 2007), comparisons between behavioural and cognitive approaches have failed to consistently identify whether one is better than the other (Siev and Chambless 2007). Around one-third of recipients fail to benefit significantly from either approach. Some recent studies have focused on this group of non-responders, exploring whether mindfulness can provide a different and more effective intervention for them. In one such study, Key et al. (2017) found participants who took part in a mindfulness intervention following unsuccessful CBT were more skilled in the use of mindfulness skills relative to a no (additional) treatment condition and achieved significant gains on measures of obsessive beliefs as well as OCD and other anxiety-related symptoms. In a more stringent comparison, Külz et al. (2019) compared a similar intervention with an active psychoeducational intervention. Both interventions achieved benefits of a similar magnitude some 6 months after the end of therapy, although the mindfulness group appeared to have achieved them more quickly.

Research box 5

Külz, A.K., Landmann, S., Cludius, B. et al. (2019) Mindfulness-based cognitive therapy (MBCT) in patients with obsessive-compulsive disorder (OCD) and residual symptoms after cognitive behavioral therapy (CBT): a randomized controlled trial, *European Archives of Psychiatry and Clinical Neuroscience*, 269: 223–33.

Up to a third of people with OCD treated with CBT fail to benefit significantly, and provide a challenge to therapists. Given the different mechanisms through which mindfulness and CBT influence outcomes, there are grounds to hypothesize that the two approaches may be synergistic and if one approach is unsuccessful, people with OCD may still benefit from the alternative. There is also encouraging work from people with depression, where mindfulness has been shown to reduce the risk of relapse after treatment with CBT. With this in mind, this study identified people who failed to benefit from CBT and explored whether subsequent treatment with mindfulness would be of benefit.

Method

Participants

Participants were 125 individuals recruited from the **primary care** system and newspaper adverts. They were accepted into the study if: (i) they met the DSM-5 criteria for a primary diagnosis of OCD based on their score on the Yale-Brown Obsessive Compulsive (Y-BOC) Scale and its related interview; (ii) they were aged between 18 and 70 years; and (iii) they had completed at least 20 sessions of CBT in the previous 3 years with at best 6 months of temporary remission. Exclusion criteria were: (i) a recent episode of severe depression or **psychosis**; (ii) a range of diagnoses including borderline personality disorder or autistic spectrum disorder; and (iii) having recently (within 12 weeks) started either pharmacological or alternative psychological treatments.

Interventions

Participants were randomly allocated to either mindfulness-based cognitive therapy (MBCT) or a psychoeducational group (OCD-EP). Both involved eight group sessions, each involving 120 minutes of therapist contact, followed by two booster sessions at 3- and 6-month follow-ups. MBCT comprised the teaching and practice of mindfulness (see Chapter 3 for details). OCD-EP comprised a series of presentations and education about the aetiology, mechanisms, and maintaince factors in OCD, including metacognitive and neurobiological perspectives, existing pharmacotherapy and psychological interventions, and relapse prevention.

Intervention sessions were videotaped to allow checks of adherence to the differing treatment protocols and supervision of therapists. Each intervention was provided by experienced clinical psychologists with specific training in MBCT or advanced training in CBT.

Outcome measures

Outcome measures included the following and were taken prior to and after therapy and at 6-month follow-up:

- *OCD* was measured using the Y-BOC, which is an interview-based questionnaire with a final diagnosis based on the questionnaire score and clinician judgement. Participants were considered to have 'improved' if their score was reduced by at least 35% together with a clinical global impression score of 1 ('very much improved') or 2 ('much improved'). A partial response was defined as 25–35% improvement in the Y-BOCS-score plus a clinical global impression score of at least 3 ('minimally improved'). Assessments were conducted by trained raters, blind to the treatment condition. A self-report assessment of OCD symptoms was measured by the revised Obsessive-Compulsive Inventory (OCI-R). Meta-cognitions (beliefs about beliefs, including issues such as controllability and danger associated with beliefs) were measured using the Meta-Cognitions Questionnaire (MCQ). Finally, dysfunctional obsessive beliefs were measured by the Obsessive Beliefs Questionnaire (OBQ).
- *Depression* was measured using the Beck Depression Inventory (BDI).
- *Quality of life* was measured by the brief World Health Organization Quality of Life (WHOQoL) measure, a widely used and well-validated measure of overall quality of life.
- *Facets of mindfulness* were measured by the Kentucky Inventory of Mindfulness Skills (KIMS).

Results

No significant differences in demographic variables were observed between participants allocated to the MBCT ($N = 61$) or OCD-EP ($N = 64$) condition. The mean age of participants was 39 years, two-thirds (61.6%) of whom were women. They had experienced OCD for an average of 11.74 years. Participants in the OCD-EP condition did have significantly higher Y-BOCS scores than those in the MBCT condition (23.1 versus 20.8).

Table 1 shows the percentage of participants in each condition to achieve differing levels of recovery following the interventions. Fisher's exact test revealed a significant difference in outcome favouring the MBCT group at the end of therapy ($p < 0.02$), but this was no longer evident at follow-up. It is noteworthy that improvements on the Y-BOCS scale scores did not differ according to treatment condition, suggesting that these differences were largely due to the clinical impressions of improvement which form part of the Y-BOCS assessment process.

Table 1 Percentage of participants to achieve differing levels of improvement at two follow-up assessments

	MBCT-post	OCD-EP-post	MBCT-follow-up	OCD-EP-follow-up
Improved	21.3	12.5	31.2	23.4
Partial improvement	13.1	4.7	9.8	9.4
No change	65.6	82.8	59.0	67.2

Other key findings focused on differences between the two conditions rather than changes over time. These were analysed using analysis of covariance to partial out any differences on each measure at baseline. The findings were consistent in that participants in the MBCT condition saw greater improvements ($p < 0.02$) on the key OCD measures of the OCI-R, OBQ, and MCQ immediately post-treatment, but not at follow-up. A similar pattern of results was found for scores on the BDI, KIMS, and WHOQoL. Table 2 presents the data underpinning the OCD-measure related findings.

Table 2 Mean scores (and standard deviations) for each of the key OCD measures at each time point.

	Pre	Post	Follow-up	p-value post	p-value follow-up
Y-BOCS total					
MBCT	20.8 (6.5)	17.1 (7.4)	15.8 (7.8)	0.353	0.263
OCD-EP	23.1 (5.8)	20.1 (7.7)	18.6 (7.4)		
OCI-R				0.018	0.398
MBCT	24.8 (10.1)	22.1 (10.4)	21.4 (12.9)		
OCD-EP	26.3 (13.0)	26.1 (13.7)	24.4 (12.6)		
OBQ				0.018	0.184
MBCT	188.7 (51.4)	155.5 (57.6)	162.6 (64.1)		
OCD-EP	199.8 (44.7)	181.2 (45.9)	178.2 (50.1)		
MCQ				0.021	0.110
MBCT	73.5 (15.5)	64.4 (15.3)	65.0 (16.2)		
OCD-EP	74.4 (14.6)	69.8 (14.2)	68.7 (15.2)		

Note: The p-values reported are for the comparisons between each measure at each time point.

Discussion

The authors note this is the first study comparing MBCT with an active psychological intervention in the treatment of OCD. They note that both treatment approaches were highly acceptable and had fewer drop-outs than is usually reported (MBCT 6.6%, OCD-EP 9.4%). Despite this high retention, though, the outcomes were modest and limited to self-report measures. The authors speculate that this may reflect greater acceptance of OCD symptoms, and less of a struggle against them – an outcome more likely to be detected by the psychometric measures than the Y-BOCS. Overall, then, while the intervention proved modestly successful in a difficult-to-treat group, there was no clear evidence to justify the routine use of mindfulness-based interventions in this population.

Pharmacological interventions

Based on data from 11 randomized controlled trials, Hirschtritt et al. (2017) concluded there was strong evidence to support the use of SSRIs as a first-line treatment for OCD, although their effectiveness can now be usefully augmented by a range of additional approaches including antipsychotic medications where these prove less than optimally effective. Due to high levels of relapse following cessation of treatment, Greist et al. (2003) suggested that a 2-year active treatment phase was required for them to be maximally effective. One way this may be obviated is by combining pharmacological and psychological treatment approaches. Meng et al. (2019), for example, found a combination of CBT plus SSRI to be more effective that SSRIs alone. After 6 months of therapy, 83% of those in the combination intervention achieved a significant benefit, compared to 52% of those who only received SSRIs. In addition, Tolin et al. (2004) explored whether CBT may be beneficial to those who fail to respond to multiple medications. The intervention proved successful with 53% of participants achieving significant clinical gains, despite many being described as 'putting low effort into CBT'. So, a combined treatment approach may be maximally effective, although the indicators of need and ultimate benefits have yet to be fully understood.

Case formulation

Mr R was a 38-year-old gentleman referred to the Lancashire Clinical Psychology Services with a diagnosis of OCD. At the time of referral, he lived alone after the end of a long-term relationship. He lived in a flat, in which he restricted himself to three rooms as he considered the other rooms to be contaminated. He held down a job as an office manager, but found it increasingly difficult to do so, as his OCD was becoming increasingly difficult to hide and/or control. His fears related to what he considered to be symbols related to death or existential nothingness. These included a wide range of stimuli, including the numbers 3, 6, and 9 (or any combination of these), blank walls (symbolizing 'nothingness'), and people he associated with religions of various types. He attempted to avoid such stimuli by, for example, avoiding looking at car registration plates, not using supermarket aisles with the key numbers, avoiding purchases which included the key numbers, and avoiding looking at a particular white wall in the entrance to the school in which he worked. If he encountered any of these stimuli, he engaged in brief safety behaviours, which were wide-ranging and involved, for example, repetition of safe numbers and thinking about alternative 'safe' people. Most safety behaviours were relatively brief, although the high frequency with which they were elicited nevertheless made them extremely problematic. Others were more disruptive. He delayed purchasing food or items he would want to keep for a long time until the purchase date did not include a key number. Likewise, he would abandon purchases or leave them unused if the bill total included a key number. If he noted a car registration that included a key number before making any purchase, he would circle the shop twice in his car before parking.

Long-term antecedents

Mr R was an anxious child, and tended to be a worrier, although there was no particular focus to his worries. His mother, to whom he was very close, tended to be obsessive, to worry, and to fuss about a variety of things. He remained very close to his parents, eating most days with them and staying overnight in their house quite frequently. As an adult, he had left school and attended a local university. He established a number of friendships, although these were based around a pub and drinking culture. He enjoyed drinking, but restricted this to one or two days a week, and did not use it as a coping strategy to help him deal with his anxiety. He had had two long-term relationships, but both had eventually collapsed, partly due to his dissatisfaction with the relationship, partly because of his somewhat rigid lifestyle. Although not dominated by obsessive or compulsive behaviour, he nevertheless led an extremely ordered and rigid lifestyle.

Short-term antecedents

His disappointment with these relationships led him to seek counselling. During this process, he was hypnotized and encouraged to read books exploring the existential meaning of life. During one period of hypnosis he reported being terrified by an image of death and existential 'nothingness'. He was unable, or unwilling, to provide any detail on this experience, but it was clearly terrifying and triggered his present problems. He developed a strong fear of death and 'detachment from life' or 'existential nothingness', and sought to avoid symbols or other factors associated with these thoughts. Key triggers to thoughts of death or nothingness included key numbers, religious icons and individuals, and certain books. The latter were easy to avoid; the first two were more problematic.

Formulation

The acute fear Mr R experienced while hypnotized triggered a strong conditioned fear to a wide variety of symbolic objects – all of which represented death, separation of the self from others, and existential 'nothingness'. He experienced, in Wells' terms, thought–event fusion, in that he feared that the experience of having a thought linked to death or existential nothingness implied that he would experience either death or its associated 'nothingness' while alive. His fear failed to habituate as he consistently engaged in safety behaviours in response to these thoughts, and never allowed himself to experience that his fears were unfounded.

Intervention

Despite the wide-ranging and, to him, terrifying, nature of his concerns, Mr R was aware that his safety behaviours were irrational and inappropriate. He had good psychological insight, and was happy to follow a psychological treatment approach. In view of the frequency and number of triggers to his compulsive behaviour, this meant that a number of target obsessions/triggers were selected as therapeutic targets rather than trying to change his response to them all simultaneously. Accordingly, he developed a hierarchy of triggers to his fearful thoughts. Easy triggers to work on included a wall in his house adjacent to a house in which a Muslim lived, and a blank wall he passed as he entered and left his school. More difficult triggers included specific individuals who were associated in some way with his fears, including work colleagues and a previous girlfriend. The most difficult triggers were those involving numbers, with the greatest difficulty associated with purchasing food or long-term purchases from aisles 6 or 9 or with dates and prices including these numbers. Each week, Mr R elected to cut out the safety behaviour associated with one or two key triggers. In the sessions between these homework tasks, he developed cognitive challenges that he could use to challenge any fears he experienced if necessary and planned and rehearsed his response to each trigger. Due to the regularity with which he encountered many triggers, he did not deliberately seek out trigger situations, but learned to respond without safety behaviours in a somewhat *ad hoc* manner. Less frequent behaviours over which he had significant control and had consistently avoided, such as purchasing food at certain prices or using aisles in the supermarket were more planned. Over a period of several months, he achieved significant gains – albeit with some weeks in which progress was better than others – and was discharged after 12 treatment sessions.

6.6 Chapter summary

1. Specific phobias are an unrealistic fear of an identifiable stimulus.
2. Psychoanalytic models suggest that phobias result from anxiety impulses when id impulses are repressed.
3. Behavioural models consider them to stem from negative conditioning experiences.

4. Cognitive behavioural models consider the condition to arise from a variety of potential causes, including conditioning and vicarious learning, and to be moderated by factors including previous experience of the feared stimulus and the use of coping strategies.

5. Seligman argued that the potential to develop some phobias may be hard-wired into our brains – preparedness theory.

6. Phobias involve high levels of autonomic system arousal. As yet, there is little evidence of more general neurotransmitter dysregulation in the condition.

7. Behavioural or cognitive behavioural treatments appear to be the most effective treatments for the condition.

8. Generalized anxiety disorder (GAD) is an excessive, long-term, diffuse, and inappropriate anxiety.

9. Levels of GAD vary according to the social and economic stress across the population and time.

10. It is partly genetically mediated via the septo-hippocampal system and Papez circuit, in the behavioural inhibition system. Activity of this system is dependent on levels of norepinephrine, serotonin, and GABA.

11. Psychoanalytic explanations consider GAD to arise from excess punishment or protection during childhood. These lead to distorted id impulses or inadequate defence mechanisms.

12. Humanists consider GAD to be the result of a deviation from the pathway to **self-actualization** as a result of conditions of worth imposed by others distorting the idealized self, and then the actual self.

13. Cognitive models of GAD emphasize the role of worry and meta-worry in maintaining anxiety.

14. Pharmacological treatment may be equally or more effective than psychological therapies in the short term. Cognitive therapies are most effective in the long term.

15. Panic disorder occurs when an individual experiences repeated unexpected panic attacks.

16. It has a modest genetic heritability, and is mediated by high levels of norepinephrine and low levels of GABA.

17. Cognitive models provide an explanation of panic in the absence of obvious triggers: people with the condition experience catastrophic cognitions in response to internal, usually physiological, stimuli.

18. Cognitive behavioural interventions appear to be the most effective treatment for the disorder.

19. Obsessive-compulsive behaviour is the result of anxiety triggers the individual is unable to avoid.

20. Psychoanalytic theories and cognitive theories agree that compulsions form part of a repertoire of safety behaviours the individual uses to reduce the threat associated with the anxiety. They disagree about their nature and causes.

21. The symptoms of OCD appear to result from lowered serotonin levels and raised dopamine levels, affecting the functioning of areas of the frontal cortex and basal ganglia.

22. Cognitive behavioural therapy combining exposure/response prevention and cognitive restructuring may prove the most effective treatment for obsessive-compulsive disorder, although many people do not benefit from this or pharmacological therapy.
23. Relapse following the cessation of pharmacological therapy is common.

6.7 For discussion

1. Which strategies may increase or decrease levels of worry in GAD?
2. Which factors would indicate either psychological or pharmacological approaches being the treatment of choice in people with an anxiety condition?
3. Combining psychological and pharmacological treatments may sound an attractive idea. But what may be the pitfalls of this approach and how likely is this to be successful?
4. How important are cognitive processes in the development and treatment of anxiety disorders?
5. Should the various anxiety disorders be seen as differing presentations of common underlying psychological processes? Or are they, in fact, unrelated disorders?

6.8 Further reading

Butler, G., Fennell, M. and Hackmann, A. (2010) *Cognitive Behavioral Therapy for Anxiety Disorders*, New York: Guilford Press.

Forsyth, J.P. and Eifert, G.H. (2016) *The Mindfulness and Acceptance Workbook for Anxiety: A Guide to Breaking Free from Anxiety, Phobias, and Worry Using Acceptance and Commitment Therapy*, Oakland, CA: New Harbinger.

Perez-Edgar, K. and Fox, N. (eds.) (2018) *Behavioral Inhibition: Integrating Theory, Research, and Clinical Perspectives*, Cham: Springer.

Wells, A. (2007) *Cognitive Therapy of Anxiety Disorders: A Practical Guide*, Chichester: Wiley-Blackwell.

Winston, S.M. and Seif, M.N. (2017) *Overcoming Unwanted Intrusive Thoughts: A CBT-Based Guide to Getting Over Frightening, Obsessive, or Disturbing Thoughts*, Oakland, CA: New Harbinger.

7 Mood disorders

Depression is a significant symptom of mood disorders. What determines the differing diagnostic categories are the causes of depression and conditions with which it co-exists. Major depression is a condition in which the individual experiences a significant degree of impairment as a result of depression. Seasonal affective disorder is a seasonal condition, usually occurring only in winter. Finally, bipolar disorder is a condition in which the individual fluctuates between periods of profound depression and manic behaviour. The chapter also considers the causes of suicide (not all of which are associated with depression) and the treatment of people who have unsuccessfully attempted suicide. By the end of the chapter, you should have an understanding of:

- The nature and **aetiology** of depression, seasonal affective disorder, and bipolar disorder from a number of theoretical perspectives
- The causes of suicidal behaviour
- The types of interventions used to treat each disorder
- The relative effectiveness of each of these interventions.

7.1 Major depressive disorder

For a **DSM**-5 diagnosis of major depressive disorder, the individual must be experiencing five or more of the following symptoms during the same 2-week period and at least one of them should be either depressed mood or loss of interest or pleasure:

- Depressed mood most of the day, and nearly every day
- Markedly diminished interest or pleasure in all, or almost all, activities most of the day, and nearly every day
- Significant weight loss in the absence of dieting or weight gain (or decreased or increased appetite nearly every day)
- Slowing down of thought processes and reduction of physical movement
- Fatigue or loss of energy nearly every day
- Feelings of worthlessness or excessive or inappropriate guilt nearly every day
- Diminished ability to think or concentrate, or indecisiveness, nearly every day
- Recurrent thoughts of death or suicidal ideation without a specific plan, or a suicide attempt or a specific plan to die by suicide.

The symptoms must be sufficiently severe to cause clinically significant distress or impairment in social, occupational or other important areas of functioning.

People who are depressed are characterized by emotional, motivational, physiological, and cognitive problems. They feel low in mood and gain no pleasure from their usual activities. They are frequently unmotivated to take voluntary action, often spending a considerable amount of time in bed or withdrawing quietly from the company of others. They may be markedly slow in their activities or speech, with confused or slow thoughts, and have difficulties retaining information or solving problems They generally hold negative views about themselves and marked pessimism about the present and future. They may feel out of control and unable to change their situation. Some, but by no means all, will experience suicidal thoughts or actions.

About 7% of the population across the world are likely to become clinically depressed in any one year, and 11% will be depressed at some time in their life (Lim et al. 2018), with rates being significantly higher in women than in men. About a quarter of depressive episodes last less than one month. Between 25% and 30% of people remain depressed one year after onset, while nearly a quarter are depressed for up to 2 years. The typical age of onset of a first episode of depression is between the ages of 24 and 29. Although there is a debate concerning an 'epidemic' of mental health problems including depression across the world, a **meta-analysis** by Baxter et al. (2014) of over 100 epidemiological studies revealed substantial stability in the **prevalence** of depression between 1990 and 2010.

Aetiology of major depressive disorder

Biological mechanisms

Both norepinephrine and serotonin have been implicated in the aetiology of depression. It was initially thought that low levels of either **neurotransmitter** impacted on mood, particularly as drugs that increase serotonin levels appear to improve mood. This simple model is now being challenged by recent data. Rampello et al. (2000), for example, argued that mood is a consequence of an imbalance between several neurotransmitters, including serotonin, norepinephrine, dopamine, and acetylcholine. It is possible that serotonin provides overall control of a variety of brain systems, and that low serotonin levels disrupt activity within these systems, resulting in depression. Some have argued that the 'type' of depression may be a function of the relative dysfunction within these various neurotransmitters, with deficits in dopamine being associated with low motivation and **psychomotor** retardation, and deficits in serotonin linked to anxious depression (Dayan and Huys 2008) – which, incidentally, is why **SSRIs** are now frequently used in the treatment of a number of anxiety disorders.

Serotoninergic and dopaminergic pathways can be found throughout the brain, although the major brain area involved in depression is the limbic system and in particular the prefrontal cortex, amygdala, and hippocampus. An interesting, emerging, theory is that these pathways may be directly affected by inflammatory processes (Lotrich 2015). In what has been termed 'inflammatory cytokine-associated depression' (ICAD), cytokines (cells which modulate the activity of the immune system) may trigger an inflammatory response in the brain that disrupts serotonin activity, and hence other neurotransmitters, leading to the intriguing possibility of treating some types of depression with anti-inflammatory drugs (Kappelmann et al. 2018).

Although there have been some negative findings, there is increasing consensus that genetic factors influence risk for major depression, although risk translates to depression through interaction with environmental triggers (Beck 2008). McGuffin et al. (1996), for example, found that **monozygotic (MZ) twins** had a concordance rate of 46%, while that for **dizygotic (DZ) twins** was 20%. Genes thought to be implicated include those involved in the synthesis of serotonin from tryptophan and the transmission of serotonin at the synapse, including 5-HTTLPR, the serotonin transporter (*SLC6A4*), dopamine transmission (*DAT1* and *DRD4*), as well as norepinephrine metabolism (e.g. Lam et al. 2018; Zahavi et al. 2016). In addition to influencing risk for disease, genes may also influence the effectiveness of medication such as SSRIs used to treat depression (Tsai et al. 2009).

Socio-cultural factors

A number of social stresses have been shown to increase risk for depression, many of which may be established early in life. Childhood abuse and neglect are strongly predictive of adult depression, with rates of depression between three and four times higher among individuals abused as a child than those with less traumatic upbringings (MacMillan et al. 2001). It is noteworthy that the link between emotional abuse and depression is consistently stronger than that between either sexual or physical abuse and depression (Gibb et al. 2001). Abuse may increase risk through the experience of attachment anxiety in adulthood (Van Assche et al. 2020), as well as through negative self-schema established as a consequence of abuse.

More proximal stresses associated with adult depression include economic deprivation (Lorant et al. 2003), poor social and/or marital relationships (e.g. Werner-Seidler et al. 2017), and the discrimination associated with being a member of an ethnic minority (Ong et al. 2009). Elder abuse is a significant risk factor for depression among older people, although good social support can moderate its effects (Dong et al. 2010). Among older adults, illness may also contribute to the onset of depression. Tsai et al. (2005), for example, found that respiratory disease, poor cognitive function, a poor social support network, dissatisfaction with their living situation, perception of poor health status, and perceived income inadequacy were significant predictors of depressive symptoms in their sample of Taiwanese older adults. Unfortunately, the experience of stress and depression whether in childhood or adulthood is thought to sensitize the individual to future stressful situations, making them subsequently more vulnerable to depression in the future.

Explanations of why more women report depression than men vary. Initially dismissed as a reporting bias, there is now good evidence that there are real gender differences in the prevalence of depression (Weich et al. 1998). Social explanations of these phenomena suggest that women experience more role limitations and responsibilities than men. In particular, they tend to have lower-status jobs and have more **spillover** between work and home – that is, when they finish work, they are more likely than men to take on domestic roles and continue working. Girls may also be more vulnerable than boys during childhood. Other potential explanations, including that women experience higher rates of adverse life events than men, or are more vulnerable to adverse events and less able to cope with them, have not been supported (see Piccinelli and Wilkinson 2000).

Psychodynamic explanations

Freud ([1917] 1957) considered depression to be similar to grieving. During grieving, the individual regresses to the oral stage of development as a **defence mechanism** against overwhelming distress. This involves complete dependence on the loved one, as a consequence of which they merge their identity with them and symbolically regain the lost relationship. In addition, through a process known as introjection, they direct their feelings for the loved one onto themselves. These feelings may include anger as a result of unresolved conflicts. This reaction is generally short-lived, but can become pathological if the individual continues to introject their feelings in the long term, leading to self-hatred and depression.

Freud suggested that 'normal' depression results from an imagined or symbolic loss. Events are seen as somehow removing the love or esteem of important individuals, and the depressed person introjects their negative feelings towards the individual they consider to be rejecting them. Those most prone to depression are people who fail to effectively progress though the oral stage of development, because they are either gratified too much or too little at the time. Such people remain dependent on others for love and approval throughout their lives, and are susceptible to events that trigger anxieties or experiences of loss.

Behavioural explanations

Behavioural theories of depression focus on **operant conditioning** processes. Lewinsohn et al. (1979), for example, suggested that depression is the result of a low rate of positive social reinforcement. This leads to low mood and reductions in behaviour intended to gain social rewards. The individual withdraws from social contacts, an action that may result in short-term increases in social contact as they gain sympathy or attention as a result of their behaviour. This establishes a further reinforcement schedule, known as secondary gain, in which the individual is rewarded for their depressive behaviours. This phase, however, is usually followed by a reduction in attention (reducing the frequency of rewards available from the environment) and lowering of mood.

From behavioural to cognitive understandings

A shift from behavioural to cognitive models of depression is exemplified by changes made to Seligman's (1975) **learned helplessness** model of depression. Seligman initially considered depression to result from the individual becoming aware that they were unable to control their physical or social environment. The term 'learned helplessness' stemmed from animal experiments in which animals were typically kept in an area from which they could escape – by jumping over a low barrier, for example. Following a mild electric shock, the animals quickly learned to jump over the barrier to avoid further shocks. However, when they were prevented from doing so by being placed in a harness, they eventually stopped trying to avoid the shock even when the possibility of escape was open to them. They had learned that they could not avoid the shock and expressed their helplessness by inertia and not trying to change the situation. These 'symptoms' are similar to those of clinically depressed individuals, including lack of motivation, passivity, and disrupted learning.

Seligman's behavioural model of depression was subsequently revised in the late 1970s by Abramson et al. (1978), partly in response to the developing paradigm of cognitive psychology. The revised learned helplessness theory suggested that depression – or more accurately, hopelessness – was the result of three key attributional processes in response to both positive and negative events:

- *Internal/external*: did the outcome arise as a result of the person or the situation?
- *Stable/unstable*: will the result happen every time, or is it changeable or random?
- *Global/specific*: does the outcome occur in all situations, or only in specific instances?

According to the revised model, individuals prone to depression tend to view negative events or outcomes as internal, stable, and having global causes ('It's my fault, it will always go wrong … and this is just typical of my life'). By contrast, positive outcomes are attributed to external, unstable, specific causes: 'Things went well, but no thanks to me. It was down to luck and won't happen again'. That is, they have a negative attributional style. Abela and Seligman (2000) stated these attributions result in depression only if they produce a sense of hopelessness; that is, a belief that the individual has no response available to them that will alter their situation and that desirable outcomes will not occur.

A second cognitive model of depression provided a template for the first generation of cognitive therapy for a range of disorders. Beck (1997) argued that depression results from inaccurate cognitive responses to events that affect us. In depression, the immediate responses to such events are what Beck termed automatic negative thoughts. These seem immediate and valid and are often accepted as true. However, they systematically misinterpret events in ways that lead to depression. Errors that typify such thinking include overgeneralization, selective abstraction, and dichotomous thinking (see Table 7.1). They influence what Beck

Table 7.1 Some examples of Beck's depressogenic thinking errors

Absolutistic thinking	Thinking in 'all-or-nothing' terms: 'If I don't succeed in this task, I am an absolute failure. I am either the best teacher, or I am nothing ...'
Overgeneralization	Drawing a general (negative) conclusion on the basis of a single incident: 'That's it – I always fail at this sort of thing ... I can't do it!'
Personalization	Interpreting events as personal affronts or obstacles: 'Why do they always pick on ME ... even when I'm not to blame?'
Arbitrary inference	Drawing a conclusion without sufficient evidence to support it: 'They don't like me ... I could tell from the moment we met ...'
Selective abstraction	Focusing on an insignificant detail taken out of context: 'I thought my lecture went well. But that student who left early may have been unhappy with it. Perhaps the others were as well but didn't show it ...'

referred to as the *cognitive triad*: beliefs about our self, events or other people that affect us and our future.

According to Beck, our conscious thoughts are distorted by underlying depressogenic schemata (schema in the singular). These are unconscious underlying beliefs about ourselves and the world that influence conscious thought and are established during childhood. Negative events in childhood, such as parental rejection, establish negative **cognitive schemata** about the self and the world. For most of the time, these beliefs are not particularly salient, or else the individual would be chronically depressed. However, when we encounter stressful circumstances in adulthood, and particularly those that echo previous childhood experiences (divorce or separation, for example, reflecting earlier experiences of parental rejection), there is an initial lowering of mood, following which underlying negative schemata are activated, influencing our surface cognitions and leading to longer-term depression (see Figure 7.1).

There is good evidence that some negative schemata are more accessible at times of low mood than at other times. Others may remain salient throughout the life course (see discussion of schema models of personality disorder in Chapter 11). However, Meichenbaum (1985) challenged the notion that schemata are irrevocably established during childhood and argued that they may change as a consequence of events over the life course. Determining which explanation is right has proven extremely difficult. Clinical practice has shown that some negative schemata beginning in childhood endure over long periods and can be difficult to change. However, this does not necessarily reflect a childhood critical period. An alternative explanation may be that childhood beliefs are maintained because nothing happens to make the individual question their initial assumption. Indeed, their own behaviour may result in these beliefs being reinforced. A girl who does not believe that her parents love her, for example, may react against them and cause them to treat her more severely or rigidly than would otherwise have been the case, providing support for the initial belief. Over time, this belief and its associated behaviours may spill over to other relationships, resulting in relationship problems that continue for many years. Here, the schemata laid down in childhood are maintained in adulthood not because of a critical period,

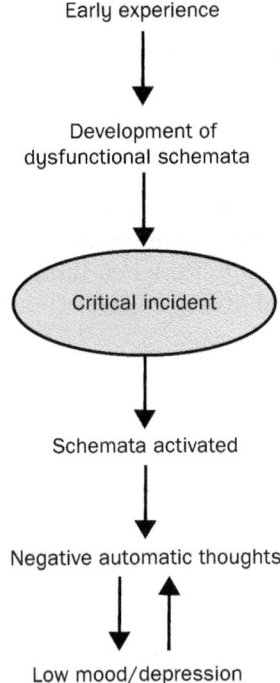

Early experience

Development of
dysfunctional schemata

Critical incident

Schemata activated

Negative automatic thoughts

Low mood/depression

Figure 7.1 Beck's developmental model of cognitive and behavioural precursors to depression

but because the woman's behaviour as an adult continued to elicit responses that reinforced her childhood beliefs.

There is a strong reciprocity between mood and cognition: negative cognitions lower mood, and low mood increases the salience of negative cognitions. However, there has been some debate as to whether cognitive distortions contribute to the *initiation* of episodes of depression or simply follow its onset, as theorized by Beck. This issue can be addressed experimentally using priming to compare the performance of non-depressed people who have or have not experienced a previous episode of depression; experimental procedures include attentional bias to negative words, rating positive and negative attributes as personally relevant, and recall of autobiographical memories. The hypothesis of such studies is that under neutral conditions the two groups would perform equally; however, following induction of low mood through processes such as listening to sad music, people who have experienced depression (and may therefore be considered to have depressogenic schema) would evidence a stronger bias towards negative beliefs/stimuli. In general, these hypotheses have been supported (Scher et al. 2005).

In a more naturalistic study of this process, Abela and D'Alessandro (2002) asked university applicants to complete measures of depressed mood and dysfunctional attitudes between 1 and 8 weeks before receiving their admissions decision. This measure was preceded by a priming task (completion of a questionnaire focusing on negative life events) designed to activate latent depressogenic schemata. Two months later, following the decision to accept or reject them from entry into the university, participants completed measures of depressed mood, negative views of the self, and negative views of the future. Consistent with Beck's theory, dysfunctional attitudes at baseline predicted negative mood immediately following a 'reject' decision. Evidence of the rigidity of such thinking can be found in the work of Deveney and Deldin (2006), who experimentally evoked either positive or negative mood in people with major depressive disorder and non-depressed controls. Following mood induction, the control group evidenced less cognitive flexibility when the trigger evoked positive emotional change, while the depressed group was less flexible following induction of negative mood.

Research box 6

Shensa, A., Escobar-Viera, C.G., Sidani, J.E. et al. (2017) Problematic social media use and depressive symptoms among U.S. young adults: a nationally-representative study, *Social Science and Medicine*, 182: 150–57.

Although the use of social media brings many benefits, it also can have its disadvantages. A recent meta-analysis by Yoon et al. (2019), for example, found greater use of social networking sites and higher levels of checking to be associated with higher levels of depression. Similarly, greater upward social comparisons were linked to depression. Accordingly, it may not be the use of social media *per se* that causes depression, but the repeated checking of social media posts. The study reported here explored this issue, distinguishing between what the authors termed 'problematic social media use' and social media use in general. Their definition of problematic social media use comes close to that of an 'addiction' (see Chapter 16): an excessive concern about social media, driven by a strong motivation to use social media, and the devotion of so much time and effort to social media use that it impairs other social activities, studies/job, interpersonal relationships, and/or psychological health and well-being.

Method

Participants

The study involved a representative population survey of US adults aged between 19 and 32 years. The sample was drawn from a previously constructed nationwide research panel of over 55,000 members who had indicated a willingness to be involved in research. The present study involved 3,048 panel members who had completed a baseline survey 18 months previously. A total of 1,796 (59%) completed this second survey. The majority were white (57.3%), in a committed relationship (55.6%), with a yearly household income of $30,000 or above (75.3%), and at least some college level education (64.4%). Forty-four per cent reported problematic social media use.

Measures

- *Depression* was measured using the 4-item Patient-Reported Outcomes Measurement System (PROMIS) depression scale for adults., which although brief has been validated against longer measures including the Beck Depression Inventory (BDI).
- *Problematic social media use* (PSMU) was measured using questions adapted from the Bergen Facebook Addiction Scale (BFAS). It has six items: (i) Spent a lot of time thinking about SM or planned use of SM?, (ii) Felt an urge to use SM more and more?, (iii) Used SM in order to forget about personal problems?, (iv) Tried to cut down on the use of SM without success?, (v) Become restless or troubled if you have been prohibited from using SM?, and (vi) Used SM so much that it has had a negative impact on your job/studies?
- *Social media use (SMU)* was measured using an open rating of hours/minutes (excluding work) spent on social media per day. Frequency of use of 11 social media platforms was assessed with a scale anchored by 'I don't use this platform' and 'More than 5 times a day'. Scale frequency scores ranging from 0 to 385 were derived from these reports.

Socio-demographic measures included age, race/ethnicity, relationship status, living situation (with parents, etc.), education level, and household income.

Results

Owing to the skewed nature of some of their data, the plan to conduct a linear regression to identify independent predictors of PROMIS depression scores was deemed inappropriate. They replaced this with ordinal regression, which is the optimal analysis to predict categorical variables. To do this, participants were identified as a 'case' for depression if they achieved a score on the PROMIS indicating a 'moderate' (a score of 5–10) or 'severe' (11–20) degree of depression or as a non-case. Logistic regression was then used to determine the association between each predictor variable and the assignment of participants at each level of caseness. The data are reported as odds ratios, with an odds ratio of 1 indicating that the variable does not discriminate between differing levels of caseness and non-case. Odds ratios >1 indicate an increased likelihood of the variable predicting being in one of the 'case' groups, and an odds ratio <1 indicating a decreased likelihood of this. Table 1 reports the bivariate odds ratios between depression and each of the measures of social media use. The first odds ratio (OR) column is the bivariate relationship. The second column, AOR (adjusted odds ratio), is the relationship after partialling out the influence of other confounding variables.

Table 1 Bivariate and multivariate associations between social media use and depressive symptoms

Measures	Depression category			
	OR [95% CI]	*p*-value	AOR [95% CI]	*p*-value
PSMU	1.11 [1.08, 1.15]	<0.001	1.09 [1.05, 1.13]	<0.001
SMU time	1.00 [1.00, 1.00]	<0.001	1.00 [0.999, 1.001]	0.43
SMU frequency	1.01 [1.01, 1.01]	<0.001	1.01 [1.00, 1.01]	<0.001

Put another way, these data indicate a 9% increase in risk for being a depression 'case' if participants are identified as engaging in problematic social media use. This compares with a 1% increase in risk for individuals who frequently check social media, and no additional risk for time spent on social media. Of the other variables measured, the only other significant predictor was household income, with higher levels of income linked to lower levels of depression (e.g. household income >$75,000 versus <$30,000: AOR: 0.55 [0.37, 0.81]).

Discussion

The results of the study indicate a high level of problematic use of social media among young adults: 44% reported some level of problematic use. In addition, the authors found that time spent on social media is not independently linked to depression; however, the degree of problematic use and also frequency of checking were. The latter may be considered a facet of problematic social media use. However, it also formed an independent predictor. It is possible to speculate that checking of social media use forms a precursor behaviour to problematic use and, as such, is an early risk behaviour. The authors note that the use of social media may indicate risk for depression rather than a single cause of depression. Individuals who engage in high levels of social media use may experience fewer face-to-face interactions and it may also facilitate more time spent in excessive (negative) self-comparison with others' idealized portrayals of themselves. An alternative explanation may be that depressed people engage more with social media as an easier way of social engagement than face-to-face communication.

Treatment of major depressive disorder

Biological interventions

There are now three types of antidepressant in general use that impact on serotonin levels: **tricylics**, SSRIs, and **SNRIs** (see Chapter 4). Other drugs, including those affecting the noradrenaline and dopamine pathways, are available but used less often (Dhillon et al. 2008). SSRIs have little therapeutic advantage over **tri-cyclics**, but are less likely to have side-effects such as blurred vision, drowsiness, and constipation, and as a consequence are tolerated better and less likely to be discontinued by those receiving them (Barbui et al. 2000). Gillman (2007) suggested that some SNRIs do not have sufficient biochemical impact on the noradrenergic system to effectively influence mood, and so their impact is likely to be no better than that of SSRIs, an argument consistent with the findings of a randomized controlled trial reported by Shelton et al. (2006), who found no clinical differences between an SSRI and SNRI. Interestingly, Herrera-Guzmán et al. (2009) found that although an SNRI proved no more effective in treating depression than an SSRI, it was more effective in one particular respect: it led to greater improvements in episodic and working memory.

Stop and think ...

Irving Kirsch researches the **placebo** effect. In his critique of the evaluation of all drugs, and in particular SSRIs, he argued that comparing the treatment of SSRIs with a no-treatment group means that any outcome is likely to be an effect of both the drug and a placebo effect. Higher-quality studies typically counter this weakness by comparing drugs, in this case an SSRI, with an inert copy of the drug – a placebo intervention. Any difference in effectiveness between the active and placebo drug, the pharmaceutical companies argue, is therefore attributable to the SSRI. On this basis, SSRIs are clearly more effective than placebo.

But, argued Kirsch, most people in drug trials can fairly quickly make a good guess whether they are taking the active or placebo drug, not because of its effectiveness but through the presence or absence of side-effects. A 'drug' with no side-effects is likely to be placebo. On this basis, trial participants and the doctors assessing their outcomes can often make a reasonable guess which condition the individual is in: an outcome that both diminishes the placebo effect and also the integrity of the research (the doctors making the assessment should be 'blind' to the treatment condition). The optimal placebo, Kirsch argued, is one that has side-effects similar to those of the drug itself. In the rare cases where this type of placebo is used, Kirsch notes the apparent benefits of SSRIs are almost nullified. To be fair to the argument, a number of commentators have questioned some of Kirsch's analyses and assumptions elsewhere in his book, but his basic premise appears sound and does question some of the assumptions made both in pharmaceutical and possibly psychological trial research. So, how do we optimally evaluate the effectiveness of specific forms of medication, and the specific psychological interventions that may be effective within the broad therapeutic approaches usually evaluated in psychological trials? It may appear easy, but it actually is more complicated!!

A more 'natural' remedy than SSRIs involves using extracts of the plant *Hypericum perforatum,* more popularly known as St. John's wort. Its mode of action is little understood, but it does seem to benefit those receiving it. Indeed, in a meta-analysis of its effectiveness and comparison with SSRIs, Cui and Zheng (2016) concluded that it was as effective as SSRIs, better tolerated by its recipients, and had fewer side-effects. That said, the drug does have some side-effects, including gastrointestinal discomfort, fatigue, dry mouth, dizziness, skin rash, and hypersensitivity to sunlight.

Electrical stimulation

The success of antidepressants in treating depression, and concern over their acceptability as a first-line treatment, have meant that ECT is increasingly used as a second-line treatment for 'treatment-resistant cases' – that is, those individuals who do not respond either to pharmacological or psychological interventions (see Chapter 4). ECT does appear to have some benefit, and given the lack of response to other treatments, any gains may be considered successful. For this reason, the UK NICE guidelines (NICE 2009a) recommend the use of ECT for people with 'severe depressive illness or catatonia, in whom an adequate trial of other treatment options has proven ineffective and/or when the condition is considered to be potentially life-threatening'. However, the guidelines also specifically state that ECT should only be used during the acute phase of any treatment and do not recommend its use over an extended period of time to maintain initial improvements in mood, despite some evidence of potential gain (e.g. Gagné et al. 2000).

More recently, there is an emerging and much less controversial treatment involving electrical stimulation of specific brain areas. Transcranial direct current stimulation (tDCS) is a minimally invasive form of brain stimulation that does not induce seizures and does not result in the profound side-effects associated with ECT. A weak direct electrical current is applied using two electrodes placed on the scalp focusing on specific brain areas: in the case of depression, typically the left and right dorsolateral prefrontal cortexes. Unfortunately, while this approach has proven beneficial, this is only at a level comparable with a low-dose SSRI in cases of mild-to-moderate depression that are not treatment-resistant (Brunoni et al. 2013), so it cannot be considered a replacement for ECT. See also discussion of transcranial magnetic stimulation in Chapter 4.

Psychological interventions

The seminal cognitive treatment of depression was developed by Beck (1976). Despite its name, cognitive therapy has its historical roots in the behavioural treatment of depression, and still maintains a strong behavioural element (see also discussion of cognitive therapy in Chapter 2). It typically involves several phases or strategies, including:

- *an education phase* in which the individual learns the relationships between cognitions, emotions, and behaviour
- *behavioural activation* and *pleasant event scheduling* to increase physiological arousal and engagement in functional, social, and other rewarding activities

- *cognitive rehearsal* to prepare participants to cope with behavioural hypothe-sis-testing or other situations that have previously been problematic
- *behavioural hypothesis testing* in which the individual deliberately tests the validity of their negative assumptions, in the hope of disproving them.

Despite Beck's emphasis on cognitive causes of depression, treatment may first involve increasing engagement in physical activities. For those who are profoundly depressed, this may involve planning times to get out of bed, go to the shops, and so on. For those who are less depressed, it may involve engaging in social or 'pleasant' activities. Cognitive factors are usually addressed only after the **client** has experi-enced some improvement in energy or mood. At this time, they are taught to identify the 'faulty thinking' that leads to low mood and to use **cognitive challenge** to counter it. In addition, the person is typically given homework to complete between sessions, usually involving some form of behavioural hypothesis-testing or practice in the use of new coping skills. Hypothesis-testing involves direct, behavioural chal-lenges of negative cognitions. Someone who is not sure they will be able to cope with a particular situation, for example, may be encouraged to enter the situation and try to cope with it. Such tasks should be selected with care. The therapist, at least, should be confident the client will be able to cope with the situation, as failure will reinforce negative expectations: the very thing the task was set up to disprove.

By the mid-1980s, the general consensus was that cognitive therapy was at least as effective as antidepressant therapy in the treatment of both moderate and severe depression. However, the publication of the results of a major trial chal-lenged this consensus. The National Institute of Mental Health (NIMH) Treatment of Depression Collaborative Research Program (Elkin et al. 1989) was a particu-larly important trial, as it was the first to compare two psychological treatments, cognitive therapy and **interpersonal psychotherapy (IPT)**, with both a tricylic and a placebo drug intervention. By the end of the 16-week treatment phase, all the active interventions appeared to be equally effective. Fifty-five per cent of participants in the IPT condition (originally considered to be a placebo interven-tion) were clinically 'improved', versus 57% in the active drug intervention, 51% in the cognitive therapy group, and 29% in the placebo group. That cognitive ther-apy proved significantly less effective than **pharmacotherapy** for severely depressed individuals, however, was of concern. It may be that this finding was specific to this study, as DeRubeis and colleagues' (1999) review of short-term outcomes for people with severe depression found cognitive therapy and pharma-cotherapy fared equally well. The evidence of effectiveness of IPT has subse-quently led it to be an empirically validated intervention in depression, and one that has been found consistently to be of similar effectiveness to cognitive therapy (e.g. Health Quality Ontario 2017).

The long-term results of the NIMH study were much more favourable to the psychological interventions (Shea et al. 1992) – and here may lie their advantage over pharmacological therapy. Relapse rates following discontinuation of drug therapy are often much higher than those following cognitive therapy, even when the initial treatment is successful. Hollon et al. (2005), for example, compared outcomes in three groups of patients over a period of one year. The first group comprised people who had been successfully treated with cognitive therapy, which was then discontinued. The second group comprised individuals successfully treated with medication, which was also discontinued. The final group comprised a group of people successfully treated with medication, which was then withdrawn and replaced with a placebo. Relapse rates in the following year were 31% following cessation of cognitive therapy, 76% of those who received neither medication nor placebo, and 47% among those who continued on placebo.

In an attempt to improve the still significant relapse rate following the cessation of CBT, Teasdale et al. (2000) implemented a programme of mindfulness (see Chapter 3) to teach participants coping skills to help them avoid relapse. A decade later, Kuyken et al. (2016) conducted a meta-analysis of nine studies utilising this approach, with over 1,250 participants. They found that people who received this intervention during full or partial remission were around 25% less likely to relapse in the year following treatment than those who did not receive it. Of note also is that mindfulness-based cognitive therapy (see Chapter 3) has proven an effective treatment for people who fail to improve following a course of antidepressant or psychological therapy and with a current episode of depression lasting at least one year – a chronic, difficult-to-treat population. Cladder-Micus et al. (2018) randomly allocated a group of such people to receive either (i) treatment as usual, which could have included health professional support, medication or psychological interventions provided routinely within the mental health services, or (ii) group sessions teaching mindfulness combined with usual care. By the end of therapy, those in the mindfulness condition achieved higher remission rates, lower levels of depressive rumination, and a higher quality of life. Of course, mindfulness is a central element of acceptance and commitment therapy (see Chapter 3), and direct comparisons of this wider approach with cognitive therapy show similar **effect sizes** (Öst 2014).

Case formulation

Mrs Jones was an extremely overweight woman who worked as a carer in a residential home for people with chronic illness (see also discussion of Mrs Jones' case in Chapter 3, Box 3.1). Some years before her referral, she had married a resident for whom she had cared who had multiple sclerosis. He had since died. Following his death, she experienced a significant period of depression and had taken long periods of time off work.

Long-term antecedents

Mrs Jones was an only child. She had been brought up in a small village in Gloucestershire. She had been sexually abused by a close friend of the family for 2–3 years from around the age of 6. She felt disgust at the abuser's behaviour, but also blamed herself for much of what happened. She believed she deserved to be abused because: (i) she was a bad person, since of all the people that he could have abused, he chose her and that must indicate that he saw something bad in her; (ii) her parents did not love her, because they did nothing to prevent the abuse;

and (iii) God did not love her. These beliefs were reinforced by the fact that occasionally her parents left her with the abuser while they went away on weekends.

Confirming her low self-esteem, Mrs Jones had not performed well at school, had a poor social life, and her relationship with her parents was poor. She did not have any boyfriends, and did not try to make herself attractive to men. She became significantly overweight, partly because she gained some pleasure from eating and partly because it made her unattractive to men.

Shorter-term antecedents

Mrs Jones met her husband-to-be while he was being cared for in a residential facility. At the time he was severely disabled by multiple sclerosis, and had a poor prognosis. As a consequence of their developing relationship, he left the home and they began living together, marrying soon after. Due to his physical infirmity, they did not have sexual relations. Indeed, she rapidly became his full-time carer, helping him to eat and drink as well as perform other basic biological functions. From her perspective, her husband provided company, and he could not leave her however unattractive she felt or how poor their relationship. And he was not a sexual threat. He provided a safe focus for her love, in that she was quite literally in control of their relationship. She perceived his death, therefore, not just as the loss of a loved one, but the loss of her feeling of safety in the world. She was unable to ask for support from her parents, whom she considered did not care for her, and the negative beliefs she held about herself came to the fore. By the time she was seen by a psychologist, she was withdrawn, disengaged from the world, spending most of her time alone in her house.

Formulation

Mrs Jones had chronic low self-esteem because of events that had occurred in her childhood, and her failure to challenge the basis of those beliefs. She felt unloved and did not love herself. She was frightened of sexual relationships, but nevertheless desired 'safe' relationships with men. The one, safe relationship with an adult she had achieved was not strong, but it had protected her against her negative self-beliefs and self-disgust. The loss of this relationship and of any support, combined with a reactivation of her negative beliefs about herself resulted in significant distress and depression.

Intervention

The enormous challenge for Mrs Jones was to confront her negative beliefs about herself, established in her childhood and reactivated following the death of her husband. These beliefs were not only depressogenic but also cut her off from her family at times when they may have been able to offer her support. These issues were addressed in therapy using the Socratic dialogue approach. One issue discussed in this context was Mrs Jones' belief that her parents knew she was being abused by her abuser, and chose to let it happen. The therapist and Mrs Jones examined the evidence related to this belief. One key issue was that Mrs Jones was occasionally left alone with the abuser. She took this as a clear sign that her parents both knew what was happening and condoned it. However, close questioning on this issue reminded Mrs Jones that she hadn't wanted her parents to worry about her or for her abuser to tell her parents what was occurring, so when he came to stay she had pretended to be looking forward to it and smiled and laughed while her parents were there. As a consequence, they could not have been aware of her concerns and distress. Through similar questioning, she began to believe that she was chosen not because of who she was, but because of her availability, that her parents were unaware of what was happening, and was less strong in her beliefs that she was a bad person and that (as a consequence) God did not love her. This recognition did not immediately transform Mrs Jones into a happy and carefree person. Nevertheless, she was able to establish a warmer and more loving relationship with her mother, and began to develop stronger acquaintanceships and then friendships with people she knew, including one man with whom she developed a strong, if non-sexual, relationship. Her mood lifted and she was able to return to work. She remained a vulnerable individual, but began to cope well with life.

7.2 Suicide

Only about half of people who die by suicide have an identified mental health problem, the most common being depression, substance-related disorders, and schizophrenia. Suicide and suicidal ideation have also been reported in people with a range of mental health problems (e.g. PTSD), as well as those affected by such issues as gender dysphoria and transition, chronic pain, and abortion. According to one of the methodologically stronger studies, around 8% of people who experience bipolar disorder will take their own life, with figures for depression of around 7% and for schizophrenia 5% (Nordentoft et al. 2011). Bronisch and Wittchen (1994) found that 56% of their sample of people with a diagnosis of depression reported thinking about death, 37% reported wishing to die, and 69% had suicidal ideas. García-Vega et al. (2018) reported that 48% of those attending a gender identity treatment clinic had reported some degree of suicidal ideation, and 23% had attempted suicide. Among the general population, suicide rates are less than 1% (Nordentoft et al. 2011), while around 8% report having suicidal ideas (Bronisch and Wittchen 1994). Among those who are depressed, suicide is more strongly associated with moderate than severe depression, as those who are severely depressed may lack the volition to act on their feelings. Indeed, some people kill themselves as their depression begins to lift because although they are still hopeless, they become more impulsive and motivated.

Aetiology of suicide

Socio-cultural factors

Suicide rates vary across countries. Russia, for example, has an annual rate as high as 26.5 per 100,000 people (down from 47.5 in 2000), while Greece has a rate of 3.8 per 100,000 (WHO 2017). Suicide rates are relatively low among people who are married or co-habiting, and higher among divorcees and social groups under particular pressure. Shahmanesh et al. (2009), for example, reported that 19% of sex workers in Goa had made at least one suicide attempt in the 3 months prior to their survey. This was linked to partner violence, violence from others, entrapment, and declining mental health. Social deprivation combined with easy access to alcohol contribute to the disturbingly high levels among native Americans and the indigenous peoples of Alaska (Jiang et al. 2015).

Men are more likely than women to die by suicide (by a ratio of around 5:1), with young men at particularly high risk. In the UK in 2016, there were 13.5 suicides per 100,000 men but in marked contrast 4.4 per 100,000 women (WHO 2017). Suicide is particularly prevalent among young people, and is the third leading cause of death among Americans aged 15–24 years (Anderson and Smith 2003). Young people may take their own life as a consequence of abuse, bullying, exam stress, and other problems in combination with catastrophic thinking, poor coping strategies, and limited social support. Gay, lesbian, and bisexual individuals are also at particular risk of suicide, with rates nearly two and a half times higher than among their heterosexual counterparts, and over four times higher among younger people (di Giacomo et al. 2018). Among older people, suicide may be attempted as a consequence of increasing disability: 44% of one sample of elderly people apparently took their own life to prevent being placed in a nursing home (Loebel et al. 1991). Suicide among those who have recently been bereaved is also frequent.

A more theoretical social model of suicide was developed by Durkheim ([1897] 1951), who identified three types of suicide: anomic, altruistic, and egoistic. According to Durkheim, *anomic suicide* occurs when the social structure in which an individual lives fails to provide them with sufficient support, leading to a loss of sense of belonging – a state known as anomie. High levels of anomie occur at times of both societal and personal change, including economic stress, immigration, and social unrest. *Altruistic suicide* occurs when an individual deliberately sacrifices him or herself for the well-being of others. Perhaps the clearest example of this can be found among suicide bombers who Grimland et al. (2006) argued are not suicidal in a despairing or negative sense, but see their behaviour as a glorious martyrdom, an act of war, bolstered by cultural and religious beliefs (and a period of indoctrination and preparation). Finally, *egoistic suicide* occurs among those not governed by the norms of society, who are outsiders or loners in a more permanent state of alienation than those who die by anomic suicide.

Psychoanalytic explanations

According to Freud ([1920] 1990), suicide represents a repressed wish to kill a lost love object, and is an act of revenge. Hendin (1992) identified a number of other **psychoanalytic** processes that may lead to suicide, including the idea of realizing a rebirth or reunion with a lost object, as well as self-punishment and atonement.

Cognitive explanations

The psychological characteristics of individuals who attempt suicide often involve feelings of hopelessness, worthlessness, guilt, despair, depressive **delusional** symptoms, inner restlessness, and agitation (Stewart et al. 2005). Individuals at risk are also likely to have pre-morbid characteristics including high levels of impulsivity, irritability, hostility, and a tendency to become aggressive, as well as a history of alcohol or drug abuse (Dumais et al. 2005). People with memory deficits and poor problem-solving skills (Arie et al. 2008) are also over-represented, perhaps reflecting a limited ability to solve problems while going through an acute life crisis or suffering from mental health problems.

A more elaborate cognitive model of suicide was developed by Rudd (2000), based on Beck's model of emotional disorders and his own clinical experience. According to Rudd, the components of the underlying cognitive triad are the *self* as worthless, unloved, incompetent, and helpless, *others* as rejecting, abusing, and judgemental, and the *future* as hopeless. In contrast to depression, where sadness predominates, the suicidal individual may experience a range of emotions including sadness, guilt, and anger. Thoughts may focus on revenge, but this will not lead directly to suicidal behaviour. Thoughts and emotions associated with suicide occur at the same time as high levels of physiological arousal and agitation: a profoundly depressed non-aroused individual will not have the motivation to attempt suicide. Risk of suicide varies over time, with periods of acute risk interspersed with lower levels of risk. High levels of risk occur when multiple risk factors converge. These may include situational stress, the activation of negative schemata, emotional confusion, and poor coping skills.

Rudd's model is entirely consistent with that of Beck (Wenzel and Beck 2008), which simply states that suicidal acts are predicted by three factors: dispositional vulnerability factors, cognitive processes associated with 'psychiatric disturbance', and cognitive processes associated with suicidal acts. In both cases, 'cognitive processes' embrace both cognitive content and cognitive processing, including attention and memory processes (much as the third-wave models considered in Chapter 3). Wenzel and Beck flesh out their theory, however, by considering a range of dispositional factors increasing risk for suicide, including:

1. Impulsivity when linked to expressed hostility and aggression in a concept they term 'disinhibitory psychopathology'
2. Poor problem-solving skills and an 'over-general' memory style that results in a failure to remember the specifics of personal memories when making judgements, and increased vulnerability to the belief that there is no escape from distress
3. A trait-like maladaptive cognitive style involving cognitive distortions such as dichotomous thinking, jumping to conclusions, and magnification.

A range of personality factors may also make someone more vulnerable to suicide, including perfectionism, neuroticism, and introversion.

Treatment of attempted suicide

It may seem obvious, but the simplest way to prevent suicide is to prohibit access to the means of doing so. Mann and Michel (2016), for example, found that in countries and states with differing laws on firearms, restricted access equates to lower levels of firearm-related suicides. The WHO (2012) supports this approach and has identified several other public health approaches, including enhancing social connections within society, gateways to support in institutions such as schools and workplaces, and adopting appropriate media reporting of suicides.

More therapeutic interventions involve working with individuals who have stated a clear intention to take their own life or have already made a suicide attempt. Clearly, such individuals may benefit from treatment of any underlying disorder. They may also benefit more directly from addressing factors that contributed to their suicide attempt. One way through which this can be achieved is by developing strategies to cope more effectively with the problems they face. The key elements of this approach include:

- both the person in crisis and therapist gaining a good understanding of the nature of the problems
- identifying in what ways the situation could be improved – the desired goal (such as better relationship with partner)
- identifying strategies by which any goals can be attained (talking more, going out together, and so on).

This approach can be used with couples or even families as well as individuals. A more 'crisis-focused' intervention known as Cognitive Reappraisal Intervention for Suicide Prevention (CRISP) has been developed by Kiosses et al. (2018). This is premised on the assumption that suicide is preceded by an overwhelming emotional crisis ('perfect storm'), which leads to suicidal ideation and an attempt at suicide. Therapy involves identifying the triggers to this crisis and providing strategies for dealing with it as well as challenging the suicidal ideation. As the name implies, cognitive reappraisal is central to the intervention, which involves a number of elements:

- *Education about the CRISP model*: identify links between triggers, emotions, and suicidal ideation and behaviours
- *Identification of situations/triggers, negative emotions, and thoughts*: triggers can be external or internal events, concerns, or problems
- *Examination of the utility of negative emotions*: exploration of the individual's motivation to change their negative mood states
- *Distancing from the emotional experience*: the therapist helps the individual to perceive a situation or the emotional experience from an objective point of view
- *Reappraisal of the emotional response to the trigger*: the therapist and individual work together to change the individual's perspective on the situation and to reduce their negative emotional response – a key question may be: 'is your emotional response proportionate to the situation?'

Evaluations of the effectiveness of these various approaches have generally supported their use. Indeed, in a meta-analysis of psychosocial interventions following suicide attempts, Van der Sande et al. (1997) found problem-focused and cognitive behavioural interventions were the only ones to prove effective in this

population. More recently, Calati and Courtet (2016) found that a range of psychotherapies, including CBT, dialectical behaviour therapy (see Chapter 11), cognitive
therapy, and IPT, reduced risk for suicide significantly more than 'treatment as
usual', although the absolute differences were relatively modest. They calculated
an overall risk for further suicide attempts in the intervention arms of the studies
they reviewed of 9.12%, and in the treatment as usual arms of 15.71%, a difference
of 6.59%. Attempts at providing interventions online have shown promise, with
ease of access being a key benefit, but there is not, as yet, sufficiently robust
evidence of effectiveness in these interventions to recommend their use (Stefanopoulou et al. 2020).

A second strand of research has focused on working with the family or partners left behind by people who die by suicide. For these individuals, there is evidence of some benefit of family therapy and bereavement groups. Linde et al.
(2017) were able to identify seven such studies in their systematic review. Interventions included bereavement support groups, cognitive behavioural interventions,
and a writing intervention, which involved writing about the emotions triggered
by the death. The authors concluded that despite the low methodological strength
of the studies, each appeared to be of some benefit, with bereavement groups
helping lower the intensity of uncomplicated grief, writing interventions lowering
suicide-specific aspects of grief, and CBT being particularly beneficial for people
who had high levels of suicidal ideation.

7.3 Seasonal affective disorder

Seasonal affective disorder was only recognized as a distinct disorder by Rosenthal and colleagues in the mid-1980s (Rosenthal et al. 1984). Despite its distinct
aetiology, considered below, DSM-5 now considers it to be a subcategory of major
depressive disorder: major depressive disorder with seasonal pattern (MDD-SP).
That is, it has the defining characteristics of depression, but these present only at
a specific time of year (e.g. autumn or winter) and full remission is seen at a characteristic time of year (e.g. spring). To be given a diagnosis of MDD-SP, an individual should demonstrate at least two episodes of depressive disturbance in the
previous two years, and seasonal episodes should substantially outnumber non-
seasonal episodes.

The primary characteristics of MDD-SP include increased appetite, weight,
and duration of sleep, as well as other depressive symptoms including sadness,
decreased activity, anxiety, work problems, decreased libido, and daytime tiredness (Magnusson and Partonen 2005). The depression is seldom severe enough to
require absence from work. Winter episodes typically begin in November and last
about 5 months. Age of onset is typically between 20 and 30 years, with women
most likely to be affected (Roecklein and Rohan 2005). It can be a chronically
recurring problem: up to 42% of people have recurring episodes for up to 11 years
following initial onset, some of which may occur in winter and some of which
may become non-seasonal (Thompson et al. 1995). National prevalence of
MDD-SP varies between <1% and >10% and is generally considered to be more
prevalent in countries furthest from the equator, which receive the least sunlight

in the winter, although this seems to hold more for US states than countries in Europe (Magnusson and Partonen 2010).

People whose symptoms are so severe that they receive a diagnosis of MDD-SP are a subset of a larger group of people who experience a variety of negative symptoms over the winter. Less dramatic seasonal changes in activity and weight occur within the general population. Terman (1988), for example, reported that 50% of the general population reported lowered energy levels, 47% reported increased weight, while 31% reported decreased social activity in the winter months. Twenty-five per cent reported that these changes were sufficient to signify a personal problem.

Aetiology of MDD-SP

Explanations for MDD-SP are almost uniquely biological.

Circadian hypothesis

According to the circadian hypothesis, the key to MDD-SP is a hormone known as melatonin. Release of melatonin from the pineal gland at the base of the brain is triggered by darkness, and it is found mainly in the midbrain and hypothalamus. It controls sleep and eating. In mammals that are living wild, the release of melatonin as the nights become longer reduces their activity, slows them down, and prepares them for winter rest or hibernation. Early melatonin models thought that MDD-SP resulted from an excess production or responsiveness to melatonin. However, evidence of differences in melatonin in people with and without MDD-SP have not proved conclusive. As a consequence, Lewy et al. (1998) suggested that rather than the *level* of melatonin being the determinant of mood, it is the times at which it is secreted that is important. They hypothesized that 'normal' depression can present due to poor sleep resulting from disruption of the circadian wake–sleep cycle. In the case of MDD-SP, changes in the times of dawn and dusk in the transition from summer to winter affect the time that melatonin is released, shifting the circadian rhythm of sleep, and disrupting its alignment with other biological rhythms. A number of studies have provided evidence of both advances and retreats in the release of melatonin in people experiencing MDD-SP. Lewy et al. (2006), for example, found that 71% of their sample began releasing melatonin later than a comparison group, while 29% released melatonin earlier than the population at large.

Light therapy trials (see below) have also provided an indirect test of the hypothesis. The goal of light therapy is to re-phase the wake–sleep cycle to that of the summer. According to Lewy and colleagues, this may be achieved through exposure to light early in the morning, which helps maintain the summer wake–sleep cycle and delays the secretion of melatonin until later in the day. This, together with earlier sleeping times in the evening, should prove an effective treatment for MDD-SP. Their own work supported this hypothesis, with findings that light therapy in the morning was more effective than if it was provided in the evening (Lewy et al. 1998). A second series of studies have directly tested the impact of light therapy on delayed melatonin release. Eastman et al. (1993), for example, found that following light therapy, 75% of recipients shifted their melatonin release to within the range of the typical population. Overall, it does appear that light therapy in the morning is effective and likely achieves its effects through the shifting of melatonin release (Rohan et al. 2009). However, the effectiveness of night or even midday light therapy, while less than morning therapy (38%, 32%, and 53% remission, respectively; Terman et al. 1989), suggests this may not be the only mechanism.

Serotonin hypothesis

A second hypothesis suggests that at least some of the mechanisms underlying MDD-SP may not be particular to this syndrome, and may be those that underpin other forms of depression. A number of factors tie serotonin to the aetiology of MDD-SP. Serotonin, which varies seasonally, is involved in the control of appetite and sleep, and is a precursor to melatonin. By reducing serotonin through the removal of one of its precursors (i.e. tryptophan) from the diet results in depressive symptoms during the summer in people who typically develop winter MDD-SP (Neumeister et al. 1997). Further evidence of a role for serotonin comes from treatment trials involving SSRIs. Both sertraline and fluoxetine have proven moderately effective in the treatment of MDD-SP. However, these are generally not as effective as light therapy (Partonen and Lonnqvist 1998) and work best with people who have not responded to light therapy (Pjerk et al. 2004), suggesting that while serotonin levels may be implicated in MDD-SP, they do not provide the entire picture. Interestingly, given the apparent different aetiology between non-seasonal depression and MDD-SP, while some biological studies have implicated genes related to serotonergic transmission in MDD-SP, these findings have been much less consistent than those linking them to major depressive disorder (Rohan et al. 2009). Genes that influence circadian rhythms have also been implicated, and may turn out to be the main controlling mechanism (Garbazza and Benedetti 2018).

A psychobiological model

Although the dominant models of MDD-SP are biological, people with MDD-SP have been found to differ from typical population controls and be similar to non-seasonal depressed individuals on a number of psychological variables, including dysfunctional attitudes and a negative attributional style (e.g. Hodges and Marks 1998). Rumination following the onset of MDD-SP and disengagement from pleasurable behaviours have also been found to be predictive of its severity (e.g. Young and Azam 2003). These and other data led Rohan (2008) to propose a psychobiological model in which individuals have two vulnerabilities: (i) a genetically mediated physiological vulnerability, including circadian rhythm dysregulation, and (ii) a psychological vulnerability that includes dysfunctional attitudes, rumination, negative attributional style, and behavioural disengagement which are triggered in the autumn in the expectation of emotional and behavioural difficulties during the winter. These combine to trigger and maintain an episode of MDD-SP, which lasts until the circadian rhythms once more become consistent with day–night hours and cognitive processes become more positive as summer approaches.

Treatment of MDD-SP

Biological interventions

The recognized treatment of MDD-SP is known as 'bright light' treatment, which lowers a person's melatonin. In this, the individual is typically exposed to high levels of artificial light, varying from 2,500 lux for a period of 2 hours to 10,000 lux for half an hour each day over a period of 1–3 weeks. For comparison, light in the house typically measures 100 lux or less. Outside lux levels vary between 2,000 lux or less on a rainy winter day to 10,000 lux in direct sunlight. Exposure is increasingly done in the morning to help shift individuals into an appropriate melatonin day–night rhythm.

These interventions have been shown to be effective. Sumaya et al. (2001) reported a trial in which depressed participants were subject to three conditions in a randomized order: (i) a therapeutic dose of 10,000 lux for 30 minutes daily for one week; (ii) a non-therapeutic dose of 300 lux over the same time period (placebo); and (iii) a no-treatment group. At the end of treatment, 50% of those receiving the therapeutic dose no longer met the criteria for depression. Levels of depression were unchanged in the non-therapeutic and no-treatment groups. Building on this success, more recent studies have tried to find the optimal wavelength of the light to improve mood. In one such study, Strong et al. (2009) compared the effects of short-wavelength light (blue light) with those of dim red LED lights. The blue light proved the more effective of the two. Despite these successes, not all studies have shown light therapy to be effective. Wileman et al. (2001) randomly allocated people with MDD-SP to either an active (4 weeks of 10,000 lux exposure) or what they considered to be a placebo (4 weeks of 300 lux) condition. At the end of treatment, 30% of those in the active treatment and 33% of those in the placebo treatment were no longer depressed; 63% of those in the active group and 57% of the placebo group showed 'significant' improvements. The authors took this to indicate either a high level of placebo response among people with MDD-SP, or that the threshold for light therapy was lower than initially thought.

More recently, a number of studies have explored whether light therapy may prevent future episodes in vulnerable individuals. However, in a recent Cochrane review, Forneris et al. (2019) concluded that just one of these studies met their criteria of methodological rigour. This study, by Meesters et al. (1999), found that both white and infrared light therapy reduced the risk for an episode of MDD-SP by around a third: 43% in the white light condition, 33% in the infrared condition, and 67% in the no-treatment control condition.

Although light therapy remains the pre-eminent treatment for MDD-SP, some people prefer to take medication. SSRIs result in greater improvement than placebos (Pjerk et al. 2005), have comparable effects to light therapy (Thaler et al. 2011), and achieve significant gains among people who have benefited little from light therapy (Pjerk et al. 2004).

Psychological interventions

Although the biological model of MDD-SP has largely driven biological treatments, the psychobiological model of Rohan allows the possibility of successful treatment using CBT approaches to change inappropriate cognitions and behaviours. And they do appear to be of benefit. Rohan et al. (2016), for example, compared long-term outcomes following either a 6-week CBT-based intervention or light therapy. In the year following treatment, both groups appeared to have benefited equally. At 2-year follow-up, those receiving light therapy were five times more likely to experience a further episode than those who received CBT.

7.4 Bipolar disorder

DSM-5 has a number of related diagnoses under the rubric of bipolar disorder. The main categories, however, are *bipolar I*, which involves episodes of severe mania and often, but not necessarily, depression; and *bipolar II*, which requires the occurrence of one or more episodes of major depressive disorder alternating with a less severe form of mania, known as hypomania:

- *Bipolar disorder I*: individuals typically experience alternating episodes of depression and mania, each lasting weeks or months. Some may experience several episodes of either mania or depression, separated by periods of 'normality'. Some people may swing between depression and mania in one day.
- *Bipolar disorder II*: depressive episodes predominate. The individual may swing between episodes of hypomania (an increase in activity over the normal, but not as excessive as mania) and severe depression. In addition, they will not experience an episode of mania.

The DSM criteria for a manic episode are:

- An episode of: (i) abnormal and persistently elevated, expansive or irritable mood, and (ii) abnormal and persistently increased goal-directed activity or energy. These should be evident for at least one week and be present most of the day or nearly every day.
- During these episodes, at least three of the following symptoms should be evident and represent a noticeable change from usual behaviour:
  - inflated self-esteem or grandiosity
  - decreased need for sleep (e.g. feeling rested after as little as 3 hours of sleep)
  - more talkative than usual or pressure to keep talking
  - flight of ideas or the experience of 'racing thoughts'
  - high levels of distractibility
  - increase in goal-directed activity or psychomotor agitation
  - excessive involvement in activities that have a high potential for problematic consequences (e.g. unrestrained spending sprees, sexual indiscretions).

Manic individuals move rapidly, talk rapidly and loudly, and their conversation is often filled with jokes and attempts at cleverness. Flamboyance is common. Their judgement is often poor, and they may engage in risky and other behaviours that they regret when less manic. They may also become extremely frustrated by the actions of others, whom they see as preventing them achieving their great plans. Of note is that while many people appear extremely happy while in a manic episode, this may not always be the case. The experience of Christina, who had experienced significant mood swings for many years, illustrates this. When she was in a manic phase, she typically wore livid-coloured clothes, used bright and excessive make-up, and was generally hyperactive, gregarious, and had difficulty in concentrating on one thing at a time. She looked like she was having fun. Talking to her about her experiences gave a different impression:

I know it looks like I'm having fun, being happy and all that. But it's not how I feel. I feel driven by things, it's like there's something in me driving me, making me do things wild. Like the make-up, it's all over my face, and I don't like it but I do it. I feel really down sometimes while I'm acting all manic. It's not like I choose to though, it's like it's happening despite how I feel – it's not happy. I really don't like it. And I don't like people around thinking I'm happy too ... it's really weird.

Between 1% and 2% of the adult population will experience bipolar disorder at any one time, with disorder I being slightly more prevalent (Clemente et al. 2015). While the overall prevalence among men and women is similar, women seem to have more depressive and fewer manic episodes than men and to cycle between these episodes more frequently (APA 2000). Episodes can last for many months, on average about 5 months for depression and 3 months for mania (Tondo et al. 2017). The first episode of bipolar disorder usually occurs between the ages of 20 and 30 years. Over half of those who have an initial episode of major depression and at least 80% of those who have an initial episode of mania will have one or more recurrences, and over 50% will experience this within the first year of the disorder (Yatham et al. 2009). The seriousness of the disorder tends to increase over time, although after about 10 years there may be a marked diminution in severity.

As with major depression, the prevalence of the condition differs according to social and cultural circumstances. Grant et al. (2005) found an overall prevalence within the US population of 2%. However, prevalence was higher among Native Americans, young adults, people who were living alone following separation or bereavement, and those in lower socio-economic groups. Prevalence was lowest among Asian and Hispanic peoples. Episodes can be triggered by negative life events and, depression in particular, maintained by low social and family support (Johnson et al. 2000).

Aetiology of bipolar disorder

Biological mechanisms

Given the role of serotonin and norepinephrine in depression, it would seem logical to assume that they also play a role in mania. However, the biological model that has emerged is not as simple as might have been expected. Data on norepinephrine

are consistent with a simple model of mood disorders. High levels of norepinephrine are typically associated with elevated mood and mania; low levels result in
depressed mood. No such relationship has been found for serotonin levels. Indeed,
mania has been associated with low levels of serotonin (Mahmood and Silverstone 2001), just as in depression. This finding is perhaps relevant to psychological studies that suggest manic behaviour may be somehow 'masking' depressed
mood. Data such as these led some researchers to suggest a *permissive theory
of bipolar disorder,* in which low serotonin levels permit the activity of norepinephrine to determine mood. Low serotonin combined with low norepinephrine
results in depression; when combined with high norepinephrine, it results in
mania. Dopamine has also been implicated, with a state of excess dopaminergic
activity in the ventral striatum and substantia nigra in mania reflecting a sensitivity to rewards. The role of dopamine in a depressed phase is less understood
(Ashok et al. 2017).

A second model of bipolar disorders moves from consideration of neurotransmitters to the electrical conduction of whole neurons. Two processes involved in
nerve transmission may be implicated: disturbances in activity of second messengers known as phosphoinositides, which instigate the firing of nerves including
those involved in moderating mood, and altered sodium and potassium activity in
the same neurons (see Chapter 4). In mania, second messenger activity or sodium
and potassium transport across the cell membrane may be excessive and result in
overactivity of the neuron system; in depression, there may be low activity in the
neurons (Lenox et al. 1998).

A third factor that may contribute to bipolar disorder involves actual damage
to the neurons. Sassi et al. (2005) found evidence of neuronal abnormalities in the
prefrontal cortex of young people with bipolar disorder, similar to those found
in adults with the disorder. Because this was observed in both groups, they
concluded that this damage was unlikely to represent long-term degenerative processes, and was more likely to reflect an underdevelopment of dendritic
connections and synaptic connections. Nugent et al. (2006) found evidence of
neuronal damage in adults in parts of the brain, including the amygdala and
hippocampus. These structures within the limbic system contribute to control
over emotions and emotional behaviour. They suggested that repeated stress and
elevated **glucocorticoid** secretion may have contributed to neuronal damage
and dysfunctional processing of these brain areas. The damage to these and other
neurons appears to lead to marked cognitive decrements in individuals with bipolar disorder, including deficits in **executive functioning** and verbal memory
(Sobczak et al. 2002). There may also be dysregulation of calcium activity within
neurones in the limbic system and frontal lobe, although any dysregulation
appears to be constant and does not vary according to the state of the individual
(Sigitova et al. 2017).

In MZ and DZ twins, concordance for bipolar disorder has been estimated to be
around 40% and 5–10%, respectively (Craddock and Jones 1999). Interestingly,
the key genes influencing risk for bipolar disorder may include those involved in
calcium regulation (e.g. *CACNA1C*; Harrison et al. 2018), although it seems that
any genetic risk is unlikely to be unique to bipolar disorder and may implicate
other disorders such as schizophrenia (O'Donovan and Owen 2016).

Psychoanalytic explanations

Psychoanalysts view mania as an extreme defence mechanism to counter unpleasant emotional states or unacceptable impulses. Katan (1953), for example, suggested that as periods of mania frequently follow states of depression, the conflict in mania may be of a similar nature to that in depression. People who pass from depression into mania maintain their preoccupation with a real or imagined loss. In the manic state, this anxiety is externalized. Aggressive drive is directed outwards, and the individual reacts to external objects in the same manner as introjection directs anger inwards in depression.

Cognitive models

The cognitive model of unipolar depression has been adapted to explain bipolar problems by two groups of researchers. Newman et al. (2002) suggested that schemata can act in a 'bidirectional' manner in people with bipolar disorder. A schema related to being loved, for example, may have two poles – 'I am totally unlovable' versus 'Everybody loves me'. Depending on mood and any relevant life events, both positive and negative, either one of these poles may be activated. A second cognitive model (Lam et al. 2003) suggests two key beliefs underpin the condition:

- The ability to achieve goals – 'If I try hard enough, I should be able to excel at anything I attempt'.
- A lack of dependence on others – 'I do not need the approval of other people to be happy'.

According to Lam et al., success in achieving goals leads to euphoria, and a positive feedback loop leading vulnerable individuals to continue trying to achieve new goals in an attempt to maintain or enhance the positive emotional state they have achieved through their initial success. In order to do so, their behaviour becomes increasingly goal-driven and the views of others are disregarded. Failure to achieve their goals results in low mood and a downward cycle of behaviour. Countering this model are the findings of Scott et al. (2000), who found people with bipolar disorder (while neither depressed nor manic) reported higher levels of interpersonal dependence and a stronger need for social approval than controls. Of course, it is possible that these needs differ at times of depression and mania.

As in the psychoanalytic models, a third cognitive model – that of Winters and Neale (1985) – suggests mania is a defence reaction against depression, and argues that a combination of low self-esteem and unrealistic standards of success may drive both depressive and manic episodes. According to Winters and Neale, when individuals with this constellation of cognitive schemata experience an adverse event, they experience either the emotions of depression and cognitions related to low self-esteem, or a defensive reaction against them, in which they adopt the *manic disguise* through which they report normal self-esteem levels. Why such individuals adopt differing strategies at different times is unclear. However, it may be a result of the acceptability of each response to those around the affected individual. Where the expression of negative emotions is unacceptable, they may adopt a manic coping style, which may be rewarded by continued or even increased social contact with important others. Despite this social reinforcement, however, the individual may eventually be unable to continue with these behaviours, and their depression may 'break through'. They then swing into a depressive episode.

In one of the few experimental tests of the manic defence hypothesis, Lyon et al. (1999) compared the attributions made by people with bipolar disorder who were either manic or depressed and 'typical' controls, in response to hypothetical positive and negative events. Both groups of people with bipolar disorder attributed personal responsibility for more negative events and for fewer positive events than those in the control group. By contrast, when asked to endorse a number of positive and negative attributes as descriptors of 'self', both controls and people with mania endorsed largely positive items. Those in the depressed group endorsed mostly negative items. On a subsequent memory test of these words, however, people who were both manic and depressed recalled more negative words than the normal controls. Lyon and colleagues took this pattern of results to indicate that while people with mania explicitly made positive attributions about themselves, underlying this was a set of negative beliefs about self: the manic defence.

Treatment of bipolar disorder

Lithium therapy

Standard antidepressants are typically not used in the treatment of bipolar disorder, as they may provoke rapid mood swings rather than stabilize mood (Keck et al. 2007) and evidence of their effectiveness is lacking (Pacchiarotti et al. 2013). Instead, lithium bicarbonate is the main treatment of choice to minimize mood swings. Lithium typically achieves this within 5–14 days in about 60% of cases, and has to be taken continually to minimize risk of the onset of depression or mania. Suppes et al. (1991) reported relapse rates 28 times higher among individuals who stopped taking lithium when not experiencing symptoms than those who continued its use. How it achieves these therapeutic gains is unclear. It may act on all three processes that appear to influence mood: increasing serotonin activity, regulating the activity of second messengers, and/or correcting sodium and potassium activity within the neuron (e.g. Huang et al. 2009).

Despite its therapeutic potential, the effectiveness of lithium in clinical practice has been less than was hoped for, possibly because of poor adherence to recommended treatment regimes. Around a quarter of people prescribed lithium stop taking it after a month (Kessing et al. 2007). Reasons for this include side-effects of weight gain, problems with coordination and tremor, excessive thirst, and memory disturbance. Psychological factors include a dislike of medication controlling mood, feeling well and seeing no need for medication, and missing the highs of hypomania. In addition, many users complain of a continuous 'damping down' of all emotions, which they find problematic. A further caution is that the window between ineffective and toxic doses of lithium is narrow. Too high a dose will result in lithium intoxication, the consequences of which include nausea, vomiting, tremors, kidney dysfunction and, potentially, death. Accordingly, levels of lithium have to be regularly monitored by blood testing, a further disincentive to adherence.

A final aspect of research into the effectiveness of lithium has revealed how a surprisingly large number of psychosocial factors moderate its effectiveness. Kleindienst et al. (2005) found that high social status, good family support, and adherence to taking the medication each contributed independently and positively to the effectiveness of lithium therapy. By contrast, living in a high expressed emotion environment (see Chapter 13), neurotic personality traits, and stressors including unemployment and other adverse life events, contributed to a poor response to lithium.

Cognitive behavioural approaches

The biological model of bipolar disorder has been dominant for some years, and it is only recently that attempts to change the course of the disorder using cognitive behavioural methods have been attempted, often in combination with some form of medication (Chiang et al. 2017). This approach does appear to be of benefit, with the meta-analysis by Chiang and colleagues of data from 19 randomized controlled trials showing modest but consistent gains, including lowered relapse rates (around half that of control groups) and improvements in symptoms of depression, mania severity, and psychosocial functioning following the use of CBT in bipolar I and bipolar II.

The main psychotherapeutic approach has involved the use of **psychoeducational** programmes to prepare people to cope with relapse. In one evaluation of this approach, Scott et al. (2001) randomly allocated people with bipolar disorder into treatment with lithium either alone or in combination with cognitive therapy. The cognitive therapy involved three elements:

- an educational phase to prepare people for the cognitive approach
- a focus on cognitive behavioural methods of symptom management, including establishing regular activity patterns and time management, as well as challenging dysfunctional thoughts
- anti-relapse techniques involving developing strategies for managing medication, coping strategies to deal with stress, or seeking help at times of the onset of signs of relapse.

Each intervention lasted 6 months. By this time, those in the combined intervention showed more improvements on measures of general functioning and depression than those in the drug treatment group. The data on relapse were equally impressive. Those who received the combined intervention were 60% less likely to relapse than those in the drug-only condition. Lam et al. (2003) also found that cognitive therapy plus drug therapy proved more effective than drug therapy alone. At one-year follow-up, those who received the additional intervention experienced fewer relapses and hospitalizations, with relapse rates of 44% in the cognitive therapy group and 75% in the drug-only group. Subsequent analysis showed a reduction of effect over time, with smaller (but still significant) gains maintained at 3-year follow-up (Lam et al. 2005). A further approach to working with individuals has involved the use of mindfulness, which has been shown to reduce anxiety and residual depressive symptoms between acute episodes over a short period (Salcedo et al. 2016). More studies are required to determine its impact on relapse rates.

A second therapeutic approach has involved working with families, based on research such as that by Kleindienst et al. (2005), who highlighted the role of family dynamics in relapse. Miklowitz et al. (2003) reported an intervention designed to improve communication, problem-solving, and coping strategies training within the family, comparing this with standard care and a brief two-session family intervention. At 2-year follow-up, those receiving the family therapy were less likely to experience a relapse than the standard care group (47% versus 71%). The benefits were greater for those living in a high expressed emotion environment. Rea et al. (2003) compared family and individual psychoeducational interventions and found that the family intervention was superior in the long term. Relapse rates were 60% among those who received the individual intervention and 28% of those who received the family intervention.

7.5 Chapter summary

1. Major depression involves significant psychological impairment lasting at least 2 weeks. About one-third of the people who become depressed will remain depressed one year later.
2. Genetic factors contribute to the risk of depression.
3. Serotonin dysregulation may result in depression as a result of a loss of control over a number of brain systems, including those mediated by norepinephrine and dopamine.
4. Socio-cultural explanations of depression focus on differences in stress and coping across social groups.
5. Psychodynamic explanations consider depression to result from the symbolic loss of love or esteem, and internalization of negative feelings towards the responsible person.
6. Behavioural theories suggest that depression is the result of a lack of social reinforcement.
7. Cognitive theories consider negative automatic thoughts and dysfunctional schemata to be causal.
8. Both pharmacological and cognitive interventions appear to be equally effective in the short-term treatment of depression. Cognitive interventions may be more effective in the long term. Mindfulness may provide an effective treatment for people with recurrent depression.
9. St. John's wort may prove an effective natural therapy.
10. ECT may be effective for some 'treatment-resistant cases', but 'maintenance ECT' remains controversial.
11. While individuals with serious mental health problems may be at increased risk of suicide, so are individuals without such disorders.
12. In adults, the primary trigger to a suicide attempt is interpersonal problems.
13. Freud considered suicide to be an attempt at revenge on a hated individual.
14. Cognitive explanations suggest that poor problem-solving skills and feelings of being worthless and rejected, combined with situational stress, emotional

confusion, and high levels of physiological arousal place an individual at risk of taking their own life.

15. Interventions that increase problem-solving skills appear to reduce the risk of suicide.
16. MDD-SP appears to result from disordered melatonin and circadian rhythms.
17. Bright light therapy appears to be the most effective treatment for MDD-SP.
18. Bipolar disorder is the result of neural mechanisms involved in the transmission of information along the neuronal axis.
19. Cognitive models provide a psychological explanation for the development of bipolar disorder.
20. The primary treatment of bipolar disorder involves lithium medication, although cognitive behavioural and family interventions also appear to be of significant benefit.

7.6 For discussion

1. Jacobson and Hollon (1996) argued that the short-term findings of the NIMH depression study were flawed as a result of the inexpert implementation of cognitive therapy. Given the spread, and possible dilution, of therapist skills away from centres of excellence, is this an argument for the use of pharmacological therapies over the psychotherapies?
2. Consider why the relapse rate among people with depression treated with antidepressants is significantly higher than that among people treated with cognitive therapy.
3. Should we be trying to treat bipolar disorder using psychological therapies if it is essentially a biological condition?
4. If MDD-SP has an aetiology involving melatonin and changes in light, why is it responsive to CBT?

7.7 Further reading

Bryan, C.J. and Rudd, D.M. (2018) *Brief Cognitive-Behavioral Therapy for Suicide Prevention*, New York: Guilford Press.

Chiang, K.J., Tsai, J.C., Liu, D. et al. (2017) Efficacy of cognitive-behavioral therapy in patients with bipolar disorder: a meta-analysis of randomized controlled trials, *PloS One*, 12: e0176849 [https://doi.org/10.1371/journal.pone.0176849].

Geddes, L. (2019) *Chasing the Sun: The New Science of Sunlight and How it Shapes Our Bodies and Minds*, London: Profile Books.

Kirsch, I. (2009) *The Emperor's New Drugs: Exploding the Antidepressant Myth*, London: Bodley Head.

Segal, Z., Williams, M. and Teasdale, J. (2018) *Mindfulness-Based Cognitive Therapy for Depression,* New York: Guilford Press.

Wells, D. (2011) *Metacognitive Therapy for Anxiety and Depression,* London: Guilford Press.

Zalsman, G., Hawton, K., Wasserman, D. et al. (2016) Suicide prevention strategies revisited: 10-year systematic review, *Lancet Psychiatry,* 3: 646–59.

Mind and body

This chapter explores some of the psychological conditions in which the relationship between psychological and physical processes is most apparent. At a quick glance, the first two, somatic symptom disorder and illness anxiety disorder, appear very similar as they both involve the reporting of inappropriately high levels of physical symptoms, and some clinicians have argued that they overlap in a number of ways. However, there are key differences between them. Somatic symptom disorder involves the experience and reporting of recurrent and frequently changing physical symptoms, which cannot be explained by any known medical condition and may raise some concern. Illness anxiety disorder is characterized by an excessive fear of illness and the belief that one has an undiagnosed physical disease. It may involve checking or seeking medical reassurance as a means of reducing fear.

The other two conditions are more easily distinguishable. The first, body dysmorphic disorder, involves an excessive dissatisfaction with one's body or particular body parts. Finally, the chapter examines one of the most intriguing psychosomatic conditions, conversion disorder (now known as functional neurological symptom disorder), in which an individual may develop extreme and disabling physical symptoms, such as paralysis or blindness, with no apparent physical cause. By the end of the chapter, you should have an understanding of:

• The nature and **aetiology** of each condition from a number of theoretical perspectives
• The types of interventions used to treat each disorder
• The relative effectiveness of each of these interventions.

8.1 Somatic symptom disorder

Somatic symptom disorder (SSD), previously known as somatoform disorder, is characterized by the experience of physical symptoms that cause distress in the absence of any known physical pathology. It is often accompanied by high levels of depression or anxiety (e.g. J. Wang et al. 2017). The **DSM**-5 criteria for the disorder are relatively simple but difficult to specify:

- One or more somatic symptoms that are distressing and result in significant disruption of daily life
- Excessive thoughts, feelings or behaviours related to somatic symptoms or associated health concerns, evidenced by:
  - disproportionate and persistent thoughts about the seriousness of these symptoms
  - persistently high levels of anxiety about health or symptoms
  - excessive time and energy devoted to these symptoms or health concerns.

An individual with the disorder typically makes repeated and frequent visits to their doctor complaining of a range of physical symptoms and is frequently referred to hospital consultants, partly to ensure there really is no organic cause for the symptoms but also, in many cases, to ease the pressure on family doctors to 'do something' about the symptoms the individual is experiencing. These may be diffuse, can cause considerable disability and distress, and include:

- *Gastrointestinal*: nausea, vomiting, abdominal pain
- *Sexual*: painful sensations, pain during sex
- *'Pseudoneurological'*: amnesia, difficulty swallowing, dizziness, difficulty walking
- *Pain*: diffuse pain throughout the body or limbs, headaches, 'pins and needles'
- *Heart and lungs*: difficulties breathing, palpitations, chest pain.

Most of us experience sensations or symptoms that are not related to an obvious illness at some time or other. Indeed, Hiller et al. (2006) reported that 82% of their general population sample had experienced such symptoms in the previous week. Symptom reporting was higher among women than men, people aged over 45 years, the less educated, those on a low household income, and rural dwellers. The most common symptoms included various types of pain, food intolerance, and 'sexual indifference'. This background of symptom reporting can make it difficult to determine the **prevalence** of clinically significant SSD within the general population, with reported rates varying between 1% and 7% (e.g. Creed and Barsky 2004; APA 2013). Among attenders of medical practitioners, rates are unsurprisingly much higher. Clarke et al. (2008), for example, estimated 20% of attenders of **primary care** physicians could be considered as having somatic complaints explained by 'psychological disturbance'. Cao et al. (2019) estimated prevalence of SSD to be high as 34% in a sample of Chinese out-patients, perhaps reflecting many Asian people's physical model of mental health problems (see Chapter 5).

Aetiology of SSD

Developmental models

Classic Freudian explanations focus on sudden, inexplicable presentations of physical symptoms – a functional disorder – and are considered later in the chapter. However, some post-Freudian analysts have considered the processes within SSD. According to Guthrie (1996), deficiencies early in the mother–child relationship leave the individual with an inability to use their imagination and the language to describe and control stress and distress. This results in a limited fantasy life, difficulties in processing emotional experiences, and a susceptibility to somatic complaints, and contributes to difficulties in developing appropriate relationships in adulthood. Any relationships the individual does develop are either chaotic or symbiotic. In the latter, they form a relationship with someone who adopts the role of carer – and they adopt the role of invalid. The physical symptoms they report therefore act both as a way of coping with intolerable emotional feelings and as a means of eliciting the care of their partner.

An alternative psychoanalytic understanding was proposed by Bucci (1997), who argued that as children we establish representations of events or 'objects' (such as people) across all modalities. These include memories of the event or object, their symbolic interpretations, and related somatic, emotional, and even motoric associations. According to Bucci, somatization occurs when dissociation arises within our emotional schema between the symbolic representation of objects and their associated somatic elements. As a consequence, the individual may experience significant emotional responses to particular individuals or situations, but not understand why these emotional responses occur or have the language to describe or resolve them. As an example of this process, an individual who was emotionally abused as a child by a parent may have experienced intense fear in the presence of that individual, but as they were totally dependent on them and could therefore not avoid them, the child could not develop appropriate links between feelings of fear, cognitive representations of fear, and behaviours typically associated with fear such as avoidance. In adulthood, interpersonal fear and discomfort is therefore felt at a somatic level only; unconnected to thoughts that would help make sense of these feelings. As a consequence, the individual cannot develop appropriate strategies to resolve the problems causing their fear, and continues to experience the somatic distress over a sustained period of time. This would eventually be interpreted as an illness or set of symptoms with no obvious psychological cause.

Other theories also implicate the role of childhood experiences in the development of SSD. A number of retrospective studies have found that adults who report high levels of somatic symptoms are more likely to have witnessed more illness, or complaints about illness, in family members than is the norm. In one study of this phenomenon, Craig et al. (2002) compared the (self-reported) history of three groups of women who were diagnosed to have SSD, had a long-term illness, or were healthy. Somatizing mothers were three times more likely than the other women to have witnessed a parent having a physical illness. The children of these somatizing mothers were, in turn, more likely to report health problems than were the children of the medically ill or healthy women, and had more consultations with family doctors. In a second study with the same women, Craig and his colleagues (2004) demonstrated the subtle way in which parents can focus on health-related issues. In this study, they observed the women playing with their 4–8-year-old children in a structured play setting. Somatizing mothers were less emotionally responsive and gave their children less attention than the other mothers during both play tasks. However, they were *more* responsive to their child than the other mothers when they played with a medical box. Integrating these various strands of evidence, Craig et al. (1993) suggested a two-stage process to the development of SSD:

- lack of care or neglect during childhood increases the risk of an emotional disorder such as anxiety or depression in adulthood
- high levels of illness behaviour among parents predispose children to interpret the emotional symptoms associated with mood states as indicative of physical illness.

More recent developmental theories have taken this basic premise and sought to develop it further. Central to these approaches is that people with these childhood experiences who go on to develop SSD may do so because of attachment insecurity, stemming from the maternal lack of sensitivity, which has been shown to predict anxiety, depression, and SSD (e.g. Maunder et al. 2017). According to Okur Güney et al. (2019), this lack of parental responsiveness may also contribute to a failure to learn effective emotional awareness and a lack of appropriate emotional regulation strategies, including understanding and reflecting on emotions, excessive autonomic responses to stress, and a rigidity of cognitive and behavioural responses that fail to adjust to any emotional experience. Thus, the individual is faced with poor emotional regulation and a tendency to somatize any distress experienced.

A psychobiological model

The simplest biological model of somatization suggests that people with the disorder have a biological sensitivity to physiological activity within the body, which they report as 'symptoms'. The biological pathways through which this may occur are not clear, and not all the evidence supports the notion of this hypersensitivity. Nevertheless, Rief et al. (2004) speculated that dysregulation of amino acids and serotonin may contribute to somatization. They compared levels of various amino acids including tryptophan (a precursor to serotonin) in patients with somatization disorder, with and without depression, and typical controls and found low levels of tryptophan were associated with high levels of somatization independently of the presence of depression. They took these data to suggest that the serotonergic system may be involved in a process of sensitization of neurons (including those in the muscles) that leads to a state of **hyperalgesia**, which forms the basis of chronic somatization.

A more complex model was developed by Rief and Barsky (2005), who noted that all our body organs continually produce sensory information that is forwarded to higher cortical structures. The healthy nervous system learns to filter out this 'sensory noise', preventing over-stimulation of the upper cortical structures with irrelevant information. We experience higher levels of physical sensations if this filtering process is distorted. Rief and Barsky contended that a number of physical and psychological factors can increase or decrease both the need for the filter to operate and its effectiveness. In their perception-filter model (see Figure 8.1), they highlight a number of factors that increase the physical signals, and thereby increase the risk of experiencing unexplained symptoms, including high levels of sympathetic activity, stress, and neural sensitization. Factors that decrease the effectiveness of the filter include high health anxiety, which may result in the individual interpreting any physical sensations in a catastrophizing manner. That is, they may misperceive body sensations as evidence of dangerous somatic processes. They also have an attentional bias to focus their attention on any sensations they experience and on previous memories of previous symptoms and medical explanations for them.

In an exploration of the latter process, Rief et al. (2006) asked people with SSD, people who were depressed, and healthy controls to listen to an audiotape providing three reports relating to a medical, social or 'neutral' situation. The medical report involved a person with abdominal pain visiting their doctor reporting the results of medical tests. After each report, participants rated the likelihood of a range of symptoms identified in the report indicating the presence of a serious illness. The people with SSD rated each symptom as more likely to be associated with a serious illness than either of the other two groups. They also rated more concern over the symptoms. Rief's model is consistent with the idea that stress or low mood can trigger somatic sensations which are difficult to control, are interpreted as symptoms of illness, and then trigger concerns about health, a focusing of attention onto the sensations, a lowering of the filter, and apparent confirmation of unexplained physical symptoms.

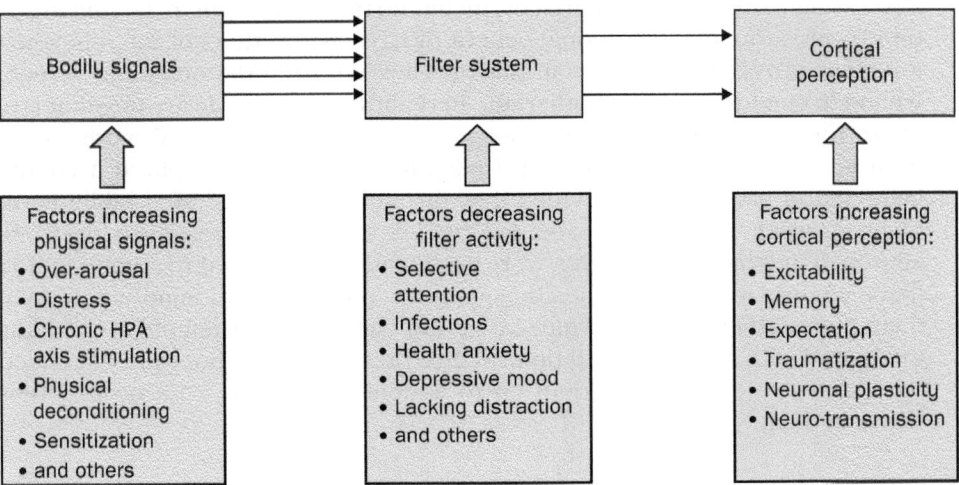

Figure 8.1 Rief and Barsky's (2005) perception-filter model. HPA, hypothalamic–pituitary–adrenal

Treatment of SSD

Pharmacological treatment

Although SSD may be treated using some form of antidepressant in clinical practice (Kurlansik and Maffei 2016), the evidence base for any such intervention is limited. A Cochrane review by Kleinstäuber et al. (2014), for example, considered evidence from 26 randomized controlled trials, many of which had 'serious shortcomings', of the use of a range of antidepressants, alone or in combination with antipsychotic medication, and found no benefit from the use of **tricyclics**, weak evidence for the use of **SSRIs** alone, and some additional benefit from combining SSRIs with antipsychotics. Overall, they concluded that there were no clear and reliable differences between active antidepressants and **placebo** interventions.

Psychological interventions

Unfortunately, relatively few studies have shown the effectiveness of psychological interventions in the treatment of SSD. The condition is often reported as difficult to treat, a statement that is justified by the findings of a Cochrane review (van Dessel et al. 2014) of 21 treatment studies involving CBT, mindfulness, psychodynamic and integrative therapies. Overall, the drop-out rate from therapy was high (often over 20%), and the **effect size** in comparison with usual care or **waiting list controls** (the weakest comparisons groups available) relatively small. Only CBT achieved any meaningful gains, but even these effects were modest and varied considerably across studies. Escobar et al. (2007), for example, examined the effectiveness of CBT targeted at people with subclinical SSD, comparing it with usual care. By the end of therapy, 60% of the intervention group reported their physical symptoms to be significantly improved versus 25% in the control condition. Unfortunately, this benefit had faded at 6-month follow-up. Van Dessel's more rigorous comparisons, including those with 'enhanced (but unstructured) care', found no additional benefit of CBT. The authors of the report make a further proviso: the studies in their review reported the outcomes of people willing to engage with psychotherapy. In reality, many people are unwilling to do so, so the overall impact of psychological therapies in the 'real world' may be even less. Despite this negativity, Hedman et al. (2016) compared a cognitive behavioural programme provided live, through the internet, and bibliotherapy. Their 12-week programme adopted an 'exposure with response prevention' approach in which participants were systematically exposed to stimuli that triggered anxiety in relation to health/symptoms, and then used mindfulness to help them cope rather than strategies involving checking or attempts at avoidance. Compared with a control condition, all three active interventions proved effective on a measure of health anxiety up to 6-month follow-up, with no differences between them.

Research box 7

Davoodi, E., Wen, A., Dobson, K.S. et al. (2018) Early maladaptive schemas in depression and somatization disorder, *Journal of Affective Disorders*, 235: 82–89.

Cognitive models of mental health disorders vary in terms of psychological processes such as attention, memory, and so on. However, a central element to them all is the notion that long-term schemata based on childhood, and perhaps subsequent, experiences drive our response to the life challenges we face. While processes such as attentional bias may be common to all disorders, there is a general consensus that the cognitive content may differ between them. The present study set out to explore this issue, comparing underlying **cognitive schemata** in people diagnosed with depression and somatization disorder, with the expectation that there would be different patterns of schema across the two groups.

Method

Participants

Participants were 30 people diagnosed with major depressive disorder and 30 diagnosed with somatization disorder according to DSM-IV criteria (approximating to somatic symptom disorder in DSM-5) following assessment by the diagnostic interview, the Structured Clinical Interview (SCID-I). They were drawn from patients in a hospital and psychiatric clinic in Tehran. Exclusion criteria were **psychosis**, current/previous manic disorder, as well as alcohol or drug abuse.

Measure

The sole measure was the Young Schema Questionnaire – Short Form (YSQ-S). This instrument comprises 75 items listing a range of schemata, to which participants respond using a scale from 1 ('completely untrue of me') to 6 ('describes me perfectly'). It measures the following *schema domains* and individual schemata:

Disconnection and rejection

- Abandonment/ instability   Significant others will not be able to provide support or protection because they are emotionally unstable and unpredictable
- Mistrust/ abuse   Others will hurt, abuse, humiliate, cheat, lie, manipulate or take advantage
- Emotional deprivation   The desire for a normal degree of emotional support will not be adequately met by others

- Defectiveness/ shame
One is defective, bad, unwanted, inferior or invalid in important respects; or that one would be unlovable to significant others if exposed

- Social isolation/ alienation
One is isolated from the rest of the world, different from other people, and/or not part of any group or community.

Impaired autonomy and performance

- Dependence/ incompetence
One is unable to handle one's everyday responsibilities in a competent manner, without considerable help from others

- Vulnerability to harm or illness
Exaggerated fear that imminent catastrophe, including illness, will strike at any time and that one will be unable to prevent it

- Enmeshment/ undeveloped self
Excessive emotional involvement and closeness with one or more significant others (often parents) at the expense of full individuation or normal social development

- Failure
One has failed or will fail in areas of achievement.

Other-directedness

- Subjugation
Surrendering of control to others to avoid negative consequences

- Self-sacrifice
Excessive focus on meeting the needs of others at one's own cost.

Over-vigilance and inhibition

- Emotional inhibition
Inhibiting spontaneous action, feelings, communication

- Unrelating standards
One must strive to meet very high standards to avoid criticism.

Impaired limits

- Entitlement/ grandiosity
One is superior to others and entitled to special rights and privileges

- Insufficient self-control/ self-discipline
Refusal to exercise sufficient self-control and frustration tolerance in order to achieve personal goals or to restrain the excessive impression of one's impulses.

Results

Differences in scores on the YSQ-S were first analysed using multivariate analysis of variance to assess whether there were overall differences between the totality of schema item scores between participants diagnosed with depression and somatization disorder. This proved significant ($F_{15,42} = 4.77$,

$p < 0.001$, $\eta_p^2 = 0.630$), permitting a series of individual analyses of variance exploring differences between each item score. These data are reported in Table 1.

Table 1 Mean scores (and standard deviations) on each schema for depressed and somatizing participants

	Depressed	Somatizing	*p*-value
Disconnection and rejection			
Abandonment/instability	18.86 (7.78)	15.83 (7.49)	NS
Mistrust/abuse	18.83 (6.49)	13.83 (6.74)	NS
Emotional deprivation	20.66 (6.27)	14.23 (8.02)	<0.05
Defectiveness/shame	16.17 (4.89)	12.20 (3.95)	<0.001
Social isolation/alienation	18.90 (6.01)	11.23 (5.44)	<0.001
Impaired autonomy/performance			
Dependence/incompetence	14.07 (7.44)	10.90 (6.14)	<0.05
Vulnerability to harm or illness	17.76 (7.68)	14.03 (7.34)	<0.05
Enmeshment/undeveloped self	14.31 (6.42)	14.50 (8.02)	NS
Failure	17.24 (7.16)	11.37 (5.74)	<0.001
Other-directedness			
Subjugation	18.72 (6.63)	13.27 (7.81)	<0.001
Self-sacrifice	19.38 (6.43)	20.20 (6.42)	NS
Over-vigilance and inhibition			
Emotional inhibition	20.24 (6.85)	13.37 (7.03)	<0.001
Unrelating standards	22.38 (4.69)	19.73 (7.20)	<0.001
Impaired limits			
Entitlement/grandiosity	18.45 (4.82)	15.63 (6.78)	NS
Insufficient self-control/self-discipline	19.45 (5.54)	14.87 (6.34)	<0.01

Discussion

The results are quite stunning, and slightly surprising. Depressed individuals score consistently higher than somatizers on virtually all these negative schemas including that relating to vulnerability to harm or illness. This may represent a wider sense of vulnerability to harm from a range of internal and external sources, and is not specifically limited to illness. Nevertheless, one would hypothesize that of all schemata, this would be significantly more evident in people whose condition is characterized by a sense of health threat. The lack of a 'typical' population comparison group restricts the interpretation of these findings. It is possible, for example, that somatizers express significantly higher levels of health vulnerability than this group.

8.2 Illness anxiety disorder

The difference between somatic symptom disorder and illness anxiety disorder (IAD), previously known as hypochondriasis, is subtle. People with SSD experience a range of unexplained 'symptoms', whereas those with IAD both experience 'symptoms' and/or consider them to indicate they have an illness. They may also believe they may develop an illness in the future, even if they have no ongoing symptoms. The DSM-5 criteria for the disorder are:

- Preoccupation with having or acquiring a serious illness
- Somatic symptoms are not present or only mild in intensity
- There is a high level of anxiety about health, and the individual is easily alarmed about their health status
- The individual either performs excessive health-checking behaviours (e.g. looking for signs of disease) or engages in maladaptive avoidance (e.g. avoiding doctors)
- The preoccupation with illness has to be present for at least 6 months, but the feared illness may change over this period.

People with IAD exaggerate the dangerousness of bodily signs and symptoms, and believe they are more likely to have or to develop an illness than is justified on the basis of any evidence. They are highly sensitive to information that suggests the possibility of them having a disease, and frequently seek confirmation of their worries from a variety of sources. By contrast, they are highly resistant to reassurance: appropriate information, education, and explanation typically fail to reduce any fears of disease (Rassin et al. 2008). Their fear seems limited to threats to health and is not found in other areas of life. Barsky et al. (2001), for example, found that hypochondriacal patients considered themselves at more risk of developing various diseases than a comparison group of patients from a primary care setting, but the two groups did not differ in their perceived risk of being involved in an accident or the subject of crime.

The prevalence of IAD has been variously estimated to lie between 2.1% and 13.1% of the general population, and between 2% and 20% of patients in medical settings (Scarella et al. 2019). The wide range in rates reflects differing sample methods and also differing definitions of IAD used in them. No differences in prevalence have been found across a range of demographic features, including age, ethnicity, and education, but women are more likely to be diagnosed with the disorder than men. Fink et al. (2004), for example, estimated the overall prevalence of IAD among people admitted into general medical wards to be 3.5%, with markedly different rates between men and women (1.5% and 6.0%, respectively). The typical age of onset appears to be around early- to mid-adulthood, and once present is likely to become long-lasting.

Aetiology of IAD

Psychoanalytic models

Illness anxiety disorder has received surprisingly little consideration within the psychoanalytic literature, which has focused on explanations for the cause of unexpected symptoms rather than worry about them. Indeed, Freud (1914) originally considered it to be an 'actual neurosis'. That is, unlike the defensive neuroses, he considered IAD to be a response to genuine symptoms; they were not generated by the unconscious as a result of some internal conflict. However, Freud (1914) subsequently developed a more psychoanalytic explanation for IAD, arguing that the libido could be divided into two dimensions. *Object libido* involves a love of external objects; *ego libido* involves love for oneself and one's body. It can also be called narcissism. According to Freud, challenges to the object libido result in neurotic anxiety; challenges to the ego libido result in IAD. One challenge may come from the individual him or herself. According to Freud, if an individual becomes absorbed by his or her ego libido, two things may happen. Their focus on external sources of love will diminish, and they will develop anxiety about their physical state. The individual focuses on their love of their body and physicality, but at the same time becomes anxious that they may lose the object of their love and attention. Thus, they focus on both the good things about their body, but also any threats to their health that may destroy the object of their love.

Developmental models

Many of the risk factors for IAD overlap with those thought to increase risk for SSD. Rates of physical and sexual abuse among people with IAD are higher than among comparison groups (e.g. Rief and Barsky 2005), as are reports of inadequate or inattentive parenting (Bass and Murphy 1995). Other studies have reported high levels of childhood sickness (Craig et al. 1993) and parental overprotection and encouragement of sick-role behaviour, particularly where the parent has high levels of health anxiety (e.g. Thorgaard et al. 2017). Just as in SSD, these parenting styles may result in insecure attachment styles, placing individuals at risk for IAD and with little faith in medical care as well as a range of interpersonal problems (Noyes et al. 2003).

Further reflecting the overlap between the two disorders, the model of IAD proposed by Anagnostopoulos and Botse (2016) is similar to the model of SSD proposed by Craig and colleagues. It proposes that as a consequence of lack of parental care or an adverse early environment, a child may come to view others as unreliable caregivers. The one way of gaining attention these children may have is through complaints of physical symptoms, as their parents are unresponsive to complaints of psychological distress. Thus, a cycle of complaints about physical symptoms, reinforced by parental attention, is established. This then becomes the primary way of gaining adult attention and feelings of attachment. This has two outcomes. First, the child learns to use complaints of physical symptoms to gain attention and perhaps love. Second, the child fails to learn other ways of eliciting care and attention from their environment. As an adult, the still insecurely attached person may communicate his or her need for care through complaints of illness. Unfortunately, these attempts at seeking support are frequently ignored, and even viewed with some suspicion, leading to an alienation from those around them, and reinforcing the original fear of lack of attachment and supportive relationships. Thus, the individual becomes locked into a vicious circle of distress, worries about health, alienation from potential support, and the frequent use of medical services as a support for both emotional and physical distress.

IAD as threat

The model developed by Warwick and Salkovskis (1990) focused on the immediate cognitive processes involved in IAD. They suggested that current life stresses or simply noticing bodily signs can activate previously latent cognitive schemata about health and disease – probably developed in childhood as a result of circumstances described above – that are faulty, unduly alarming or pessimistic. This leads to a number of sequelae:

- *Selective attention to information supporting this schema*: an increased focus on internal physiological factors such as heart rate, gastric motility, and so on. People with IAD may also focus on observable bodily signs such as lumps, bumps and moles, and bodily products such as sputum, faeces, and so on.
- *Cognitive errors*: disconfirmatory information, such as medical reassurance (even when sought) is ignored. By contrast, rumination about the consequences of illness may occur, usually in some catastrophic form.
- *Physiological changes*: autonomic activity may increase due to anxiety, resulting in change in bowel habits, sleeping, and so on. Each will confirm the health problem.
- *Behavioural responses*: these may involve safety behaviours such as repeated checking, taking unnecessary preventive medication, and so on. People with IAD may avoid activities that trigger health rumination or seek family or medical reassurance that 'all is well'. Safety behaviours, like those in obsessive-compulsive disorder (OCD), maintain the problem, as the individual feels emotionally more secure following their execution and never learns that a failure to engage in them will not lead to disastrous outcomes.

This link with OCD (see Chapter 6) is not coincidental. There are high levels of co-morbidity between the two conditions, they have similar checking rituals and goals related to them (the security they are 'safe'), and both respond to SSRIs (see below). On this basis, Hartmann et al. (2019) called for a transdiagnostic approach linking a number of anxiety disorders including OCD and IAD through a range of common psychological processes rather than domains of concern. Despite these commonalities, though, people with IAD typically have less insight than those with OCD and are more fixed in their beliefs.

A psychobiological variant of the threat model

A variant of the threat model is one of threat combined with symptom sensitivity. That is, people with IAD do actually experience more physical sensations than most people due to a physiological sensitivity, and are more likely to label these sensations as symptoms of some underlying medical condition (Marcus et al. 2006). Some data favouring this model may be found in genetic studies of IAD, in which specific pathways to IAD have been found. Gillespie et al. (2000), for example, examined the genetic risk for developing what they termed somatic distress.

They gave measures of anxiety, depression, phobic anxiety, and somatic distress to 3,469 Australian twins aged 18–28 years, and found that 33% of the variance in somatic distress appeared to be due to a genetic influence unrelated to depression or phobic anxiety. Accordingly, their data suggest a unique genetic contribution to the reporting of somatic distress, and that this is not a manifestation of a more general propensity to anxiety or depression. Whether any genetic influence translates into a high sensitivity to physical sensations is less clear, however. Krautwurst et al. (2016), for example, reported two of several studies to find either no, or even a negative relationship between levels of health anxiety and accuracy of detection of one's own pulse rate and 'non-specific skin conductance fluctuations'.

Stop and think ...

One of the comments often made about medical students as they go through their training is that they develop every illness they encounter – or at least they think they do. Luckily, most of them recover from these non-existent illnesses before developing the next. But this reaction to health and health risk information may have implications for many more people. We are increasingly made aware of our health and the health risks associated with our behaviour, our genetic make-up, and the environment in which we live. Unfortunately, it seems that for some vulnerable people, just being made aware of potential health problems evokes high levels of health anxiety. So, while some may benefit from health advice, others simply become worried about their health. As well as creating a health-conscious society, are we also creating a health-anxious one? Conversely, does ready access to information about alternative treatments of dubious merit and websites providing detailed and (sometimes inaccurate) data on side-effects of 'legitimate' medications and other therapies make us more reluctant to seek help from appropriate formal sources? And is the combination of these processes resulting in increased levels of health anxiety within the general population?

Treatment of IAD

Psychological treatment

Psychological treatment for IAD can be difficult, particularly where individuals hold a strong belief in their having a physical disease. One way this has been addressed is through the use of a variety of CBT interventions, including:

- *Behavioural hypothesis-testing*: this can involve working with a **client** to investigate the reality of their symptoms. If someone has a fear of a muscle-wasting disease, for example, they may predict they would become extremely weak if they engage in even light exercise. With some encouragement, this hypothesis can be tested – and hopefully found to be inaccurate.

- *Reducing checking and medical consultation*: in order to reduce safety behaviours in general, and use of medical support in particular, the individual may reduce checking behaviour and medical consultations – or at least delay them. This is similar to the approach taken in OCD and phobias – that is, exposure plus response prevention (see Chapter 6). They may also develop a realistic strategy for when to seek medical help.
- *Cognitive challenge*: this involves techniques to counter some of the catastrophic thoughts that an individual may have about their symptoms. Thus, fear that one has a serious heart problem may be based on the experience of chest discomfort, heart missing a beat, and breathlessness. These experiences may be contextualized and made less threatening by reframing:

'Most heart beats change rhythm from minute to minute'.
'It's normal to become breathless following exertion – especially if you are unfit'.
'I've had these symptoms before, and although they made me worried, they did not lead to any problems'.

A number of studies have shown cognitive behavioural interventions based on the Salkovskis model to be effective when compared with usual care. Barsky and Ahern (2004), for example, found benefits following a six-session CBT intervention including lower levels of hypochondriacal symptoms, beliefs, and health-related anxiety at 6- and 12-month follow-up compared to a no-treatment control group. Arguing that people with illness anxiety disorder may have very fixed illness beliefs that are difficult to address using cognitive challenge, McManus et al. (2012) explored the impact of a mindfulness-based cognitive therapy intervention. Immediately following the intervention, 47% of the intervention group and 78% of the usual care group met the criteria for a diagnosis of illness anxiety disorder. The gains in the intervention group were even greater at one-year follow-up, with 28% of the intervention group and 75% of the usual care group meeting the same criteria.

A further way in which interventions in IAD have developed is through the use of the internet. Newby et al. (2018), for example, compared the effectiveness of an internet-delivered CBT programme, with support from a remote clinician, and a live **psychoeducation** control group. Using an intention-to-treat analysis (which assumes drop-outs from therapy have made no improvements), they found participants in both conditions showed some improvement, with the internet group achieving higher levels of 'clinically reliable change' on a self-report health anxiety measure: 84% versus 34%. Newby and McElroy (2019) went on to examine a very specific issue related to health anxiety within this intervention study, what they term 'cyberchondria': excessive health-related online searches, leading to increased anxiety in relation to health status. Again, their internet-based CBT appeared to be of some benefit, achieving significant reductions in online activity and the distress associated with it.

Pharmacological treatment

Until the late 1980s, the general consensus among clinicians was that **pharmacotherapy** would not benefit people who experienced IAD. However, the similarities between IAD and OCD have led to the use of SSRIs in an attempt to treat it, with some success, although large trials of their effectiveness are still lacking. In one study, Fallon et al. (2008) reported a small placebo-controlled trial of fluoxetine and found significant benefits during the 24 weeks in which patients were receiving the drug. Unfortunately, they were not able to report outcomes following discontinuation. In a study comparing psychological and pharmacological treatments, Greeven et al. (2007) reported a better response to cognitive behavioural intervention than to medication. Using an intention-to-treat analysis, they found that after 16 weeks treatment, 45% of people in the psychological group achieved significant reductions in symptoms, compared with 30% of those treated with paroxetine (an SSRI) and 14% given placebo. Of those who completed treatment, the equivalent percentages were 54%, 38%, and 12% respectively.

Case formulation

Mrs T was a woman in her sixties. She lived with her son in a working-class area of Bristol. At the time she was seen by a clinical psychologist, she had been seen by the psychiatric services for many years complaining of various physical symptoms which had no obvious physical cause. These changed over the course of the years, but included a tingling down both sides of her body, dizziness, feeling weak, headaches, and episodic collapsing.

By the time she was referred to the psychology services, every general practitioner (GP) in her local area had struck her off their list of patients, because she was visiting them once or twice every week complaining of various symptoms and requesting treatment. She had been given multiple diagnostic tests, none of which found any evidence of disease. The GPs felt unable to treat her and had become increasingly frustrated and then frankly annoyed by her repeated visits. The situation had become so bad that the GP service had organized for her medical care to be provided by the GPs on a rolling basis, for 3 months each – something that they adhered to, albeit reluctantly. In addition to medical help, she had sought treatment from a variety of alternative practitioners including herbalists, chiropractors, reflexologists, and shiatsu practitioners, none of whom had been of help. She denied any psychological element to her symptoms. She lived with her 40-year-old son, who spent much of his time out of the house or in his own room. She socialized with one or two long-term psychiatric patients she had met through her contact with the psychiatric services. She rarely left her house, and then only to go shopping in her local shops.

When first seen by a psychologist, she complained of long-standing physical symptoms, and was able to provide a diary of her symptoms, recorded on an hourly basis, over many months. She talked incessantly of her symptoms, and it was extremely difficult to divert her from them. Investigation of relevant psychological issues proved difficult, as sessions were, at least initially, somewhat overwhelmed by her repeated descriptions of her physical symptoms. However, a time line of key issues did emerge.

Long-term antecedents

Mrs T came from a working-class family. She had three siblings and a history of illness within the family. Her father worked long hours, and competition for parental attention was strong. She was unhappy at times, as she felt neglected and estranged from her parents, and did not socialize well with other children from the neighbourhood. There was little emotional warmth in the family. She was often sick as a child, and gained some attention within the family at these times. She left school with no qualifications, but did meet a man who she married and with whom she had a baby. Unfortunately, the marriage was unhappy, and she described him as a 'little odd'. She divorced him after a few years and brought up the child on her own. She stated that she had some physical health problems at the time of her marriage, and that they gradually grew worse in the following years.

Short-term antecedents

Her son, who was in his forties, did not marry and continued to live with her until the time she was seen by the psychiatric services. He was relatively happy, did not work, and had minimal social relationships, but was keen to move out of the house and develop on his own. However, he was concerned about his mother's health and had continued to live at home in case she became acutely ill and he was unable to help her. He was very worried about his mother and would not forgive himself were anything to happen to her and he was not there to help. He coped with living at home by spending much of his time in his own room, to avoid her constant complaints of physical problems.

Formulation

Mrs T was brought up in a family of little emotional warmth, in which the emotional needs of the children were not recognized and certainly not responded to. One way in which she could gain some parental attention was through 'being ill'. It is possible that she learned to signal emotional distress through the reporting of physical symptoms. Her experience and reporting of such symptoms had varied across her life, with the distress associated with a poor marriage and subsequent divorce being obvious triggers. The latest cause of her symptoms was her worry that her son would leave home and she would be alone, with relatively little social contact. Her symptoms could therefore be seen as both her typical response to stress and a means of keeping her son close to home and as a source of companionship. The style of her attachment to him could be described as anxious attachment, as she feared that if he left home he would also leave her. Her total focus on her symptoms increased her awareness of her bodily experiences, and increased their impact on her.

Intervention

Mrs T did not recognize that her symptoms might be associated with any psychological issues. She certainly did not recognize the formulation as relevant to her. Nevertheless, it was possible to negotiate some form of intervention. The ideal intervention might be:

- Help Mrs T and her son gain insight into the psychological factors contributing to her problems.
- Teach her cognitive strategies to challenge her worries.
- Teach her strategies such as mindfulness to help her tolerate her distress. Identify other ways of distracting from distress and worries.
- Negotiate with her son a mutually agreeable plan in which he were to leave home, but maintain contact with his mother.

The actual intervention was in some ways more complex and involved more people:

- Regular and pre-arranged appointments with a GP during which she could discuss her symptoms. It was acknowledged both by Mrs T and the doctors that they would not expect these to result in a 'cure' for her symptoms but this would help her limit her repeated, consistent, and increasingly fractious appointments with her doctors.
- Regular meetings with a community mental health nurse, to discuss issues of a psychological nature and to gain support and help in her keeping to the plan.
- She was unwilling to practise strategies such as mindfulness. However, she agreed to leave the house more often and to engage in things to distract her from her worries – this included going out with one of her friends and attending a day hospital one or two days a week, joining in the activities there.
- Her son agreed to consider negotiating leaving home but only after he could see some improvement in his mother's health.

The intervention worked reasonably well, but was not without its problems. While she stuck to her agreement to limit her visits to her GPs, for example, she began to attend her local A&E departments: at one time attending three hospitals in one week. We negotiated this issue by noting that her symptoms had lasted many years without becoming so serious that she had required medical treatment and that her visits to any doctor (including A&E departments) did not result in any effective treatment. Accordingly, delaying seeing a doctor by, say, a week would be unlikely to either result in a sudden deterioration of her health or stop her accessing an effective cure. She could see the logic of this argument, and agreed to try and reduce her visits to the hospitals. To help her cope with the consequent anxiety, she would try and talk with her friends on the phone about non-health-related issues or do other things to distract her from her worries.

This proved an effective approach. Over the following 6 months, she showed significant improvements. Her mood lifted, she was more social, and went on day trips with friends. She focused less on her symptoms and did not let them dominate her life as much as before. She still experienced her symptoms, but was better able to cope with them. Her son continued to live at home, but life was better as (by mutual agreement in a joint session with the psychologist) Mrs T had agreed to talk less about her symptoms and he had agreed to be more social around the house and to spend more time with her. So, their relationship had improved, and he no longer felt the need to leave home.

8.3 Body dysmorphic disorder

Many of us have some degree of dissatisfaction with our body. Fallon et al. (2014), for example, found that up to a quarter of men and a third of women express significant body dissatisfaction. Significantly fewer of us are so unhappy that this dissatisfaction reaches pathological proportions and meet the criteria for body dysmorphic disorder (BDD). People with BDD experience a preoccupation with an imagined defect in appearance as well as significant levels of negative thinking, self-criticism, anxiety, and depression. According to DSM-5, the following criteria must be met for its diagnosis:

- Preoccupation with one or more perceived deficits or flaws in physical appearance that are not observable or appear slight.
- At some point, the individual has performed repetitive behaviours (e.g. seeking reassurance, mirror checking) or mental acts (e.g. comparing self with others) in response to these concerns.
- Concerns can involve preoccupations with the face (such as scars, spots, acne, or the shape or size of the nose, mouth, etc.), the hair (fears of receding hairlines), or the size and shape of any other body part, including hips, buttocks, legs, and hands. Men tend to be concerned about their body build, genitals, and hair. Women focus on their hips, breasts, and legs (Phillips et al. 2006a). Typical behaviours include:
  - frequent checking of appearance in mirrors
  - camouflaging the perceived defect with clothing, make-up or posture
  - seeking surgery or other medical treatment
  - attempts to convince other people of the deformity
  - skin picking
  - measuring the disliked body part
  - excessive dieting or exercise
  - avoiding social situations in which the perceived defect may be exposed
  - feeling very anxious and self-conscious around other people because of the perceived defect.

As a result of their concerns, people with BDD frequently hide their perceived defect by camouflaging it (clothing, make-up) or changing it through excessive exercise, dieting or surgery. Levels of distress can be such that many people with BDD experience major depression, social phobia, and substance abuse (Sobanski and Schmidt 2000). Up to 80% experience suicidal ideation at some time in their life, and around a quarter will attempt suicide (Phillips 2004). Less dramatically, the condition may prevent normal social, economic, and sexual relationships. Didie et al. (2008), for example, found that 80% of their sample of people with BDD reported some degree of impairment in work: 39% claimed not to have worked in the previous month as a result of their disorder. Among the general population, the prevalence of BDD is about 2.5% in women and 2.2% in men (Koran et al. 2008). Not surprisingly, perhaps, rates are higher among people seeking plastic surgery, where they are around 10% (Aouizerate et al. 2003). Sadly, for these people, surgery rarely improves their feelings about themselves. Rates of spontaneous remission are low (Phillips et al. 2008), while perhaps unsurprisingly, around a third of people with BDD will also have some form of eating disorder (Ruffolo et al. 2006).

Clinicians have considered whether BDD is significantly different to other diagnoses, and whether it can be subsumed within them. Phillips et al. (2006b) adopted a dimensional view (see Chapter 1), arguing that people with extremely strong beliefs are no different from people with a 'non-delusional' disorder, except in the strength of their belief and should therefore not be considered under a separate diagnosis. A second suggestion is that BDD may be considered a variant of OCD (see Chapter 6), and it does now sit within the DSM-5 classification group of obsessive and related disorders. The preoccupations held by people with BDD resemble obsessions, in that they are anxiety-producing, recurrent, and difficult to control. Repeated checking or other procedures to reduce anxiety are also similar to OCD. In addition, family members with BDD are more likely to have a relative with OCD than the general population. Despite these similarities, a number of important differences have been found between the two disorders (e.g. Phillips et al. 2012). Compared to people with OCD, those with BDD experience poorer insight, higher co-morbidity with major depression, social phobia and **psychotic** disorders, and higher suicide attempt rates

A third approach has argued that BDD is a form of eating disorder – or that BDD and eating disorders lie on a continuum of disorders relating to body image distortion. Cororve and Gleaves (2001) identified the key driver of both BDD and eating disorders as excessive concerns about physical appearance. Perhaps the most problematic issue for this model is that it assumes eating disorders are primarily driven by weight or appearance concerns. While this is generally true of bulimia, these may form only part of the clinical picture in anorexia (see Chapter 12). In addition, the appearance concerns of people with BDD may be unrelated to their weight. People with anorexia, for example, may focus on body areas typically linked to weight concerns, whereas people with BDD frequently fixate on facial features, hair, and skin (Toh et al. 2020). Accordingly, there may be significant overlap between the conditions, but they cannot be considered synonymous (Phillipou et al. 2019).

Aetiology of BDD

Socio-cultural factors

There has been little systematic research into the social and cultural factors associated with the development of BDD *per se*, although much more has focused on non-clinical levels of body dissatisfaction and eating disorders. Unsurprisingly, perhaps, both mainstream and social media appear to have a significant influence on these outcomes. Fardouly and Vartanian (2015), for example, found a positive correlation between use of Facebook and body image concerns, which appeared to enhance pre-existing appearance concerns through negative comparisons with peers and celebrities. Such issues are not limited to Western countries. In a sample of Taiwanese adolescents, Kaewpradub et al. (2017) found use of the internet and social networks was associated with low body image satisfaction and either inappropriate eating behaviours, including bingeing and purging, or a drive for muscularity (particular in males). Of particular concern is that these attitudes may be affecting even younger children. Tatangelo et al. (2016) reviewed the relevant literature and found consistent evidence of body dissatisfaction in children under the age of 6 years (with rates across studies varying between 20% and 70%), largely driven by their parents' attitudes and behaviour. Despite these societal influences, most people do not become as obsessed or concerned about their appearance as people with BDD. Other factors may give rise to a specific vulnerability to such influences, although what contributes to this vulnerability is largely speculative at present.

Psychoanalytic models

A psychoanalytic view suggests that BDD arises from an individual's unconscious displacement of sexual or emotional conflict or feelings of guilt and poor self-image to specific parts of the body (Sobanski and Schmidt 2000). The displacement is thought to occur because the underlying problem is so threatening to the **ego** that it is unconsciously displaced into the more psychologically manageable issue of appearance. The body part of concern, such as the nose, may represent another, more emotionally threatening body part, such as the penis (Phillips 1996).

A psychological model

A key factor in the development of BDD appears to be critical events or traumatic incidents that involve an individual's appearance. The most common example is being teased about weight or size (Buhlmann et al. 2007), with many people with the disorder reporting repeated criticism about their appearance from members of their own family. More general vulnerability factors may involve being neglected as a child, leading to feelings of being unloved, insecure, and rejected. Didie et al. (2006), for example, found that over three-quarters of individuals in their sample of people with BDD reported some level of maltreatment during childhood, including emotional neglect (68%) and emotional abuse (56%). Other trauma, such as sexual abuse or assault, may also be implicated, although rates of this experience were significantly lower (28%). Many people with BDD also report having experienced a physical injury or illness. According to Veale (2004), these critical events activate dysfunctional assumptions about the normality of physical appearance and the implications of appearance for self-worth and acceptance. In one exploration of this phenomenon, Osman et al. (2004) conducted a semi-structured interview with people with BDD and 'typical' controls. During the interview, the people with BDD evidenced more spontaneously occurring negative appearance-related images than did control participants. These images were linked to early stressful memories.

Veale (2004) argues that once established, the disorder may be maintained by selective attention to perceived physical problems or information that supports this belief. Jin et al. (2018), for example, found that men at risk of muscle dysmorphia paid more attention to, and found it more difficult to pull away from, strong muscularity features in photographs of males than those not at risk. In addition, Rosen (1996) suggested that rehearsal of negative and distorted self-statements about physical appearance results in them becoming automatic and believable. Finally, the positive emotional responses associated with avoidance, checking, and reassurance-seeking behaviours reinforce and maintain the condition, just as in OCD. Buhlmann et al. (2006) provided experimental evidence of some of the cognitive distortions held by many people with BDD. In their study, people with BDD and a 'typical' control group completed two questionnaires accompanying facial photographs of people in various everyday situations. One questionnaire included self-referent scenarios ('Imagine that the bank teller is looking at you. What is his facial expression like?'), while the other included other-referent scenarios ('Imagine that the bank teller is looking at a friend of yours ...'). They were asked to identify the emotion evident in each face. Overall, people with BDD had more difficulty identifying emotional expressions in self-referent scenarios than did the comparison group. They also misinterpreted more expressions as contemptuous and angry in self-referent scenarios than did controls.

Treatment of BDD

Psychological treatment

The most common psychological treatment for BDD involves CBT. Exposure with response prevention to previously avoided situations can include exposure to the sight of the individual's own body or showing their perceived defect in social situations. Often, exposure programmes follow hierarchies of increasingly distressing body parts or avoided situations. Prevention of checking or self-reassuring behaviours is used to counteract checking rituals. Finally, cognitive restructuring, in which dysfunctional thoughts are identified and then challenged, as well as other coping methods (such as relaxation) may be used as participants work through the hierarchy. This approach does appear to be effective. In a **meta-analysis** of the data then available, Harrison et al. (2016) reviewed evidence from seven randomized controlled trials of CBT for BDD. Of these, all achieved significantly greater improvements in BDD symptoms than either a waiting list control or placebo intervention condition, with gains lasting up to 4 months following the cessation of treatment. It is noteworthy that the severity of BDD was not predictive of outcome, a finding also evident in subsequent studies. Since this review, Krebs et al. (2017) have provided evidence of a longer-term benefit. They followed up a group of young adults with a primary diagnosis of BDD for one year following the cessation of a CBT programme. Immediately at the end of therapy, 40% of those receiving CBT achieved clinically significant reductions in symptoms; 7% of those in the control condition who received a psychoeducational and weekly telephone monitoring intervention achieved the same criteria.

At 12-month follow-up, 50% of the participants in the CBT group were clinically improved. Interventions have also moved to the internet, with similar benefits (e.g. Enander et al. 2016).

Pharmacological treatment

Although it is generally acknowledged that treatment with SSRIs is the pharmacological treatment of choice for BDD (e.g. Dong et al. 2019), randomized controlled trials are generally lacking. In one such study, Phillips and Rasmussen (2004) found fluoxetine was more effective than placebo over a period of 12 weeks. The same research group (Phillips et al. 2016) compared the effects of 14 weeks of treatment with another SSRI (escitalopram) against those of a placebo intervention. By the end of this treatment phase, 67% of those who initiated but did not complete treatment with the SSRI (30% of the original sample) evidenced significant clinical improvements; 81% of those who completed the whole intervention achieved this criterion. Full remission was achieved by 20% and 26% of these groups, respectively (no data were presented for the placebo intervention). Over the next 6 months, 18% of those who achieved the clinically relevant gains relapsed. Drop-out was associated with the experience of side-effects including fatigue, nausea, sexual dysfunction, insomnia, and headache. Similar effects have also been found in a small open trial of venlafaxine, an **SNRI** (Allen et al. 2008).

8.4 Functional neurological symptom disorder

Long known as hysteria or **hysterical disorder**, the American Psychiatric Association (APA 2013) now calls this condition functional neurological symptom disorder (FNSD). 'Functional' here implies that the neurological symptoms have a psychological function, such as avoidance of, or a means of expressing, distress. The DSM-5 criteria for the disorder are the presence of:

- one or more symptoms of altered voluntary motor or sensory functions
- clinical evidence of incompatibility between these symptoms and recognized neurological or medical conditions.

People with functional disorder often present with striking neurological symptoms such as weakness, lack of coordination, paralysis, sensory disorders or memory loss, in the absence of any medical pathology. Less common symptoms include somatosensory disorders and skin changes. Many people appear unconcerned about their symptoms, a characteristic sometimes labelled *la belle indifférence*. Initially termed hysteria, from the Greek word for uterus, the condition was thought to occur as a result of the uterus literally wandering through the body, resulting in symptoms as varied as feelings of suffocation, dramatic fits, paralysis of the limbs, fainting spells, a sudden inability to speak, and an inability to take in food. Treatment involved encouraging the womb back to its proper place through physical manipulation.

More recently, the condition came to prominence in the First World War, when many soldiers in the trenches developed a condition known as 'shell shock', of which the most prominent features were blindness, paralysis, contractures, **aphonia**, anaesthesias, and profound amnesias. The initial interpretation of these symptoms was that they resulted from micro-haemorrhaging in the brain, as a consequence of the shock created by exploding shells: hence the term 'shell shock'. Subsequently, doctors noted that the majority of soldiers with the condition had not been close to any explosions, there was no evidence of any brain haemorrhages at autopsy in those who died, and the condition occurred among recruits who had not yet been in battle. As a result, it became considered a psychological rather than a physical condition. Interestingly, social and cultural factors appear to have influenced both the development and treatment of shell shock. Officers were less likely to develop these problems than enlisted men, but when they did, they were more likely to be taken from the trenches and receive long-term treatment, even when their symptoms were relatively minor.

Within medical settings, the condition can be surprisingly prevalent. Stone et al. (2010) estimated the prevalence of functional disorders among patients referred to a Scottish neurological service to be around 16%. Jones et al. (2020) estimated that 25% of people admitted to hospital with a possible stroke were actually what they termed 'functional stroke mimics'. Individuals with this condition were most likely to be female and to report weakness and numbness more than language problems or reduced consciousness. Finally, Benbadis and Allen Hauser (2000) estimated that 10–20% of patients referred for treatment of epilepsy in the USA had what they termed 'psychogenic non-epileptic seizures'. The prevalence of functional disorders within the general population is harder to estimate. However, Favarelli et al. (1997) reported a rate of 0.3% among a relatively small sample of 673 individuals. It has high co-morbidity, with Malik et al. (2010) finding rates of 60% for both depression and anxiety in their sample of patients. It also has a poor prognosis. For example, Crimlisk et al. (1998) followed 73 people with medically unexplained motor symptoms for 6 years. Over this time, only three people were given a medical diagnosis, indicating an initial misdiagnosis, 75% were diagnosed with a 'psychiatric disorder', and 45% were diagnosed with a personality disorder. The presenting symptom was unchanged in 14%, and had worsened in 38%. Interestingly, Ahmad et al. (2008) found the rate of admissions to hospital with a diagnosis of medically unexplainable stroke symptoms varied according to the phase of the moon. Over a period of 13 years, admissions were higher during a full moon than at other times. The authors offered no explanation for this. On an equally bizarre note, Burneo et al. (2003) noted that a key diagnostic feature of the disorder was what they termed 'the teddy bear' sign: 87% of the 903 cases they reported brought a teddy bear to the diagnostic testing process. Incredibly, their findings were replicated by Cervenka et al. (2013), who observed a smaller association then Burneo and colleagues, but still found that patients aged 18 or over who brought a stuffed animal to their assessment for epilepsy were three times more like to be diagnosed with psychogenic non-epileptic seizures than those who did not.

Aetiology of FNSD

Social processes

Social factors are involved in the development of FNSD, at least on some occasions. The condition has been described as contagious, in that the sight or knowledge of one person with unexplained symptoms may trigger similar symptoms in others, particularly when many people are grouped together and placed under some form of stress. One such incident among US Army recruits occurred over a 12-hour period following the evacuation of 1,800 men from their barracks owing to a suspected toxic gas exposure, which turned out to be a false alarm (Struewing and Gray 1990). Despite the lack of toxin in the atmosphere, over two-thirds of the recruits developed at least one respiratory symptom, and 375 were evacuated by air ambulance for immediate medical investigation; eight were kept in hospital. Two weeks after the incident, 55% of a sample of this group reported developing at least one symptom, including cough, light-headedness, chest pain, shortness of breath, headache, sore throat or dizziness. Those who reported the most – or the most severe – problems reported high levels of physical stress, mental stress, and awareness of rumours of odours, gases, and/or smoke. Another famous incident involved the so-called 'toxic lady' in California. Admitted for cervical cancer, it was claimed that her body and breath exuded an odd garlicky smell. Unfortunately, the woman became acutely ill while in hospital, and during her unsuccessful treatment one of her physicians felt faint and left the room. A member of staff who checked on the health of this physician also fainted, as did a second clinician. Over the next few days several other staff members developed symptoms that included loss of consciousness, shortness of breath, and muscle spasms. Findings that subsequent blood tests in these individuals were normal led to the conclusion that the symptoms were essentially 'hysterical'. Explanations for these mass events focus on the so-called nocebo effect, in which individuals experience sensations usually due to increased sympathetic arousal, believe these are evidence of an illness, which leads to further symptoms and the experience of an 'illness'.

Psychoanalytic explanations

Early psychoanalytic explanations of functional disorders considered the condition to reflect anxiety aroused by unconscious conflict being converted into physical symptoms. Freud (Freud and Breuer 2004) thought that one ego **defence mechanism** against high levels of distress was to convert this distress from psychic to physical symptoms. Perhaps the most famous case he reported was that of Anna O, who was initially treated by Joseph Breuer. Anna O was a 21-year-old woman who became ill while nursing her terminally ill father. Her own illness began with a severe cough, and subsequently included paralysis of the extremities of the right side of her body, contractures, disturbances of vision, hearing, and language, lapses of consciousness, and **hallucinations**. Breuer noticed that when Anna told him the content of her daytime hallucinations, while under hypnosis, she became calm and tranquil. He considered this to be a way of expressing the 'products' of her 'bad self': a process of emotional **catharsis**. Breuer further developed his understanding of her symptoms following a period of time when Anna O stopped drinking, and quenched her thirst by eating fruit and melons. At this time, she recounted in one of her sessions how she had been disgusted by the sight of a dog drinking out of a glass. Soon after this revelation she asked for a drink. Breuer took this to indicate that insight into the factors associated with the beginning of symptoms was a key issue in relieving them. This became a focus of later hypnotic sessions.

The twist in the story came from Freud's analysis of the situation. He noted that Anna specifically required Breuer to provide the therapy, and that when she was in a hypnotic state, she needed to feel his hands to ensure he was there. In addition, one of the symptoms she developed was believing that she was pregnant with his child. Freud took this as an indication that she was in love with Breuer and that her hysterical symptoms were the result of these secret sexual desires. In fact, Freud considered functional disorders to result from an unresolved Electra complex (see Chapter 2). In this, the young girl is sexually attracted to her father. If her parents' responses to this are harsh or disapproving, the girl's feelings are repressed. This leads to a preoccupation with sex, at the same time as an avoidance of it. If these sexual urges occur later in life, the defence mechanism evoked can involve conversion of the sexual impulses into physical symptoms.

Behavioural explanations

The behavioural explanation of the symptoms of FNSD is that they are functional and under the control of the individual expressing them. They are functional in the sense that they lead to some sort of benefit or reinforcement: the obvious one in the case of Anna O being the attention given to her by Breuer, while the men in the trenches potentially avoided being killed. In arguing this case, Miller (1999) suggested that it is very difficult to determine from an external standpoint what is motivated, controllable, voluntary behaviour and what is not. However, he argued that some notable cases of functional disorders seem to be faked and under voluntary control, albeit it in a rather clumsy way.

One example of this was reported by Zimmerman and Grosz (1966), who asked a patient with functional blindness to identify which one of three visual stimuli was being presented to them. The patient performed this task at a level consistently below chance: a finding that may be considered unusual, because if he was unable to see, he should have performed at chance levels. Zimmerman and Grosz then presented the stimuli in a non-random order (left-centre-right, left-centre-right, etc.), and the person was informed of which stimulus had been presented on each trial following their attempt to identify it. This is a task for which one would expect a blind person to learn the sequence and perform at above-chance levels. The participant in their study did not. Finally, when he was allowed to overhear a comment by a confederate of the experimenter that 'the doctors reckon that the patient can see because he makes fewer correct responses by chance than a blind man would make' (1966: 259), his performance improved to chance levels. Miller speculated that this indicated the individual was dissimilating.

This argument can also be made from an anatomical perspective. Merskey (1995) noted, for example, that patients with functional aphonia (inability to speak) may be able to cough, yet both processes require the vocal cords to function normally. If an individual can cough, there are no anatomical reasons for them not being able to talk. Similarly, some patients with an inability to move their limbs may show evidence of tensing both the apparently affected muscles and those which prevent movement of the limb. Again, this suggests that some sort of voluntary processes are at work. Despite these cases, Miller (1999) acknowledged these findings do not necessarily mean that all people with these phenomena are faking.

Functional disorders as a form of hypnosis

An opposing interpretation of functional symptoms, proposed by Oakley (1999), suggested that they are evidence of some form of hypnotic processes at work. He noted a number of similarities between functional disorders and hypnosis:

- *Similarities in 'symptoms'*: many conditions that can be established in hypnosis are similar to frequently reported functional symptoms – motor paralysis (inability to rise from a chair, move an arm, etc.), loss of touch or pain sensation, blindness, and the generation of pain sensations.
- *Lack of concern over symptoms*: both hypnotized individuals and many people with FNSD express a lack of concern over their strange symptoms.
- *Involuntariness*: the deficits or physical states that are associated with both FNSD and hypnosis involve a degree of involuntariness. People report that they would like to, for example, move their hand, but cannot. 'They say "I cannot"; it looks like "I will not"; but it is "I cannot will"' (cited in Oakley 1999).
- *Apparent malingering and display of 'implicit knowledge'*: both functional disorders and hypnosis can appear as if the individual is deliberately faking their symptoms. They may respond as if they do not have the deficit while still reporting it. People who are deaf as a result of hypnosis and functional disorder, for example, have both been shown to alter their speech in response to external noise, implying some sort of knowledge of stimuli that they apparently cannot sense. The performance of the functionally blind individual reported by Zimmerman and Grosz (1966) provides further evidence of this implicit knowledge. Miller suggests this could be evidence of faking. However, Oakley had a different explanation. He proposed that these examples could suggest that any mechanisms responsible for both functional and hypnotic blindness occur at a late stage in processing of visual material. Becoming aware of visual stimuli involves a series of processes before we become consciously aware of any stimulus: reception of information in the visual cortex, transmission of this information to the temporal and parietal lobes where the location and type of stimulus are determined, and then to the prefrontal cortex where this information is integrated with memories. All this occurs before we are aware of having seen a stimulus. It is possible that processes/deficits associated with hypnosis or functional disorder occur before we become consciously aware of the stimulus, but allow some form of apparently conscious response to stimuli.

Oakley suggested that if we accept that there are some commonalities between functional disorders and hypnosis, there may also be common neurological processes. In one study of functional disorder, Marshall et al. (1997) investigated the neural processes that occurred in a lady with FNSD when asked to move her paralysed left leg, using functional magnetic resonance imaging (fMRI):

- *Preparing* to move her leg resulted in activation of her left premotor cortex and both cerebellar hemispheres: the same processes that occurred when she was preparing to move her non-paralysed right leg. The authors interpreted this as an indication of her 'genuine' preparation to move her left leg.

- When *trying* to move her leg, there was activation of the normal movement-related brain areas including the left dorsolateral prefrontal cortex and both cerebellar hemispheres. There was no activation of the right premotor areas or the right primary sensorimotor cortex necessary for movement. However, areas of the brain not usually involved in movement – the right cingulated cortex and right orbitofrontal cortex – *did* show activation. The authors proposed that this activation somehow inhibited movement of her left leg.

Marshall et al. suggested that the desire to move was evidenced by the activation of the movement-related areas of the brain. However, this activation was somehow overridden by other neurological activity: not 'I cannot' or 'I will not' but 'I cannot will'.

Tangential evidence for the hypnosis hypothesis can be found in the findings of Roelofs et al. (2002), who found that people diagnosed with FNSD were more susceptible to hypnosis than those with other emotional disorders, and greater susceptibility was associated with higher symptom reporting. More direct evidence is the similarity between patterns of neurological activation in people who are given hypnotic commands under hypnosis and those with a functional disorder. Vuilleumier (2014) summarized the neurological data and identified significant overlap between the activation patterns in hypnosis and FNSD, although they are not identical. In functional disorders, the key neurological structures involved are the primary motor and/or sensory pathways, as well as the ventromedial prefrontal cortex (VMPFC), precuneus, and perhaps other limbic structures. Accordingly, the brain regions involved in functional disorders are those that access internal representations about the self, integrate information from memory and imagery with affective relevance (in VMPFC), hold information about sensory or agency representations (the precuneus), and process emotions (the limbic system).

These neurological processes can be explained by cognitive models. Oakley (1999) suggested that our decision-making involves a hierarchical cognitive system, controlled by a supervisory control system. The overarching control of responses to environmental events is provided by a central executive. At a lower level, mental functioning comprises a series of learned behavioural sequences. These are guided by action schema stored in long-term memory. They enable routine behaviours, and are relatively uncontrolled by the central executive. Action at this level is guided by processes which we are not aware of – they are unconscious. The executive becomes involved in active planning and decision-making only when the learned behavioural sequences are insufficient to cope with our responses: when there are no pre-existing action schemata. A major function of the executive is to exert attentional control: to focus attention on demanding tasks, and away from distracting stimuli. According to Shallice (1988), any mental processing involving the central executive becomes part of our conscious awareness, and any actions that follow its activation are thought of as voluntary. Processing below this level (the learned behavioural sequences) is unconscious. These processes explain, for example, the commonly reported phenomenon of having driven a car for many miles, and yet having no real recollection of the journey. The process of driving can be relatively automatic and, if the driver focuses their attention on other things, may happen at an unconscious level and be filtered out from conscious awareness.

Oakley (1999) went further to suggest that not all those elements being processed by the central executive come into consciousness. Indeed, one of the functions of the executive is to select from a range of processing which ones come into awareness: those that are relevant to current actions or concerns are selected, those less relevant remain unconscious. He also suggested that so-called negative hypnotic phenomena, such as analgesia, blindness, and paralysis, may occur under hypnosis as a result of the executive system withholding sensory information from our awareness following suggestions from an external source. Because we are unaware of this selection, any failure to move or lack of sensation is thought of as involuntary. By contrast, action sequences may occur as a result of processing the executive does not allow into awareness; so an individual may make apparently 'involuntary' movements which they consider to have been out of their control. In this way, hypnotic phenomena are the result of selective awareness governed by the central executive. Oakley suggests that functional symptoms may result from the same processes. In this case, the executive 'chooses' in some way to allow or disallow various information into awareness. This may be the result of a variety of unconscious 'internal dynamics and motivations in the interests of providing a solution to what may be an otherwise insoluble psychological problem' (Oakely 1999: 260).

The role of stress

Oakley's concept of FNSD as a consequence of individuals facing an otherwise insoluble problem hints at the role that stress may have as a precipitant to this disorder. Evidence does partially support this contention. Duncan and Oto (2008), for example, reported high levels of trauma in their population of 'psychogenic non-epileptic attacks': 32.5% reported sexual abuse, 26% reported physical abuse, while 19% reported a traumatic bereavement. In a novel development of this literature, Nicholson et al. (2016) compared the frequency of recent severe life events in people diagnosed with depression, functional disorders, and 'healthy controls'. In addition, they measured the degree to which the conditions provided a form of 'escape' from each stressor. Fifty-six per cent of people with a functional disorder reported at least one serious life event in the month prior to its onset; this compared to 21% of those with depression and the controls. Fifty-three per cent of the functional disorder group rated the event as a 'high escape event', compared with 14% in those with depression and none of the control group. Those with a functional disorder were also most likely to report sexual abuse in the past that was relevant to the present stressor and the onset of symptoms. While these findings are impressive, a meta-analysis of all such studies (Ludwig et al. 2018) confirmed the findings: while many people with the disorder will report significant stress triggers, many do not.

Treatment of FNSD

Empirical evidence of the outcomes of treating functional disorders is still relatively sparse. Nevertheless, a range of interventions has been used, including physiotherapy, CBT, and hypnosis. The first of these is clearly most relevant where movement or gait problems dominate. This approach involves demonstrating that participants can achieve normal movement, educating them about their condition, and training them in previously normal movements while minimizing maladaptive motor responses. On the basis of a limited, but relatively successful, number of intervention studies, a British expert consensus group (Nielsen et al. 2015) concluded this was an appropriate and likely effective intervention. This approach may be enhanced by the addition of a behavioural component. LaFrance et al. (2014) examined the effectiveness of an SSRI, 'cognitive behavioural therapy informed psychotherapy' for a 12-week period, or a combination of the two in the treatment of non-epileptic seizures. The key outcome measure was the number of seizures participants reported. The combined intervention proved most effective (a 68% reduction), with the SSRI and CBT being equally effective (a 56% reduction each) at the end of therapy. In a direct comparison of CBT against standard medical treatment, Goldstein et al. (2010) randomly allocated participants with non-epileptic seizures to these two conditions. The CBT comprised 12 sessions of six phases: (i) treatment engagement, (ii) reinforcement of independence, (iii) distraction, relaxation, and refocusing techniques at the earliest signs of an event, (iv) graded exposure to avoided situations, (v) cognitive restructuring, and (vi) relapse prevention. By the end of therapy, participants in the CBT condition were experiencing a modest but statistically significantly reduction in the frequency of seizures per month; however, this was no longer evident at 6-month follow-up.

A very different approach was taken by Ataoglu et al. (2003). They used a therapeutic technique called paradoxical intention (see Chapter 5), in which individuals are encouraged to maintain or even exacerbate their symptoms. They compared this approach with the use of an anxiolytic, diazepam, in 30 patients diagnosed with pseudoseizures. Of the 15 patients who completed paradoxical intention treatment, 14 showed some improvement; of the 15 treated with diazepam, 9 showed improvements after 6 weeks of treatment. Finally, Moene et al. (2003) assigned patients with motor disorders with symptoms including paralysis, gait disturbance, coordination problems, aphonia, and non-epileptic seizures either to a waiting list control or active treatment using hypnosis. Treatment involved ten sessions, focusing on suggestions of symptom reduction and age regression to enable emotional insight. The waiting list control group design did not allow long-term follow-up measures to be taken. However, at the end of therapy, patients in the intervention condition showed significantly more improvement on video-based measures of their disorder than those in the control group.

8.5 Chapter summary

1. SSD is characterized by the experience and reporting of physical symptoms that cause distress but lack corresponding physical pathology.
2. Up to 0.7% of the general population could be diagnosed with SSD.
3. Biological models of the disorder suggest it results from a sensitivity to physical sensations perhaps due to dysregulation in the serotonergic system. This may be added to by catastrophic interpretation of these sensations.

4. Psychological models suggest SSD results from modelling of somatic complaints by parents and gaining attention of parents by reporting physical problems. In time, individuals may come to express emotional distress through reporting physical symptoms.

5. There are relatively few reported treatment studies, although there is preliminary evidence that treatment with SSRIs or CBT may be of benefit.

6. The key symptom of IAD is a preoccupation with the fear of having a serious illness – in the absence of contrary medical evidence.

7. Warwick and Salkovskis considered IAD to be a response to immediate threat that triggers health concerns established earlier in life. These become the focus of attention and cause considerable distress.

8. The main treatment for IAD is generally cognitive behavioural, although there is some evidence that SSRIs may be effective.

9. Body dysmorphic disorder involves a preoccupation with an imagined defect in appearance, often with high levels of negative thinking, self-criticism, anxiety, and depression.

10. Developmental psychological theories suggest that the condition is triggered by critical or traumatic incidents that involve an individual's appearance, and is maintained by selective attention to perceived physical limitations.

11. Low levels of serotonin may also be implicated in the disorder.

12. Treatment studies are few and usually involve cognitive behavioural therapy.

13. FNSD presents as a neurological or sensory disorder that is disabling but has no physical cause.

14. Aetiological explanations vary from it being a deliberate behaviour under the control of the affected individual to being a form of hypnosis. Both may be precipitated by stress, although why this should lead to functional symptoms in particular is not understood.

15. Treatment studies suggest that cognitive behavioural and hypnotic treatments may be of some benefit.

8.6 For discussion

1. How may childhood factors translate into somatization disorders, and what factors may maintain them once established?

2. Why are somatization disorders hard to treat?

3. Are the somatization disorders distinct disorders or simply the end of a spectrum of health or appearance concern most of us experience at some time?

4. What factors may contribute specifically to the onset of a FSND? Do these differ from those that trigger a variety of other mental health disorders? What other factors may contribute to the disorder?

5. Why are people with FNSD likely to present accompanied by a teddy bear?

8.7 Further reading

Brown, R.J. (2004) Psychological mechanisms of medically unexplained symptoms: an integrative conceptual model, *Psychological Bulletin*, 130: 793–812.

Liu, J., Gill, N.S., Teodorczuk, A. et al. (2019) The efficacy of cognitive behavioural therapy in somatoform disorders and medically unexplained physical symptoms: a meta-analysis of randomized controlled trials, *Journal of Affective Disorders*, 245: 98–112.

Phillips, K.A. (2005) *The Broken Mirror: Understanding and Treating Body Dysmorphic Disorder*, New York: Oxford University Press.

Scarella, T.M., Laferton, J.A., Ahern, D.K et al. (2016). The relationship of hypochondriasis to anxiety, depressive, and somatoform disorders, *Psychosomatics*, 57: 200–7.

van Dessel N., den Boeft M., van der Wouden, J.C. et al. (2014) Non-pharmacological interventions for somatoform disorders and medically unexplained physical symptoms (MUPS) in adults, *Cochrane Database of Systematic Reviews*, 11: CD011142 [https://doi.org/10.1002/14651858.CD011142.pub2].

Wilhelm. S., Philips, K.A. and Steketee, G. (2013) *Cognitive-Behavioral Therapy for Body Dysmorphic Disorder: A Treatment Manual*, New York: Guilford Press.

9 Trauma-related conditions

This chapter focuses on three types of problems that may occur as a result of trauma experienced by the individual either as an adult or as a child. The first, post-traumatic stress disorder (PTSD), is widely acknowledged as a natural response to being involved in or seeing highly traumatic events. The other two conditions are more controversial. Indeed, their very existence has been called into question. The chapter explores evidence relating to two apparent responses to childhood trauma: hidden and recovered memories, and dissociative identity disorder (DID), previously known as multiple personality disorder. By the end of the chapter, you should have an understanding of:

- The nature and treatment of post-traumatic stress disorder
- The controversy surrounding 'recovered memories'
- The controversy surrounding dissociative identity disorder
- Treatment approaches used in DID.

9.1 Post-traumatic stress disorder

The **DSM**-5 criteria for a diagnosis of post-traumatic stress disorder (PTSD) are the most complex of the entire manual, allowing for over half a million combinations of symptoms that can be diagnosed as PTSD (Galatzer-Levy and Bryant 2013). The individual must experience the following:

- *Exposure to death, threatened death, actual or threatened serious injury, or actual or threatened sexual violence through*: (i) direct exposure, (ii) learning a relative or close friend was exposed to trauma, or (iii) indirect exposure to details of the trauma, as a consequence of professional duties.

- *The traumatic event is persistently re-experienced* through at least one of: (i) unwanted upsetting memories, (ii) nightmares, (iii) flashbacks, and (iv) emotional distress or (v) physical reactivity after exposure to reminders of the trauma.
- *Avoidance of trauma-related stimuli* involving trauma-related thoughts or feelings, or external reminders of the trauma.
- *Negative changes in cognitions and mood,* including at least two of: an inability to remember key features of the trauma event, overly negative beliefs about oneself or the world, exaggerated self- or other-blame, negative affect, decreased interest in activities, feeling isolated, difficulties experiencing positive affect.
- *Trauma-related arousal and reactivity* that began or worsened after the trauma, evident through irritability or aggression, risky or destructive behaviour, hypervigilance, heightened startle reaction, difficulty concentrating, difficulty sleeping.

Finally, symptoms must last at least one month and create distress or functional impairment. More descriptively, the condition involves three psychological processes:

- *Intrusive memories*: the trauma is re-experienced through intrusive thoughts, flashbacks or nightmares. The individual may choose to ruminate about the traumatic event or its consequences, sometimes for many hours a day. Images and other sensations (smell, sound) of the trauma may also spring unbidden to mind, in the form of flashbacks. These can feel as real as the event but may be fragmentary or partial. Emotions associated with the trauma may be relived with similar intensity to those felt at the time. Images have been described as if being in a film of the incident. Initially, the person may feel they are actually 'in' the film: as they recover, they feel they are watching the film as an outside observer. That is, they begin, almost literally, to feel more detached from the trauma. Nightmares can be intense and severely disruptive of sleep.
- *Avoidance*: this may involve mental **defence mechanisms** including being unable to recall aspects of the trauma, emotional numbness, or detachment from others, as well as physically avoiding reminders of the trauma.
- *Arousal*: persistent feelings of over-arousal that may be evidenced by irritability, being easily startled or hypervigilant, suffering insomnia, or having difficulty concentrating.

Triggers to PTSD are wide-ranging, and include war experiences, childhood sexual and physical abuse, adult rape, and natural and technological disasters. Perhaps the most frequent cause of PTSD is road traffic accidents: about 22% of people involved in such an accident go on to develop some degree of PTSD (Lin et al. 2018). Around 4% of the US population are likely to be experiencing some degree of PTSD at any one time (Kilpatrick et al. 2013). Rates among groups that regularly encounter traumatic events are higher. Bennett et al. (2004), for example, found a **prevalence** of 22% among emergency ambulance personnel. Rates among combat veterans from Vietnam are as high as 30% for men and 27% for women (Kulka et al. 1990), while rates of PTSD among child soldiers in Africa approached 60% (Ovuga et al. 2008). PTSD is not only a consequence of the experience of external events. Data is accumulating to show that PTSD occurs following acute and frightening life-threatening health problems, such as heart attacks or diagnoses of cancer (e.g. Tulloch et al. 2015).

PTSD often begins within a few weeks of the precipitating event, but can be triggered by further trauma or life events as diverse as trauma anniversaries, interpersonal losses, or changes in health status sometime after the originating event. Of the three key symptoms, re-experiencing appears to decrease most rapidly. People in whom hyperarousal is the dominant symptom appear to have the worst prognosis (Schell et al. 2004). According to Sareen (2014), an adult's risk for distress will increase as the number of the following 'risk' factors increases:

- multiple exposures to traumatic events
- traumatic events that are either very severe and/or long-lasting
- being female
- exposure to other serious but not traumatic life stresses either as a child (e.g. childhood maltreatment) or adult
- personal factors of neuroticism or trait-avoidance coping
- low levels of social support.

Here is the story of Ron, which shows how both the situation and the reaction of the people around him can contribute to the development of PTSD.

At the time this happened, I was working in a small hut on an industrial estate. They had been building some more units and had a crane on a lorry to lift things around the site. This was right next to our office. You couldn't see it, because there were no windows on that side of the hut, but you knew it was there ... I don't know why, but on the day of the accident they were using the crane without stabilizing it by putting the legs onto the ground. The upshot of this was that the crane toppled over and fell onto the building I was in. The first we were aware of things was a lot of shouting and mechanical noises we now know were it toppling. Then there was a great crash and the arm of the crane smashed through the building. I was in there with my mate. Amazingly, neither of us were actually hit by the thing. But we were both trapped by debris from the building. I think I was knocked out for a while because I cannot remember in detail what happened, but it could only have been for a minute or two. I wasn't hurt too badly, but I was trapped. The worst part of it all, was just having to wait to get out. I was frightened that the gas pipes were fractured and the image of dying in a fire went through my mind. I hate being unable to move and all sorts of things went through my head about what would happen to me while I couldn't move. I felt really frightened until I could hear people coming to dig us out, and they lifted the heavy stuff off me and I could move ...

Once I was out, I went to the sick bay and was sent home. I told them I was OK, just 'cos I wanted to get home and get out of it. I was driven home and spent the rest of the day like a zombie. I just phased out. I didn't want to talk about it. Kept myself to myself. I slept OK. I hate missing work so I went in the next day. My mates took me to look at the hut, and they were saying how lucky we were to get out alive.

Everyone I met said the same thing! I know they were being friendly, but that made things worse, and I began to think about things more and more. I felt shaky and sick … In the end, I had to go home.

The nightmares began a couple of days later. I dreamt that I was in the building – this time I was watching the crane fall even though I didn't in real life and felt trapped as it hit. Each dream was terrifying and I woke up sweating and breathing hard. I could dream two or three times a night. I had to get up and watch TV, have a cup of tea and a fag to help me calm down after them … I couldn't go back to sleep. I took about eight or nine weeks off work because of all this. I was just too knackered to work.

I was also pretty uptight during this time. I'm usually very easy going. But I ran into problems with the wife because I was so difficult to live with … The dreams gradually got better and I forced myself to go back to work. I had a few panic attacks when I went back to start with because I was working in a temporary building which had no windows, so I panicked at the thought of things that were happening outside. The new office has large windows, and that's OK for me now.

World events and PTSD

Until 2020, the most widely experienced trigger to PTSD was the destruction of the World Trade Center buildings by Al Qaeda on 9 September 2001, which was watched by hundreds of thousands if not millions of people live on television. To investigate its impact, Galea et al. (2003) conducted psychiatric telephone surveys 1, 4, and 6 months after the event across the population of New York. The prevalence of 'probable PTSD' directly related to the attacks immediately following the event was understandably high but declined from 7.5% one month after the event to 0.6% 5 months later. Symptoms were highest among people who were directly affected by the attacks; but a significant number of people not directly affected also met the criteria for a diagnosis. Predictors of PTSD included worries about future terrorist attacks, reduced self-confidence and perceptions of personal control, guilt/shame and helplessness/anger, and low levels of social support (e.g. Simeon et al. 2005). More frequent viewing of television images was also associated with a higher risk for PTSD and depression (Ahern et al. 2002). One key image that influenced rates of PTSD was that of people 'falling or jumping' from the building. The prevalence of PTSD among individuals who repeatedly saw this image was 17.4%, while 6.2% of viewers who did not see this image developed PTSD. The attack also increased risk for PTSD among children. In New York itself, direct exposure to events, exposure of a family member, and a prior history of trauma increased the risk of problems (Hoven et al. 2005). However, simply watching events on television also contributed to risk. Lengua et al. (2005) found that 8% of their sample of children from Seattle who had only seen events on television met the criteria 'consistent with PTSD'. As in Hoven and colleagues' study, girls experienced more emotional problems than boys.

Now, sadly, another world event has taken over at the top of the league of world traumas. Covid-19, and its treatment, is now contributing significantly to a range of mental health problems across the population. Rates of depression and anxiety are high as a function of lockdown and health concerns among the general population. However, specific traumatic outcomes are also being reported. One aspect of treatment that may significantly contribute to trauma is the long-term airway ventilation experienced by the sickest of patients. Data from Covid-19 patients is lacking at the time of writing, but there is clear evidence that this will contribute to significant trauma symptoms. On ventilation, patients are typically sedated and in and out of consciousness. Many experience nightmares as a consequence of their physical experiences, sensory deprivation, and dream-like psychological experiences of care by alien-looking creatures in masks and gowns, which they are unable to reality check. Previous studies have shown that up to two-thirds of patients and their carers are likely to experience PTSD following long-term ventilation (see Garrouste-Orgeas et al. 2019). Add to this the fear of dying, symptoms including chronic shortness of breath even when ventilated, and long-term symptoms following discharge from hospital, the likelihood is of even higher levels of psychopathology in Covid-19 patients and their families. Indeed, the one set of data published at the time of writing is a Chinese study indicating 96.2% of patients discharged from hospital following treatment for Covid-19 had 'significant post-traumatic stress symptoms'. More generally, evidence from the SARS outbreak, some years previously, indicates that hospital workers as well as the general population are at increased risk of PTSD following lockdown, particularly when this is imposed due to potential contact with people who are infected with the virus (Brooks et al. 2020)

Aetiology of PTSD

Neurological factors

The brain systems involved in PTSD are those involved in processing emotions and memory and our behavioural responses to them: the amygdala, hippocampus, and ventral medial prefrontal cortex. The hippocampus is responsible for storing and retrieving memories. It is linked to the amygdala, the area of the brain particularly associated with the formation of conditioned fear responses. The prefrontal lobe is responsible for controlling our behaviour in response to emotions triggered by activation of the amygdala and hippocampus.

Two stress hormones are particularly implicated in PTSD: norepinephrine and cortisol. Increases in these hormones generally enhance memory. However, the levels that may occur at times of traumatic stress may actually be toxic to brain tissue and result in neuronal death, damaging the memory systems. The hippocampus, in particular, may be vulnerable to damage following severe trauma, leading to reductions in its size, which may recover following treatment or resolution of the trauma (Apfel et al. 2011). Damage to differing parts of the fear processing system can result in a number of problems:

- Damage to the *hippocampus* may cause problems in working memory (Shaw et al. 2009) and an exaggerated conditioned fear response. The latter may be an outcome of difficulties in differentiating between present and past experiences. As a consequence, contexts that resemble those of the trauma event can trigger fear and hypervigilance as the fear system is activated, as if the initiating event is ongoing.

- In contrast to the hippocampus, the *amygdala* may increase in size following a traumatic event (Morey et al. 2012). Activity of the enlarged amygdala contributes to the core symptoms of PTSD: flashbacks, negative mood alterations, an extreme startle response, and avoidance of anything that triggers memories of the trauma. Brewin (2001) speculated that flashbacks occur when information is transferred from the amygdala to the hippocampus.
- Damage to the *prefrontal lobe* leads to difficulties in controlling behavioural responses to the strong and fearful emotions the individual may experience.
- Finally, the *sympathetic nervous system* (see Chapter 4), controlled by the hypothalamus and levels of norepinephrine, is responsible for the high levels of physiological arousal associated with the condition.

These neurological changes contribute not only to the symptoms of PTSD but may confuse those experiencing them, as they feel out of control of their strong emotional responses to often relatively benign situations. These individuals may experience rage or distress as a consequence of trivial incidents as well as heart palpitations, memory loss, shaking, insomnia, nightmares, and difficulty concentrating.

Conditioning models

The conditioning model of PTSD (Foa and Kozak 1986) considers PTSD to be a classically conditioned emotional response. According to Foa and Kozak, associations are stored in neural networks, linking emotions, cognitions, and perceptual memories. As such, re-exposure to similar contexts or stimuli evokes memories of the event and the conditioned fear response. Avoidance of reminders of the trauma not only prevents distress, but also prevents habituation of the fear response to stimuli associated with the event (Mowrer 1947). As a result, occasional and accidental encounters with relevant stimuli result in flashbacks and other cued memories. Chemtob et al. (1988) proposed a similar model to that of Foa and Kozak, but suggested that memories of the incident are maintained within a neural network which is permanently activated (as opposed to being activated by environmental and emotional cues) and causes the individual to function in 'survival mode', resulting in the hyperarousal symptoms of PTSD.

A schema model of PTSD

The first schema model of PTSD, developed by Horowitz (1986), was strongly influenced by psychoanalytic theory. He proposed that PTSD occurs when the individual is involved in events that are so horrific, they cannot be reconciled with their view (schema) of the world. The belief that one may die in an incident, for example, may shatter previous beliefs of invulnerability. The individual feels unsafe and vulnerable. To avoid this ego-damaging discrepancy, defence mechanisms of numbing or denial are evoked. However, these compete with a second innate drive, known as the completion tendency. This requires the individual to integrate memories of trauma into existing world models or schemata: either to make sense of the memories according to currently held beliefs about the world or to change those beliefs.

The completion tendency maintains trauma-related information in active memory in an attempt to process it. Defence mechanisms try to stop these memories entering consciousness. The symptoms the individual experiences result from the fluctuating strengths of these competing processes. When the completion tendency breaks through the defence mechanisms, memories intrude into consciousness in the form of flashbacks, nightmares, and unwanted thoughts or emotional memories. When defence mechanisms are effective, the individual experiences periods of numbness or denial. Once trauma-related information is integrated into general belief systems, the symptoms cease.

Research box 8

Johnson, R.A., Albright, D.L., Marzolf, J.R. et al. (2018) Effects of therapeutic horseback riding on post-traumatic stress disorder in military veterans, *Military Medical Research*, 5: 3.

Most interventions focused on the treatment of PTSD have involved the core elements of exposure and coping with traumatic memories. These address the core underpinnings of the disorder. However, there are other ways in which rehabilitation of individuals with PTSD can take other paths, some of which may not immediately be obvious. This study takes one of these paths. It addresses a highly traumatized population, US military veterans, using a somewhat unusual intervention that had shown some benefit in a number of reported case studies, but had yet to be formally evaluated in a randomized controlled trial. The authors predicted the programme would reduce PTSD symptoms, loneliness and social isolation, and increase coping self-efficacy and emotional regulation.

Method

Participants

Participants were 42 of 57 people contacted through letters of invitation sent to veterans whose electronic records suggested they met the criteria for a diagnosis of PTSD and who lived within a 50-mile radius of the Therapeutic Horse Riding Center (which was based within the College of Veterinary Science, University of Missouri). Of the 57 contacted, 13 did not meet the criteria for entry into the study, and others dropped out of the recruitment process for a number of personal reasons.

Participants were randomly allocated to the therapeutic horse riding (THR) condition or a **waiting list control**. The intervention comprised six, weekly, small group riding lessons led by an occupational therapist and riding instructor. Participants spent time learning to ride and grooming skills. There was no formal therapeutic element.

Measures

Background measures including a range of demographic variables and a physical health history were taken at baseline. Repeated measures were:

- *PTSD Checklist – Military Version* (PTSD-M): a 17-item measure of PTSD based on 'stressful military experiences' and DSM-IV-TR criteria for PTSD. The measure gives a cut-off score of 50 as 'indicative' of a PTSD diagnosis.
- *Coping Self-Efficacy Scale* (CSES): measures perceived ability to cope with life's challenges or threats by using problem-focused and avoidance coping, and support from family and friends.
- *Difficulties in Emotion Regulation Scale* (DERS): measures modulation of emotional arousal; awareness, understanding, and acceptance of emotions; and ability to act in desired ways regardless of the emotional state.
- *Social and Emotional Loneliness Scale for Adults* (SELSA): measures emotional, family, and romantic loneliness.

Process

For veterans in the THR condition, measures were taken at baseline and 3 and 6 weeks into the intervention. For the waiting list control condition, measures were at baseline, and then 3 and 6 weeks into the control condition (the equivalent time-frame to the THR group) and again 3 and 6 weeks into their intervention phase.

Results

The reported sample characteristics were of 32 males and 6 females (presumably 4 did not report their gender), with a mean age of 54 years and with the range of deployments ranging from zero to ten. Table 1 reports the outcome data during the active intervention and equivalent control condition phase.

Table 1 Mean scores (and standard deviations) on key measures over time-frame of the intervention

	Baseline	**Week 3**	**Week 6**
PTSD symptoms			
Wait list	58.36 (16.40)	57.62 (13.15)	59.23 (14.29)
THR	57.72 (14.63)	53.22 (13.8)	47.00 (14.67)

	Baseline	Week 3	Week 6
Coping self-efficacy			
Wait list	114.43(64.02)	103.38(61.08)	115.00 (48.17)
THR	115.59(50.55)	116.09(50.68)	130.21 (51.84)
Emotion regulation			
Wait list	113.50(27.80)	109.46 (24.33)	110.00 (32.07)
THR	106.00(29.60)	108.65 (21.46)	99.42 (18.31)
Social and emotional loneliness			
Wait list	49.35 (5.06)	52.08 (12.40)	53.61 (8.03)
THR	50.38 (11.92)	53.52 (13.70)	57.00 (10.29)

Repeated-measures analysis of variance revealed a significant reduction in PTSD scores over the course of the study, and between each measurement occasion ($F_{1,17}$ = 10.678, p = 0.005; $F_{1,17}$ = 8.750, p = 0.009) in the THR but not the waiting list condition. Overall, participants had an 81.8% likelihood of improvement in their PTSD. Further detailed examination showed that participants had a 66.7% likelihood of having lower PTSD scores at 3 weeks, and an 87.5% likelihood at 6 weeks. No other consistent changes were found.

Discussion

This was a seriously under-powered study, with only 13 waiting list and 19 intervention participants providing data at week 6. In addition, although there was evidence of a reduction in PTSD scores in the riding group, no interaction term is reported, so while the data seem to show more marked changes in the riding group than in the control condition, this was not statistically confirmed. Finally, the longevity of any changes was not measured. Accordingly, the study really should be considered a successful pilot intervention that would benefit from a larger confirmatory trial. Despite these provisos, while this type of intervention may never replace a formal therapeutic approach, this and similar interventions may prove effective adjuncts to them.

A process model of PTSD

Brewin (2001) added a second level of information processing to the model proposed by Horowitz. According to Brewin, the individual can both deliberately choose to address their traumatic memories, and memories may come to consciousness without deliberate recall. These processes involve two differing memory systems:

• *Verbally accessible memories (VAMs)*: this system involves memories of the incident that can be deliberately accessed. They tend to be fragmented, based on normal recall processes, and can be changed as the person processes information about the traumatic incident. They may, for example, become less traumatic as the individual reframes the incident as being less threatening than they initially thought; they may become more traumatic if they later consider the event to have been more personally threatening.

- *Situationally accessible memories (SAMs)*: these flashback memories cannot be deliberately accessed but come to consciousness in response to cues that remind the individual of the incident – including activation of the VAM system. They may also occur when the brain is not actively processing information – most commonly at night in the form of nightmares. They feel as if they are 'in the event' and cannot be deliberately changed.

According to Brewin, resolution of PTSD requires both sets of memories to enter the normal memory system. By this time, they are still accessible but do not carry the high levels of emotional content associated with both VAMs and SAMs. Resolution of VAMs involves deliberate recall and reframing of information. This leads to an integration of the VAMs with pre-existing beliefs and models of the world, and restores a sense of safety and control over both self and the world. Activation of the SAMs is also required, and the SAMs gradually change over time and become less emotion-laden and frightening. Changes in SAM representations may occur through the integration of new, non-threatening information or, more frequently, through the creation of new SAMs. As SAMs may be triggered through conscious processing of VAMs, this process may occur naturally. Both these processes are similar to the completion tendency described by Horowitz. Thus, the model includes elements of the schema theory of Horowitz, as PTSD resolves when memories of the event are integrated within pre-existing memory structures and elements of Foa and Kozak's fear network in terms of the representation of memories.

Empirical investigation of these processes can be difficult. However, Brewin and colleagues have been able to find differences in the types of memories people provide from VAMs and SAMs. Hellawell and Brewin (2004), for example, asked people to recall and write a narrative of the trauma that led to their PTSD and then to identify which parts of the narrative were based on flashback memories (SAMs) and which were based on 'ordinary' memories (VAMs). They found narrative involving flashback memory was associated with higher levels of autonomic and behavioural arousal (as observed by a researcher) than writing based on ordinary memories. In addition, writing based on flashback memories was more detailed, and made more mentions of death, fear, helplessness, and horror. It was also more likely to be written in the present tense than memory sections written from ordinary memory. By contrast, sections written from ordinary memory tended to mention more 'secondary' emotions such as guilt and anger, which may have been experienced following the incident rather than at the time of its occurrence.

Brewin suggested that the hippocampus is the neural centre involved in processing VAMs. The amygdala may be involved in processing the more emotionally laden SAMs. Brewin, like Horowitz, suggested that emotional processing results from a drive towards resolution of conflict between previously held schemata and new information. The activation of SAMs provides the detailed information needed to allow cognitive readjustment to the trauma. Once integration has been achieved, the symptoms of PTSD will resolve.

A psychosocial model

Extending the work of Brewin to include a wider set of psychosocial factors, Joseph and colleagues' (1995) model of PTSD included:

- *Event stimuli*: iconic representations of the event held in immediate memory.
- *Event cognitions*: memories that provide the basis for re-experiencing phenomena or intrusive memories – Brewin's SAMs.
- *Appraisals and reappraisals*: the individual's thoughts about the incident – Brewin's VAMs. These involve interpretation of information relevant to the incident, drawing on past representations and experiences. They may comprise automatic thoughts triggered by stimuli associated with the trauma or more considered attempts to think through and perhaps reappraise the meaning of the event. Key appraisals are those related to guilt, control, and self-blame.
- *Coping attempts*: flashbacks and emotional memories of the event may result in coping attempts intended to minimize emotional distress. These usually take the form of avoidance of reminders, memories or similar emotions and activities associated with the event. They may also involve attempts at inhibiting unwanted memories.
- *Personality*: this will influence the type of cognitions and emotions experienced at the time of a traumatic incident, the appraisals made in response to it, and subsequent coping strategies.
- *Social support*: an important moderator of the response to trauma, perhaps because talking to other people helps the individual assign new meanings to the event and provides support for the expression of negative emotions.

According to Joseph et al., traumatic events result in immediate cognitions that trigger extreme emotional arousal ('I'm going to die!'). This arousal interferes with the processing of these cognitions. As a consequence, they are held in specific memory networks and form the basis of the re-experiencing phenomena. They are influenced by the nature of the trauma, the core assumptions and beliefs an individual has about the world, elements of the situation which presented the most threat, and the personality of the individual.

Subsequent reappraisal of the situation may also influence outcome. If an individual reflects on events and thinks they were less threatening than they appeared at the time, they may experience fewer symptoms over a shorter duration than if they do not reduce, or even increase, the level of perceived threat. Attributions of failing to take control of an event ('I could have done something to stop it – and I didn't') are linked to the emotions of shame and guilt, and increased risk for PTSD. Andrews et al. (2000), for example, found shame and anger to be key predictors of levels of trauma one month after experiencing a violent crime, and shame to be predictive of symptoms 6 months following the incident. Similar findings have been reported following sexual abuse (Feiring et al. 2002) and being stalked (Kamphuis et al. 2003). Together with feelings of loss of self, distrust, alienation from others, and a sense of being permanently damaged, these responses have been termed the 'experience of mental death', which Ebert and Dyck (2004) labelled the core feature of PTSD. Beliefs that an individual is unable to cope with strong emotions may also lead to avoidance of potentially stressful situations and prevent the individual from learning that they can, indeed, cope with them. Finally, good social support will generally lessen the symptoms of PTSD, partly perhaps because this supports rehearsal and positive reappraisal of event-related cognitions. In one study of this phenomenon, Dworkin et al. (2018) followed up survivors of sexual assault and found that social support was associated with greater reductions in PTSD symptoms over time – with the proviso that substance abuse appeared to reduce the benefits of this support.

Stop and think ...

The outcomes of traumatic events are not all negative. Calhoun and Tedeschi (1999) identified a more positive outcome they termed 'post-traumatic growth'. These changes include improved relationships, new possibilities and a greater appreciation for life, a greater sense of personal strength and spiritual development. People who experience post-traumatic growth frequently report an increased sense of their own capacities to survive and cope with whatever life throws at them. They also may find themselves becoming more comfortable with intimacy and having a greater sense of compassion for others who experience life difficulties. A commonly reported change is that people begin to value the smaller things in life more and also to consider important changes in the religious, spiritual, and existential beliefs they may hold. They may also change their life goals in the light of their traumatic experience. Rather than focusing on relief from the negative outcomes of trauma, should therapy focus more on fostering these more positive outcomes?

Treatment of PTSD

Preventing PTSD by psychological debriefing

Psychological debriefing is a single-session interview conducted immediately following a traumatic event intended to prevent the development of PTSD. It involves encouraging the individual to talk through the event and their emotional reactions to it in a detailed and systematic manner. It is thought to aid integration of incident memories into the general memory system.

Debriefing is now regularly offered following traumatic incidents, despite increasing questions about its effectiveness. Rose et al. (2002), for example, concluded from their **meta-analysis** of four well-conducted randomized controlled trials that debriefing may not only be ineffective in preventing PTSD, it can actually increase risk for the disorder. None of the studies they reviewed found a reduced risk for PTSD in the 3–4 months following the incident. The two studies that reported longer-term findings found that those who received debriefing had nearly twice the risk of developing PTSD than those who did not receive the intervention. That is, debriefing seemed to inhibit long-term recovery from psychological trauma. A number of explanations have been proposed for these findings, although each remains speculative:

- 'Secondary traumatization' may occur as a result of further imaginal exposure to a traumatic incident within a short time of the event
- Debriefing may 'medicalize' normal distress and increase the expectancy of developing psychological symptoms in those who would otherwise not have done so
- Debriefing may prevent the potentially protective responses of denial and distancing that may occur in the immediate aftermath of a traumatic incident.

In a robust counter-argument to these criticisms, Hawker et al. (2011) contended that the studies showing debriefing to be potentially problematic failed to follow appropriate debriefing protocols, used debriefing with individuals for whom it was not intended, and those who received debriefing tended to have more severe initial symptoms that those who did not. They argued that where conducted appropriately, debriefing can be of significant benefit, and called for more research of this issue. An alternative, low-key and unstructured emotional venting into a remote website while telling 'stories' about the experience of caring for Covid-19 patients, has been shown to be of benefit to healthcare workers (Bennett et al. 2020). Accordingly, there may be variants of debriefing that can be of benefit.

Pharmacological treatment

A variety of drug types, including antidepressant **MAOIs**, **SSRIs**, and **tricyclics**, have been used in the treatment of PTSD. However, SSRIs are now considered the pharmacological treatment of choice (Sullivan and Neria 2009) due to their relatively few side-effects and comparative effectiveness with other drugs. Nevertheless, psychological therapy is more frequently the first-line treatment of the disorder. This was supported by the findings of Chen et al. (2013), who found a preference for exposure-based intervention among a sample of 'treatment-seeking' individuals with chronic PTSD.

Exposure techniques

The principles underpinning exposure methods in the treatment of PTSD are that the individual will ultimately benefit from exposure to memories of the event and their associated emotions. The conditioning model suggests that this involves a process of habituation. A more neurocognitive explanation is that exposure leads to reconciliation between memories and the meaning of the traumatic event and pre-existing world schemata. Only by accessing and processing these memories will resolution be possible.

Trauma-focused CBT may lead to an initial exacerbation of distress as upsetting images, previously avoided where possible, are deliberately recalled. To minimize this distress and prevent drop-out from therapy, a graded exposure process may be adopted in which the individual initially talks about elements of the traumatic event at a level of detail that does not overwhelm them. More distressing memories are avoided at this time, and become the focus of the next levels of intervention. Reactivation of memories by this procedure involves describing the experience in detail, focusing on what happened, the thoughts and emotions experienced at the time, and any memories that the incident triggered. This approach may be augmented by a variety of cognitive behavioural techniques, including relaxation training and cognitive restructuring. Relaxation may help the individual control their arousal at the time of recalling the event or at other times in the day when they are feeling tense or on edge. Cognitive restructuring may help them address any distorted cognitions they had in response to the event and make those thoughts less threatening ('I'm going to die! ... It felt like I was going to die, but actually that was more my panic than reality ...'). Wells and Sembi (2004) focused on teaching people to minimize the rumination that can be a particularly distressing element of PTSD by using active distraction techniques.

Several studies have shown trauma-focused therapy to be better than no treatment or alternative interventions, including supportive counselling and relaxation therapy without exposure, as both an early intervention (Roberts et al. 2019) and for those with more chronic PTSD (Bisson et al. 2013). In one such study, Marks et al. (1996) compared relaxation, exposure alone, cognitive restructuring alone, and exposure plus cognitive restructuring. By the end of the intervention, all treatments proved better than relaxation, with no differences in effectiveness between them. At 3- and 6-month follow-up, however, the exposure programme proved superior. It seems that cognitive restructuring may help participants cope with the anxiety and other emotions evoked in the early stages of exposure programmes, but exposure to traumatic memories is critical to long-term benefit. The optimal treatment seems to involve a combination of cognitive strategies in the early stages of therapy combined with gradual exposure to traumatic memories. Deblinger et al. (2016) argued, further, that group-based trauma-focused CBT may be of particular benefit because it may reduce the feelings of shame, isolation, and stigma experienced by many people with PTSD.

Interestingly, treating people with PTSD may not require a great deal of specialist training. Gillespie et al. (2002) taught healthcare staff to provide an exposure-based intervention for PTSD in response to a large bomb which exploded in the small Northern Irish town of Omagh in 1998. Staff received a 2-day workshop plus telephone contact with an expert in the treatment of PTSD and therapy supervision. The effectiveness of their intervention was similar to that reported in previous studies involving expert therapists.

Eye movement desensitization and reprocessing

The most recent treatment of PTSD, known as eye movement desensitization and reprocessing (EMDR), was discovered by chance by Shapiro (1995). She noticed that while walking in the woods her disturbing thoughts began to disappear, and when recalled were less upsetting than previously. She associated this change with her eyes spontaneously moving rapidly backwards and forwards in an upward diagonal due to changes in light shining through the trees. Subsequently, this process has been developed into a standardized intervention and subject to a number of clinical trials in the treatment of PTSD.

Treatment involves participants recalling target memories as single visual images, which are combined with a negative cognition associated with the image, framed in the present tense ('I am terrified') and held in memory. They are then asked to track the therapist's finger as it is moved increasingly quickly back and forth across their line of vision. After 24 such movements, the **client** is instructed to 'Blank it out' or 'Let it go'. This procedure is repeated until the client experiences minimal distress to the presence of the image and negative cognition. If no changes occur, the direction of eye movements is changed.

EMDR incorporates controlled exposure to elements of the trauma stimulus. An important question is therefore whether the addition of the eye movements enhances the effect of exposure. This does not seem to be the case. Bisson et al. (2013) conducted a meta-analysis to examine the effectiveness of EMDR in the treatment of PTSD versus no treatment, non-specific treatment, and the exposure methods described above. Their analyses indicated a benefit for EMDR when compared with no treatment or non-specific treatments, but no difference in effectiveness compared with other interventions, primarily trauma-focused CBT, which involved exposure to trauma memories. That said, from a clinical perspective EMDR may be of particular benefit to individuals who have difficulty in detailed recall or the ability to provide accounts of complex memories relating to the traumatic event.

Case formulation

Mr F was a prison officer in a small town in the west of England. At six feet four inches, he was a big strong man, fond of playing rugby for a local team and drinking with his mates. He was happily married with two young children. He had no history of mental health problems, and looking at him one would imagine him as an archetypal 'good coper'. However, his history of PTSD showed that even 'good copers' may develop significant mental health problems.

Long-term antecedents

As is often the case with PTSD, there were very few long-term antecedents for Mr F's development of PTSD. He had no history of mental health problems and was happily married with his wider family also around for support. He was happy at work, and had no work or home-related problems.

Short-term antecedents

The trigger to Mr F's PTSD was a simple event. He was walking a group of prisoners down a flight of steps in an isolated stairwell, when he slipped and fell. Against prison regulations (as a result of his shift being short-staffed), he was on his own in the stairwell with no fellow prison officers. As a consequence, the prisoners took the opportunity to knock him to the ground, and began to beat and kick him around the body and head. The force of his beating was such that he was briefly knocked unconscious. The last thought he remembers before losing consciousness was that he was going to die. He was taken to the prison wing, before being sent home to recover from his injuries.

Over the next few months he experienced a significant number of flashbacks to the incident, feeling the force of the blows to him and experiencing the fear of dying. Many occurred at night, while in bed. Every flashback was terrifying, and in the hour following them he had to get out of bed and try and watch television or read a book to help him calm down. He regularly had two or more flashbacks per night. As a consequence, he became increasingly exhausted. In addition, he spent much of the day mulling over the causes and consequence of the attack. He would spend many hours ('A day may disappear') looking out of a house window dwelling on the attack. He believed that both the prisoners were to blame – as they had, he believed, tried to kill him – as well as his fellow prison officers, who had allowed the incident to occur. The prison service was unsympathetic to his condition, writing frequent letters asking when he would return to see the prison occupational health physician, threatening to reduce his pay, and so on. He began to believe that these letters were a deliberate form of harassment.

As a result of these various processes, his mood became increasingly depressed. He was able to engage with his wife and son for brief periods in the day – helping prepare breakfast, for example – but found these times increasingly difficult to manage and he became increasingly isolated even within the family home. He also isolated himself from the home, spending hours away in peaceful places dwelling on the events and their consequences. He was unable to go into any area where he believed there would be prison officers or ex-prisoners, as he was unsure whether he would be able to cope with the sight of them, expecting to be extremely frightened, but also angry and possibly expressing his anger. In a relatively small town, this severely limited where he was able to go.

Formulation

Mr F had a significant post-traumatic response. The critical factor in its development was his belief that he was going to die as a result of his beating. He continued to hold this belief, believing that it was only the somewhat late intervention by his colleagues that prevented him dying in the incident. This continued catastrophic belief helped maintain his anxieties. His response to the incident was typical, if rather stronger than, most responses to PTSD. He experienced the three key symptoms of PTSD: flashbacks when his mind was unoccupied, pre-occupation and rumination on the originating incident, and heightened arousal. His depression stemmed from the nature of his beliefs, including the belief that some prisoners wanted him dead and that the institution for whom he worked and his work colleagues cared little for his well-being. These beliefs were maintained by his avoidance of colleagues who *did* try to visit him at home following the incident: visits which tailed off over time as they were apparently unwanted. In addition, his rumination constantly focused on his negative beliefs about the incident and how close to death he had been, and his anger towards the prison service. Accordingly, although he chronically ruminated about the incident, he had failed to normalize or reappraise it into something less threatening, both of which may have reduced the frequency and severity of his flashbacks. The time spent dwelling on these negative thoughts combined with exhaustion due to lack of sleep and his dislocation from his family and friends led to depression, and a vicious cycle of rumination, flashbacks, avoidance of positive aspects of life, low mood, rumination … and so on.

Intervention

Mr F had severe PTSD and depression (a relatively common co-morbidity). The usual treatment for PTSD involves either exposure or EMDR. Some individuals prefer the latter, particularly as if they find it difficult to focus on the distressing issues for a prolonged time or to verbalize their thoughts. However, Mr F was unwilling to utilize either approach. In addition, his belief that he could have died in the incident was unshakeable. Accordingly, initially, he and his therapist took another approach. Instead of focusing on the PTSD symptoms, they focused on reducing his rumination, his depression, and avoidance of feared situations. One strategy for this was to plan things to do that broke him out of his ruminations and began to normalize his day. His daily plans, for example, involved sitting with his family watching television, walking the dog with his wife, and going out for drives or (when they occurred) watching rugby matches with his brother. The aim was to reduce the time he spent ruminating and provide a number of rewarding/enjoyable experiences each day. In addition, he began a graded exposure to places in the town that he had begun to avoid for fear of meeting ex-cons or colleagues. In preparing for this, he rehearsed how he would respond to seeing such individuals – using relaxation and breathing techniques he was taught, and using **self-instruction** to calm himself. He also used the relaxation and breathing exercises to help him calm down following any flashbacks he had, particularly at night. This approach took several weeks before he began to feel less depressed and more able to go into town. He also experienced several setbacks when he received letters from the prison service, which he now considered to be a form of harassment. Once he began to feel less depressed and more engaged with his family, therapy began to focus on reducing the trauma-related symptoms. As he was already ruminating frequently on the trauma (and he had successfully reduced the time spent ruminating), therapy involved EMDR rather than an exposure programme. This was gradually introduced as his tolerance to the images increased. In addition, he engaged in cognitive therapy, reappraising the role of his colleagues more positively (some had, for example, visited him at home after the incident – so they had shown concern for him). In addition, while he continued to believe that the prisoners who attacked him had wanted him dead, he was able to defuse some of these thoughts, entertaining the idea that they perhaps wanted to hurt rather than kill him, and that the attack was not personal but one which any officer might have experienced if the occasion presented. Depersonalizing the attack was important as it reduced his feelings of threat and shame ('I was so hated by the prisoners that they wanted to kill me') that had been triggered by the attack. He did recover, but not quickly, and despite normalizing his life away from the prison, Mr F was unable to work at the prison.

9.2 Dissociative amnesia

Since the late 1980s, it has been argued that many women who were sexually abused as children had repressed all memories of those events, and that repressed memories could only be recovered in the course of psychological therapy. Initially called repressed or recovered memory, DSM-5 now calls this phenomenon dissociative amnesia; the inability to recall autobiographical information that is usually of a traumatic or stressful nature, is inconsistent with normal forgetting, and is potentially reversible.

In a seminal text, Bass and Davis (1988) advised therapists to accept accounts of these 'recovered memories' at face value, and to suspend disbelief even if they found some parts of their history doubtful. Subsequently, several surveys of therapists revealed that 20–60% of their female clients had reported previously forgotten abuse during the course of therapy (e.g. Loftus and Ketcham 1994). Individuals identified as abusers, often parents or other family members, frequently denied these events, claiming they had been wrongfully accused; that is, the recovered memories of abuse were false memories. Since this time, arguments surrounding the nature of recovered memory have been vociferous and often emotional – so much so, they have been termed 'memory wars'. The arguments of the various 'camps' are outlined below.

Explanations of recovered memory

Accurate accounts

Recovered memories are accurate accounts of previously forgotten events and should be accepted as such even in the absence of corroborative evidence. Explanations for these apparent failures of memory involve the experience of dissociation as a defence against the trauma at the time the individual experienced it. This is an altered state of consciousness in which ordinary perceptual and cognitive functioning is impaired: events feel unreal and distant from the individual. Retrieval of associated memories is poor, as little if any processing takes place at encoding. What memories there are may be fragmented, yet vivid and intense. Hunter (1997) described three forms of dissociation that have been reported by child abuse victims: (i) out-of-body experiences in which events were seen as happening to someone else who looked like the victim; (ii) conscious attempts to 'blank out' memories of the assaults during or after they had happened; and (iii) the creation of an imaginary world into which the respondent could escape and feel safe during or after the abuse. Failure to recall events may be the result of denial and long-term dissociation that prevents the retrieval of any memories that do enter into memory stores.

Illusions

Recovered memories are illusions – false memories resulting from the therapy process itself (Zola 1998). Such memories are 'implanted' by therapists who believe the client is an abuse victim and use therapeutic techniques to persuade the client to remember these 'forgotten' episodes of abuse in order to 'recover'. The likelihood of suggestive influences leading to memory errors is increased by the perceived authority and trustworthiness of the therapist, and their repetition and plausibility. Perhaps the least plausible accounts are the recovery of memories of alien abduction (McNally et al. 2004), although memories of long-term ritual and satanic abuse involving gang rape and ritual (child) murders have proven equally untenable (e.g. Noblitt and Perskin 2000).

Normal forgetting

Recovered memories are not 'special', but are the result of normal forgetting (Loftus and Ketcham 1994). This explanation may be particularly relevant to single traumatic episodes but has more difficulty in accounting for the forgetting of repeated traumatic episodes.

Evidence of recovered memory

Protagonists on each side of the debate have interpreted research findings both to support their case and question those who disagree with them. The debate has drawn on research related to normal memory processes as well as more clinical issues.

Age at time of incident

Recovered memories are sometimes described from before the age of 2, and often in significant detail. Morton et al. (1995), for example, reported that 26% of allegations involving abuse began when the claimant was aged between 0 and 2 years old. This, argue opponents of recovered memory, makes such memories unlikely to be accurate. Most people are unable to recollect experiences from the first 2–3 years of their lives, as the cortical areas that eventually become the sites for permanent memory storage are undergoing a process of maturation at this time that makes them unable to process and store information needed for long-term recall.

Corroboration

Gaining corroborative evidence of child sexual abuse is clearly problematic, and the majority of research focusing on false memories relies on uncorroborated evidence (Loftus and Davis 2006). Nevertheless, Feldman-Summers and Pope (1994) found some degree of corroborative evidence in 47% of the cases they examined, including the abuser acknowledging some or all of the remembered abuse or someone else reporting abuse by the same perpetrator. Similar levels of corroboration, 41%, were reported in an unrelated survey of British clinical psychologists (see Brewin and Andrews 1998).

Conditions of recall

Clearly, if recovered memory is a therapy-generated phenomenon, the majority of memories should reappear during therapy. This does not always appear to be the case. Feldman-Summers and Pope (1994) found that while over half such memories were recovered in the context of therapy, 44% of their respondents stated that recovery had been triggered exclusively in other contexts. By contrast, Goodyear-Smith et al. (1997) reported summary data from several papers indicating that in over 80% of cases of sexual abuse, memories had emerged while complainants were undergoing psychotherapy. It is noteworthy that memories that occur outside therapy are usually triggered by events that remind the individual of the abuse, are of single incidents, and the memories are instantly recalled in full (Brenneis 2000). By contrast, memories stemming from therapy tend to be fragmented, vague, and lacking in detail. In addition, the majority of incidents recalled in this way (multiple events beginning in early childhood, involving bodily penetration by male family members) are rarely reported among verified recovered memory cases (Brenneis 2000). Of note also are the findings of Geraerts et al. (2009), who identified two different subgroups of people who recover memories in different contexts. Those who recalled memories within therapy were found on psychological testing to evidence a heightened susceptibility to the construction of false memories and no tendency to underestimate their prior remembering. By contrast, those who spontaneously recall such events appeared highly susceptible to forgetting prior incidents but showed no susceptibility to suggestion. They took this to indicate that spontaneous memories were more likely to be reliable than memories that emerged from therapy.

Attempts to forget

A key factor in the repressed memory debate is the assumption that those who remember childhood trauma as an adult have used unconscious coping mechanisms to 'forget' their trauma. If this is the case, then one would assume that a significant percentage of people who undergo other (non-abuse) traumas as a child would engage in similar coping strategies and have similar problems of recall. Evidence of accurate recall in adults who experienced being kidnapped, the Holocaust or parental murder as children suggests this does not typically occur (see Zola 1998).

Proponents of the repressed memory hypothesis counter these data by suggesting that sexual abuse is different from other trauma and that it has specific and unique consequences for coping. They argue that because abuse is usually carried out by parents or significant others rather than strangers and occurs in isolation rather than with companions, the effects are unique. One proponent of this argument, Freyd (1996), argued that sexual abuse of children is more than a trauma, it is a betrayal, and that 'betrayal trauma' is more prone to repression than other types of trauma. According to her model, sexual abuse by a trusted caretaker will be more likely to be repressed than sexual abuse by a stranger. Some evidence in support of this hypothesis was reported by Pope and Feldman-Summers (1992), who surveyed a representative population of US psychologists. Of those who responded, 24% reported having been abused at some time, and of these 40% reported forgetting this abuse for a period of time. Of this smaller group, 56% reported that it involved sexual abuse by a relative, while only 37% reported that it involved sexual abuse by a non-relative. The data provides only modest support for Freyd's contentions, and have not always been replicated, including in a sample of adults with documented abuse as children (Goodman et al. 2003).

Evidence of the creation of false traumatic memories

The central argument of those claiming traumatic memories are false is that they result from therapists planting suggestions of childhood abuse in people to whom this has not happened. This is certainly possible and there are many examples of this process occurring outside therapy. Piaget, for example, was able to recall being kidnapped as a 2-year-old in some detail, despite the fact the event never occurred: it was a childhood story told to him by his nurse. A more experimental example of the phenomenon is provided by Loftus and Coan (1998), who asked adults about childhood events, one of which had never occurred, in the presence of other family members who 'reminded' them of the event during the interview. Subsequently, 6 of the 24 participants in the study 'remembered' the false episode as real and provided additional details about it. Using a similar method, Hyman et al. (1995) asked college students about various childhood events that had never happened, including spending a night in hospital for treatment of an ear infection. At the end of the first interview, in which no participants 'recalled' the false events, they were encouraged to try to remember more information about them before a subsequent interview. During this second interview, a quarter of the participants 'recalled' detailed information about this false event.

More specifically, Loftus and Davis (2006) highlighted a number of processes that may combine to allow or even encourage the construction of false memories within therapy, often in the absence of deliberate or malicious bias by either therapist or client:

- *A priori expectations of abuse*: many clients and therapists may have *a priori* assumptions that abuse has occurred, even in the absence of direct evidence. Confirmatory bias may lead both to a search for evidence or to interpret information in the light of these expectations.
- *Motivated cognition*: many, if not most, people enter therapy with the hope of finding the 'cause' of their problems. They are therefore motivated to explore potential routes to their distress. If a therapist is also so motivated, then evidence may be sought to identify abuse. Therapists may even suggest the possibility of abuse and search for evidence of it.
- *Identity maintenance*: once a client has begun to admit the possibility of abuse, they may take on the identity of an abused person (which may provide validation of their distress) and look for evidence to support this new identity.

- *Therapeutic techniques*: hypnosis, regression, guided imagery, and dream interpretation all permit and may facilitate the development of false memories.
- *Repeated attempts at recall*: even in the absence of specific therapeutic techniques, repeated attempts at recall increase the number of both true and false memories recalled.
- *Abuse-related images and misattribution as memories*: repeated discussion of abuse may evoke images of abuse, which become increasingly prone to being attributed as memories.

These processes were seen by Loftus and Davis as deliberate therapeutic attempts to trigger, what they would consider, false memories; and these processes may still be reasonably prevalent. Patihis and Pendergast (2019), for example, found that of more than 2,000 US citizens who had received therapy, 9% reported actively being questioned about repressed memories of childhood abuse. However, a more neutral process may also be at work. McNally (2012), for example, considered a number of cases in which a 'normal' memory of abuse as non-traumatic was subsequently revised as an outcome of therapy and came to be seen as traumatic. This change in 'meta-awareness', a new *interpretation* of a memory, may be experienced as recovery of a memory, but does not require the process of 'recovery'.

Retraction

Although the prevalence is unknown, many people who recall traumatic memories eventually retract and claim that the events never actually occurred: that they are a consequence of within-therapy processes (e.g. Laney and Loftus 2005). Here, for example, is the testimony of Clare, who retracted her claims of sexual abuse by a family member. Her story focuses on the power that her therapist had over her, how he shaped her 'memories', and how she came to recognize his negative influence over her:

Looking back, it's difficult to see how things could have got this far, and been so destructive. How could a relationship with a therapist become the only – the total – focus of my life for three years? How could I have sold my soul, my very self, to another human being? How could I have fallen under the spell of a man who, it turns out, had problems in his own life; a man so inadequate himself that he needed me and others to be 'sick' in order for him to be powerful and strong? I trusted this man with my life – my soul. I shared everything with him – my dreams, the desires of my life. I confessed my sins to him. He was my partner, mother, father, sister, best friend, and teacher. My role model. He was everything to me. Whatever he said, I agreed with. How could he be wrong? My life became so linked with his life, my ability to think for myself disappeared. I thought what he wanted me to think. I believed what he wanted me to believe. I became what he wanted me to become.

Overview of the evidence

While some commentators (e.g. Loftus and Davis 2006) have been extremely sceptical about the nature of recalled memories, Brewin and Andrews (e.g. 2017) take a more cautious and conciliatory view, and suggest the present state of evidence is as follows:

- The age at which the majority of events are said to have occurred extends beyond the period of infant amnesia
- Corroboration occurs with reasonable frequency given the nature of the alleged incidents
- The content of most recovered memories concerns a variety of events known to occur with reasonable frequency, and is not limited to child sexual abuse
- Well-trained therapists not using inappropriate techniques have reported clients recovering memories
- The context of recall is not limited to the therapist's office
- In analogue studies, involving similar processes to those in the therapy sessions, implanted memories have been induced in nearly 50% of participants, but only 15% of individuals experience memories sufficiently robust to warrant being rated as 'full memories.

On this basis, Brewin and Andrews suggested that the evidence is not sufficient to rule out the possibility that recovered memory may genuinely occur, at least in some cases, and that each case should be taken on its own merit. Indeed, even Otgaar et al. (2019), who argued strongly against the concept of dissociative amnesia, which they believed allowed wholesale inaccessibility of entire autobiographical experiences, conceded that 'trauma can sometimes lead to feelings of depersonalization and that, probably because of accompanying stress levels, memory problems might arise'.

9.3 Dissociative identity disorder

Another phenomenon closely related to childhood trauma, previously called multiple personality disorder, is now known as dissociative identify disorder (DID). A defining characteristic of individuals with a diagnosis of DID is that they appear to possess two or more distinct identities or personalities, known as 'alters'. As the phenomenon emerged, people with DID reported relatively few alter personalities. Now, the average number of alters reported is as many as 15, and some individuals report more than 100. According to DSM-5, the key diagnostic criteria for DID are:

- Disruption of identity characterized by having two or more distinct personality states (described in some cultures as an experience of possession). The disruption in identity involves marked discontinuity in the sense of self, and is accompanied by different moods, behaviour, consciousness, memory, perception, cognition, and/or sensory-motor functioning across personalities. These may be observed by others or reported by the individual.
- Recurrent gaps in the recall of everyday events, important personal information, and/or traumatic events that are inconsistent with ordinary forgetting.

Multiple alters can live in a complex ecosystem in which each has a role, of which the central one is to protect the host personality from memories of trauma. It is common for each alter to guard a particular memory. Some alters are aware of other alters; others do not know of their existence. Most alters do not see themselves in the physical body they are in: children see themselves as four feet tall, women see themselves as girls, and so on. They may be of different nationalities and races. Some may speak different languages. Alters may have different facial expressions and different mannerisms. There are many different kinds of alters and all systems are different, but the following are some of the more common types of alter described by people with such experience (http://traumadissociation.com/alters):

- *Host*: this person can either be the original birth child, or an alter that is the main personality presented to the outside world.
- *Original birth child*: this person may be awake and functioning or said to be asleep. This person is sometimes referred to as the core personality.
- *Child alters*: child alters (or 'littles') can range from the age of an infant upwards. These are the alters that took much of the abuse, and often carry a large number of memories. They display behaviour that is appropriate for their age. Often, they carry much pain, both physical and emotional.
- *Gatekeepers*: some systems have a gatekeeper, who directs and has control of the body. They may also control the length of time an alter is in body. They do not often come out themselves but seem happy to observe and direct the others.
- *Internal self-helpers*: these keep the alters safe. They usually know all the alters and the details of the abuse they endured. They are very helpful in therapy, and help the therapist understand why a particular alter feels the way they do or decide the action of a particular alter. They also decide what information is passed to other alters and to the host.
- *Protectors*: protectors protect (!) the system from outside threats. They can usually talk hard, or fight, or do whatever is necessary to keep the system safe. They often use anger as a defence. They are especially protective of the child alters.

Switches between alters often results from some sort of stress or upset, which causes another alter, usually a protector alter, to emerge. Stresses can include comments by others, seeing the abuser, an unexpected touch, arguments and aggression – even having sex. Sel (1997) suggested that the individual has an ecosystem of alters who compete with each other to gain control over the output channels. The alter that most successfully maintains an emotional equilibrium is most likely to be adopted. When the individual moves to a different context, different **cognitive schemata** may be more adaptive and the dominant alter will switch. Based on formal diagnostic interview and DSM-5 diagnostic criteria, prevalence levels of DID within the general population are around 1.0–1.5% (Brand et al. 2016).

Aetiology of DID

The nature and, indeed, existence of 'true' DID, have been as hotly debated as the existence of recovered memories, and the arguments are very similar (see, for example, Piper and Merskey 2004). Such is the level of debate that even some researchers of this disorder remain neutral about its nature and **aetiology**. Elzinga et al. (2003) stated, for example, that they adopted a 'pragmatic stance ... without making *a priori* claims about the nature of so-called "identities"' (2003: 237). Some researchers (e.g. Gleaves et al. 2001) have contended that its existence is self-evident, there are too many people experiencing these symptoms to deny the reality of the problem, and that it is a consequence of childhood trauma. Others (e.g. Spanos 1994) have rejected the concept, arguing that the symptoms are invented by the individuals reporting them, or even implanted in their consciousness through the use of hypnosis by over-zealous therapists.

This social model contends that DID is a set of beliefs and behaviours constructed by the individual in response to personal stress, therapist pressure, and societal legitimization of the construct of 'multiple personality'; and that DID forms a legitimate way for many people to understand and express their failures and frustrations, as well as a tactic for the manipulation of others. Twenty years on, the controversy persists, although it has become rather more nuanced. Dalenberg et al. (2012), for example, still contended that DID is a legitimate diagnosis stemming directly from childhood trauma. Others (e.g. Lynn et al. 2014), while accepting a role for trauma, have argued that other factors may also contribute to the experiences of people with DID and that it may not necessarily be central to its development.

Childhood trauma

There are at least two alternative childhood trauma models of DID. In one, Gleaves (1996) argued that the experience of severe trauma during childhood produces a mental 'splitting' or dissociation during the trauma as part of a defensive reaction. The abused child learns to dissociate, or enter a self-induced hypnotic state, placing the memory of the abuse in the subconscious as a means of coping with the trauma. These dissociated parts of the individual 'split' into alter personalities, which, in adulthood, manifest themselves to help the individual cope with stressful situations and express resentments or other feelings that are unacceptable to the primary personality. This model fits well with the model of hypnosis in psychosomatic disorders outlined in Chapter 8. Taking a similar approach, Putnam (1997) proposed that traumatic environments prevent children from completing the developmental task of consolidating an integrated sense of self from what he termed the 'discrete behavioural states' – involving cognitive and emotional functioning – which predominate in infancy. He suggested that normal caregiving environments facilitate integration of these differing states into a single integrated whole. Trauma actively inhibits this integration. Instead, the child develops a series of separate states that are adaptive to their parental behaviours.

Support for the childhood trauma model can be found in the increasing numbers of studies in adult and child populations showing a link between an adult diagnosis of DID and childhood trauma. Dalenberg et al. (2012) identified 38 studies exploring this relationship which met a set of methodological criteria including a good sample size, the use of a community sample or clinical samples including non-DID diagnoses and people with no evidence of previous trauma. They excluded studies which consisted entirely of people diagnosed with DID.

Their summary results identified moderate **effect sizes** for risk linked to sexual abuse, physical abuse, and overall trauma scores. Rates of trauma within the DID samples varied between 18% and 84%. Accordingly, trauma appears to have a role in the development of DID, but other factors are clearly relevant. Disorganized attachment appears to be a particularly important influence on risk, as (oddly, but consistently) are painful medical procedures or hospitalizations. Lynn et al. (2014) pointed out that despite the care taken by Dalenberg to identify methodologically strong studies, most studies of adults lack corroboration of the childhood events, and both groups agreed that more longitudinal studies of at-risk groups are needed to provide definitive evidence.

Experimental evidence

Experimental studies of memory provide an interesting second strand of evidence. A key requirement for the 'strong' explanation of DID is that memories remain 'locked' within certain alters and do not leak out into other states. In this way, some alters, at least, are protected against memories of traumatic events; memories of events that occurred in childhood are thought to remain within the memory system of the alter that experienced them, and not spread into other memory systems. This phenomenon could provide a test of the DID diagnosis, as it allows experimental testing with clear hypotheses: memories should not pass between alters.

In one study of this issue, Elzinga et al. (2003) assessed both implicit and explicit memory performance in 12 people with DID. They presented participants with 96 words, half of which had a threatening or sexual connotation, and half of which were neutral. Participants were instructed after each presentation to either remember or forget the presented word, as forgetting it would aid their recall of the other words in a subsequent memory test. They then completed an interference task, following which they were instructed to change state. All participants reported they achieved this change, and the new state (alter) reported that they had no conscious recall of the words they had previously been exposed to. They then took part in an implicit memory test in which 48 words were flashed 'briefly' on a computer screen followed by a mask of letters for one second. They were then asked to guess what word had been presented. Following a second interference task, participants were then presented with the stems of the previously presented words and asked to complete them. Finally, participants were asked to switch back to their original state and this sequence of testing was repeated. Their findings indicated a significant reduction of explicit memory between states. Participants were more likely to recall words they had been asked to recall when in the same state than when in a different state from the state in which they were presented with the words. However, the second alter still remembered significant numbers of words. Levels of recall of emotional to-be-remembered words, for example, were 36% in the same state and 21% in the second state. In addition, there was no evidence of any differences across states on their measure of implicit memory. These data show some transfer of information between states, and counter the argument of a compartmentalized memory, with each memory system specific to a different personality, leading the authors to conclude that the problems reported by people with DID did not reflect actual memory retrieval inability. Instead, they were better characterized as a meta-memory disorder, in that they held inaccurate beliefs about their own memory functioning.

A second type of experimental research involves the study of how susceptible people with DID are to the inculcation of false beliefs. Both Dalenberg et al. (2012) and Lynn et al. (2014) explored this issue. Dalenberg et al. reviewed the evidence based on one particular measure of DID and contended that the strength of association between measures of false memory/susceptibility and DID were modest, with almost half the studies exploring this association reporting correlations less than 0.1: a small effect size. Lynn et al. widened the scope of their review to include other (related) measures, and concluded that DID *was* associated with a range of measures of false memory/susceptibility, including imagination inflation, and false recall of trauma stimuli, including a 'bus explosion' and childhood events that had not occurred. Clearly, the 'personality war' continues, albeit with acknowledgement by sceptics such as Lynn et al. that childhood trauma may be one potential pathway to DID, but that this may be just one of several mechanisms.

Treatment of DID

Not surprisingly, protagonists for and against the concept of DID have differing ideas about its treatment. Spanos (1994), for example, contended that the goal of treatment is to help clients accept that their alter identities are real personalities rather than self-generated fantasies. By contrast, Gleaves (1996) contended that the opposite is true. He argued that the central goal of treatment should be to help the individual understand that the alters are in fact self-generated, not to convince them that they are real people. He argued that therapists working with people with DID should emphasize the fundamental nature of the disorder as a difficulty in integrating various aspects of the personality rather than a profusion of personalities.

For most therapists working with people diagnosed with DID, the ultimate goal of therapy is to integrate the various alters into one cohesive personality, a process known as fusion. In this state, the person is aware of all their behaviours and thoughts and accepts them as their own. Oke and Kanigsberg (1991) used a combination of play, guided imagery, life skills teaching, projective techniques, and group therapy to help bring awareness and understanding of other selves, and through this eventually achieve cohesion between all alters. Unfortunately, the effectiveness of this and similar types of intervention (e.g. Kellett 2005) remains limited to descriptions of interventions with no outcome data, or case reports, which by their very nature tend to be positive (few therapists like to broadcast their failures widely, and most journals are biased against publishing 'negative results'). Their efficacy or otherwise has yet to be fully investigated. Nevertheless, the International Society for the Study of Trauma and Dissociation (2011) has argued that trauma-focused psychotherapy is likely to be of benefit if it follows consensus guidelines, which largely focus on treating the individual as a holistic entity rather than working separately with different alters, with the goal of gradual integration.

A fundamental cautionary note about such efforts has come from people with DID. Many sub-personalities reject integration as a therapeutic goal, as they see integration as a form of death. Rossel (1998) argued that in a disintegrating post-modern world, it is of little benefit to attempt to achieve integration. Instead, the individual should be open to the experience of shifting between alters, which should be construed as a positive and comfortable experience, not a negative, destructive one.

9.4 Chapter summary

1. PTSD has three central symptoms: (i) intrusive memories; (ii) attempts at avoidance of these memories; and (iii) high levels of arousal.
2. The neurological substrates of PTSD are the amygdala and hippocampus that together mediate fear and memory, and link the two together. High arousal is mediated by the sympathetic nervous system.
3. The conditioning model of PTSD provides a partial explanation of the phenomenon, but cognitive models such as that of Brewin provide a more in-depth understanding.
4. Clinical incident debriefing is often provided at traumatic incidents. Evidence is mounting that this may actually inhibit long-term recovery from psychological trauma.
5. Exposure methods may prove the best intervention for PTSD, particularly when combined with strategies to help clients cope with any emotional distress triggered by the therapeutic process.
6. EMDR appears to be of benefit, but no more than exposure methods.
7. Since the 1980s, an increasing number of people have begun to report recovered memories of trauma, usually sexual trauma, experienced in childhood.
8. Three explanations have been proposed to account for this phenomenon: (i) the memories are real and have been hidden as a result of a number of unconscious self-protective mechanisms; (ii) they are the result of therapists shaping clients' apparent recall of past events that did not in reality occur; and (iii) they are incidents forgotten as a result of normal forgetting processes.
9. Arguments about which of these explanations is correct have focused on a number of issues: the age at the time of the incident, distortions in memory over time, mixed levels of corroboration of events, and experimental evocation of false memories.
10. Brewin and others have suggested that while some memories may be false, others may be truly repressed and recovered. Each case should be considered on its own merits.
11. The clinical model suggests that DID is a response to repeated childhood sexual trauma involving severe dissociation at the time of the trauma, resulting in the development of 'alters' or alternative personalities.
12. The socio-cognitive model suggests this is a response to therapist and social pressure to behave in a way that suggests multiple personalities.

13. Debate about which of these models is the better has focused on differing explanations of the prevalence of the disorder, whether therapists can 'teach multiplicity', social and therapist pressures to present with DID, and the relationship between childhood abuse and DID.
14. While some cases of DID may be created by the process of therapy, others may represent a 'real' clinical condition. Each case should be considered on its own merits.

9.5 For discussion

1. How should we support or treat people immediately and in the weeks following exposure to a highly traumatic event?
2. Which factors may contribute to the development of PTSD?
3. Should therapists continue to explore issues of childhood sexual abuse if an individual with long-term mental health problems says this did not take place?
4. Some therapists have identified sexual trauma to have occurred in substantial numbers of women they have worked with. Others find virtually none. Why may this be the case, and how should any healthcare service respond to such differences if they occur among their therapists?
5. If an individual presents with the multiple altars associated with DID, what should be the goals of therapy, and how may you set about achieving them?

9.6 Further reading

Boyd, J.E., Lanius, R.A. and McKinnon, M.C. (2018) Mindfulness-based treatments for posttraumatic stress disorder: a review of the treatment literature and neurobiological evidence, *Journal of Psychiatry and Neuroscience*, 43: 7–25.

Brand, B.L., Sar, V., Stavropoulos, P. et al. (2016) Separating fact from fiction: an empirical examination of six myths about dissociative identity disorder, *Harvard Review of Psychiatry*, 24: 257–70.

Brewin, C.R., Gregory, J.D., Lipton, M. et al. (2010) Intrusive images in psychological disorders: characteristics, neural mechanisms, and treatment implications, *Psychological Review*, 117: 210–32.

Brewin, C.R. and Holmes, E.A. (2003) Psychological theories of posttraumatic stress disorder, *Clinical Psychology Review*, 23: 339–76.

Otgaar, H., Howe, M.L., Patihis, L. et al. (2019) The return of the repressed: the persistent and problematic claims of long-forgotten trauma, *Perspectives on Psychological Science*, 14: 1072–95.

Pendergast, M. (2014) *The Repressed Memory Epidemic: How It Happened and What We Need to Learn from It*, Cham: Springer.

10 Sexual disorders

There are two categories of sexual disorders: *sexual dysfunctions*, which involve a problem in sexual response, and *paraphilias*, which involve repeated and intense sexual urges, behaviour or fantasies in response to objects or situations that society deems inappropriate. This chapter examines both types of problems. It considers problems that some people experience during the sexual act, focusing on the male problem of failing to achieve an erection and its female 'equivalent', previously known as vaginismus and now known as genito-pelvic pain/penetration disorder (GPPD), and considers how these may be treated. It then describes the **aetiology** and treatment of paedophilia and transvestism. Finally, the chapter considers the problems faced when an individual questions their very sexual identity and wishes to change it: gender identity disorder. By the end of the chapter, you should have an understanding of:

- The nature and aetiology of erectile dysfunction, vaginismus, paedophilia, transvestism, and gender identity disorder
- The types of interventions used to treat each disorder, and their relative effectiveness.

10.1 Sexual dysfunctions

The sexual dysfunctions are those that involve a problem with the sexual response. They include disorders of desire, such as an aversion to sexual activity and low sexual drive, and problems of orgasm including premature ejaculation in men and a failure to achieve orgasm in both men and women. Here, two conditions are considered: erectile dysfunction in men and genito-pelvic pain/penetration disorder in women. Both problems markedly interfere with, or may prevent, the sexual act. Both are treatable using relatively simple behavioural and pharmacological interventions.

Erectile disorder

DSM-5 (APA 2013) states that a diagnosis of erectile disorder will involve one of three symptoms experienced on all or almost all (75–100%) occasions of sexual activity:

- marked difficulty in obtaining an erection
- marked difficulty in maintaining an erection until the completion of sexual activity
- marked decrease in erectile rigidity.

The diagnosis requires persistence of these symptoms for approximately 6 months. Other factors that must be taken into consideration include whether the condition is generalized or situational, and whether it is a mild, moderate or severe case (APA 2013). It is a fairly common disorder, particularly among older men, although younger men are not immune. Kessler et al. (2019) summarized the data from around the world, with studies reporting overall frequencies within the male population of between 13% and 70%, when 'mild' cases of the condition were included. The **prevalence** rises as men get older. In an Australian study, Chew et al. (2008) found that the lowest rates of significant problems in adults were among men aged 30–39 years (9%) and highest among men aged 70–79 years (69%). Among older men, contributors to erectile dysfunction are more likely to be physical, including high blood pressure and cardiovascular disease, prostate disease, and diabetes. Among younger men, psychological factors may be more important (Kessler et al. 2019), although the exact mix of physical and psychological causes is unclear.

Aetiology of erectile disorder

Psychodynamic explanations

According to Janssen (1985), erectile failure results from an oedipal conflict constellation involving fear of castration or incest, uncertainties in sexual identity, incestuous object choices, latent homosexual tendencies, and a fear of aggressive-phallic impulses. These may develop as a result of factors that inhibit appropriate passage through the oedipal stage of psychosexual development (see Chapter 2). In a case example, Janssen described one man who reported that as a child his mother had turned to him to discuss matters relating to her relationship with his father. When his father became aware of this, he became angry and abused his mother. The **client** feared that he too would become the focus of his father's wrath and experienced a conflict in wanting to defend his mother, but to avoid confrontation with his father. This prevented his successful resolution of the oedipal conflict. In adulthood, the fear of his aggressive father prevented him developing appropriate emotional and sexual relationships with women. Treatment involved dealing with his relationship with his father, not any explicit sexual function.

Psychobiological explanations

Erectile dysfunction can be caused by a range of hormonal and vascular problems, including low levels of testosterone, conditions which affect blood flow including diabetes and atherosclerosis, and nitric oxide dysfunction. The latter is critical to the link between psychological and biological processes. Nitric oxide, released from nerve endings in the penis and the smooth muscle surrounding blood vessels in the penis, results in a relaxation of the blood vessels within the penis, increasing blood flow and resulting in an erection. The activity of nitric oxide is influenced by both sympathetic and parasympathetic nervous systems. Sympathetic arousal inhibits the release of nitric oxide; parasympathetic activation facilitates its release. Put another way, the stress response inhibits release and prevents arousal; relaxation facilitates it. Accordingly, stress related to both the sexual act and potentially beyond may significantly contribute to dysfunction. An example of the wider effect of stress can be seen in the findings of Aghighi et al. (2015), who found both general anxiety and depression to be associated with erectile dysfunction in a sample of middle-aged men with the disorder. Longer-term contributors may be negative beliefs about the self, arising from childhood experiences including disrupted childhood attachment (Rajkumar et al. 2015).

More closely linked to sex itself, Bancroft (1999) noted that sexual anxiety adversely affects sexual performance as a result of cognitive and perceptual factors. He suggested that men's sexual excitement depends on a delicate balance between excitatory and inhibitory mechanisms. Two key inhibitory processes are performance anxiety and fear of negative outcomes, both of which reduce parasympathetic activity and interfere with the sexual act. Both may lead to a process coined by Masters and Johnson (1970) as 'spectatoring', in which the individual becomes so concerned by the adequacy of their penis or their performance that they distract from sexually arousing cues, and lose their erection (Wyatt et al. 2019). Difficulties in sexual performance may also lead to pre-sexual anxiety or a focusing on anxiety-related cognitions during subsequent sex, which will further interfere with sexual performance. Performance anxiety may be particularly high if men set themselves inappropriately high performance expectations. Zilbergeld (1992), for example, noted that men frequently buy into the fantasy that their performance is the 'cornerstone' of every sexual experience and that a firm erection is the key element of every sexual encounter: views not necessarily subscribed to by their female partners. According to Zilbergeld, a failure to achieve this ideal results in fears of dysfunction, loss of masculinity, and declining interest in their partner.

Treatment of erectile disorder

Anxiety reduction and desensitization

The classic treatment programme for erectile disorder, known as *sensate focusing*, was developed by Masters and Johnson (1970). It involves a structured approach, designed to take the stress out of the sexual act. It begins with the couple learning to touch each other in pleasurable ways, but with a mandate not to touch each other's genitals. Their goal is to enjoy the intimacy of touch, not to give or receive sexual pleasure. Once couples are comfortable with non-genital sensate focusing, they are directed to gradually make genital contact and to give and receive pleasure doing so. At this time, they are still mandated not to attempt intercourse, nor for the male to try to achieve or maintain an erection (although this typically occurs). Finally, when the couple are comfortable with this level of intimacy, they may progress to full intercourse. This is a frequently applied intervention; although there are relatively few studies of its effectiveness, it is generally considered to be highly effective when conducted appropriately (Weiner and Avery-Clark 2014).

Hawton et al. (1992) considered the most important predictor of outcome following a programme of sensate focusing and graduated stimulation techniques was the couple's ratings of marital communication before treatment, which can be intervention targets within a programme of sensate focusing: (i) status and dominance issues; (ii) intimacy and trust; and (iii) loss of sexual attraction. Each of these may be more or less salient in the lifetime of a sexual relationship. Status and dominance issues may be salient when one partner loses a job or achieves promotion; intimacy or trust issues may be salient following an affair, while loss of sexual attraction may follow weight gain or some other physical or psychological changes. Following an intervention addressing these factors, Hawton and colleagues reported that 70% of couples reported a positive outcome.

Medical approaches

Perhaps the best-known pharmacological treatment for erectile failure is sildenafil, more popularly known as Viagra. Now just one of a number of drugs known as PDE5 inhibitors, Viagra was originally developed as a drug to treat angina, but accidentally proved equally or more effective in inducing erections: an interesting side-effect for those testing it out! It works on the smooth muscle of the penis. Inhibition of the enzyme phosphodiesterase type 5 (PDE5), which breaks down cyclic guanosine monophosphate (cGMP), results in smooth muscle relaxation, and maintains the erectile response. As a consequence, PDE5 inhibitors enhance the sexual response rather than initiate it, and erection therefore follows sexual stimulation, and does not immediately follow taking the drug, as is the case in some alternatives.

PDE5 inhibitors are generally effective in treating erectile dysfunction, whatever the cause. Goldstein et al. (1998), for example, reported that 70% of men treated with Viagra reported improvements in the quality and frequency of erections; 70% of attempts at intercourse were successful, compared with 22% of attempts by those treated with **placebo**. PDE5 is predominantly found in the penis. However, it is also found in other areas of the body. As a consequence, about 16% of users experience headaches, 10% experience facial flushing, with other effects such as gastrointestinal upset and alterations in colour vision being somewhat rarer. One of the more dramatic side-effects was thought to be the onset of a heart attack, but this is now thought to be a result of exercise, not the drug (Holmes 2000). Of note also in this context is the finding by Khan et al. (2019) that combining Viagra with a programme involving sensate focusing and **cognitive challenge** of inappropriate cognitions proved more effective than drug treatment alone.

Genito-pelvic pain/penetration disorder

Vaginismus, now less succinctly termed 'genito-pelvic pain disorder/penetration disorder' (GPPD) by DSM-5 was thought to be a consequence of persistent involuntary spasm of the musculature of the outer third of the vagina that prevented sexual intercourse. However, this focus on vaginal spasm has proved erroneous, as only around a quarter of women who have difficulties that prevent intercourse experience this symptom (Lahaie et al. 2014). The APA has therefore extended the diagnostic criteria to include persistent or recurrent difficulties relating to intercourse involving one (or more) of the following:

- marked vulvovaginal or pelvic pain during vaginal intercourse or penetration attempts
- marked fear or anxiety about vulvovaginal or pelvic pain in anticipation of, during, or as a result of vaginal penetration
- marked tensing or tightening of the pelvic floor muscles during attempted vaginal penetration
- symptoms need to be present for at least 6 months and to cause significant distress.

The disorder can cause considerable distress or interpersonal difficulties. It is thought to be one of the most common of the female psychosexual dysfunctions, although its exact prevalence among the general population is unknown. An estimated 10–34% of women are thought to be affected by GPPD (Dias-Amaral and Marques-Pinto 2018).

Aetiology of GPPD

Psychoanalytic explanations

Classic psychoanalytic theory considers GPPD to result from unresolved psychosexual conflicts in early childhood. Women with the condition have been characterized as fixated or regressed to the pre-oedipal or oedipal stages. According to Abraham (1956), in less severe cases, women are not able to transfer their libidinal energy from their father to their husband/partner. In more severe cases, women remain fixated on their mothers, and have a poor prognosis.

Cognitive behavioural explanations

Women with a diagnosis of GPPD are more likely to have a positive history of sexual, physical or emotional abuse than those without these difficulties (e.g. Meana et al. 2017). Sexual pain complaints are also more frequent in women with a history of depressive or anxious disorders, and are associated with low affective involvement, avoidance of intimacy, and higher levels of anticipatory anxiety about abandonment (Dias-Amaral and Marques-Pinto 2018). This anxiety may lead to difficulties in intercourse, with an initial painful experience leading to fearful and catastrophic thoughts about pain and its meaning. These, in turn, lead to somatic hypervigilance at the time or during subsequent attempts at intercourse. This serves to amplify any negative physical sensations, which may be exacerbated by low levels of lubrication and increased risk of pain. These experiences serve to confirm catastrophic thoughts, increase anxiety, and lead to the avoidance of sexual activity (Anderson et al. 2016).

Treatment of GPPD

Psychological approaches

Just as in erectile disorder, an important way of reducing anxiety associated with the sexual act has been through the use of sensate focusing techniques, with a gradual progression to genital touching; although given the more elaborate model of GPPD now proposed, a wider cognitive behavioural intervention may be of benefit. In one study of the effectiveness of this latter approach, van Lankveld et al. (2006) examined the effectiveness of a manualized approach within a group therapy format focusing on: (i) education concerning the biological and physiological mechanisms of GPPD; (ii) learning relaxation skills; (iii) a graded sensate focusing programme including use of a dilator to penetrate the vagina leading to penile penetration as homework; (iv) optional guided imagery exercises; and (v) use of cognitive restructuring to reframe self-defeating cognitions. This approach was compared with a no-treatment control, and 'minimal contact bibliotherapy' in which participants received the same manual as the 'live' participants, but briefer contact by telephone with the therapists. Participants in the control condition made no gains, while those in both intervention conditions made gains. At one-year follow-up, 21% of the 'live' therapy participants and 15% of the bibliotherapy participants reported successful intercourse.

10.2 The paraphilias

Defining which of the various forms of sexual activity is 'normal' and 'abnormal' is not unproblematic. However, a number of sexual behaviours are generally considered to be 'abnormal'. These are referred to as the paraphilias, which include behaviours that are legal, such as fetishism and transvestism, and some that are illegal, in particular, paedophilia (see Table 10.1).

Table 10.1 Some of the more prevalent paraphilias

Fetishism	Recurrent intense sexual urges, sexually arousing fantasies or behaviours that involve the use of non-living objects, often to the exclusion of all other stimuli; common fetishes are to women's underwear, boots, and shoes
Exhibitionism	Recurrent urges to expose the genitals to another person of the opposite sex – often while having sexually arousing fantasies
Voyeurism	Recurrent and intense urges to secretly observe unsuspecting people as they undress or have intercourse
Sadomasochism	Sexual stimulation through the act of being humiliated, beaten, bound or otherwise made to suffer, or being the one to inflict such acts
Frotteurism	Repeated and intense sexual urges to touch and rub against non-consenting others

Many people who engage in paraphilic behaviour neither experience distress as a result, nor do they seek help to change the nature of their sexual interest. As a consequence, people who engage in unusual sexual behaviour may be considered as at the edge of the distribution of sexual interests rather than disordered. With this in mind, DSM-III (APA 1987) stated that any paraphilic behaviour had to result in personal distress before a diagnosis of a 'disorder' be assigned. However, following strong criticism of this *laissez-faire* approach, DSM-IV-TR (APA 2000) stated that a range of sexual interests including paedophilia, sexual sadism, and voyeurism were considered to be 'disorders' if the person acted on their desires, even though their behaviour may neither cause personal distress nor 'impaired functioning'. This approach is largely continued in DSM-5, which now differentiates between the experience of 'atypical sexual interests', which do not indicate a 'mental disorder', and the consequences of that interest, which may. For any sexual behaviour to be labelled as a disorder, it has both to be atypical and lead to the following consequences:

- the individual feels personal distress about their interest, not merely distress resulting from society's disapproval; or
- the individual has a sexual desire or behaviour that involves another person's psychological distress, injury or death, or a desire for sexual behaviours involving unwilling persons or persons unable to give legal consent.

The latter requirement emphasizes the overlap between psychopathology and legal and social norms in relation to the relevant behaviour.

Paedophilic disorder

DSM-5 defines paedophilia as:

- recurrent intense sexual urges and sexually arousing fantasies involving sexual activity with a prepubescent child or children, and
- the person has acted on these urges, or the sexual urges or fantasies cause marked distress or interpersonal difficulty.

The individual may be further identified as: (i) exclusive, with only an attraction to children; (ii) non-exclusive, where there is an attraction to both children and adults; and (iii) limited to incest. In addition, the perpetrator has to be at least 16 years old and at least 5 years older than the child or children involved. Note the emphasis on the victim's sexual maturity, not age. Legal definitions lay clear boundaries as to the age at which consenting couples may have intercourse. Violation of these limits will result in an individual being termed a sex offender, but not a paedophile unless the other child is prepubescent.

Paedophilic behaviours vary. Some paedophiles may look at and not touch a child. Others may want to touch or undress them. When sexual activity occurs, it often involves oral sex or touching the genitals of the child. In most cases, except incest, there is no penetration. Where sex is penetrative, it is usually with older children and may involve threats or force. More typically, however, paedophilic individuals depend on persuasion, guile, and 'friendship' (Murray 2000). Most perpetrators are relatives, friends or neighbours of the child involved. Men who are sexually attracted to pubescent children tend to be gender specific in their attraction; men who are particularly attracted to prepubescent children are likely to be less gender-bound, and the attraction is more likely to be bisexual. Prevalence levels of paedophilia are extremely difficult to determine. However, the APA (2013) estimated a population prevalence of between 3% and 5%, with an estimated 10-to-1 ratio of men to women, although this figure may be an underestimate of the number of women involved (Vandiver 2006).

Aetiology of paedophilic disorder

Neurological models

A recent study by Långström et al. (2015) found a strong genetic link with child abuse within families. They estimated genetic factors contributed to 46% of the cases of such behaviour, leaving 54% to be explained by environmental factors. Any genetic processes are likely to be mediated through neurological mechanisms, and although these remain unclear a number of neurological models have been proposed, including:

- *The frontal lobe theory*: anomalies of function or volume in the orbitofrontal and left and right dorsolateral prefrontal cortex have been detected in paedophilic men (e.g. Schiffer et al. 2008) The orbitofrontal cortex is responsible for behavioural control, in particular inhibiting sexual behaviour. Accordingly, these differences are better at explaining a lack of control over sexual behaviour more than the object of that behaviour.
- *The temporal lobe theory*: disturbance in activation of the temporal lobes, parts of which are involved in the sensory processing of sexual activity, can result in an increase in paedophilic behaviours (Mendez et al. 2000). An interesting case study provides some context here. Mendez et al. (2000) reported the case of a 60-year-old man who developed frontotemporal dementia and presented with increased sexual drive and recent sexual abuse of young children. Treatment with antidepressants, thought to reduce temporal cortex dysfunction, banished this behaviour. However, the case is considered to provide an example of the expression of latent paedophilic tendencies which are released due to hypersexual drive rather than the development of attraction towards children *per se*. Accordingly, as with the frontal lobe theory, the temporal lobe theory may better explain the drive for sexual pleasure, and a degree of hypersexuality, rather than the object of that pleasure.

Long-term risk factors

These neurological findings are consistent with findings that paedophiles are more likely to have deficits in **executive function** (the brain areas associated with this include the dorsolateral prefrontal cortex and orbitofrontal cortex) in general, and perform relatively poorly on tasks that require sustained attention and inhibition of behaviour (e.g. Suchy et al. 2014). Thus, they may have difficulties in inhibiting sexual urges and be more impetuous in their sexual decision-making. The object of their desire may be more determined by social and sexual experiences.

Many child sex offenders report that their early relationships with their parents were disruptive and/or that they had experienced childhood sexual abuse. In one study involving a matched comparison between male paedophile and 'healthy' individuals, for example, Cohen et al. (2002) found 60% of paedophiles reported experiencing adult sexual advances as a child. This compared with 4% of the comparison group. These data are extremely difficult to validate. Many people who engage in paedophilic behaviour have a vested interest in reporting such events as a way of minimizing their own responsibility for their actions or gaining the sympathy of others. In an attempt to minimize these problems, Dhawan and Marshall (1996) used detailed interviews and questionnaire methods to try to corroborate or challenge any misreporting. They concluded that 50% of imprisoned paedophiles had been sexually abused as children. What this, of course, does not explain is why such episodes predict later sexual offences. A number of authors have speculated why this may be the case, with various suggestions that the abused child is trying to gain a new identity by becoming the abuser, they are engaged in an imprinted sexual arousal pattern established by early abuse, or that early abuse leads to hypersexual behaviour (e.g. Cohen et al. 2002).

Behavioural theories (e.g. Barbaree 1990) suggest that child offenders develop a strong sexual attraction to children following pairings of sexual arousal and images of children. These associations typically occur in early adolescence, and may initially be accidental. However, they may be strengthened by masturbation to images of children and the use of pornography. In a partial test of this model, Barbaree and Marshall (1989) measured the sexual response to pictures of female children and mature women among men who had either sexually abused children not in their family, committed incest, or claimed to have no sexual interest in children. Their findings were somewhat surprising. Less than half of the non-familial offenders and only 28% of those who had committed incest were more sexually stimulated by pictures of young women than those of mature women. In addition, 15% of men who reported no sexual interest in children were more sexually aroused by pictures of children than of mature women. While the conditioning model may hold for some individuals, it does not hold for all. In addition, a study by Klucken et al. (2009) showed that men are more easily conditioned through exposure to sexual stimuli than are women, further challenging the conditioning theory, particularly as it applies to female paedophiles.

These data indicate that sexual interest is not the only factor that influences the sexual choices of paedophiles. Another important factor may be a failure to develop satisfying psychological and sexual relationships with adults. Many paedophiles report high levels of loneliness, associated with insecure attachments as a child and avoidant or anxious-ambivalent attachments as an adult (Bogaerts et al. 2005). As a result, some seek out intimacy with children, with whom they find it easier to instigate both physical and non-physical relationships, and who are easier to control. However, this is certainly not the case for all paedophiles, emphasizing that the route to paedophilia differs widely between individuals. Nevertheless, Finkelhor's (1984) 'preconditions theory' of paedophilia identified these factors as key to the condition. He suggested that paedophilia is the result of four factors:

- the belief that sex with children is emotionally satisfying
- the belief that sex with children is sexually satisfying
- an inability to meet sexual needs in a more socially appropriate manner
- disinhibited behaviour at times of stress.

Pithers (1990) provided a useful description of the process of disinhibition at times of low mood. He noted that the desire to engage in paedophile behaviour is frequently triggered by low mood as a result of stress or conflict. As a result, individuals seek some way of decreasing these negative feelings, and allow themselves to enter a high-risk situation. This may appear the result of seemingly irrelevant decisions that place them in increasing proximity to potential victims. Once in this situation, they are overwhelmed by the potentially powerfully rewarding feelings associated with paedophile acts. They focus on these rather than the long-term negative outcomes to the situation, and as a result engage in some form of paedophile behaviour. Once the immediate 'rush' has receded, they may once more experience remorse, but feel out of control of their behaviour, a negative mood state that may trigger the cycle again.

These factors are added to by cognitive distortions that support sexual acts with children. Common cognitive distortions are that children are as interested in sex as adults, that they seek out sex with adults, and that they enjoy and benefit from the experience. Some of these may be truly believed by the individual. Others may be deliberate falsification, to minimize negative reactions from others. Implicit tests of attitudes are particularly revealing in this context. In one study, using the Implicit Association Test, Mihailides et al. (2004) found that child sex offenders were more likely to implicitly endorse 'children as sexual beings', 'uncontrollability of sexuality', and 'sexual entitlement' beliefs than other types of offender and non-offenders. Paedophiles also frequently have a repertoire of beliefs/justifications used in their defence within the justice system. Malesky and Ennis (2004) explored the occurrence of a number of beliefs evident on posts on a pro-paedophile internet message board:

- *Justification of reprehensible conduct*: including moral justification (e.g. the act was beneficial to the child), psychological justification (the individual has an innate sexual orientation), and palliative comparison (downgrading the behaviour by comparing it to other more heinous behaviours)
- *Misperception of consequences*: including minimizing (the child did not suffer), misattributing blame (it's the parents' fault) or ignoring (I don't care)
- *Devaluating and attributing blame to the victim*: including dehumanization of the victim (she's a slut anyway) and attribution of blame (dressed like that she was asking for it).

Cognitive distortions were found in 36% of posts, with by far the most frequent (34%) involving some form of justification of conduct.

Pulling these various strands together, Ward and Siegert's (2002) pathways model identified a number of pathways to paedophile behaviour, including:

- *Intimacy deficits*: the individual possesses normal 'sexual scripts' (i.e. they know and can conform to the rules of appropriate sexual acts), and only offends at certain times such as when a partner is unavailable or during a period of sustained loneliness.

- *Deviant sexual scripts*: the individual has 'subtle' distortions in their sexual scripts and dysfunctional schema about the nature of relationships. Paedophiles in this category prefer adult sexual partners. However, they fear intimacy and rejection from adults, and equate sexual relationships with emotionally intimate relationships. They therefore experience their emotional needs as sexual needs, and seek sexual relationships obsessively, particularly when they feel lonely. Sex with children may occur simply because 'they are in the right place at the right time' (Gannon et al. 2004).
- *Antisocial cognitions*: men in this pathway hold strong antisocial beliefs and do not feel the need to conform to societal norms. They may enjoy inappropriate sexual activity as an exciting statement of their antisocial attitudes.
- *Multiple dysfunction*: these individuals may be considered 'classic' paedophiles. They choose children as their preferred sexual partners. They are characterized by intimacy and social skills deficits, engage in sexual acts as a means of emotional regulation, and have cognitive distortions supportive of paedophile acts. They usually consider children as sexual beings who have the capacity to make their own decisions about when, where, and with whom to have sex.

Three of these pathways, intimacy deficits, antisocial cognitions, and multiple dysfunction, have subsequently been confirmed using a cluster analysis of data from 97 UK child offenders by Gannon et al. (2012), who also provide support for novel clusters of 'impulsivity' (with largely normative functioning on most measures, but high levels of impulsivity and targeting of older children aged between 10 and 17 years) and 'boy predators', who almost fitted within the multiple dysfunction cluster, but did not hold intimacy deficits and reported a preference for impersonal and sadomasochistic tendencies. The multiple dysfunction cluster, although clearly distinguishable, had the lowest number of members.

Case formulation

Mr J was a 30-year-old man, admitted to hospital as a result of a period of severe depression. Prior to his depression he had been a teacher in a school in the North of England. Although there was no evidence that he had engaged in paedophile acts with any children, his name was found on a distribution list for child pornography kept by a paedophile ring. His house was raided, and paedophile materials were found in it. He was therefore charged by the police, and found guilty of using child pornography. The school at which he worked was notified of this outcome and he was immediately dismissed from his job. He was married at the time that this occurred, but was immediately asked to leave the marital home and his wife began divorce proceedings. He moved to London, where he could be 'lost among the crowd' and had some family contacts. There he became profoundly depressed, and was admitted to hospital where he entered into therapy for his depression.

Long-term antecedents

Mr J was homosexual, and had experienced a sexual preference for males since he became sexually aware. During his adolescence he had no sexual relationships with either boys or girls. However, while masturbating, his imagery focused on young adolescent boys. As he grew older and left home to go to university, he found both his homosexuality and sexual interest in young boys shaming and inappropriate. He therefore did not seek sex with young men, but did have a number of age-appropriate homosexual relationships prior to his marriage, but these had generally ended disastrously. As a consequence, in an attempt to conform to both his and his parents' perceived norms, he began to date women towards the end of his university studies and was able to establish a long-term relationship with a woman with a low sex drive. He later married this woman. They lived together from the time he was at university to the time he was identified as a paedophile. His marriage had been functional and pleasant, but not sexually satisfying. During this time, he had regularly used child pornography (with a particular interest in young adolescent boys) unknown to his wife. He taught physical education (and mathematics) at school so clearly had the possibility of seeing young boys with little or no clothing. He denied ever having abused this possibility, and no complaints had been made against him at school. Of course, the truth of his claims is difficult to determine, as however motivated he was to change, there is little benefit to admitting behaviours that could be both embarrassing and put him at risk of legal action.

Formulation

Mr J did not fit the 'classic' profile of a paedophile. He was able to develop age-appropriate social (and to a more limited extent sexual) relationships both with men and women. He was not 'driven' to paedophilia as a consequence of an inability to engage with age-appropriate individuals. In addition, he did not condone his behaviour, and considered his sexual interest to be inappropriate and felt ashamed by it. He thought that while he claimed to have had no physical contact with young boys, even using photographs in this way was exploitative and morally unacceptable. His depression was a consequence of the loss of his job and his marriage, the probability that he would never find work again, and the shame he felt as his behaviour had been made public. His interest in young boys was maintained by masturbation to their images.

Intervention

Mr J was motivated to engage in therapy because he found his sexual interests inappropriate and shaming. He began a programme of masturbatory reorientation. In this, he began to masturbate to images of young children to achieve sexual excitement, before shifting the focus of his images to those of more mature boys or young-looking men. He found the image of one young-looking male Hollywood star (who will remain nameless!) particularly exciting. This programme worked very well, and over time he found that he could become sexually excited by the images of age-appropriate men.

Despite these gains and the claims he made about only using child pornography to provoke sexual excitement, his behaviour followed the pattern suggested by Pithers (1990) on at least one occasion. At this time he was feeling depressed, and decided to go for a walk, which drew him 'accidentally' to a shopping area frequented by local schoolchildren, and 'he happened to pass by a [public] toilet' when a young boy walked into it. At this point, he was excited by the thought of seeing the young child expose himself, and followed him into the toilet. There, he watched him use the urinal. The child was unaware of his presence, and there was no social or physical contact with him. Nevertheless, this reinforced the need to set up a relapse prevention programme, in which he drew up a list of alternative behaviours to do when he felt depressed or the need for sexual excitement. The alternative behaviours he engaged in were fairly limited, and included calling his family on the telephone or visiting them, and focusing on chores or tasks about the house. The one thing that he determined not to do was to leave the house at such times, as this would inevitably lead to him 'accidentally' walking into high-risk areas. In addition, when leaving the house at all times he walked routes that did not pass schools or other places where young people might congregate, to reduce the likelihood of temptation. Despite this setback, both interventions appeared to progress well after this point, and Mr J was able to avoid putting himself at risk of offending for several months. He was eventually discharged, although with regular follow-up appointments in an attempt to monitor and prevent future problems.

Treatment of paedophilic disorder

Social constraints

One way in which society has dealt with issues of paedophilia has been to try to control – not treat – the actions of paedophiles. A number of laws have been instituted to facilitate this process in the UK, including:

- *The Sex Offenders Act 1997*: established a list of all people convicted of acts 'of a sexual nature involving an abuse of power, where the victim is unable to give informed or true consent'. It covers a range of offences, including rape, incest, child abuse, and indecent assault. Offenders have to register with the police and notify them of any changes in their name and address. People who do not register can be imprisoned or receive a £5,000 fine. People stay on the register for differing times, depending on the nature of their conviction. People who receive a non-custodial sentence or caution stay on the list for 5 years; those given sentences of 30 months or over stay on indefinitely.
- *Crime Sentence Act 1997*: allows for sex offenders who are convicted of a second serious sex offence to be automatically given a life sentence.

- *Crime and Disorder Act 1998*: gives police particular powers against sex offenders, allowing them to apply for a 'Sex Offenders Order' for any offender who can reasonably be considered a public risk. Courts can impose conditions on offenders, such as banning them from places where children are likely to come together, such as parks and schools.

Stop and think ...

In some states in the USA, a law unofficially called Megan's Law provides information about the presence of a child sex offender in the neighbourhood. This may involve the individual involved telling his neighbours that he is a paedophile and leaving a notice in their window with this information on. In addition, websites with names, addresses and photographs of offenders are publicly accessible. This does not happen in the UK at present, although schools or youth clubs can be made aware of the presence of a convicted offender by the police. When names have been publicized, as in a series of photographs in the now defunct *News of the World* newspaper, the high publicity given to these issues apparently led to attacks on people suspected of being paedophiles. In one instance, in South Wales, the house of a doctor who worked with children – a paediatrician – was mistakenly attacked. Clearly, there are a number of issues raised by these facts:

- How do we ensure that the risk of paedophiles accessing and assaulting children is minimized?
- How do we counter the need to ensure the safety of children with the physical safety and rights of people who may or may not have committed paedophile acts?

Treatment programmes for paedophilic disorder

As sexual activity with young persons is against the law, treatment is usually initiated in a prison or a secure forensic facility. Even here, engagement in treatment programmes is not compulsory, and only about 25% of those offered treatment choose to engage in treatment programmes while up to 86% drop out from treatment (Larochelle et al. 2011).

Physical treatments

Physical treatments suppress sexual urges and behaviour, but do not change the object of sexual desire. Two surgical procedures, castration and neurosurgery, are no longer considered ethically acceptable. However, chemical approaches involving administration of drugs that block the production or action of androgens, hormones that influence the male sexual response, remain in use. Androgen blocking drugs have proven moderately successful, although quality data is lacking.

In one of relatively few studies, Rösler and Witztum (1998) examined the impact of monthly drug injections of a gonadotrophin-releasing hormone combined with supportive psychotherapy for up to $3\frac{1}{2}$ years in a series of 30 patients. All participants reported a reduction in inappropriate sexual fantasies and a reduction to zero 'incidents' per month while taking the medication. An alternative drug medication involves the use of luteinizing hormone-releasing hormone (LHRH) **agonists**, which also prevent the production of testosterone, and have similar levels of effect. Briken et al. (2003) identified four case reports, seven uncontrolled studies, and only one study comparing LHRH agonists with an androgen **antagonist**. Thus, the total sample of patients treated (often in an uncontrolled study) was 118, and all outcomes were self-report. With these cautions in mind, they concluded that the LHRH was an effective form of treatment.

A major problem for antiandrogen treatments is that between 30% and 100% of the people prescribed these drugs do not take them (Seto and Barbaree 1999). Many of those who stop taking them presumably do so because they want to reoffend, as they do not change any of the beliefs or attitudes that drive deviant sexual behaviours. Nor does treatment come without its problems, which as well as sexual dysfunction include loss of body hair, hot flushes, mood swings, breast growth, and weight gain. For these reasons, as well as the desire to reoffend, many individuals choose not to receive this treatment or stop taking it once initiated, and Turner and Briken (2017) recommended their use only for individuals at the highest risk of offending.

Behaviour therapy

Both aversion therapy and masturbatory reconditioning methods have been used in the treatment of paedophilia. In aversion therapy, an inappropriate sexual stimulus is paired with an aversive event such as mild electric shock or strong aversive odour. This process is thought to condition a negative emotional state to the presence of the sexual stimulus. Most studies show some reduction of arousal to stimuli of young children. However, this may not result in reductions in offences. Rice et al. (1991), for example, followed 136 non-familial child molesters, 50 of whom received aversion therapy, following their discharge from a maximum security prison. Over a period of about 6 years, 31% were convicted of a new offence. Recidivism rates were no lower among those who received aversion therapy than those who did not.

Masturbatory reconditioning involves the individual initiating a sexual response through the use of their favoured sexual images. Once they have achieved an erection, they switch to more appropriate images, such as a naked woman or man. They continue to masturbate to orgasm, when they concentrate deeply on this image. This approach may be combined with a graded series of 'normal' images, from less to more typical of the desired sexual focus. This approach has a number of advantages over aversion therapy. First, it is less ethically challenging and more acceptable to potential recipients. Second, it does not involve laboratory equipment and can be practised between therapy sessions. There is little empirical evidence of its effects and it is considered to be relatively ineffective and is now not widely used (Fagan et al. 2002).

Relapse prevention

Relapse prevention involves teaching the individual to do the following:

- identify situations in which they are at high risk of offending behaviour
- get out of the risky situation
- consider lapses as something to be learned from
- identify factors that led to relapse and plan how these could be avoided in the future.

The relapse prevention programme described by Marques et al. (2005) was an early large study of its effectiveness, involving over 700 participants. It involved an intensive in-patient programme conducted in a secure forensic hospital and a one-year support programme following discharge. Participants were given sexual education and taught general coping skills such as relaxation, stress and anger management, as well as social skills. More specific interventions included identifying the behaviours that preceded offending behaviour and addressing how these may be interrupted. It also dealt with issues of responsibility and minimization. Over a 5-year follow-up, this intervention had a known reoffence rate of 10.8% in contrast to the 13% rate among those who did not receive the intervention – a modest difference. The programme was most successful with offenders who had male victims, and less successful with those who had female victims, although why is not clear. Unfortunately, by its 8-year follow-up assessment, there were no differences in outcome between those people who took part in the programme and those that did not.

This failure to prove benefit has been echoed following a similar intervention in the UK. The SOTEP (Sex Offenders Treatment Programme) is the standard approach used by the English and Welsh prison systems, and was evaluated in a population of over 2,500 treated and more than 1,300 untreated sex offenders. Participants could enter the programme if they evidenced apparent motivation to change, were at risk of recidivism, and were able to engage with the programme. The programme included 20 'blocks' including the following:

- Identifying and challenging pro-offending thinking
- Learning positive coping strategies and developing an action plan for practising positive coping
- Identifying factors contributing to their sexual offending
- Group members reporting an accurate account of offending behaviour, identifying triggering events, relevant emotions, behaviours, and cognitions present in the offence pathway
- Increasing awareness of the relevance of deviant sexual fantasy to offending, increasing motivation to abandon deviant fantasy, and developing non-deviant fantasy material
- Building on insights and to formally begin the process of change: set targets for new behaviours and ways of thinking
- Undermine any beliefs that the experience of being abused was harmless or positive for group members' victims.

Despite this impressive programme, participants had worse outcomes than those who did not take part (Mews et al. 2017). Following an average 8.2 years follow-up period, the sexual offending rate was 2% higher in the intervention than in the comparison group (10% versus 8%). Those who took part in the programme were also more likely to be identified as using child sexual imagery than those who did not (5% versus 3%). These data add to the systematic review by Långström et al. (2013), which reached similar negative conclusions. One ray of hope for interventions has been the Dunkelfeld Project in Germany, which offered a combination of pharmacological and psychotherapy for self-referred and anonymous paedophiles that had not entered the legal system. Unfortunately, although initial analyses suggested their intervention may have been of benefit, subsequent analysis (Mokros and Banse 2019) found this conclusion to be too optimistic and the intervention did not reduce 'proneness to commit sexual offenses against children'.

Research box 9

Eke, A.W., Helmus, M. and Seto, M.C. (2019) A validation study of the Child Pornography Offender Risk Tool, *Sexual Abuse*, 32: 456–76.

One of the most difficult things in sexual offending is identifying and measuring recidivism, and identifying those people most likely to reoffend. With this intent, a number of studies have evaluated the ability of a number of risk assessment tools to identify future risk of offending. Self-report intentions are clearly highly suspect in any risk indication. Accordingly, the Child Pornography Offender Risk Tool (CPORT) comprises seven verifiable offender characteristics that can be put into a risk equation. Each item is categorically rated as present or not present:

- age at the time of the index investigation of 35 years of less
- any prior criminal history
- any failure on conditional release
- any contact sexual offending
- indication (admission or diagnosis) of sexual interest in prepubescent or pubescent children
- more boy than girl content in child pornography
- more boy than girl content in other child-related materials.

In the initial development sample of 266 men convicted of child pornography offences followed for a period of 5 years, the CPORT was found to have an area under the receiver operating characteristic (ROC) curve of 0.74, which indicates a 'fair' degree of discrimination (e.g. acceptable levels of accurate prediction and few false-positives and false-negatives). An area under the ROC curve of 0.80–0.90 would be classified as 'good', 0.90–1.00 as excellent. Eke et al.'s 2019 study added to these data in order to validate these findings in a larger sample of offenders, comparing them with the predictive ability of an alternative and well-validated assessment, the Correlates of Admission of Sexual Interest in Children (CASIC).

Method

Participants

Participants were 86 first-time child pornography cases provided by a 'large Canadian provincial police force'. Over half (59%) were detected due to online activity, while 41% were detected through other routes including being discovered by others in use of porn. Most looked at porn online, with only a small minority (9%) using offline material including material they made themselves. The majority of the sample (97%) had at least one index charge for possession of child pornography (an average of 2.4 offences), almost half (45%) had distribution charges, while fewer had production charges (16%).

Measures

- *Child Pornography Offender Risk Tool* (CPORT) items were coded such that a score of 0–7 was possible. The mean score was 1.81 among those completed assessments with no missing data. Frequencies for the seven CPORT items were : (i) age 35 years or younger, 44%; (ii) prior criminal history, 42%; (iii) failure on conditional release, 17%; (iv) any contact sexual offending, 26%; (v) indication (admission or diagnosis) of sexual interest in children, 13%; (vi) more boy than girl content in child pornography, 17%; and (vii) more boy than girl content in other child-related materials, 17%. Inter-rater reliability of the assessments was high.
- *Correlates of Admission of Sexual Interest in Children* (CASIC) measures six items associated with paedophilic or hebephilic disorder: (i) never married, 49%; (ii) child pornography content included videos, 67%; (iii) child pornography content included sex stories involving children, 9%; (iv) evidence of interest in child pornography over 2 or more years, 36%; (v) volunteered in a role with high access to children, 13%; and (vi) engaged in online sexual communication with a minor or officer posing as a minor, 12%.

Procedure

Participants were identified through information provided by two Canadian services. Information was coded from police files, interviews, and police officer notes. Coding took a half to full day per case. Follow-up was determined as the time following the first point of release from detention to the date when criminal records were checked, 5 years after the start of the study. Any time in custody since the starting point was subtracted from the calculated time.

Findings

Data from this study were added to those of a previous study, involving 266 participants that followed the same procedure, allowing analysis to be based on a total of 346 offenders at baseline. Overall recidivism rates over the follow-up period in this total population were 11.6% for any sexual crime and 8.4% for offences involving recidivism. Among subgroups of offenders, the highest rates of recidivism were among those with both pornography and contact offences. Rates for any sexual offence within this group were 25%, and for use of child pornography, 18%.

ROC analyses of the area under the curve to determine the accuracy of prediction (assessing accurate, false-positive, and false-negative predictions) were generally within the upper range of the 'fair' category, and generally slightly outperformed the CASIC.

Table 1 Area under the (ROC) curve scores for the CPORT and CASIC, with data from assessments that were complete and those with missing data

	All offenders	Porn/no contact offenders	Porn + contact offenders
	AUC [95% CI]	AUC [95% CI]	AUC [95% CI]
Any sexual recidivism			
CPORT (all cases)	0.742 [0.631–0.843]	0.671 [0.529–0.813]	0.794 [0.626–0.961]
CPORT (no missing info)	0.759 [0.660–0.859]	0.704 [0.571–0.863]	0.795 [0.629–0.962]
CASIC (no missing info)		0.564 [0.427–0.701]	0.787 [0.559–0.974]
Any child porn recidivism			
CPORT (all cases)	0.740 [0.637–0.844]	0.685 [0.538–0.832]	0.767 [0.592–0.943]
CPORT (no missing info)	0.771 [0.657–0.885]	0.705 [0.550–0.861]	0.896 [0.767–1.00]
CASIC (no missing info)		0.553 [0.374–0.692]	0.707 [0.540–0.876]

Discussion

The CPORT proved an effective risk assessment tool for all offender groups and also appeared robust in the context of missing data: a likely reality of 'real-world' use. The authors note that the study was underpowered to assess the predictive strength of individual items (which were also reported) but had sufficient power to assess the strength of prediction of the whole measure. As well as forming part of a risk assessment process, the tool also identifies risk factors that should form the basis of any assessment of offenders and key information that should be shared amongst those involved in working with them.

Transvestic disorder

DSM-5 defines transvestic disorder as:

- the experience of intense sexual arousal from cross-dressing, as manifested by fantasies, urges, or acts, for at least 6 months
- these fantasies, sexual urges or behaviours cause clinically significant distress or impairment in social, occupational or other important areas of functioning.

The term disorder and its link to distress or impairment are important here. As the leader of the working group for DSM-5, Blanchard (2010) noted that transvestism is a form of behaviour; it only becomes a disorder if the individual finds it personally problematic in some way. As phrased in the report: *An ego-syntonic, well-adjusted transvestite could be classified as a transvestite for research or descriptive purposes without being diagnosed with a disorder.* Around 3% of men and 0.4% of women reported at least one episode of transvestic fetishism in a Swedish population survey (Långström and Zucker 2005).

Boys who grow up to engage in transvestite behaviour neither engage in 'feminine' behaviours before puberty, nor do they cross-dress. Similarly, men who are transvestites are unremarkably masculine in their adult hobbies and career choices. Transvestites usually begin cross-dressing at puberty, and rarely later than mid-adolescence. This typically results in sexual excitement, although many people report that they dress in this way because they like the feel of the clothes and that there is no sexual motivation to their behaviour. Some adolescents wear feminine clothes occasionally; others compulsively wear them under their masculine clothes. Attempts at passing off as a woman are rare in adolescence. However, cross-dressing is frequently accompanied by fantasies of being female, and these fantasies may form the nucleus of sexual fantasies. In a survey of over 1,000 adult transvestite men, Docter and Prince (1997) reported that 40% of their sample experienced sexual excitement and orgasm 'always' or 'often' when they cross-dressed. Only 9% of the sample said they never experienced this. Cross-dressing frequently elicits less and less sexual excitement as the individual grows older and may eventually have no discernible sexual association. However, the desire to cross-dress may remain the same or even grow stronger, and may be accompanied by feelings of comfort and well-being. Lack of opportunity to cross-dress can result in a lowering of mood and marked irritability. As a result, many transvestites continue to wear women's undergarments beneath their normal male clothes.

Among Docter and Prince's respondents, 87% reported being exclusively heterosexual; 83% were either married at the time of the survey or had been married; 32% of their wives knew they cross-dressed before marriage; 28% were completely accepting of the behaviour once they became aware of it, while 19% were 'completely antagonistic'. It is common for transvestite men to stop cross-dressing in the early months or years of relationships with a new partner, although many revert to cross-dressing in time. Many enjoy 'normal' heterosexual intercourse. Others need props such as wearing feminine attire to achieve sexual pleasure.

As social reaction can be very negative to transvestic behaviour, cross-dressing usually takes place in arenas where such behaviour is acceptable, including the home and transvestite clubs or organizations. Nevertheless, Docter and Prince reported that 71% of their sample had cross-dressed in public: 10% had been on a bus or train while cross-dressed, 28% had eaten in restaurants, 26% used the ladies' toilet, and 22% had tried on feminine clothing in stores. When asked their preferred gender identity, 11% preferred their masculine self, 28% preferred their feminine self, and 60% had an equal preference for the two.

Some people experience guilt and shame as a result of their feelings and behaviour. Such individuals may make repeated, frequently unsuccessful, efforts to overcome their perceived anomaly. They may rid their wardrobe of feminine clothes, before acquiring new ones in the following weeks and months. This cycle may occur repeatedly in younger people who later become more accepting of their feelings. In Docter and Prince's sample, 70% reported having purged their wardrobe on at least one occasion, and 45% reported seeking counselling as a result of their feelings.

Aetiology of transvestic fetishism

Biological factors

There are surprisingly few studies of a biological cause of transvestism, and most are case studies rather than formal scientific studies. One such case, reported by Riley (2002), involved a 72-year-old man who was treated with a drug known as selegiline, an **MAOI** (see Chapter 4), which, among other actions, increases serotonin and dopamine activity. Following this treatment, the man developed a frequent impulse to wear women's clothing despite never having had this desire previously. The drug was withdrawn, and his urge to wear women's clothing stopped. This remains one of the very few studies of biological mechanisms.

Parental relationships

Various, often contradictory, family theories of transvestism have been proposed. Newcomb (1985) found that transvestite men were more likely than other heterosexual men to characterize their parents as less sex-typed and more sex-reversed in terms of dependence and affiliation. This suggested some form of modelling process may be involved. However, men who become transvestites tend to adopt typical masculine roles as a young child, countering this type of theory. A second theory has suggested that the principal maternal influence in transvestism is one of hostility and anger towards males. Zucker and Bradley (1995) noted evidence that boys who develop transvestism have higher separation rates from their mothers than is the norm, suggesting this reflected their mothers' aggressive attitudes towards men, and that transvestites are avoiding this hostility by dressing as women.

Behavioural condition

More conventional reinforcement models (Crawford et al. 1993) suggest that if a child is exposed to women's clothing and enjoys the feel of them or masturbates while wearing them, this may establish a reinforcement process that results in the continuation of this behaviour.

Psychoanalytic processes

Ovesey and Person (1973) suggested that the psychoanalytic processes that lead to transvestism occur after an individual has consolidated their sense of maleness. Their mother is typically warm and supportive, their father distant and threatening, even verbally or physically abusive. As a result, the mother turns towards her son for gratification not forthcoming from her marriage. She is seductive towards the boy, but at the same time encourages his cross-dressing either overtly or covertly. In doing so, she is thought to be gratifying herself sexually, but repressing her real (sexual) interest by denying his masculinity. The child is gratified by her intimacy, but also feels guilty. He assumes that his mother wishes to dress him as a girl in order to placate his father. The intimacy of his mother and the perceived rivalry of his father prevent a successful resolution of the oedipal complex (see Chapter 2).

After childhood, the individual seeks to preserve the mother as a dependence object, and is attracted to women like his mother who will accept or even encourage cross-dressing. Adult transvestites resort to cross-dressing under periods of stress and wear female underclothing as a protective device. Female clothes provide protection in three ways:

- they symbolize the mother and perpetuate dependence and continued need for her protection
- they symbolize auto-castration, a token submission to male competitors, which wards off their retaliation
- they disguise masculinity to disarm rivals.

The clothes conceal the penis, the symbol of masculine power, and deny hostile intent. They allow the individual to avoid detection by their rivals, which not only allays anxiety, but even confers on the individual an inflated sense of masculinity. Ovesey and Person went so far to suggest that 'the transvestite is Superman in drag!'

Treatment of transvestic fetishism

Transvestism is not a 'condition' that requires treatment. Nevertheless, people whose behaviour is affecting their relationships or who find their behaviour unacceptable may seek treatment. Marital problems often lead to attempts at behavioural change and the initiation of therapy. Treatment usually focuses on the sexual elements of transvestic behaviour and includes aversion therapy and modification of sexual fantasy. Some aversion programmes have proven moderately successful. Marks et al. (1970) reported that two-thirds of participants in electrical aversion therapy 'improved' with treatment, up to a follow-up period of 2 years. This compared with one-quarter of a control group who did not receive the intervention. A second approach to the treatment of transvestism involves masturbatory retraining. Here, the individual masturbates using his preferred sexual object, including female props worn either by the individual or his partner, before reverting to images of more 'normal' sex objects immediately before and at orgasm. Again, a number of case descriptions and uncontrolled studies have shown this method to have been used with good effect (Laws and Marshall 1991).

More recently, Chiang et al. reported significant changes following a cognitive behavioural programme instituted following an individual developing 'severe moral anxiety' (1999: 299). The individual involved did not respond to psychodynamic therapy, but a combination of supportive and cognitive therapy proved of some value, at least in the short term.

10.3 Gender dysphoria

In contrast to transvestism, where men dress as women, but accept their male identity, individuals with gender dysphoria believe themselves to have been born the wrong sex. DSM-5 now emphasizes the fact that this state is not a psychiatric 'disorder' by changing its name from gender identify *disorder* in DSM-IV to gender *dysphoria*, implying a non-pathological state of unhappiness with one's gender. That said, it remains a 'diagnosis' within a framework of psychiatric illness, so does not escape this implication entirely. In order to achieve this 'diagnosis', DSM states the individual must experience, for a period of 6 months or more, at least two of:

- a marked incongruence between their experienced/expressed gender and primary and/or secondary sex characteristics
- a consequential strong desire to be rid of one's primary and/or secondary sex characteristics
- a strong desire for the primary and/or secondary sex characteristics of the other gender
- a strong desire to be of the other gender (or some alternative gender different from one's assigned gender)
- a strong desire to be treated as the other gender (or some alternative gender different from one's assigned gender)
- a strong conviction that one has the typical feelings and reactions of the other gender (or some alternative gender different from one's assigned gender).

Critically, the condition must be associated with clinically significant distress or impairment in social, occupational or other important areas of functioning

In adolescents and adults, gender dysphoria is manifested by a preoccupation with the belief that the individual is born 'the wrong sex', and a desire for the removal of primary and secondary sex characteristics. Many opt for surgery to change their body to what they consider their appropriate sex. They become transsexuals. Others do not take such a radical step, but dress and try to pass themselves off as a member of their desired sex. People with gender dysphoria are often sexually attracted to people of the same sex, which they interpret as conventional heterosexual preference.

Most adults with gender dysphoria report a history of consistent cross-gender behaviour in childhood. Boys may reject the rough-and-tumble play and prefer the company of girls. They frequently dress in women's clothing and insist they will grow up to be a girl. Some claim their penis and testes are disgusting and hope they will somehow change into female genitalia as they grow older. Girls may reject urinating in the sitting position, and assert that they do not want to grow breasts or menstruate. They may reject typical girls' clothing. Hoshiai et al. (2010) found that 90% of Japanese female-to-male (FtM) individuals started to feel discomfort with their gender identity before graduation from elementary school. By contrast, about half the male-to-female (MtF) individuals started to feel discomfort with their gender identity after graduation from elementary school. Among the FtMs, almost all were sexually attracted to females, while MtF individuals were much more varied in their interests: 35% were attracted to males, 22% to females, 16% to both, and 27% felt no attraction to either males or females. Gender identity may also change over time in young people. Wallien and Cohen-Kettenis (2008), for example, followed a cohort of 77 children referred to a clinic as a result of gender dysphoria. At 10 years follow-up, 43% of their sample were no longer gender **dysphoric**. Of note was that the stronger the cross-gender behaviour, the more likely the child was to remain gender dysphoric. Some adults may also spontaneously change their gender identity (Marks et al. 2000), although such cases are rare.

The prevalence of gender dysphoria is difficult to determine, as some individuals may remain hidden. However, a recent Irish survey (Judge et al. 2014) determined that one MtF individual per 10,000 head of population became known to the medical services; the prevalence of FtM individuals was 1 in 28,000. More population-based surveys have found rates of incongruent gender identity and a desire to undergo sex reassignment of around 0.6% of men and 0.2% of women (Zucker 2017). Rates of gender dysphoria among young people appear relatively high, with estimates of between 0.5% and 1.3% of this generation experiencing a transgender identity. The stability of this orientation is unknown. Rates of co-morbidity with emotional disorders are high. Judge et al. (2014), for example, found that 35% of their sample of people diagnosed with gender dysphoria were clinically depressed, while an overall rate of 19% for co-morbidity with any psychiatric disorder was reported by Hoshiai et al. (2010) in their Japanese population. These high rates of psychopathology may be the consequence of both individuals' unhappiness with their assigned gender and a frequent negative societal response to them (see below).

Aetiology of gender dysphoria

In a blunt summary of our understanding, or lack of understanding, of gender dysphoria, Kaltiala-Heino et al. (2018) described the causes of the condition to be 'unknown'. A number of theories have been posited, but fail to provide an unequivocal explanation for gender dysphoria.

Genetic factors

In one of the few studies of the genetic processes in gender dysphoria, Coolidge et al. (2002) found that 2% of their sample of over 300 **monozygotic (MZ)** and **dizygotic (DZ)** twins showed some evidence of gender identity disorder symptomatology based on self-report measures. Applying statistical modelling to their data, they found that 62% of the variance in reported symptoms could be attributed to biological factors, while 38% was attributable to environmental factors. These data led the investigators to suggest that the causes of gender dysphoria were primarily biological, not psychological. Since then, a number of studies have attempted to identify gene alleles associated with the condition, with mixed and contradictory findings, although some degree of replication has been found in relation to genes that control both androgen and oestrogen pathways (e.g. Foreman et al. 2019).

Biological factors

Although most commentators, and the genetic data, suggest that gender dysphoria is primarily the result of biological processes, what these are is far from clear. Studies of sex hormonal disturbance in adulthood are surprisingly difficult to conduct, because many people with gender dysphoria take hormones of the opposite sex either as part of a treatment programme or by purchasing them on the black market. Despite these interpretive difficulties, what evidence there is does not support a simple hormonal explanation, with few if any differences between both men and women with gender dysphoria and those without (e.g. Gladue 1985). A variant of the hormonal theory, that abnormal levels of prenatal hormones may influence gender identity, has also not been supported (e.g. Yalom et al. 1973).

Although several studies have failed to find any differences between the brains of people with and without gender dysphoria, a small number have found evidence to suggest a neurological substrate to the experience of these individuals. Zhou et al. (1995) conducted autopsies on the brains of six people who had changed their sex from male to female. They found an area of the brain, known as the bed nucleus of stria terminalis (BST), within the hypothalamus to be much smaller than is typically found in men. Indeed, the size of the BST matched that typically found in women, which is usually about half the size of that found in men. In a further investigation of this phenomenon, Kruijver et al. (2000) examined the number of somatostatin-expressing neurons in the BST. They found the same pattern of neurological findings. The number of these neurons in the BSTs of male-to-female transsexuals was similar to those in the females' BST, while the number of these neurons in a female-to-male transsexual was in the male range. What this difference actually means is not clearly understood, although the BST is known to regulate sexual activity in male rats. It is possible, therefore, that this may contribute in some way to gender dysphoria. Unfortunately, the theory is not without its challenges. Chung et al. (2002) found that differences in BST structure do not emerge until adulthood, while the experience of gender dysmorphia typically arises in childhood. A second challenge comes from findings that hormonal treatments similar to those taken by participants in both the Zhou and Krujver studies change the size of the BST (Hulshoff Pol et al. 2006), allowing the possibility that any brain differences were a consequence of hormonal therapy rather than innate biological differences.

A second strand of research has explored gender-related performance on neuropsychological tasks known to differ between males and females. A biological model would suggest that males who want to change their sex to female would perform better on neuropsychological tests that favour women, and vice versa. Unfortunately, as with the brain studies, a clear picture is lacking. Haraldsen et al. (2003), for example, found that untreated people with gender dysphoria performed on cognitive tests in ways that were predicted by their biological sex, not their gender identity, suggesting few neurological differences between people with gender dysphoria and those without.

Psychoanalytic explanations

Psychoanalytic explanations suggest that male transsexuals have an ambiguous core gender identity. According to Ovesey and Person (1973), male transsexualism originates from extreme separation anxiety early in life before the individual has fully established his own sexual identity. To alleviate this anxiety, the individual resorts to fantasy of symbiotic fusion with the mother. In this way, mother and child become one and the danger of separation is nullified. In the transsexual's mind, he literally becomes the mother, and to sustain this fantasy attempts to revert his core identity from male to female.

To explain the desire for the removal of the penis, Ovesey and Person noted that the transsexual does not experience castration anxiety, as do most boys. Instead, they experience anxiety that continues until they *are* castrated. The penis is clear evidence that they have failed to psychically fuse with the mother. For the same reason, they reject the act of homosexuality, as this would also acknowledge them as male. They prefer to reject any sexual experience, and generally have little or no experience of sex, even masturbation. In sum, the motivation for security takes priority over motivation for sexuality, as a result of fear of early maternal abandonment.

Early life conditioning

Girls who exhibit high levels of tomboy behaviour tend to have parents who do the same, and to choose their father as their favourite parent. This allows the possibility of learning such behaviours from their parents and being rewarded for expressing them (Zucker et al. 1994). Early life experiences are dominated by family. However, as an individual grows up, they are subject to influences of a wider range of people: peers, school teachers, and so on. It is likely that such exposure results in differing and opposing reinforcement processes in which the individual may be punished for behaving in 'inappropriate' ways. Indeed, around half of children referred to gender clinics report significant bullying at school by their peers. Clark et al. (2014), for example, found that trans-gender-identifying adolescents were over four times more likely to have been bullied and twice as likely to have been afraid for their personal safety or in a serious physical fight than their typical peers. Thus, it seems that many young people experience significantly adverse conditioning experiences as a consequence of their behaviour and apparent sexual orientation. A simple conditioning theory struggles to explain the extremely strongly held beliefs about their gender that such people hold in the face of these experiences.

Treatment of gender dysphoria

Physical treatment

Many people with gender identity disorder request sex reassignment surgery. This involves a complex, staged process. For male-to-female transitions, treatment starts at least a year before surgery (see Box 10.1). First, the individual starts taking the female hormone oestrogen that results in a number of physical changes, including the development of breasts and a softening of the skin. Fat may shift from the shoulders to the hips in feminine fashion.

Box 10.1 Problems of gender dysphoria

Access to sex change surgery in Britain is limited. At times of inadequate resources for healthcare, this type of surgery is given a low priority, and many people with gender identity disorder can find it extremely difficult, if not impossible, to obtain this treatment from the National Health Service. Many people who choose to have surgery do so by paying privately for it, through specialist private companies such as TRANSFORM, who provide an assessment of the individual's suitability for gender reassignment, hormone therapy, support for a year while they await surgery and try to live as someone of the opposite sex, and then surgery and post-surgery support.

Simon was a 30-year-old man just beginning this process. He had been to the initial assessment and accepted as a possible 'case', and had begun hormone therapy at the time of the interview in which he described what led him to seek gender reassignment and the frustrations he had experienced on the way:

I am so angry. I know I have the wrong body, and no one can convince me that I am wrong. As long as I can remember, I have felt this way. I wanted breasts, to be a girl, to have a period – to get rid of my penis. I envy them so much ... I have tried to go along with things, not to be as I am. It's really pretty frightening admitting it and having to go the whole way like I want to. But it's what I want ...

I married someone just to try and conform. I love her as well. Not in a physical way, though. We don't have sex ... she isn't really a sexual person so that's all right. That's why I began to see her. She isn't very attractive, but she's a good person, so it feels good that she's with someone like me, where sex isn't a big deal. It doesn't feel right, but we are good friends and we get on well. I tried to keep things a secret. I have – had – a place in my wardrobe where I keep women's clothing. I put it on when she is at work. It feels so natural and fantastic. It's the only time I felt I was really me, and how I wanted to be. I had a wig, make-up and stuff so I could really feel like a woman. It was secret, but she came home when I was wearing it one day, and so I had to explain some of how I feel and what I want. She knows I want to change my sex. We're going to live together until I do, even though my body is going to change with the hormones. But she wants to live with me despite it. I don't know what will happen and how we'll feel in time, though ... I wear the clothing and the wig at home all the time now, now she knows. She's OK about it ... I'm not a 'trannie' [transvestite] though, because I want more – just dressing up isn't enough. They are just men playing at being women. I want and have always wanted to be a proper woman.

It has been so frustrating getting so far. I went for an interview at Charing Cross Hospital and they agreed to put me on their programme, but the local health people wouldn't pay for it, even though I had letters from my GP and a psychiatrist saying I needed it. So I had to go to TRANSFORM. I went to see them and they agreed to give me an assessment by a psychologist, and he agreed to put me on the programme. And that was great ... but I had no money, so I couldn't do it straight away. I felt so low at the time ... very depressed. I really needed it, but no one would let me get on with things. I was pretty close to suicidal ... I thought things would never change ... and I couldn't tell my wife why I was so low ... I'm still on antidepressants now ... I think they're the only thing keeping me going ... I still don't know how I'm going to pay for surgery ... I would sell the house but that's not fair on my wife, so I'm happy I'm on the hormones and beginning to see changes, but I can't see how I will go the whole way ... but I won't be happy unless I do, because emotionally it all feels so right.

Once initiated, hormones are taken indefinitely. This itself appears to bring benefit. Eighty per cent of those treated with hormones report less gender dysphoria and improvements in quality of life (Murad et al. 2010). At the same time, the person will undergo electrolysis to rid them of masculine hair patterns. They are also trained to raise the timbre of their voice. At this early stage, some people may also have cosmetic surgery to alter facial features such as their chin or larynx to make them appear more feminine. Most of these changes are reversible. More enduring changes are usually held back for at least a year during which the individual is required to live as a woman. Only if this 'trial period' is completed successfully will the final surgery be conducted. This involves amputation of the penis and construction of an artificial vagina. This will permit normal sexual intercourse.

For female-to-male reassignment, a similar process is followed. Hormone therapy changes body shape, redistributing fat, as well as deepening the voice. However, surgery is more arduous, and the end results are less successful. The penis that can be constructed is generally small and not capable of a normal erection. Accordingly, sexual intercourse is not possible without the use of artificial supports. Surgery may also include bilateral mastectomy and hysterectomy.

The social and psychological outcomes of surgery are generally good. Weyers et al. (2009), for example, reported that transsexual women compared favourably with the general population on measures of both physical and mental quality of life. In addition, they reported high levels of satisfaction with their self-image as women. They were less satisfied with their sexual functioning, which while they can achieve and enjoy intercourse, was less satisfying than the comparison group. This dissatisfaction with physical limitations was echoed in the findings of Kuhn et al. (2008), who found low levels of regret and emotional difficulties in transsexual men and women, but that they did report more physical and role limitations than a comparison group. Of particular concern are the outcomes of young people who have changed gender. However, the findings here are relatively reassuring. Durwood et al. (2017), for example, found that transsexual children aged between 3 and 12 years who received appropriate social support following transition did not differ from gender-matched control children and their siblings on measures of depression or self-worth, although they showed marginally elevated levels of anxiety. The authors do note, however, that unsupported children are likely to experience significantly more mental health problems than the norm.

Psychological therapies

Although in the past, psychological approaches were used in attempts to shift young people away from their cross-gender identity beliefs, there is now a consensus that psychological therapy should be used to support individuals with any mental health problems as a consequence of their desire for, or experience of, sexual transition (American Psychological Association 2008). Despite this consensus, data to show the effectiveness of such support is still lacking. Indeed, as recently as 2017, Bechard et al. were still feeling the need to argue for this support to be made consistently available.

10.4 Chapter summary

1. There are two broad categories of sexual disorder: disorders of response (including erectile dysfunction and vaginismus) and disorders of desire, the paraphilias.
2. Erectile disorder can be the result of physical factors, but is frequently the result of psychological ones. Common factors include anxiety, often as a result of distorted beliefs about sexual performance, and 'spectatoring'.
3. Genito-pelvic pain disorder/penetration disorder is also triggered by anxiety.
4. Treatment using sensate focusing and graded exposure methods is effective in both disorders.
5. The paraphilias are generally considered to be the result of conditioning processes in childhood, although specific paraphilias may have multiple casual factors.
6. Paedophilic disorder may result from conditioning processes, poor adult attachment and sexual relationships, an emotional congruence with children, and processes such as justifying cognitions that support the behaviour.
7. Many people imprisoned as a result of paedophile behaviour do not enter treatment programmes. For those that do, cognitive behavioural programmes that address the cognitions supporting the behaviour and develop strategies for dealing with high-risk situations appear the most effective treatment, although no treatment appears to be of consistent benefit. Masturbatory reconditioning may also alter the object of sexual pleasure. Hormonal therapies may be effective as long as the drug is taken, but compliance is low and relapse, once the drug is stopped, is high.
8. Transvestism is not a 'disorder' that requires treatment, but some people choose to seek treatment due to social and marital pressures.

9. Transvestic disorder is usually considered to be the consequence of conditioning processes, and treatment involves reconditioning using masturbatory retraining techniques. Aversive approaches are rarely used for ethical reasons.
10. Gender dysphoria occurs when an individual feels that they are the incorrect gender and wishes to change it.
11. Gender dysphoria is poorly understood. No evidence of biological determinants has been found, and psychological models struggle to provide adequate explanations of the condition.
12. People with gender dysphoria are generally resistant to psychological therapy and most eventually seek surgery and hormonal treatments, following which most enjoy a better quality of life.

10.5 For discussion

1. Rates of recidivism among sexual offenders are relatively low, despite the lack of effectiveness of formal rehabilitation programmes. Why may this be the case? And should we provide what are now known to be ineffective rehabilitation programmes?
2. Given the difficulties of treating high-risk individuals who engage in paedophilic behaviour, should these people remain in hospital or some other institution to protect society from them? If they are released into society, should the public be made aware of where they live?
3. How can we best ensure that young people undergoing gender reassignment surgery are appropriately supported in the decision-making process and beyond.
4. Can enforced biological treatments be the ultimate treatment for recidivist paedophiles?

10.6 Further reading

Dennis, J.A., Khan, O., Ferriter, M. et al. (2012) Psychological interventions for adults who have sexually offended or are at risk of offending, *Cochrane Database of Systematic Reviews*, 12: CD007507 [https://doi.org/10.1002/14651858.CD007507.pub2].

Feinberg, L. (1997) *Transgender Warriors*, Boston, MA: Beacon Press.

Knack, N., Winder, B., Murphy, L. et al. (2019) Primary and secondary prevention of child sexual abuse, *International Review of Psychiatry*, 31: 181–94.

Shumer, D.E., Nokoff, N.J. and Spack, N.P. (2016) Advances in the care of transgender children and adolescents, *Advances in Pediatrics*, 63: 79–102.

Thomas, T. (2015) *Sex Crime: Sex Offending and Society*, Abingdon: Routledge.

Zucker, K.J., Lawrence, A.A. and Kreukels, B.P. (2016) Gender dysphoria in adults, *Annual Review of Clinical Psychology*, 12: 217–47.

11 Personality disorders

Personality disorders can affect an individual for much of their life. A number of these disorders have been identified, some of which, such as the schizoid or schizotypal disorders, have some of the features of other, more disabling, conditions – but not to such a degree that a formal diagnosis can be assigned. Others, including borderline personality or psychopathy, differ markedly from any other **DSM** diagnoses. The chapter begins with a discussion of the validity of the concept of personality disorders as distinct 'disorders', before considering a general theory explaining their development. The chapter then considers each of three clusters of personality disorders, with a particular focus on two conditions that have received the most attention from psychologists: borderline personality disorder and the associated diagnoses of antisocial behaviour and psychopathy. By the end of the chapter, you should have an understanding of:

- Issues related to all personality disorders
- Challenges to the diagnostic category of personality disorder
- A general theory of personality disorders
- The type A, B, and C personality disorder clusters, with particular focus on:
  - borderline personality and its treatment
  - the **aetiology** and treatment of antisocial behaviour and psychopathy.

11.1 Introduction

DSM IV-TR defined personality disorders as an enduring pattern of inner experience and behaviour that deviates markedly from the expectations of the individual's culture in at least two of the following: cognition, mood, interpersonal functioning, and impulse control. The pattern is inflexible and pervasive across a range of personal or social situations and is long-lasting. DSM-5 simplified this categorization by defining personality disorders as deficits in two domains: identity and interpersonal functioning. A poorly integrated sense of identify reflects the difficulty an individual may experience in maintaining a constant sense of self, and they may experience shifting internal states. Difficulties in interpersonal functioning may arise from a lack of empathy or ability to understand the internal states of other people. In addition, these impairments are relatively stable across time and context. Despite this conceptual change, the DSM continued to identify ten specific personality disorders in three clusters within this broad category, although there is considerable overlap between them (Tyrer et al. 2015):

- Cluster A: *Odd or eccentric* – paranoid, schizoid, schizotypal
- Cluster B: *Flamboyant or dramatic* – antisocial, histrionic, narcissistic, borderline
- Cluster C: *Fearful or anxious* – avoidant, dependent, obsessive-compulsive.

Around 6% of the world's population could be diagnosed with a personality disorder, with the highest rates in North and South America, and the lowest in Europe (Huang et al. 2006). Rates are similar in men and women (Coid et al. 2006). Depending on the study, between 24% and 74% of people diagnosed with a personality disorder also have major depression, and between 4% and 20% have bipolar depression. Co-morbidity with anxiety disorders is also very common (e.g. Newton-Howes et al. 2010). Antisocial and narcissistic disorders are generally thought to be more prevalent in men, and histrionic and borderline disorders more prevalent among women (APA 2000).

By definition, personality disorders are relatively stable over time. However, they may be more mutable than first thought, and a number of studies have shown significant changes over time in the experiences of people diagnosed with them. In one of the longest follow-ups yet conducted, Paris and Zweig-Frank (2001) reported the 27-year outcomes of a cohort of individuals diagnosed with borderline personality disorder. At this time, only 5 out of 64 individuals in the cohort met the criteria for the diagnosis. A more fine-grained analysis was reported by Shea et al. (2009), who followed a cohort of men and women with the same diagnosis for a period of 6 years, with yearly assessments. Encouragingly, they found gradual and consistent year-on-year improvement, with the exception of some study participants in their late thirties and early forties, who showed a deterioration in functioning over time.

Another challenge to the concept of the DSM personality disorders has been their somewhat arbitrary definitions. Ralevski et al. (2005) suggested that avoidant personality disorder and social phobia are 'alternative conceptualizations of the same disorder'. In addition, while Zanarini et al. (2002) reported high levels of inter-rater reliability in the diagnosis of borderline personality disorder using an interview schedule based on DSM-IV, test–retest reliability was not so strong. Although one-third of their symptom dimensions achieved excellent levels of reliability (based on Cohen's kappa statistic), two-thirds were only in the fair-to-good range. Tyrer et al. (2015) gave some interesting insight into the real-world diagnosis of personality disorder, noting that clinicians rarely make this diagnosis, typically diagnosing as borderline, antisocial, or not otherwise specified. They further note 'few clinicians tak[e] the trouble to assess personality status in all its components ... probably show stereotyped thinking, wherein those who repeatedly self-harm are automatically given a diagnosis of borderline personality disorder and those who are aggressive and have a history of offending behaviour are given a diagnosis of antisocial personality disorder' (2015: 720).

A dimensional approach

The concept of personality disorders may also be challenged at a more fundamental level. Personality disorders may be considered as distinct 'disorders' – a binary outcome. You either 'have' the diagnosis or you do not: the model taken by DSM. However, a number of commentators (e.g. Widiger et al. 2009) have argued that people with these traits should not be assigned a categorical diagnosis identifying them as 'disordered' or mentally ill. They may better be considered as being at the extreme of the distribution of personality characteristics rather than categorically different from the norm. Widiger (2011) noted there are 18 variants of this dimensional approach, including a variant of the DSM approach which identifies the degree to which each diagnostic criterion is present and assigns a diagnosis if the number present *and* their severity achieve a certain criterion. This is the preferred approach of most clinicians (Morey and Hopwood 2019). An alternative approach, focusing on key psychological attributes was suggested by Lynam et al. (2005) derived from the five-factor model of personality (Costa and McCrae 1992). They provide an example of antisocial personality disorder:

- *Low neuroticism*: lack of appropriate concern for potential problems in health or social adjustment emotional blandness.
- *Low extraversion*: social isolation, interpersonal detachment, and lack of support networks; **flattened mood**; lack of joy and zest for life; reluctance to assert self or assume leadership roles, even when qualified; social inhibition and shyness.
- *Low openness*: difficulty adapting to social or personal change; low tolerance or understanding of different points of view or lifestyles; emotional blandness and inability to understand and verbalize own feelings; **alexithymia**; constricted range of interests; insensitivity to art and beauty; excessive conformity to authority.
- *Low agreeableness*: cynicism and paranoid thinking; inability to trust even friends or family; quarrelsomeness; ready to pick fights; exploitive and manipulative; lying; rude and inconsiderate manner alienates friends, limits social support; lack of respect for social conventions can lead to trouble with the law; inflated and grandiose sense of self; arrogance.
- *Low conscientiousness*: underachievement: not fulfilling intellectual or artistic potential; poor academic performance relative to ability; disregard of rules and responsibilities can lead to trouble with the law; unable to discipline self (such as stick to diet or exercise plan) even when required for medical reasons; personal and occupational aimlessness.

Not only can the dimensional view be argued on theoretical and philosophical grounds, it also may be better at predicting outcome than the DSM categorical approach. Ullrich et al. (2001), for example, found that scores on personality tests were better able to predict subsequent offending behaviour than categorical diagnoses of antisocial personality disorder. In addition, a number of other studies, including that of Zanarini et al. (2002), have reported higher levels of diagnostic agreement using the dimensional approach than the more traditional diagnostic criteria.

A cognitive model of personality disorders

Although DSM identifies ten personality disorders, they have significant overlap in their characteristics (Samuel and Widiger 2008). With this in mind, Beck et al. (2016) adopted a trans-diagnostic approach (see Chapter 3) to develop a single, unitary, explanatory model for their development. In doing so, they adopted an evolutionary perspective. They suggested that key neurocognitive responses, including those affecting perception, mood, and behaviour, are genetically pre-programmed and that these responses may be adaptive in some evolutionary times, but less adaptive in others. Competitive behaviour, for example, may be of benefit at times of scarcity but not at times of social cohesion and mutual cooperation.

According to Beck et al. (2016), what we term personality disorders are the inappropriate expression of these pre-programmed responses. They suggested that it is not the behaviour *per se* that is problematic, but the individual's lack of adaptability and responsiveness to the environment. Most of us learn to adapt our behaviour as a result of life experiences, particularly those in childhood. For some people, however, childhood experiences may maintain or reinforce inappropriate pre-programmed responses. The naturally shy child, for example, whose parents' responses are to be over-protective, may not experience any other way of dealing with the world. As a result, they may fail to develop alternative coping skills and come to believe that the only way to survive in the adult world is to be dependent and subservient. Adult personality is the combined result of these pre-programmed responses and childhood experiences. Rigid **cognitive schemata** develop over time, each of which governs behaviour. Beliefs of 'being bad', for example, will lead to self-punishment; beliefs of 'not being worthy of love' will result in the avoidance of closeness, and so on.

As in his model of depression, Beck considered the core schema that drive personality disorders to be the cognitive triad concerning the self, others, and the future. Instead of being episodically activated as in the case of depression, however, these underlying schemata are chronically activated in people with personality disorders. Placing these schemata as the central driving factor in all personality disorders provides an explanation for an apparently diverse set of attributes and behaviours. The content of the schemata may vary, as a result of different child and adult experiences (and perhaps the pre-programmed neurocognitive responses), but the underlying structures are the same. Some of the key beliefs for the different personality 'types' include:

- Avoidant personality
  - *self*: socially inept and incompetent
  - *others*: potentially critical, uninterested, and demeaning

o *beliefs*: the self as worthless and unlovable: 'If people get close to me, they will discover the real me and reject me – that would be intolerable'.
- Dependent personality
  o *self*: needy, weak, helpless, and incompetent
  o *others*: need a strong 'caretaker' in an idealized way; can function well in their presence, but not without them
  o *beliefs*: 'I need other people – specifically a strong person – in order to survive'.
- Schizoid personality disorder
  o *self*: self-sufficient and a loner
  o *others*: intrusive; closeness provides an opportunity for others to fence the individual in
  o *beliefs*: 'I am basically alone'; 'I can do things better when I am unencumbered by other people'.

According to Young et al. (2003), the schemata most involved in personality disorders are those that relate to the need for security, autonomy, desirability, self-expression, gratification, and self-control. Once formed, they become self-fulfilling, and are maintained through three different processes: schema maintenance, schema avoidance, and schema compensation:

- *Schema maintenance* involves resistance to information or evidence that would disconfirm the schema through cognitive distortions and self-defeating behavioural patterns.
- *Avoidance* involves avoiding situations that may test or provide information counter to the schema.
- *Schema compensation* involves over-compensating for a negative schema by acting in the direction opposite to the schema's content. A shy woman, who believes herself unattractive to men, yet acts flirtatiously, for example, may find herself in situations in which she feels unsafe, or hurt by men drawn to her flirtatiousness who reject her when they find her withdrawn and quiet, thus supporting her schema of being unattractive.

Although a great deal of successful clinical work has been based on the schema model, until recently there have been few experimental studies of the phenomenon. However, what studies that have been conducted support the schema models developed by both Beck and Young (e.g. Arntz et al. 2005; Wenzel et al. 2007).

11.2 Cluster A diagnoses: paranoid, schizoid, and schizotypal

Each of the cluster A diagnoses involves some of the manifestations of schizophrenia. As such, they fit into a range of conditions known as the schizophrenia spectrum disorders; a linkage stemming from relatively high rates of cluster A personality disorder among the relatives of people diagnosed with schizophrenia (Nigg and Goldsmith 1994). Interestingly, though, few people diagnosed with these disorders go on to be diagnosed as having schizophrenia.

According to DSM-5, paranoid disorder involves a pervasive distrust and suspiciousness of others such that their motives are interpreted as malevolent. It begins in early adulthood. To be assigned a diagnosis, four of the following need to be present. The individual:

- suspects, with insufficient evidence, that others are exploiting, harming or deceiving them
- is preoccupied with unjustified doubts about the loyalty or trustworthiness of friends or associates
- is reluctant to confide in others due to unwarranted fear that any confidences will be used maliciously against them
- reads hidden demeaning or threatening meanings into benign remarks or events
- persistently bears grudges and slights
- sees attacks on their character or reputation not apparent to others, and is quick to react angrily or to counterattack
- has recurrent suspicions, without justification, regarding fidelity of spouse or sexual partner.

Schizoid disorder presents as a pervasive pattern of detachment from social relationships and a restricted range of expression of emotions in interpersonal settings, beginning in early adulthood. Four of the following have to be present for a diagnosis to be assigned. The individual:

- neither desires nor enjoys close relationships, including being part of a family
- favours solitary activities
- has little, if any, interest in sexual experiences with another person
- takes pleasure in few, if any, activities
- lacks close friends or confidants other than first-degree relatives
- appears indifferent to praise or criticism of others
- shows emotional coldness, detachment or flattened affect.

Finally, schizotypal personality disorder is defined as a pervasive pattern of social and interpersonal deficits marked by acute discomfort with, and reduced capacity for, close relationships. In addition, individuals may experience cognitive or perceptual distortions and show eccentricities of behaviour. A diagnosis requires the presence of five or more of the following:

- **ideas of reference**: false beliefs that random or irrelevant occurrences in the world directly relate to the individual
- odd beliefs or magical thinking that are inconsistent with subcultural norms
- unusual perceptual experiences, including bodily illusions
- odd thinking and speech (e.g. vague, metaphorical, over-elaborate or stereotyped)
- suspicious or paranoid ideation
- inappropriate or restricted affect
- behaviour or appearance that is odd or eccentric
- lack of close friends or confidants other than first-degree relatives
- excessive social anxiety that does not diminish with familiarity and is associated with paranoid fears rather than negative judgements about self.

The **prevalence** of these various disorders within the general community varies across studies, lying between zero and 4.5% for paranoid personality disorder, zero and 4.1% for schizoid personality disorder, and zero and 5.1% for schizotypal personality disorder (Torgersen et al. 2001). Five psychosocial and medical factors appear to be predictive: childhood adversities, cannabis use, history of obstetric complications, stressful events during adulthood, and serum folate levels (Belbasis et al. 2018). Perhaps not surprisingly, given the linkage with schizophrenia, factors associated with the development of schizophrenia, including prenatal exposure to famine, influenza, and even cold temperatures, have also been considered in the development of these disorders (see Chapter 13).

There is also a clear genetic component to the personality type. One of several longitudinal studies, the Copenhagen High-Risk genetic risk study (Parnas et al. 1995), followed the offspring of women with a diagnosis of schizophrenia and those of a 'typical' comparison group of children from the age of 15 to 42 years. Twenty-one per cent of the children of mothers diagnosed with schizophrenia were assigned a cluster A personality diagnosis, compared with 5% of the children in the comparison group. Of particular note is that among the children of the women diagnosed with schizophrenia, those exposed to a particularly stressful environment in childhood were most likely to be subsequently diagnosed with schizophrenia. Those who were exposed to a moderately stressful environment were more likely to be assigned a diagnosis of personality disorder, suggesting a gradient of risk based on both genetic factors and the degree of exposure to stress. Data such as these have led genetic theorists such as Meehl (1990) to suggest that the core personality disorder is genetically mediated, while risk for schizophrenia involves further genetic influences and environmental stress factors. Treatment studies of cluster A disorders are relatively rare – perhaps because people who could be assigned these diagnoses rarely seek treatment, and when they do, this may be related to associated problems such as depression.

11.3 Cluster B diagnoses: borderline personality disorder

DSM-5 considers borderline personality disorder (BPD) to involve impairments in personality (self and interpersonal) functioning and the presence of pathological personality traits. The condition is characterized by intense short-term relationships which become too demanding of those involved, and frequently self-destruct. The relationship is often seen in black and white terms, with high expectations of the other person, alternating with deep fears of being rejected, leading to feelings of perfection and anxious attachment, until the relationship becomes too demanding, and then collapses leading to catastrophic self-defeating thoughts and intense negative emotions. Unfortunately, the individual is unable to manage these emotions, and frequently engages in a number of maladaptive ways to reduce their intensity, often involving self-destructive behaviour which leads to feelings of dissociation and short-term relief. At such times, thoughts of suicide and suicide attempts are common: up to 10% of people with this disorder eventually die by suicide (e.g. Zanarini et al. 2005). Self-harm, in particular cutting of arms, legs or torso, burning or other acts of mutilation, is also common. These behaviours may also be used in a manipulative manner, to control relationships or the behaviour of others around them ('If you leave, I will hurt myself …').

About 2% of the US population is thought to have this cluster of traits (Grant et al. 2008). In population studies, the gender mix is relatively even, but significantly more women than men are found among clinic populations, leading Kulacaoglu and Kose (2018) to speculate that women are more likely than men to seek help for their difficulties. It typically begins in adolescence and continues through adulthood. As with other personality disorders, BPD is not as immutable as was once thought. Zanarini et al. (2005), for example, found that only three-quarters of a cohort of people initially given this diagnosis warranted the diagnosis 6 years later. In addition, only 6% of those people who improved experienced a 'relapse'.

For a DSM-5 diagnosis to be given, the individual must evidence a pervasive pattern of instability of interpersonal relationships, self-image and mood, and marked impulsivity beginning by early adulthood and present in a variety of contexts, as indicated by five (or more) of:

- frantic efforts to avoid real or imagined abandonment
- a history of unstable and intense interpersonal relationships, alternating between extremes of idealization and devaluation
- identity disturbance: markedly and persistently unstable self-image or sense of self
- impulsivity in at least two areas, including substance abuse and binge eating, that are potentially self-damaging
- recurrent suicidal behaviour, gestures or threats, or self-mutilating behaviour
- a marked reactivity of mood
- chronic feelings of emptiness
- inappropriate, intense anger or difficulty controlling anger
- transient, stress-related paranoid ideation or severe dissociative symptoms.

These 'official' criteria are unchanged from the previous version of DSM. However, DSM-5 also includes a 'proposed alternative' set of criteria more in line with their new model of personality disorders, including:

- Impairments in self functioning (a or b):
  a) *Identity*: markedly impoverished, poorly developed or unstable self-image, often associated with excessive self-criticism; chronic feelings of emptiness; dissociative states under stress.
  b) *Self-direction*: instability in goals, aspirations, values or career plans.
- Impairments in interpersonal functioning (a or b):
  a) *Empathy*: compromised ability to recognize the feelings and needs of others combined with interpersonal hypersensitivity (i.e. prone to feel slighted or insulted); perceptions of others selectively biased towards negative attributes or vulnerabilities.
  b) *Intimacy*: intense, unstable, and conflicted close relationships, marked by mistrust, neediness, and anxious preoccupation with real or imagined abandonment; close relationships often viewed in extremes of idealization and devaluation and alternating between over-involvement and withdrawal.

Aetiology of borderline personality disorder

Biological factors

There have been relatively few studies of the family/genetic influences on borderline personality disorders. However, a number are now emerging. Distel et al.

(2008), for example, studied a total of 3,644 twins aged between 18 and 86 years across the Netherlands, Belgium, and Australia. They estimated 42% of the variation in borderline personality features was attributable to genetic factors, with similar levels of heritability across all three countries. Similarly, Gunderson et al. (2011) found genetic influences explained 42% of the risk for BPD. Although any genetic mediators are still far from clear, risk for the condition may involve interactions between genes controlling both the dopaminergic and noradrenergic systems (Kulacaoglu and Kose 2018).

Other studies have investigated neural and neurochemical mediators of the condition. A number of imaging studies have found that the hippocampus and amygdala of people diagnosed with BPD are significantly smaller than those of typical population comparison groups (Ruocco et al. 2013). There is also evidence of damaged or poorly functioning frontal cortices (De la Fuente et al. 1997), which may be related to the dysregulation of serotonin (New et al. 2004). Functional MRI (Schulze et al. 2016) has also shown heightened activation of the limbic system (amygdala, hippocampus, and posterior cingulate cortex) combined with diminished activation of prefrontal regions during the processing of negative emotional stimuli, indicating the presence of strong negative emotions with little control of them. Reports of the effectiveness of antipsychotic medication in the treatment of at least some cases of BPD (e.g. Rocca et al. 2002) suggest that low levels of dopamine may also be implicated in its presentation.

A very different view on possible biological mechanisms in borderline personality stems involves dysregulation, and low levels of a hormone and **neurotransmitter** called oxytocin. This is perhaps best known for its role in birth and breastfeeding. However, there is also increasing evidence that within brain structures including the amygdala and hypothalamus, oxytocin is involved in empathy and social bonding. In addition, oxytocin encourage socially positive behaviour, has links to strong attachment, and may protect against early life adversity, as well as enhance encoding and conceptual recognition of positive social stimuli over social-threat stimuli (Brüne 2016). Low levels of the neurotransmitter negatively impact on each of these processes.

Psychological processes

Risk for personality disorder is increased by a number of childhood factors. People with borderline personality are more likely than the general population to have been neglected by their parents, to have been hospitalized, to have had multiple caregivers, and to have experienced parental divorce, death or significant childhood trauma such as sexual abuse or incest (Bandelow et al. 2005). One significant outcome may be poor or anxious attachment and bonding with parents, both of which may contribute to the development of the disorder (e.g. Ramos et al. 2016). Of interest in relation to these findings are those of Zweig-Frank and Paris (2002), who followed a cohort of people diagnosed with BPD for 27 years and found that while reports of parenting quality and childhood abuse or trauma did not predict the long-term outcome of the condition, a measure of parental bonding did.

From a psychoanalytic viewpoint, object relations theorists (e.g. Kernberg 1985) suggest that as a result of negative childhood experiences, the individual develops a weak **ego** and needs constant reassuring. They frequently engage in a **defence mechanism** known as *splitting*, dichotomizing objects into 'all good' or 'all bad', and fail to integrate the positive and negative aspects of self or other people into a whole (Klein 1927; see also Chapter 2). This inability to make sense of contradictory elements of self or others causes extreme difficulty in regulating emotions as the world is constantly viewed as either 'perfect' or 'disastrous'.

Cognitive theorists (e.g. Young and Lindemann 1992) argue that negative childhood experiences translate into maladaptive schemata about self-identity and relationships with others. These include beliefs that 'I am bad', leading to self-punishment; 'No one will ever love me', leading to avoidance of closeness; and 'I cannot cope on my own', leading to over-dependence. Young and colleagues (e.g. Kellogg and Young 2006) identified a number of archetypal maladaptive schema 'modes' that operate in BPD and drive its associated behaviours, including:

- *The abandoned and abused child*: one of the most painful modes, which results in the individual thinking and behaving like an abandoned child, feeling very frightened, helpless, alone, and completely unable to cope.
- *The angry and impulsive child*: involves feeling and expressing anger or rage in response to unmet core needs and is typically a response to perceived unfairness or injustice. It is evident to others usually as uncontrolled, or poorly controlled, expressions of anger.
- *The detached protector*: a form of dissociation evoked when the individual is confronted by psychologically challenging circumstances. It involves detaching emotionally from people, withdrawal, and self-soothing.
- *The punitive parent* or 'inner critic': involves punitive self-talk, focusing on perfectionism and guilt: 'I'll never get anywhere in life; I'm worthless, I'm not as good as others; no one could love me; I'm useless if I make mistakes; If I don't put other's first I'm a selfish person'.
- *The healthy adult*: a more adaptive and appropriate mode, involving nurturing the child schema, setting limits to the expression of anger, and generally moderating the impact of negative modes. It is the positive adult, taking responsibility, committing, and engaging in adult pursuits.

Individuals may switch between schema: for example, the individual may engage with the abandoned child schema when faced with interpersonal rejection, and then shift to angry impulsive child in responding to it in a self-defeating and harmful way. Strong negative emotions experienced as a consequence of catastrophic or other negative beliefs may lead to episodes of self-harm. Many people with borderline personality feel numbness or dissociation immediately before or while they harm themselves. Self-harm may therefore provide a means of escape from unbearable emotions, trigger the detached protector mode, and may not be accompanied with feelings of physical pain. Self-harm may also be maintained by operant processes: successful control of other people's behaviour by threats of self-harm reinforces its use as a means of coping. According to the cognitive model, this use of self-harm is indicative of high interpersonal anxiety, low self-esteem, and a lack of alternative coping strategies to deal with personal stress.

Cognitive processing deficits may also underpin some of the traits of borderline personality. Sala et al. (2008), for example, noted that hippocampal and frontal cortex deficiencies may be related to poor memory control. To investigate this phenomenon, they explored the capacity of people with borderline personality to first learn and then to inhibit memories of various word pairs and found both processes to be impaired. They took this to indicate that people with BPD may be less able than others to inhibit the emergence of unwanted memories and dissociative symptoms. In another cognitive deficit model of the condition, Wupperman et al. (2008) correlated measures of mindfulness with core features of BPD including interpersonal problem-solving abilities, and impulsive and passive emotion-regulation strategies in a sample of young adults. They found that deficits in mindfulness were linked to difficulties in attention, awareness, and discrimination between 'internal and external experience', factors that they saw as central to the disorder. People with BPD also experience difficulty in the rapid discrimination of both neutral and negative emotional expressions, even when these are overt and strong expressions related to anger and disgust (Daros et al. 2013) – factors likely to result in the underlying difficulties in social interaction central to the disorder.

Treatment of borderline personality disorder

Psychological approaches

Treatment of people with borderline personality is not easy, though fortunately the number of trials examining the effects of therapy is increasing. Roth and Fonagy (1998) tried to establish some overall goals of therapy and guidelines for who may benefit from it most. They suggested the following:

- Psychotherapy is more likely to be effective for less severe personality disorders.
- In individuals under the age of 30 years, the greatest risk comes from suicide. Prevention of this, rather than 'cure', may form a legitimate therapeutic target.
- Individuals with good social support, chronic depression, who are psychologically minded, and with low impulsivity are most likely to benefit from 'talking therapies'.
- People who have high impulsivity are most likely to benefit from a 'limit-setting' group or a therapist who is supportive of their attempts to struggle with uncontrollable impulses.
- Commitment and enthusiasm of the therapist may be of special significance and finding the 'right' therapist for the 'right' patient is particularly important.

One of the most important therapeutic aims is to minimize risk of self-harm. This involves identifying the antecedents to episodes of self-harm, the thoughts and feelings that accompany them, and their consequences. Each of these forms a potential point of intervention. Alternatives to self-harm often involve a high-intensity action, such as listening to loud music, or painful but not damaging behaviours such as squeezing a ball until the muscles ache. Where there is risk that an episode of self-harm will escalate into a serious attempt at suicide, specific strategies may be used to minimize this risk, including problem-solving and identifying reasons for living (see Chapter 7). The progress of therapy may also be governed by risk for self-harm, as it focuses on psychologically challenging issues. It may be useful, for example, for some people to stay in hospital during the early stages of therapy, as they may find therapy sessions so stressful that they either drop out or harm themselves in some way. The hospital can provide a safe environment, where their behaviour can be observed and controlled, and both therapist and **client** have the security of knowing that any impulsive self-harming behaviour will be seen and dealt with should it occur.

Cognitive therapy

The core of cognitive therapy is the identification and modification of cognitive schemata that drive inappropriate behaviours, using approaches such as schema-focused therapy (SFT: Young 1999) or cognitive analytic therapy (Ryle and Kerr 2002). These approaches may combine with a number of other strategies, including developing problem-focused plans to cope with urges to self-harm, mood disturbances and suicidal feelings, improving relationships, and so on. The issues addressed in therapy and the strategies used are dependent on the most pressing and problematic behaviour at the time (Davidson 2000). The central element of SFT is that the individual's behaviour and emotions are governed by maladaptive schemata. Schema-focused therapy aims to identify and change these modes of thinking, using standard cognitive techniques including cognitive restructuring. However, these are augmented by a range of other strategies, including 'limited re-parenting' in which the therapist provides an atmosphere of acceptance and safety within the therapeutic relationship. This quasi-parental relationship, in which the individual can feel safe and wanted, is seen as central to the therapy. Other intervention strategies include direct attempts at changing maladaptive behaviour and re-experiencing the emotions associated with early dysfunctional relationships. This complex intervention might last as long as 3 years, with two sessions per week.

Dialectical behaviour therapy

A second key therapeutic approach to the treatment of borderline personality disorder involves a form of therapy called dialectical behaviour therapy (DBT: Linehan 1993). This can be considered a third-wave approach (see Chapter 3), as it has a strong behavioural component (and many similarities with acceptance and commitment therapy) and does not focus on cognitive change as a key contributor to change. Therapy involves the client working individually with a therapist and in therapy groups. As with schema therapy, self-injurious and suicidal behaviours are key targets. Therapy involves teaching four sets of skills: interpersonal effectiveness, core mindfulness, emotion regulation, and distress tolerance. Interpersonal effectiveness involves learning the skills necessary to develop and negotiate interpersonal relationships. The other skills allow the individual to cope with the emotional consequences of these relationships, whether good or bad. Emotional regulation includes learning to identify and label emotions, increasing positive emotional events, and being mindful of emotions and their associated thoughts without necessarily having to respond to them. Distraction involves learning to temporarily distract from negative emotions. This may involve the use of strategies that mimic the effects of self-damaging behaviours such as cutting, but in a more benign manner. This often involves physical sensations such as a cold shower or squeezing a squeeze ball until it hurts.

Evidence of effectiveness

There is some evidence of the effectiveness of SFT and similar therapies. Blum et al. (2008), for example, compared outcomes of a cognitive behavioural programme similar to schema therapy with 'treatment as usual'. In addition to working with individuals, they included what they termed a systems approach, involving a 2-hour session to which family members or other significant individuals were invited. During this session, these people were taught about the nature of the problems their relative was experiencing. In the year following the intervention, participants in the cognitive behavioural intervention experienced greater improvements on measures of impulsivity, negative affect, and global functioning. They were no better on measures of the frequency of self-harm or suicide attempts, which are generally considered key outcomes of any intervention. However, they did make fewer visits to hospital emergency departments. Giesen-Bloo et al. (2006) compared two interventions, each of which was conducted over a 3-year period: schema therapy and psychodynamically based **transference**-focused psychotherapy. They found that more people remained in schema therapy over this time, presumably indicating the degree to which they felt they were gaining some benefit from attending. In addition, participants in the schema therapy intervention were most likely to recover, to have better improvement scores, and to report better overall quality of life.

More studies have shown DBT to be an effective intervention on key measures of self-harm and suicide risk. In one of the early randomized controlled trials of its effectiveness, Van den Bosch et al. (2005) evaluated treatment outcomes, comparing one year of DBT versus usual care, and found lower levels of parasuicidal and impulsive behaviours, sustained for 6 months after the completion of treatment. In a comparison between a similar programme and non-behavioural psychotherapy, Linehan et al. (2006) found one-year follow-up outcomes were again supportive of DBT: participants receiving DBT were half as likely to make a suicide attempt and required less hospitalization for suicide ideation than those in the psychotherapy intervention. In their Cochrane review of the impact of psychological therapies, Stoffers-Winterling et al. (2012) found that DBT was the most researched approach, and there was good evidence of effectiveness when compared with treatment as usual, in that it achieved significant gains on measures of anger, parasuicide, and mental health. It was not clear how well it compared with **placebo** or alternative therapies. Subsequently, Cristea et al. (2017) found DBT to be one of only two therapies (the other being psychodynamic therapy) to be consistently more effective than control conditions, with gains on measure of self-harm, suicide, and general psychopathology. Schema therapy, as in Stoffers-Winterling's review also, did not achieve this criterion.

Case formulation

Ms H was a 26-year-old single woman. She presented with a history of self-harm including cutting her wrists and arms, overdosing on prescription medication, and stabbing herself in the abdomen. On more than one occasion these and other harming behaviours were intended to end her life. She had previously been seen by a clinical psychologist but had dropped out of therapy after only a few sessions. She had also not taken the opportunity for therapy offered after hospital admissions following episodes of further self-harm. She had few acquaintances, and no close friends, living on her own in a bedsit in a large town in South Wales. She was unemployed at the time she was seen by a clinical psychologist.

Long-term antecedents

Ms H reported being sexually abused by her father as a young girl. This was initially denied by her family. However, once this was acknowledged (after several months of abuse), her mother left the relationship, bringing Ms H up alone (or in the company of a succession of uncaring and occasionally verbally and physically abusive 'boyfriends') from the age of 11 years. The relationship between Ms H and her mother was not good, and although she lived with her mother until aged 19 years, she felt unloved and uncared for. She was often ignored, and at best tolerated – not loved or respected. However, she learned to keep a 'good face' on her experiences and hide any distress she felt. When she did express any upset as a result of her mother or her mother's boyfriends' behaviour, the only way she could gain attention was through engaging in extremes of behaviour. She learned that self-harming behaviour such as cutting would lead to her having some attention, although it was also related to subsequent conflict and eventually led her to leave home. Episodes of low mood, related to her poor self-esteem, memories of abuse, and difficulties in relationships would also form triggers to episodes of self-harm such as overdosing, with an intent if not to die, at least to provide a time out from the distress she was experiencing. She had a succession of short-term relationships, each of which was typified as 'stormy'. She was 'claustrophobically needy', demanding her boyfriends' full attention and became upset and threatened self-harm if they were away too long. The relationships typically ended in a dramatic argument followed by her self-harming in some way. She was offered psychiatric treatment following two of these episodes but chose not to take this up. However, on a third episode she agreed to see a psychiatric nurse before being referred to a clinical psychologist.

Formulation

As a consequence of her early history, Ms H had low self-esteem and a strong sense of shame. She had not learned to tolerate or express negative emotions in a meaningful and appropriate way. Indeed, she had learned to express any negative emotion in a histrionic and overly expressive manner. When things were stressful in her life (for example, relationships failing), she felt extremely vulnerable and anxious and experienced high levels of negative affect. She had not learned to manage these emotions appropriately, and frequently did so by becoming overly reliant on support from anyone willing to provide it (usually her boyfriends), or, when this support was not available, she resorted to self-harm as a means of expressing distress, trying to manage this distress, and manipulating others ('Stay with me or I will really hurt myself'). She found therapy challenging and distressing because it addressed issues she was unable to cope with effectively. She had therefore dropped out or refused to engage in it.

Intervention

The intervention with Ms H lasted many months and involved both individual and group sessions. The first aim of treatment was to reduce her likelihood of self-harming. This involved identifying factors likely to precipitate self-harming, in order to understand and possibly avoid them happening, and learning skills including mindfulness and distraction techniques such as squeezing a ball in her hand to the point of pain to help her control her strong emotions in a more positive manner. In addition, she was taught interpersonal skills (including appropriate assertiveness and talking to people about her emotions) in order to learn to express any emotional distress in a more appropriate and acceptable manner. While these reduced the risk of self-harm, they did not entirely prevent some incidents. Nevertheless, Ms H reduced her self-harm significantly. Once she was better able to monitor and manage her negative emotions, the therapist examined some of the inappropriate beliefs related to her shame and low self-esteem ('It was my fault I was sexually abused'; 'My parents did not love me, so I am unworthy of love', etc.) using the Socratic approach of cognitive behaviour therapy. This was conducted carefully and slowly, and because the distress this process may evoke could potentially trigger self-harm, there was some debate between her therapist and the ward nursing team about whether Ms H should stay in hospital at this time. However, she and her therapist made a joint decision that she would not come into hospital, but that the therapist could be contacted at agreed times (not 'randomly', as this may increase dependency on the therapist) should contact be necessary. Ms H found this process stressful but was able to confront some of her beliefs and she became less shamed and her episodes of low mood became less frequent. She was also able to develop appropriate (non-dependent) relationships with some members of the group sessions she attended. These became a source of long-term support and reinforced changes in her approach to others – in particular learning to become less dependent and demanding. Over a period of many months, Ms H became more independent and confident. She remained fragile but was able to cope with difficult emotions without consistently harming herself (although this did not stop completely), and was able to use a number of coping mechanisms should this occur. She was able to develop supportive relationships with a number of people (all of whom themselves had a history of mental health problems). She was discharged after around one year of gradually decreasingly frequent sessions with her therapist and therapy group. However, she was given regular follow-up sessions every 3–4 months for some time to support her in her changes and, in particular, if she were to begin to experience more significant problems in the future.

Pharmacological treatment

There have been relatively few controlled trials of the effectiveness of drug therapy in borderline personality. Most studies have been relatively small, and evidence of any effectiveness is 'weak' (Paris 2008). Rinne et al. (2002), for example, found that treatment with the **SSRI**, fluvoxamine, proved successful in reducing rapid mood shifts, but not impulsivity and aggression in women with a diagnosis of borderline personality. Roepke et al. (2008) found an atypical antipsychotic, quetiapine, achieved modest gains on measures of depression but not impulsivity in 12 of the 15 people who took the drug for an 8-week period. Linehan et al. (2008) assessed whether treatment with another atypical antipsychotic, olanzapine, improved the outcome of individuals already receiving DBT. In a small study of women who either received placebo or active treatment, irritability and aggression scores tended to decrease more quickly for the olanzapine group than for the placebo group. However, self-inflicted injury tended to decrease more for the placebo group than for the olanzapine group. Although the role of oxytocin in the aetiology has opened up a new avenue for treatment, the impact of treatment with oxytocin is mixed, with gains on reducing emotional responses to stress matched by apparently paradoxical increases in interpersonal anxiety and decreased 'cooperative behaviour' (Amad et al. 2015). Overall, therefore, the evidence for the effectiveness of **pharmacotherapy** is weak, leading Starcevic and Janca (2018) to conclude that clinicians should either avoid its use or administer specific medications for specific problems the individual is facing.

Research box 10

Linehan, M.M., Korslund, K.E., Harned, M.S. et al. (2015) Dialectical behavior therapy for high suicide risk in individuals with borderline personality disorder: a randomized clinical trial and component analysis, *JAMA Psychiatry*, 72: 475–82.

Dialectical behaviour therapy (DBT) is the most strongly validated therapeutic approach to the treatment of borderline personality disorder. It is a complex package of skills and other forms of support, which requires significant therapeutic skills and training. As a consequence, Linehan and colleagues argue, there is some benefit in 'dismantling' the intervention to identify its key therapeutic elements to allow the optimal combination to be identified and used. As a consequence, they compared three variants of DBT: (i) group skills training plus 'case management', (ii) individual therapy plus activities, and (iii) standard group DBT, including skills therapy and some individual therapy. They assessed the effectiveness of these various combinations in people diagnosed with BPD and at risk of suicide.

Method

The study comprised a three-arm randomized trial, comparing three variants of DBT.

Participants

Participants were 99 women, aged 18–60 years, who met the diagnostic criteria for BPD on two clinical assessments, including the International Personality Disorder Examination, had at least one suicide attempt or episode of self-harm in the previous year and two in the previous 5 years, and at least one suicide attempt in the previous year. Participants in each condition were matched for age, number of suicide attempts, severity of depression, and number of in-patient admissions to a mental health facility over the previous year.

Measures

- *Suicide Attempt Self-injury Interview* (SASI): measured the frequency and severity of suicide attempts
- *Suicidal Behaviors Questionnaire* (SBQ): assessed suicide ideation
- *Hamilton Rating Scale for Depression* (HR-D) and *Anxiety* (HR-A): measured depression and anxiety respectively
- *Treatment History Interview* (THI): measured use of crisis services and **psychotropic medications**.

Interventions

Key aspects of the three interventions, which took place over a period of one year, are outlined in Table 1.

- *Standard DBT (DBT)*: involved four, weekly, components: individual therapy, group skills training, therapist consultation, as-needed between-session telephone coaching. Strategies included cognitive and behavioural interventions (e.g. behavioural assessment, contingency management, exposure, cognitive restructuring, and skills training), dialectics, and the acceptance practices of validation and mindfulness (see also the description of DBT in the chapter).
- *DBT skills training (DBT-S)*: provided education and practice in the skills element of the DBT intervention package, but removed the individual therapy component. Individual therapy was replaced by a 'manualized case management intervention', which involved contact as necessary, with an upper limit of once a week and a lower limit of once a month. This focused on managing suicidal crises and general problem-solving.
- *DBT individual therapy (DBT-I)*: eliminated all DBT skills training, by removing group skills training and prohibiting individual therapists from teaching DBT skills such as mindfulness. Instead, participants were encouraged to use their existing problem-solving skills in dealing with any issues they faced.

Eighteen therapists, most of whom had a doctoral degree, provided the therapy.

Table 1 The three variants of DBT compared in the three conditions of the study

	'Standard' DBT	Skills training + case management (DBT-S)	Individual DBT plus activities (DBT-I)
Individual sessions	1 hour per week, therapy	Contact as necessary via phone (min = 1 contact per month, max = 1 contact per week)	1 hour per week, no teaching/ coaching in DBT skills
Group sessions	2½ hours of skills training per week	2½ hours of skills training per week	Activity-based support group
Approach to learning skills	Coaching in new skills and development and practice of old skills	Coaching in new skills and development and practice of old skills	Coaching in use of previously acquired skills

Results

Participants in the three treatment groups did not differ significantly on pre-treatment measures, and drop-out from treatment also did not differ significantly (DBT, 18%; DBT-I, 33%; DBT-S, 27%). Rates of suicide attempts reduced across all conditions, with no between-group differences. Similarly, all groups evidenced significant reductions in self-harm, with the only between-group difference being a significantly higher number of events in the DBT-I group compared with the other two groups during the treatment year. The DBT-I intervention was less effective in treating depression than the other two conditions. Levels of suicidal ideation and suicide-related visits to the emergency department fell equally across all conditions.

Table 2 Percentage of participants and mean number of suicide and self-harm episodes over time and condition

	Pre-treatment	Treatment year	Follow-up year	Significance
	% (mean)	% (mean)	% (mean)	
Suicide attempts				
DBT	97 (3.6)	36 (3.4)	7 (2.0)	Time <0.001
DBT-I	97 (6.4)	44 (2.9)	22 (3.6)	
DBT-S	100 (2.0)	26 (2.6)	17 (1.5)	
Self-harm				
DBT	81 (19.0)	58 (10.2)	45 (7.9)	Time <0.001
DBT-I	90 (23.5)	63 (20.6)	40 (16.0)	Condition
DBT-S	82 (24.7)	56 (9.9)	46 (9.4)	Treat year <0.001

	Pre-treatment	Treatment year	Follow-up year	Significance
	% (mean)	% (mean)	% (mean)	
DBT	33	5	1	Time <0.01
DBT-I	24	6	1	
DBT-S	36	9	1	

Table 3 Mean scores (and standard deviations) on key outcomes over time and condition

	Pre-treatment	Treatment year	Follow-up year	Significance
Depression				
DBT	22.1 (11.7)	12.3 (8.0)	15.2 (8.6)	Time <0.001
DBT-I	23.8 (6.4)	18.2 (7.9)	13.9 (9.6)	Time × condition
DBT-S	23.5 (5.4)	10.4 (6.4)	11.9 (8.8)	<0.02 treatment year
				<0.001 follow-up year
Suicide ideation				
DBT	50.9 (20.3)	32.0 (21.6)	28.9 (16.6)	Time <0.001
DBT-I	58.4 (17.9)	30.3 (27.5)	25.5 (20.8)	
DBT-S	51.8 (17.3)	27.5 (19.1)	21.2 (19.2)	

Discussion

All three conditions resulted in significantly fewer suicide attempts, less suicide ideation, and fewer emergency department visits as a result of suicide attempts. Critically, all the variants of DBT were similarly effective at reducing suicidality among individuals at high risk for suicide. More fine-grain analysis indicated that the interventions including DBT skills training were more effective in reducing self-harm and improving levels of depression, suggesting that DBT skills training is a necessary component to achieve optimal outcomes.

Antisocial personality disorder and psychopathy

Antisocial personality disorder (APD) and psychopathy describe closely aligned but differing concepts. Antisocial personality disorder is a diagnosis developed by the APA; psychopathy was originally defined by Cleckley (1941) and now championed by Hare (e.g. Hare et al. 2000). According to Hare, the DSM describes an individual who is criminally antisocial, but not a true psychopath. Psychopathy, according to Hare, refers to an individual who not only has these characteristics, but also experiences a poverty of both positive and negative emotions, and is motivated by thrill-seeking as much as by any other gain. DSM-5 defines APD as a pervasive pattern of disregard for, and violation of, the rights of others occurring from the age of 15 years. Its core characteristics include:

- *Failure to conform to social norms in relation to lawful behaviours*: repeatedly engaging in behaviours that are grounds for arrest
- *Deceitfulness*: repeated lying, use of aliases, or conning others for profit or pleasure
- *High levels of impulsivity or failures to plan ahead*
- *Irritability and aggressiveness*: repeated physical fights or assaults
- *Reckless disregard for safety of self or others*
- *Consistent irresponsibility*: repeated failure to sustain consistent work or honour financial obligations
- *Lack of remorse*: indifference to, or rationalization of, harmful outcomes to others.

Those who distinguish between antisocial behaviour and psychopathy generally use Hare's (1991) Psychopathy Checklist (PCL) to diagnose psychopathy. This identifies two sets of factors associated with psychopathy: emotional detachment and an antisocial lifestyle. Emotional detachment involves a lack of capacity to process emotional information, and a consequent lack of understanding and disregard for the emotions of others. It is Hare's defining characteristic of psychopathy. Using the PCL to diagnose psychopathology, Hare found that up to 80% of criminals could be categorized as having APD; only 20% met the criteria for psychopathy (Hare et al. 2000).

The prevalence of antisocial behaviour is increasing over time in many countries, virtually doubling over a period of 15 years in the USA to about 3.6% of the general population. There are also marked differences in its prevalence across countries, ranging from about 0.14% in Taiwan to over 3% in countries such as New Zealand. These various findings led Paris (1996) to speculate that Asian cultures are protective against antisocial personality as a result of their family structure, which is typically highly cohesive and has clear limits on acceptable behaviour; the opposite constellation of characteristics to those implicated in the development of antisocial behaviour.

Aetiology of APD and psychopathy

The apparent confusion between antisocial personality and psychopathy has meant that the relevant literature often confuses the two concepts. Some studies of antisocial personality include within them what Hare and others would consider to be psychopathy. Other studies specifically focus on psychopathy as defined by Hare. As psychopathy is linked to an 'antisocial lifestyle', it is perhaps not surprising that many of the factors that predispose to antisocial behaviour are also associated with psychopathy. What distinguishes psychopathy from the antisocial personality are distinct neurological factors that are uniquely associated with the emotional detachment and limited range or depth of emotions central to the condition. Accordingly, this section first considers the neurological underpinnings of antisocial behaviour or APD, before considering the neurological factors that contribute uniquely to the development of psychopathy.

The neurobiology of APD

One important risk factor for APD may be low levels of sympathetic nervous system activity at times of stress (Raine et al. 1998), perhaps because the individual is driven to fearlessness and thrill-seeking as a means of increasing arousal to an optimal level achieved by others using less 'thrilling' experiences. More centrally, low levels of serotonin within the limbic system and associated brain areas are also strongly implicated and linked to high levels of impulsivity, aggression, irritability, and sensation-seeking. Moul et al. (2013), for example, found that low levels of serotonin were linked to high levels of callous-unemotional traits in antisocial boys aged 3–16 years; this in turn was associated with polymorphisms from the serotonin 1b receptor gene (*HTR1B*) and 2a receptor gene (*HTR2A*) which control serotonin levels. Siegel and Crockett (2013), among others, have argued that low serotonin levels within brain areas including the anterior cingulate cortex, ventromedial prefrontal cortex, amygdala, and striatum are also associated with impaired moral judgement and are genetically mediated through serotonin-metabolism related genes (*5-HTTLPR*; Yang et al. 2019).

These genetic influences may be mitigated by a number of factors. Legrand et al. (2008), for example, found that antisocial behaviour was substantially influenced by genetic factors in urban environments; in contrast, environmental factors were more influential in rural environments. The apparent lack of influence of the urban environment may reflect the lack of variation and universally challenging nature of many urban environments. Such is the influence of environment on risk, Viding et al. (2008) went as far as to suggest that the risk factors for APD are primarily environmental, and genetic factors moderate the influence of this risk (as opposed to the biopsychosocial model which typically assumes environmental factors moderate the impact of genetic factors).

Neurological mechanisms in psychopathy

Converging evidence also indicates that the deficits in emotional processing associated with psychopathy are linked to neuronal damage to the limbic system inhibiting the processing of emotional information, in what has been called a 'low fear' state. Laakso et al. (2001), for example, used brain imaging techniques to gain accurate data on the brain anatomy of 18 habitually violent psychopathic offenders. They found a strong negative association between the size of the hippocampus and scores on Hare's (1991) PCL, suggesting that damage in this area, which is involved in the acquisition of conditioned fear, may explain the lack of fear associated with psychopathic behaviour.

These data are added to by the findings of Kiehl et al. (2001), who used brain imaging to study activity within the limbic system in response to an 'affective memory task'. In this study, three groups of participants (criminal psychopaths, criminal non-psychopaths, and 'normal' controls) were asked to rehearse and remember lists of either neutral words or words describing negative emotions, and to identify these words in a subsequent recognition task. Psychopaths displayed significantly less activity within their limbic systems and greater activation of the frontal lobes while processing negative emotional words than the other groups, suggesting that the psychopaths and non-psychopaths use quite different brain systems to process emotional information. Birbaumer et al. (2005) extended this work to examine neurological processes while participants received painful pressure following presentation of various stimuli. The presentation of these stimuli before the pain meant that 'normal' participants learned to expect pain, reported some anxiety about these expectations, and developed a conditioned 'pain' response to these stimuli – evident through increased sweat gland activity when presented with the stimuli. During the acquisition phase of the study, they showed enhanced differential activation in the limbic-prefrontal circuit (amygdala, orbitofrontal cortex, insula, and anterior cingulate). By contrast, psychopaths displayed no significant activity in this circuit, no conditioned 'pain' response, and reported no anxiety. Even when psychopaths *do* show a neural response when asked to consider photographs of bodily injuries (including in the somatosensory cortex and right amygdala; Decety et al. 2013) from their own perspective, they do not show the same response when asked to imagine others in pain. In one genetic study adding strength to Hare's distinction between antisocial personality and psychopathy, Larsson et al. (2007) found that psychopathic behaviour was largely driven by genetic factors, while the impact of genetic factors on antisocial behaviour was significantly moderated by environmental factors.

Socio-cultural factors

Social factors clearly influence the probability of an individual engaging in antisocial behaviour and being diagnosed with APD. Dargis et al. (2016), for example, in a retrospective study of nearly 200 offenders found that the severity of maltreatment as a child was linked to the severity of both psychopathy and APD. The strongest link was between physical abuse and the antisocial facet of psychopathy. Sexual abuse, by contrast, was not associated with either psychopathy or APD. More powerful than these retrospective studies are those that follow cohorts of individuals over time prior to the onset of problems, to avoid the sampling and recall bias of retrospective studies. Perhaps the longest study of this kind is the Cambridge Study in Delinquent Development (Farrington et al. 2016). This followed over 400 boys, initially aged 8–9 years, for nearly 40 years and was able to identify childhood factors that were predictive of antisocial personality and adult convictions. The most important childhood predictors were a convicted parent, large family size, low intelligence or school attainment, a young mother and disrupted family. Family factors may also contribute to the lack of emotion associated with psychopathy. It has been suggested that the sustained experience of negative emotional events during childhood results in the individual learning to 'switch off' their emotions in response both to negative events that occur to them and to their behaviours that affect others.

While family influences are clearly important, external influences may also impact on the individual. Henry et al. (2001) found that having violent peers was predictive of later violent and non-violent delinquency. Similarly, Eamon and Mulder (2005) found that impoverished neighbourhood and school environments, exposure to deviant peer pressure, and parenting practices involving physical punishment and excessive monitoring of behaviour (perhaps as a consequence rather than cause of the antisocial behaviour) were related to antisocial behaviour among Latino adolescents in the USA. In an attempt to quantify the degree to which family and peer factors contribute to antisocial behaviour, Eddy and Chamberlain (2000) followed a group of offenders over a 2-year period. Family management skills and deviant peer association accounted for 32% of the variance in antisocial behaviour over this period. Borduin (1999) summarized the non-family antecedents of antisocial behaviour as:

- *Peer relations*: high involvement with deviant peers, poor social skills, low involvement with pro-social peers
- *School factors*: poor academic performance, drop-out and low commitment to education
- *Neighbourhood and community*: criminal subculture, low organizational participation among residents, low social support and high mobility.

By contrast, Burt and Klump (2014) found that a strong pro-social peer affiliation moderated the genetic influences on non-aggressive antisocial behaviour during childhood. These data accord with the rather more anecdotal story of James Fallon, a married 'normal guy' and neuroscientist investigating psychopathy, who had a PET (positron emission tomography) scan in order to act as a 'normal' comparison to those of his subjects, psychopaths – only to discover that his scan was identical to the extreme psychopaths he was studying, as was his genotype. Conversations with his family revealed their views on his behaviour, which was that it was rather odd at times and they could see the 'psychopath within him'. Nevertheless, he had been able to form relationships, to have and to engage with a family, and to lead a relatively normal life, an outcome he attributed to the loving, caring relationship he grew up in as a child (Fallon 2014).

Cognitive models

Children within family systems that increase risk of antisocial behaviour frequently do not have clear limits set to their behaviour. As a result, they fail to internalize the controls on their behaviour that other children adopt. These types of environment may also foster beliefs about the individual and the world that support antisocial behaviour. Lopez and Emmer (2002), for example, found that adolescents who engaged in crime believed aggression to be an effective and appropriate response to threat. Sukhodolsky and Ruchkin (2004) found that specific beliefs led to specific behaviours: beliefs concerning overt antisocial behaviour ('People need to be roughed up once in a while') were associated with overt but not covert antisocial behaviour. Conversely, beliefs related to covert behaviour ('If someone is careless enough to lose a wallet, they deserve to have it stolen') led to covert but not overt antisocial behaviour. Aggressive acts were significantly associated with high levels of anger and beliefs that physical aggression is an appropriate course of action in conflicts. Non-aggressive antisocial behaviour was associated with approval of deviancy, but not with anger or beliefs legitimizing aggression. Similar scripts may underpin adult behaviour of psychopaths. Beck et al. (1990), for example, identified their core beliefs as 'people are there to be taken', and the strategy derived from this to be one of attack. Other core beliefs included:

- Force or cunning is the best way to get things done
- We live in a jungle and the strong person is the one who survives
- People will get at me if I don't get them first
- I have been unfairly treated and am entitled to get my fair share by whatever means I can
- If people can't take care of themselves, that's their problem.

As well as these belief structures, there may be more fundamental differences in cognitive processing between psychopaths and typical individuals. The previous section considered deficits in how psychopaths process emotional information. However, Sadeh and Verona (2008) found other cognitive processes may be involved. In an experimental study, they found that participants who scored highly on traits indicating primary psychopathy (low anxiety, dominance, callousness) were more focused and less distracted by task-irrelevant stimuli than those without these characteristics. They took this to indicate that such individuals had reduced attentional capacity and had to focus more on tasks and less on peripheral issues. They also found that some characteristics of what they termed secondary psychopathy (social alienation, cynicism) were associated with poor working memory.

Treatment of antisocial behaviour

Psychological interventions

Interventions to reduce antisocial behaviour have focused almost exclusively on young people within the criminal system – fortuitously perhaps, as attempts at change in older people may prove more difficult (Davidson et al. 2008). As such, they may be better considered as programmes designed to change criminal behaviour than antisocial personality *per se*. The consensus of these studies is that the classic 'boot camp' or incarceration does not work. More effective interventions appear to be those targeting the family. Borduin (1999), for example, described a multi-systemic, family-based approach, the goal of which was to provide participants with the skills to help them cope with family and other problems. Family interventions aimed to improve parenting skills, encourage parents to support their child, and reduce levels of parental stress within the household. Parents were encouraged to develop strategies to monitor and reward progress at school, and to establish homework routines. Peer-oriented interventions were designed to increase affiliation with pro-social peers through participation in youth group meetings, organized athletics, and after-school activities. Sanctions were applied following associations with deviant peers. Cognitive behavioural interventions focused on teaching social and problem-solving skills. Interventions generally lasted up to 5 months, with initial sessions occurring as frequently as once a day, tailing off to weekly as therapy progressed.

This approach achieved significant success. Henggeler et al. (1992), for example, compared it with monitoring and general counselling in a group of 'serious juvenile offenders', most of whom had committed some form of violent crime. Immediately following the intervention, participants in the multi-systemic intervention had improved their family and peer relationships more than those in the comparison condition. By one-year follow-up, they had also been arrested less frequently and had spent less time in prison: an effect that was maintained at 2-year follow-up. In a later follow-up of a similar trial by the same group, Borduin et al. (1995) reported a halving of the known recidivism rate among those who received the intervention compared with a control group (21% versus 47%) 4 years after the intervention.

One problem faced by this type of intervention is that many parents choose not to engage with any therapy. With this in mind, Nock and Kazdin (2005) examined how a brief intervention could enhance parent participation. They used a technique they called a 'participation enhancement intervention', which involved giving parents information about the importance of attendance and engaging with the programme, eliciting motivational statements about attending and adhering to any strategies of change, and helping parents to identify and develop plans for overcoming problems that may have occurred over the period of treatment. The total time taken by the intervention was up to 45 minutes and formed part of the first three therapy sessions. It also proved effective. Parents who received the intervention reported higher levels of treatment motivation, attended more treatment sessions, and engaged more in the intervention than those in a control group.

A different approach to the treatment of antisocial behaviour does not involve the identification of particular individuals with particular problems. Instead, preventive programmes are used to target all 'at-risk' individuals. The best place to run such programmes may be within the normal day-to-day running of schools. An example of this approach is the 'good behaviour game', a widely used classroom management approach in the USA that rewards children for engaging in appropriate on-task behaviour during teaching. In it, the class is divided into two teams and a point is awarded to each team for any inappropriate behaviour involving one of its members. The team with the fewest points at the end of each day wins a group reward. If both teams keep their points below a pre-set level, they share the reward. The intervention therefore both reinforces, and establishes group pressure and norms supporting, appropriate behaviour. In one study of the effectiveness of this approach, Petras et al. (2008) compared rates of antisocial, violent, and criminal behaviour in young men aged 19–21 years who had attended schools in poor to lower middle-class areas of the US which had either implemented the programme or were in control areas. Those who had shown signs of early problems at baseline, the key target group of the programme, were significantly less likely to engage in any of these outcomes if they attended the schools in which the programme had been implemented.

Pharmacological interventions

A number of pharmacological interventions have been used to treat individuals who present with delinquent or antisocial behaviour. Some have proven effective, particularly in the treatment of aggression. Lithium or other treatments for bipolar disorder, for example, has been shown to reduce the number of impulsive aggressive episodes. Hollander et al. (2003) found greater reductions than those achieved by placebo on measures of irritability, verbal assault, and assault against objects following treatment with divalproex (used elsewhere to treat bipolar disorder and epilepsy). SSRIs have also been suggested as a means of controlling impulsive aggression, but there are as yet no large controlled trials of their efficacy (Tcheremissine and Lieving 2006), and one small study of 26 participants found no benefit to their use (Lee et al. 2008). How these interventions would compare with psychological programmes in which individuals are taught to control their anger is not known.

Treatment of psychopathy

Psychopathic individuals do not seek treatment, and most interventions are conducted within prison or other custodial settings. As a result of their lack of motivation to change, psychopathy has often been considered an untreatable condition, although there have been some voices of dissent from this somewhat negative viewpoint. Of interest are three review papers of the treatment of psychopathy published within 2 years of each other and reviewing essentially the same literature. Salekin (2002) conducted a **meta-analysis** on data from 42 treatment studies and concluded that while **electroconvulsive therapy (ECT)** and therapeutic communities were relatively ineffective interventions, good results could be achieved following psychoanalytic and cognitive therapy. Evaluating much the same literature, Reid and Gacono (2000) were more pessimistic in their conclusions and could find no evidence of consistent therapeutic gain following any form of treatment. Similarly, Wong and Hare (2002) concluded that, of the 74 empirical studies they could identify, only 2 were adequately conducted, and that the evidence was so weak that it remained unclear whether any intervention could be effective. Such was their pessimism relating to treatment outcomes, Maibom concluded that psychopathy is 'unlikely to be treatable in a piecemeal fashion' and that it is unrealistic to expect to replace 'problematic views of the world with more socially desirable ones' (2014: 31).

Measuring the effectiveness of programmes to treat psychopathy is problematic. A defining characteristic of psychopathic individuals is that they tell lies and are manipulative. Self-report measures should therefore be treated with considerable caution. Even behavioural measures cannot be relied on. The results of a study by Seto and Barbaree (1999) illustrate the problem. They examined the impact of a relapse prevention programme for sexual offenders. Participants included a range of people, not just psychopathic individuals. Their report focused on the relationship between apparent progress made within therapy as a function of in-session behaviour, homework quality, and therapist ratings of motivation and 'progress', and the frequency of reoffending following treatment. Among non-psychopathic individuals, greater within-therapy improvements were predictive of fewer offences following discharge from prison. By contrast, there was a *positive* association between apparent progress in therapy and the frequency of offences committed by the psychopathic individuals who took part in the programme. It seems that these people were able to learn the responses that the therapists considered indicative of progress and were able to simulate them. Those that were best at this simulation were also the most likely to reoffend. Therapy did nothing to change the underlying motivation of their behaviour.

Stop and think ...

Psychopathy appears to be untreatable, certainly using any psychotherapeutic approaches presently available. Should psychopaths therefore remain the target of any attempt at rehabilitation designed to change their behaviour or should society shift its approach, and work at 'rehabilitation' through working with them to identify roles within society they can best fulfil? Indeed, as their behaviour is a result of neurological deficits that inhibit the experience of empathy and responding to 'punishment', should they be seen as having a disability to which society should more widely accommodate (as with any other disability) rather than expecting them to change their behaviour?

Psychoanalysis

A number of early studies of the treatment of psychopathic individuals involved psychoanalytic methods (Salekin 2002). These were virtually all case studies, and none compared the intervention with any other form of treatment or changes within a control group. Case histories are generally considered with some caution, as clinicians typically report their treatment successes, not their failures, so they represent a biased sample of cases. The successes reported in these studies may therefore not indicate the likely success rates among an unselected group of individuals, and do not provide strong evidence for the effectiveness of **psychoanalysis** in this population.

Therapeutic communities

Therapeutic communities were first developed under the leadership of Maxwell Jones in the UK in the late 1940s. These provided an intensive 24-hour-a-day intervention to change psychopathic behaviour. Members were made responsible for the physical and emotional care of others within the community. The group itself established acceptable and unacceptable behaviours. Members were required to accept the authority of the group, and to submit to its sanctions if they disobeyed the rules. Communities were loosely based on Rogerian principles (see Chapter 2), and tried to inculcate high levels of honesty, sincerity, and empathy. Early evidence suggested this approach might be beneficial, with apparent reductions in recidivism following periods of stay in such communities and empathy. Early evidence suggested this approach may be beneficial, with apparent reductions in recidivism following periods of stay in such communities. However, this optimism might have been misplaced. In a study of the effectiveness of Grendon Prison in the UK, now advertised as the only operating therapeutic community in Europe, Gunn et al. (1978) found 70% of its psychopaths were known to reoffend, compared to 62% of a matched group of men incarcerated in a normal prison.

A more widely cited study of the effectiveness of this approach was reported by Rice et al. (1992), although the community it assessed was significantly more authoritarian than the UK model. The authors focused on a therapeutic community situated within a maximum-security prison in the USA. The programme comprised 80 hours of intensive group therapy each week, intended to help participants develop empathy and responsibility for their peers. Those who responded well led therapeutic groups and became involved in administering the programme. All participants were involved in decisions about who was released or transferred from the programme. Participants had little contact with professional staff. Nor did they have much opportunity for diversion: access to television or even informal social encounters were severely limited. Participation in the programme was compulsory: disruptive behaviour resulted in entry into a sub-programme in which the individual discussed their reasons for not wanting to be in the programme, but they were ultimately expected to resume participation. The authors noted that some of these programme characteristics would now not be ethically acceptable, but that the programme was well regarded at the time it took place in the 1960s and 1970s.

The programme accepted both psychopaths and non-psychopaths, who were followed up for an average of 10 years after discharge. Analyses compared the outcomes on psychopathic individuals, non-psychopathic participants, and a matched control group who did not enter the community. Their results were similar to those reported by Seto and Barbaree (1999). Non-psychopathic individuals were less likely to offend following discharge than those in the control group. By contrast, psychopathic individuals who participated in the programme were more likely to engage in violent crime following discharge than those in the control group, with known recidivism rates of 78% and 55%, respectively. The therapeutic community approach may actually have taught psychopathic individuals how to manipulate others more effectively: an unexpected and unwanted result.

Cognitive Interventions

Cognitive behavioural interventions may not be immune from this paradoxical outcome. Hare et al. (2000) examined the outcome of a number of short-term, prison-based, cognitive behavioural programmes including anger management and social skills training. Their data revealed that the interventions had little effect on reoffence rates of most psychopathic individuals. However, among offenders who were highly psychopathic, reoffence rates rose following treatment. Again, it seems that these courses taught these people how to be 'better psychopaths'.

Despite these negative results, a number of research groups have considered how the goals and strategies of cognitive behavioural therapy (CBT) could be adapted to treat psychopathic individuals. Beck et al. (1990) attempted to define the realistic goals of such interventions. They noted that the individual will continue to act primarily out of self-interest, and that the goal of therapy should therefore be to help them act in ways that are functional and adaptive within these limits. **Cognitive challenge**, which lies at the heart of the intervention, may therefore not only address core schemata such as 'I am always right', or 'Other people should see things my way', but also question whether antisocial behaviour is in the individual's own interest. Participants in therapy may, for example, be encouraged to question whether behaving in a way that assumes 'other people should see things my way' causes interpersonal friction that interferes with their own goals, and to change their behaviour if this is the case. This approach allows client and therapist to work together towards agreed goals.

Wong and Hare (2002) developed a substantial cognitive behavioural approach to the treatment of psychopathy, involving interventions at both an institutional (prison) and individual level. Their intervention was problem-focused and addressed issues specific to psychopathic individuals. Key elements of the programme included the following:

- *Support of pro-social attitudes and behaviour*: many psychopathic individuals within an institution seek out others with similar views who will reinforce their own beliefs. To minimize the risk of this happening, Wong and Hare suggest that a 'pro-social milieu' is established within the institution. This may be achieved by high-status individuals within the programme modelling positive attitudes and encouraging them in others and encouraging group reinforcement of pro-social behaviours. Note that the results of Rice et al. (1992) suggest that this may not be easy to establish.
- *Changing dysfunctional behaviours – aggression, manipulation, intimidation*: strategies to achieve change include the use of self-talk to prevent over-reacting to situations in which the individual feels inappropriately threatened or angry, and interpersonal skills training where these are lacking and contributing to the use of intimidation or other dysfunctional behaviours. These may be taught through role play and reinforcement of appropriate behaviour.
- *Learning to take responsibility for one's actions*: the intervention here involves a detailed analysis of the factors that lead up to offences, and identifying where the individual made choices that ultimately led to their offending. This also forms the core of relapse prevention training (see Chapter 10), as information here both encourages the individual to take responsibility for the actions that led to the offending behaviour and to identify strategies to avoid them in the future.

The programme also examined strategies for minimizing substance misuse and helping participants gain work skills or develop leisure activities to help avoid boredom once discharged, as this may trigger antisocial behaviour. Finally, the programme addressed the social network into which the individual is discharged following their stay in prison. Attempts to maintain or re-establish links with supportive family or other means of social support were recommended, although family contacts may be conducted with some caution, as relationships with family members are frequently poor. Evidence of the effectiveness of these therapeutic approaches has yet to be reported.

11.4 Cluster C diagnoses: avoidant, dependent, and obsessive personalities

Cluster C diagnoses subsume what may be termed neurotic disorders. According to DSM-5, avoidant personality disorder is characterized by social inhibition, feelings of inadequacy and hypersensitivity to negative evaluation. It begins in early adulthood and the individual has at least four of the following features:

- avoidance of occupational activities involving significant interpersonal contact, due to fears of criticism, disapproval or rejection
- unwillingness to be involved with people unless certain of being liked
- restraint within intimate relationships due to the fear of being shamed or ridiculed
- preoccupation with being criticized or rejected in social situations
- inhibition in new interpersonal situations as a result of perceptions of inadequacy
- viewing oneself as socially inept, unappealing or inferior to others
- reluctance to take personal risks or to engage in new activities because they may prove embarrassing.

A person with a dependent personality has the following characteristics. They:

- have difficulty making everyday decisions without excessive advice and reassurance from others
- need others to take responsibility for most major areas of their life
- have difficulty expressing disagreement with others for fear of loss of support or approval
- have difficulty initiating projects or doing things on their own due to a lack of self-confidence in judgement or abilities
- go to excessive lengths to obtain nurturance and support from others
- feel uncomfortable or helpless when alone
- urgently seek a new relationship as a source of care and support when a close relationship ends
- are unrealistically preoccupied with fears of being left to take care of themselves.

Finally, the characteristics of the obsessive-compulsive personality are that the individual:

- is preoccupied with details, rules, lists, order, schedules, etc. to the extent that the major point of any activity is lost
- shows perfectionism that significantly interferes with task completion
- is excessively focused on work and productivity to the exclusion of leisure activities and friendships
- is over-conscientious, and inflexible about matters of morality, ethics or values
- is unable to throw away worn-out or worthless objects even when they have no sentimental value
- is reluctant to delegate tasks or work with others unless they are completed to their standards in their preferred manner
- adopts a miserly spending style – money is hoarded for future catastrophes
- shows rigidity and stubbornness.

The prevalence of cluster C disorders in the general population typically varies between 1% and 8% depending on the disorder and study (Tyrer et al. 2015), although a prevalence as high as 17.5% was reported in a representative sample of Australian women (Quirk et al. 2017). The linkage between the conditions is not as strong as that within the cluster A group, and a number of factor analyses have found little or no overlap between the characteristics of obsessive-compulsive personality disorder and the others (e.g. Costa and McCrae 1992). There is, however, considerable overlap between the diagnostic criteria for the anxious personality types and diagnoses such as social phobia, depression, and generalized anxiety disorder, making differential diagnoses difficult to achieve at times. So close are these diagnoses that Ralevski et al. (2005) suggested that avoidant personality disorder and social phobia are 'alternative conceptualizations of the same disorder'. Certainly, these personality types place individuals at significant risk of developing diagnoses of anxiety or depression, although once developed the outcome is mixed, with some evidence of both a poorer prognosis (Viinamäki et al. 2003) and no impact on time to recovery (George et al. 2018).

Relatively few studies have explored the origins of cluster C personality disorders. However, Reichborn-Kjennerud et al. (2007) found that heritability ranged between 27% and 35% across the disorders. In addition, work by Torgersen et al. (2000) modelled the role of genetic and environmental factors in the development of a variety of personality disorders and found a significant genetic contribution to the development of dependent, avoidant, and obsessive-compulsive disorders. Their analyses excluded a role for a familial environment in cases of avoidant and obsessive-compulsive disorders, but a mixture of both genetic and environmental factors contributed to the development of dependent personality. By contrast, Myhr et al. (2004) found associations between retrospective ratings of parents as uncaring and higher attachment insecurity to be associated with anxious, cluster C, personality types. Similarly, Nordahl and Stiles (1997) found that people diagnosed with obsessive-compulsive personality disorder reported lower levels of parental care and higher levels of paternal over-protection than a typical population control group. By contrast, avoidant, dependent, and cluster A personality disorders were not associated with abnormal parental bonding.

There have also been very few studies of treatment research related to the cluster C disorders. There is some evidence of a short-term benefit of treatment by SSRIs (Fahlen 1995), although placebo-controlled, definitive studies are still lacking. Studies of the effectiveness of psychological therapies have involved subanalyses of people with both personality and clinical disorders in larger treatment trials or uncontrolled trials of CBT. Using the former approach, Tyrer et al. (1993) compared the impact of **tricyclic** antidepressants and CBT in patients with anxiety and depressive disorders, including some with cluster C personality types. Over a 2-year follow-up period, tricyclics proved the most effective intervention in this group. Gude and Vaglum (2001) found some benefit at one-year follow-up following brief treatment using schema-focused therapy, which attempted to change the core beliefs underpinning the personality, but there was no control group against which to measure progress. Subsequently, Svartberg et al. (2004) compared the effectiveness of two active therapies (short-term dynamic psychotherapy and cognitive therapy) in the treatment of a variety of cluster C disorders. Two years after treatment, 54% of the people who received short-term dynamic psychotherapy and 42% of those who received cognitive therapy showed clinically significant improvements. Finally, Emmelkamp et al. (2006) compared brief dynamic therapy and CBT in the treatment of people diagnosed with avoidant personality disorder and a **waiting list control**. Those in the CBT fared best. There is also evidence that cluster C diagnoses may influence the outcomes of treatment of other conditions. Hansen et al. (2007), for example, found that individuals with type C personality benefited more than individuals of differing personalities from a cognitive behavioural treatment of OCD.

11.5 Chapter summary

1. DSM identifies ten types of personality disorder in three clusters: A – odd or eccentric; B – flamboyant or dramatic; and C – fearful or anxious.
2. These may be better considered as extremes on a continuum of personality factors rather than distinct 'diagnoses'.
3. Beck's evolutionary model of personality disorders suggests they are the inappropriate maladaptive pre-programmed responses to environmental events, that result from an interaction between genetic and childhood factors.
4. Cluster A diagnoses are also known as the schizophrenia spectrum disorders, and include paranoid, schizoid, and schizotypal disorders.
5. Meehl suggested that the core personality disorder is genetically mediated, while risk for schizophrenia involves further genetic influences and high environmental stress factors.
6. Borderline personality disorder belongs to the cluster B group. Its core elements are an intense fear of abandonment, difficulties in coping with strong emotions, and the use of self-harm as a means of coping with strong emotions.
7. The origins of the disorder seem largely linked to experiences of childhood rejections and trauma that translate into strong negative self-schemata and dissociation as a means of coping with distress.
8. Borderline personality disorder is difficult to treat, although significant therapeutic gains have been made using cognitive behavioural techniques. The optimal intervention appears to be Linehan's dialectical behaviour therapy, although other approaches may also be effective. The disorder seems to be resistant to pharmacological therapy.
9. Although DSM tried to combine psychopathy and antisocial behaviour under one diagnostic umbrella, critics such as Hare have argued that they are different conditions. The DSM diagnostic criteria describe someone who is criminally antisocial. Psychopathic individuals experience a poverty of emotions as well as engage in antisocial behaviour.
10. Antisocial behaviour seems primarily to be the result of adverse social circumstances.
11. Psychopathic individuals also have neurological deficits within the limbic system that inhibit emotional processing.
12. Family or systemic interventions appear to be effective in the treatment of antisocial behaviour.

13. Finding effective treatments of psychopathic behaviour has proven more difficult. Standard interventions may actually increase psychopathic behaviour. Beck and Wong have been developing cognitive therapeutic interventions that may prove more effective – although there is no data yet concerning their effectiveness.
14. Cluster C diagnoses include those of avoidant, dependent, and obsessive-compulsive personalities.
15. These personalities appear to be the product of both genetic and family factors – although the role of family may be less than that of genetics according to Torgersen and colleagues.
16. Although there are few studies of the effectiveness of interventions for cluster C personalities, cognitive therapy and psychodynamic therapy both appear to be of benefit.

11.6 For discussion

1. Are the 'personality disorders' categorically different from the personalities of 'normal' people?
2. Should families whose dynamics increase the risk of their children developing personality (or other) disorders be routinely offered some form of therapeutic support?
3. Therapeutic interventions for borderline personality disorder can last for a year or more. Given the economic constraints on many healthcare providers, is this a good use of resources?
4. Should psychopaths be treated, punished, or accommodated to?

11.7 Further reading

Beck. A.T., Davis, D.D. and Freeman, A. (eds.) (2016) *Cognitive Therapy for Personality Disorders: A Guide for Clinicians*, New York: Guilford Press.

Cristea, I.A., Gentili, C., Cotet, C.D. et al. (2017) Efficacy of psychotherapies for borderline personality disorder: a systematic review and meta-analysis, *JAMA Psychiatry*, 74: 319–28.

Fallon, J. (2014) *The Psychopath Inside: A Neuroscientist's Personal Journey into the Dark Side of the Brain*, New York: Current.

Koener, K. (2012) *Doing Dialectical Behavior Therapy: A Practical Guide*, New York: Guilford Press.

NICE (2017) *Antisocial Behaviour and Conduct Disorders in Children and Young People: Recognition and Management*, London: National Institute for Health and Care Excellence.

Patrick, C.J. (ed.) (2018) *Handbook of Psychopathy*, New York: Guilford Press.

Siever, L.J. and Weinstein, L.N. (2009) The neurobiology of personality disorders: implications for psychoanalysis, *Journal of the American Psychoanalytic Association*, 57: 361–98.

12 **Eating disorders**

Chapter contents

Most of us have 'gone on a diet' at some time in our lives or wished to change our shape. Many of us succeed, at least in the short term, although we often experience a gradual increase in weight as we get older. For some, the imperative to diet or change shape may be more extreme than the norm, and may be diagnosed as an eating disorder. Two eating disorders are considered in this chapter: anorexia nervosa and bulimia nervosa. These are actually the least common eating disorders, with roughly half of all people with eating disorders fitting into a wider diagnosis of 'eating disorder, not otherwise specified' (EDNOS; Thomas et al. 2009). Nevertheless, they are the most clearly defined and treated disorders, and will therefore be the primary issues considered here. By the end of the chapter, you should have an understanding of:

- The nature of anorexia and bulimia
- The various **aetiological** explanations of both disorders, including neurological, social, familial, and cognitive factors
- The nature and effectiveness of interventions conducted with people who have eating disorders.

Although the two disorders present in quite different ways, they have a number of elements in common. Both involve prioritizing weight control, and many people with anorexia may shift into bulimic eating patterns at some time. There are also significant differences between the conditions. People with bulimia, for example, are rarely underweight and they value being sexually attractive, unlike most people with anorexia. The chapter first describes the two conditions. Then, it discusses the aetiological factors that the conditions have in common and those on which they differ. It finally considers the treatment of the two conditions.

12.1 Anorexia nervosa

First identified in the late nineteenth century, anorexia nervosa involves behaviours intended to keep the individual as thin as possible. For a **DSM**-5 diagnosis of anorexia, the individual must meet the following criteria:

- A consistent reduction in energy intake below that required, leading to a significantly low body weight inconsistent with age, developmental stage, gender, and physical health
- An intense fear of gaining weight or becoming fat, or persistent behaviour that prevents weight gain and maintains a significantly low weight
- A distorted view of their body weight and shape, or persistent failure to recognize the seriousness of their low body weight.

In addition, anorexia may be split into one of two subtypes:

1. *Restricting type*: the person does not regularly engage in binge eating or purging. Weight is lost by restrictive diet or excessive exercising. This is the stereotypical view of anorexia nervosa.
2. *Binge-eating/purging type*: the person regularly binges and purges, through self-induced vomiting and/or the misuse of laxatives or diuretics over a period of 3 months.

Across the world, between 0.5% and 2% of the population are likely to develop anorexia in their lifetime (e.g. Preti et al. 2009), with up to 90% of those affected being female, and a typical age of onset of between 14 and 18 years (Smink et al. 2012). It can be a life-threatening condition, with the highest mortality rate of any mental health disorder, and a nearly six-fold higher death rate than the general population. The most common cause of death is suicide (Arcelus et al. 2011), possibly as a result of half those affected being co-morbid for mood disorders (Ulfvebrand et al. 2015), although health complications are also strongly implicated. Psychological problems, including depression, obsessive-compulsive disorder, and anxiety, are common among people with anorexia (Jagielska and Kacperska 2017). In contrast to many mental health disorders, the **prevalence** of anorexia is highest among women in the higher socio-economic groups, and among those with high academic achievement.

For most people with anorexia, weight control is a long-term issue. Loewe et al. (2001), for example, found that 21 years after their initial admission, just over half a cohort of women diagnosed as anorexic were 'fully recovered', 21% were 'partially recovered', and 10% still met the full diagnostic criteria for anorexia. Few had sought help or any form of treatment, and 16% had died of causes related to anorexia. Even when they 'recover', many people with anorexia go on to develop eating habits typical of bulimia nervosa (e.g. Eddy et al. 2008) – that is, maintenance of normal weight while still having abnormal eating and vomiting patterns, leading some (e.g. Fairburn et al. 2003) to argue that both conditions share significant common elements. This is discussed later in the chapter.

Despite their avoidance of eating, most people with anorexia are preoccupied with thoughts of food. They may spend much of their time thinking about food, preparing it for themselves or others, or watching others eat. They may report dreaming about food, experience hunger pains, and retain an appetite for food. High levels of exercise or other behaviours that consume calories are common weight-loss strategies. Most, but not all, people with anorexia have a distorted body image, considerably overestimating their body proportions, and have a low opinion of their body shape (Dakanalis et al. 2016).

The control and reduction in weight associated with anorexia can result in a number of health consequences. The most immediate is the absence of menstruation (or amenorrhoea). Less obvious problems include anaemia, increased tooth cavities and gum infections, high blood pressure, reduced bone mineral density, low blood pressure, rough and cracked skin, and dry and brittle hair. Health problems may move to crisis in the form of metabolic and electrolyte imbalances that can be life-threatening, with up to one-third of deaths in anorexia being linked to cardiac problems (Jáuregui-Garrido and Jáuregui-Lobera 2012). The brain may also show evidence of changes at times of severe starvation, with reductions in brain volume and increases in the amount of cerebrospinal fluid. Thankfully, Wagner et al. (2006) found these changes to be reversible in people recovered for over one year.

12.2 Bulimia nervosa

The DSM-5 criteria for bulimia nervosa are:

- Recurrent episodes of binge eating, characterized by:
  - Eating within any 2-hour period, an amount of food that is 'definitely' larger than most people would eat during a similar period of time and under similar circumstances.
  - A feeling that one cannot stop eating or control the amount eaten
- Recurrent inappropriate compensatory behaviour to prevent weight gain, including self-induced vomiting, misuse of laxatives, diuretics, fasting, or excessive exercise.
- Both binge eating and compensatory behaviours that occur, on average, at least once a week for 3 months.
- Self-evaluation is unduly influenced by body shape and weight.
- The 'disturbance' does not occur during episodes of anorexia nervosa.

In addition, DSM-5 identifies two types of bulimia:

1. *Purging type*: the person regularly engages in self-induced vomiting or the misuse of laxatives, diuretics or enemas.
2. *Non-purging type*: the person uses inappropriate compensatory behaviours, such as fasting or excessive exercise, but not purging.

Many people with bulimia feel unattractive, have a fear of becoming fat, and consider themselves to be heavier than they actually are (Striegel-Moore et al. 2004). Their attempts to avoid being overweight are more chaotic than in anorexia, and periods of controlled eating are frequently interrupted by repeated, relatively short episodes of uncontrollable eating, followed by behaviours designed to counteract their consequences. The amount of food consumed in binges can be vast: up to and beyond 5,000 calories at any one time. Food is not eaten for pleasure; indeed, it is usually eaten secretly, rapidly, and barely tasted. Episodes are usually preceded by periods of considerable physical and psychological tension, and eating serves to reduce this tension. While bingeing, the individual may feel out of control, and episodes are typically followed by feelings of guilt, self-blame, and depression.

The weight of people with bulimia usually remains within the normal range, although it may fluctuate considerably over time. Between 80% and 90% of people with bulimia vomit after eating in an attempt to control their weight, up to 60% abuse laxatives, while others may exercise excessively (e.g. Roerig et al. 2010). Compensatory behaviours reduce discomfort and feelings of anxiety, self-disgust or lack of control associated with bingeing. Ironically, however, they frequently fail to prevent the calorific uptake from much of the ingested food. Bulimia involves some risk to health. Repeated vomiting and laxative abuse can lead to problems including abdominal pain, digestive problems, dehydration, damage to the stomach lining and to the back of the teeth, where regurgitated acid can do permanent damage to the tooth enamel. The most serious outcome can be an electrolyte imbalance leading to renal damage and potentially fatal cardiac arrhythmias.

Up to 50% of female students surveyed by Schwitzer et al. (2001) reported periodic binges; 6% had tried vomiting and 8% had used laxatives on at least one occasion. Few, however, engaged in these behaviours sufficiently frequently for them to be considered a disorder. Only between 1% and 3% of women will be formally diagnosed with bulimia in their lifetime (e.g. Preti et al. 2009), although among groups in which weight control is seen as particularly important, such as dancers and athletes, the prevalence may be significantly higher. The majority of those diagnosed with bulimia will no longer be bulimic 5 years after diagnosis, although nearly a half will revert back to bulimic behaviours at some point (Grilo et al. 2007).

Aetiology of anorexia and bulimia

Biochemical mechanisms

The main brain area involved in the regulation of appetite is the hypothalamus, although other brain areas and features in the gut also influence hunger and satiety. The lateral hypothalamus produces hunger when stimulated, while activation of the ventromedial hypothalamus triggers feelings of satiation and reduces hunger: for this reason it has been called the satiety centre. Activity within the hypothalamus is largely mediated by two **neurotransmitters**: dopamine and serotonin, which initiate, maintain, and then inhibit eating.

At the onset of or when anticipating eating, dopamine activity increases in both the lateral hypothalamus and the mesolimbic dopamine system – the primary reward system (see Chapter 4). Thus, the early stages of eating are both triggered and maintained by a direct effect on hunger and a feeling of pleasure. As eating continues, the dopaminergic activity is replaced by serotinergic activity, which reduces appetite and inhibits eating. Broft et al. (2012) considered people prone to binge eating may experience low levels of dopamine release (or be insensitive to the dopamine that is released) when they start eating. This may lead to binge eating as they attempt to achieve previous levels of satisfaction/reward from eating. Such speculation is supported by findings of low levels of HVA (a metabolite of dopamine) in the cerebrospinal fluid of people with bulimia (Kaye and Weltzin 1991). By contrast, people with anorexia may have an over-production of dopamine, which leads to anxiety and also an ability to go without pleasurable activities and sensations such as eating food (Kontis and Theochari 2012).

People who are currently suffering from anorexia have significantly lower levels of serotonin metabolites in their cerebrospinal fluid than individuals without an eating disorder. This is likely a sign of starvation, since the body synthesizes serotonin from the food we eat. After recovery from anorexia, however, such individuals experience significantly elevated serotonin levels (Kaye et al. 1991). Unfortunately, these higher levels of serotonin are associated with increases in anxiety and obsessive behaviour. As a consequence, Kaye et al. (2009) argued the reduced intake of food in anorexia serves to reduce anxiety and obsessive behaviour. Unfortunately, in response to this lowering of serotonin, the numbers of serotonin receptors increase in order to utilize the available serotonin. This then requires the individual to eat even less to avoid the emotional consequences of this serotoninergic activity. If an individual with anorexia does not reduce their food intake or even increases consumption, serotonin levels may spike, causing extreme anxiety and emotional chaos, with a consequent risk of further reductions in food intake to moderate their aversive mood state. These neurological data are consistent with more subjective findings that people with anorexia experience significant difficulties in emotional regulation and tend to suppress emotions and avoid conflict (e.g. Oldershaw et al. 2015).

By contrast, people with bulimia experience larger decreases in serotonin levels when going without food than typical people, and therefore binge eat to increase them (Steiger et al. 2005). Abnormalities in the serotonin system persist after recovery, suggesting these differences may have contributed to the development of the disorder and are not just a consequence (Kaye et al. 2001a).

Genetic factors may contribute to risk for both anorexia and bulimia. Klump et al. (2001) estimated that 74% of the variance in anorexic behaviours to be attributable to genetic factors, following a twin study in which they found 50% of **monozygotic (MZ) twins** but no **dizygotic (DZ) twins** to be concordant for anorexia. Keel et al. (2005) found evidence of shared genetic risk for both eating and anxiety disorders in a large-scale study involving nearly 700 twins. Bulik et al. (2019) concluded that the genes contributing to risk of anorexia are yet to be fully understood. However, they are likely to involve genes influencing serotonin metabolism, with particular attention given to various alleles of the serotonin 5-HT(2A) receptor gene, which is thought to increase serotonin levels in the non-starved state. The dopamine receptor genes *D2/D3* and *DRD4* may also be be implicated. Genetic influences on bulimia have proven more difficult to identify.

Gut microbiome

While most research related to eating disorders has focused on the brain, new research is identifying how the gut itself, or more specifically the microbiome within the gut, may also contribute to eating disorders. The gut is not a passive organ simply digesting food. It has links to the central nervous system, providing sensory information (such as fullness) to the hypothalamus, which allows the gut to respond to the various excitatory or inhibitory processes of the autonomic nervous system; hence, in another context, the feeling of butterflies when we are anxious. The microbiota within the gut may have a powerful influence on the range of processes that affect appetite, food intake and utilisation. Breton et al. (2016), for example, found ClpB protein (made of bacteria such as *Escherichia coli* found within the gut) concentrations to be significantly associated with sub-scale scores on measures of mood and dysregulated eating. The exact pathways involved, which are complex and yet to be fully determined, are likely to include the following processes:

- Microbiota are largely responsible for the production of serotonin and GABA within the body. Changes in microbiota associated with starvation may reduce the production of these neurotransmitters, thus influencing mood and food intake.
- The production of short-chain peptides within the microbiome may facilitate the secretion of satiety hormones (e.g. peptide YY) (Alcock et al. 2014).
- Enterobacteriaceae within the gut produce ClpB, which is an anorexigenic protein. Levels of ClpB correlate with α melanocyte-stimulating hormone, which is also known to be involved in satiety (Adan and Vink 2001).

Socio-cultural factors

'Thin is attractive'. People with anorexia and bulimia place a high premium on shape and weight, probably because of a more general cultural emphasis placed on physical appearance within Western society, and women with anorexia rate extremely underweight individuals as more attractive than 'typical' people (Horndasch et al. 2015). Images of femininity and female attractiveness have shifted since the 1960s to a slimmer, less 'hour-glass' shape. The classic 'figure' portrayed in *Playboy* magazine, for example, slimmed during the 1990s, with smaller hips, waist, and bust measurements (Rubinstein and Caballero 2000). Not surprisingly, the prevalence of low body weight and eating disorders is particularly high among those groups where physical attractiveness or performance is paramount, such as models, dancers, and athletes (e.g. Joy et al. 2016). In addition, as social groups develop positive attitudes towards thinness, levels of eating disorders rise within them. In the USA, for example, as a high value on thinness has shifted from white upper-class women to those in other socio-economic and ethnic groups, so has the prevalence of dieting and eating disorders (Striegel-Moore and Smolak 2000),

Judgements based on weight are not only aesthetic; attributions of a variety of personal attributes can be based on the appearance of the individual. Food, eating, and weight are seen by many as moral issues, and body shape can be a major criterion of self- and other-evaluation (Lantz et al. 2018). Many people, including health professionals and others working with overweight individuals (FitzGerald and Hurst 2017), hold prejudicial views against them (Brewis 2014).

Over half the families in which an individual develops an eating disorder are likely to place a strong emphasis on weight and shape (Haworth-Hoeppner 2000).

Such individuals are also likely to come from families with high levels of negative affect and discord and have mothers who are perfectionist (Jacobs et al. 2009). Successful dieting may be one way of gaining acceptance from parents with high aspirations, particularly where the child has not 'succeeded' in other life domains. Not eating may make an individual important within the family and give them some degree of control over other family members ('I'll eat if you …'). It may also provide a means of punishing them ('I'm not eating because you …'). A second consequence of anorexia is that it can lead the individual to be treated as a child, and allow them to avoid the responsibilities they would otherwise have to face; again, this may be most influential in families where there is a high emphasis on achievement.

A completely different model of anorexia is afforded by some family therapists, in which the person with anorexia is viewed as a symptom of a dysfunctional family. Minuchin et al. (1978) defined the characteristic of 'anorexic families' as being enmeshed, over-protective, rigid, and conflict-avoidant. That is, there is conflict between parents which is controlled and hidden. According to Minuchin et al., adolescence is a stressful time for such families, as the adolescent's push for their independence within the family increases the risk of the parental conflict being exposed. The development of anorexia prevents total dissension within the family and may even hold it together as the family unites around the 'identified patient'. The presentation of the young person as weak and in need of family support ensures that they become the focus of family attention and deflects it away from parental conflict. Evidence for this specific theory is mainly based on the clinical experience of the Minuchin group of family therapists. However, there *is* consistent evidence that family processes varying from over-protection to criticism of the person with anorexia may in different ways adversely affect the outcome of therapy (e.g. Salerno et al. 2016).

A final socio-cultural model suggests that both anorexia and bulimia may occur as a result of sexual abuse (Oppenheimer et al. 1985). According to this model, abuse results in the adolescent girl having strong negative attitudes towards her femininity, resulting in a rejection of the typical feminine shape and attempts to avoid it. This is most likely to occur around puberty. The evidence for this is not strong, and clearly only of relevance to female anorexics. Even though rates of sexual abuse are relatively high among people with eating disorders (e.g. Caslini et al. 2016), it is not a defining characteristic, as they are no higher than those among people with mood, anxiety, and other psychological disorders. More important may be insecure patterns of attachment established over childhood, as a consequence of poor parenting styles, which continue into adulthood (e.g. Tasca and Balfour 2014), and may lead to perfectionism and poor therapy outcomes (e.g. Keating et al. 2015).

Psychological explanations

Social factors translate into behaviour through cognitive processes. Despite the differences in presenting problems, Fairburn's (e.g. Fairburn et al. 2003) cognitive model proposed a similar cognitive disturbance in both anorexia and bulimia: a set of distorted beliefs and attitudes towards body shape and weight. Thinness and weight loss are prioritized, perhaps because of the high status given to looking thin and attractive, and the individual works to avoid weight gain and becoming fat. The underlying schemata involve judging one's self-worth on the basis of achieving a low body weight and being thin – so-called weight-related self-schemata.

Once weight-related schemata are established, they distort the way the individual perceives and interprets their experiences. Other people are evaluated not on the basis of personal qualities, but in terms of being thinner or fatter than the individual. All activities are assessed in terms of weight control, and any situation that leads to self-evaluation also results in an intensified focus on weight and shape. Any weight fluctuation has a profound effect on thoughts and feelings. For some people, their concerns and prioritizing control over their weight reflect a wider lack of self-esteem, a vulnerability to cultural messages about body weight (Stein and Corte 2003), and the desire to gain control over one aspect of their life. They hope to feel better about themselves if they are thinner, a process that leads them to be perpetually dissatisfied with their appearance and to be continually working to lose weight. Depression that may result from anorexic behaviour may intensify feelings of low self-esteem and increase dependence on controlling weight as a means of maintaining self-worth.

Anorexia and bulimia may reflect different ways of coping with the same underlying cognitions. According to Fairburn et al. (2003), people with anorexia are more able to sustain long-term control over their eating than those with bulimia, who are more chaotic and less consistent. He suggested that because of their restrictive dietary habits, individuals with both bulimia and anorexia are under significant psychological and physiological pressure to binge eat. To cope with these demands, both groups set a series of rules to govern their eating: when they should eat, what they can and cannot eat, and so on. These rules are typically perfectionist and difficult to achieve. Despite this, people with anorexia have sufficient self-control to be able to follow the rules they have set. By contrast, individuals with bulimia may on occasion fail to do so. This type of analysis is supported by personality studies (e.g. Levinson et al. 2019) that have found both anorexia and bulimia to be consistently characterized by perfectionism, obsessive-compulsiveness, neuroticism, negative emotionality, and harm avoidance. However, anorexia is typically associated with traits of high constraint and persistence, while people with bulimia are more impulsive and sensation-seeking (e.g. Lavender and Mitchell 2015).

Once an individual with bulimia starts to eat, Fairburn et al. (2003) suggest that they typically engage in dichotomous thinking ('I've eaten, so that's the end of my diet. What's the point of even trying to diet?') and a binge occurs. Binge eating also tends to improve low mood, and is thus in itself reinforcing. This is due to several effects, including drowsiness that follows eating large quantities of food and, in those who vomit, the feeling of relief and release of tension. These initial positive feelings are typically followed by feelings of disgust and shame at overeating, which results in a determined effort to follow the dietary rules set, which places the individual at risk of bingeing, and so the cycle continues.

Initial attempts at weight loss may be triggered by a variety of factors, including critical comments about weight or appearance, teasing, and role confusion at the time of transition from child to woman. As well as cognitive processes, dietary changes may also be maintained by a number of reinforcement processes. Positive reinforcement may initially be experienced in the form of compliments on looking slim. As these comments turn to concern, they may still provide positive reinforcement as the individual gains attention from their family. One specific form of feedback may be particularly important: the daily or weekly reinforcement of the bathroom scales. These provide unequivocal feedback on performance. For people with low self-esteem, weight loss may provide one element of control and success in their life. Weight loss becomes equated with self-esteem and self-worth, perhaps more so than any other factor in life. Anorexic behaviours may also be driven by negative reinforcement processes. People with anorexia experience an intense fear of gaining weight. Avoidance of this fear, by restrictive eating, provides relief and is negatively reinforcing.

Fairburn et al. (2003) identified a number of other factors that can exacerbate these processes:

- *Perfectionism*: the over-evaluation of, and striving for, attainment of personally demanding standards, despite potentially adverse consequences across a range of life contexts. These characteristics are highly prevalent among people with eating disorders and intensify disordered eating when applied to control weight and body shape.
- *Mood intolerance*: an inability to tolerate intense mood states, or a particular sensitivity to such states. Binge eating, vomiting, and 'driven exercising' are maintained by their role in modulating such mood states.
- *Core low self-esteem*: this results in low efficacy beliefs in relation to change, and undermines engagement with treatment.
- *Interpersonal difficulties*: these may precipitate binge episodes and undermine self-confidence and self-esteem. Family tensions may increase resistance to changes in eating patterns, particularly in younger people and those who are resisting eating.

A second cognitive model, involving a distorted body image, applies only to people with anorexia. This suggests that such people feel 'fat' even when their weight is actually clinically subnormal. Summarizing a plethora of research studies, Gupta and Johnson (2000) suggested that many people with anorexia considerably overestimate their body proportions, have a low opinion of their body shape, and consider themselves to be unattractive. By contrast, Gadsby (2017) concluded that many of these reports represent an *emotional* reaction to one's body shape rather than a perceptual experience. He suggested that those who experience an eating disorder are uncertain about their body size and shape, and only when they are compelled to make a judgement about these issues do they err on the side of reporting an overestimated body size. Skrzypek et al. (2001) reached a similar conclusion, that body image disturbance is not due to any perceptual deficit, but is based on 'cognitive-evaluative dissatisfaction'.

The restricted food intake of people with anorexia may have biological effects unrelated to body size or shape that serves to perpetuate any cognitive distortions. Starvation affects a number of cognitive processes, resulting in poor concentration, concrete thinking, rigidity, withdrawal, obsessive-compulsive behaviour, and depression. As a result, starvation may lead to a positive feedback loop in which people with anorexia become increasingly rigid in their beliefs and are unable to consider other ways of looking at their problem (Whittal and Zaretsky 1996).

Psychoanalytic explanations

Classic **psychoanalytic** theory provides a number of explanations for anorexia (Zerbe 2001). One explanation is that it stems from an unconscious confusion between eating and the sexual instinct. Some women may avoid eating as a means of, symbolically, avoiding sex. Another interpretation suggests that women with anorexia have fantasies of oral impregnation and confuse fatness with pregnancy. Starvation reduces the risk of pregnancy. Yet another explanation is that anorexia reflects a regression to an earlier stage of development: the individual literally 'shrinks' in size. This, and the cessation of menstruation, are an unconscious rejection of adulthood and a wish to revert to a childhood state. Finally, anorexia is considered by some to be the result of an arrested psychosexual development. If the child is fixated in the oral stage, sexual anxieties and obsessions are likely to be expressed as disturbances of eating.

Integrating psychoanalytical and cognitive processes, Bruch (1982) saw anorexia as the result of disturbed mother–child interactions that lead to ego deficiencies including a poor sense of autonomy and control, manifest through disordered eating patterns. According to Bruch, some mothers fail to attend appropriately to their young child's needs, perhaps as a result of prioritizing their own needs over those of the child or misunderstanding their behaviour. They may, for example, provide food and intimacy at times that suit them rather than the child, or misinterpret the child's emotions or needs. As a result, the child may grow up confused and unaware of their own internal needs, not knowing for themselves when they are hungry or full, and unable to identify their own emotions. As a consequence of their confusion, they turn to external guides such as their parents and appear to be 'model children'. However, they fail to develop genuine self-reliance and the experience of being in control of their behaviour, needs, and impulses. They feel as if they do not own their own bodies. Adolescence increases their innate need to establish autonomy, but they feel unable to achieve this. To overcome their sense of helplessness, they seek excessive control over their body size and shape and eating habits. A number of studies have provided some support for Bruch's assertions. Steiner et al. (1991), for example, reported that many parents of young girls with anorexia tended to have fed them as a baby based on their schedule rather than that of the child. Fukunishi (1997) reported that many people with bulimia mistake emotions such as anxiety or upset as signs of hunger and respond to them by eating.

Attachment theory suggests that some of these behaviours may be interpreted in terms of insecure attachment with a mother figure, leading to insecurity and anxiety at times of independence (Troisi et al. 2005). Ward et al. (2001) went further and suggested that the mothers of adolescent girls with anorexia may transmit their anxious attachment patterns with their mother to their daughters.

Box 12.1 Bulimia and anorexia

Here are a couple of accounts of people with bulimia and anorexia. Despite both being concerned with eating-related disorders, the two discourses are completely different. The account of the person with bulimia centres on the drive to eat and the guilt and discomfort associated with it. That of the person with anorexia focuses on wider issues, in particular, issues of revenge and control. The pathways to each disorder differ across people, so although these may be considered 'typical' accounts in some ways, the accounts of other people with the same disorder may differ markedly.

Bulimia

I think it's easier not to drink or take drugs than to eat normally. You can either take them or not. If you don't want to – you just avoid them. But eating is so different. You have to eat … and once you – well, I – start, it's so difficult to stop. I want to be slim and look good. And I like my food. So I say to myself OK. Today you will not eat till 6 o'clock and you will eat a healthy meal. So I start the day with good intentions.

But then I live for food. I can avoid eating at lunchtime – it's almost easy with people around me. But as the day goes on, I want food!! I don't feel hungry. But what happens when I get home, I just want to eat. It's on my mind, and I know there's food in the fridge – lovely ice cream … chocolate. God, I love chocolate! Why can't I like something healthy and low calorie?! I sit and watch the TV, but I'm thinking of food. I am now! Anyway, some nights I can get by, cook myself something reasonable – nights when I'm busy or interested in what's on TV or something. But other nights, I just go straight to the fridge and have a snack. Unfortunately, it's never a small one – what does that do to you? A couple of biscuits just doesn't work for me. So, I tend to snack on something big and calorific. Even that would be OK if I could stop there. But I tend to think, 'I've blown it now … I've begun to eat, so what's the point of stopping now?' Once I've blown away my good intentions, then I just give in to eating I suppose. So I eat and eat. I don't stop when I am full. I eat till I am bursting. I feel uncomfortable, and I know I'm bound to put on weight. I feel really guilty – another day when I haven't kept my good intentions. So, I make myself sick. I'm good at it. It's not difficult now. Then I feel better. At least I can relax and know that I won't put on weight. It feels such a relief. But I also know that I shouldn't have had to do it, so I feel guilty and vow that tomorrow I will control my eating and not need to do it. But, of course, tomorrow never comes …

Anorexia

My anorexia kicked in at age 13. I battled food issues for years before that. Mum was always on a diet – and I was often hooked into being her dieting partner, and sometimes competitor. Both our food struggles – I see now – only diverted our and the family's attention from the emotional turmoil permeating our household. I became the convenient whipping post of my parents' outbursts of anger, insecurities … I was hit a lot and verbally abused. At age 13, my parents cracked down and tried to totally control my life – friends, boyfriends – everything. That control pushed me over the edge ... Dieting became an obsession for me. I dropped two stone in a month! The hunger was still there. Some days, all I thought about was food. But I was determined to conquer it. I strove for complete control – perhaps the only control I had. I felt repulsed if I ate – I had let myself down, lost control. I wanted to look good, to fit the ideal of womanhood. But a large part of the drive was revenge! I loved to see my parents' reactions to me starving. Dieting was no longer good, something to do with my mother ... it was a weapon. Turning her own behaviour on her. They were partly angry because they could not control this part of me, and partly fear and worry. But I had control. They ranted, they shouted, and tried to get me to eat. But I wouldn't – not for them. I began to lose contact with my feelings. I wanted to starve to be in control, to prove I could do it, but also because I deserved to ... because I hated myself.

Interventions in anorexia

Given the multiple routes to anorexia, the emphasis of treatment may vary considerably across individuals. Potential interventions include cognitive behavioural therapy, family therapy, and insight-oriented psychotherapy, with the three being complementary rather than competing interventions. Interventions can be considered in two stages: (i) initial treatment, usually in hospital, focusing on weight gain; and (ii) longer-term outpatient treatment focusing on sustained cognitive and behavioural change.

Promoting weight gain

In-patient care may be necessary where an individual's weight is seriously compromised – that is, less than 75% of 'normal' for an individual's height and age. Interventions in hospital usually focus on providing extrinsic rewards for weight gain. This operant-based process involves gaining pre-specified rewards for pre-specified gains in weight, the most valued of which may be discharge from hospital on achieving a target weight. This avoids the danger of rewarding food intake, which may be subsequently vomited up and is therefore ineffective.

Some years ago, the nature of these rewards included access to a telephone or television. These are now considered to be basic rights, and removal of them would infringe such rights. Accordingly, the 'rewards' for eating are now typically defined by the individual and are more than the basic elements available to all in-patients. They may include increased social privileges, access to visitors, and exercise privileges. Caloric intake is gradually increased over time. Too high an initial calorie intake may result in refusal to consume the calories and, in the light of the previous discussion of neurological underpinnings of anorexia, result in emotional crises which the individual may find difficult to manage. Health professionals may also educate the individual about anorexia and provide more informal support and encouragement. Critical here is the reassurance that weight gains made at this time will not be translated into becoming overweight in the longer term. In a recent study of this approach, from a research group in Milan, Gentile et al. (2008) reported that of 99 individuals, 18 prematurely interrupted their treatment and 75 continued intensive in-patient treatment until they achieved their required weight. Thirty-two people with severe malnutrition were fed through a nasogastric tube until their weight increased and 'they started to cooperate with treatment'.

Stop and think ...

Most people with anorexia are intelligent and capable individuals. They choose to stop or minimize their eating. Do health professionals or others have the right to force them to eat, to prevent them engaging in what is their choice of behaviour? If someone is actively wishing not to have nutrition, should we force them to have food or put intravenous drips into their arm to improve their nutritional status? Or should we hope that they will eventually eat if their health becomes seriously compromised? It can be frightening to watch someone literally starving him or herself to death. But do we have the right to force them to eat or receive nutrition through drips or nasogastric tube in the knowledge that this will be distressing to the individual . . . and once it stops, the person is likely to continue to starve themselves?

Whether people should in essence be 'force fed' is a very live issue in anorexia and is particularly associated with the risk to health of continued starvation as well as other psychological co-morbidities (Carney et al. 2008). The debate has focused, in particular, on the competence or otherwise of people with anorexia to make what are truly life and death decisions. Some clinicians (e.g. Russon and Alison 1998) have argued that the majority of people with anorexia are mentally competent to make decisions about whether or not to eat. As a result, they suggest that it is inappropriate to treat them against their wishes, even if this leads to their death. Others (e.g. Treasure 2001), while accepting that force-feeding, usually through a nasogastric tube, is inhumane and unacceptable, have pointed out that both it and other active treatments can be legally used with people with anorexia *in extremis*, as they are not mentally competent to make decisions that may result in their death.

Treasure (2001) identified four general principles that define whether an individual is competent under the law to make therapeutic choices or to refuse treatment. They must be able to do the following:

1. Take in and retain information relevant to their decision and understand the likely consequences of having or not having the treatment
2. Believe the information
3. Weigh the information in the balance as part of the process of arriving at a decision
4. Recognize they have a health problem and take action to remedy their condition.

According to Treasure, individuals with anorexia do not conform to these criteria and are therefore deemed, under law, incompetent to make medical decisions that may endanger their life. Accordingly, doctors have the right to treat the individual without their consent. This argument is in accord with legal precedents (Jackson 2012) that have stated compulsory treatment of people with anorexia, including force-feeding, is both legal and may be necessary on occasion. However, the requirement for legal judgment in each individual case highlights the contentious nature of this process. What may also be relevant here is that while feeding through a nasogastric tubing may increase weight in the short term, it does not address the underlying psychopathology (Kells and Kelly-Weeder 2016).

Cognitive behavioural approaches

The second phase of treatment involves interventions aimed at achieving and maintaining long-term behavioural change. Perhaps the most widely used cognitive behavioural approach known as CBT-E (enhanced) developed by Fairburn (e.g. 2008), which can take as many as 40 or more therapy sessions, is designed to target the problems experienced by people diagnosed with either anorexia or bulimia following appropriate formulation rather than 'treating the diagnosis'. In anorexia, the approach has been divided into a number of phases, the first of which is intended to establish a working alliance with the individual. Garner and Bemis (1985) stated that at this time, it is critical that the individual's core beliefs are not directly challenged, as this is likely to result in a withdrawal from therapy. Instead, the therapist needs to align with the individual, recognize how their weight-control strategies are intended to fulfil important functions for them, and appreciate that these strategies have been partly successful. This may be linked to questioning whether they have achieved everything the individual intended and evaluating the emotional and physical costs of extreme dieting. The first few sessions may be spent developing a list of the advantages and costs of their anorexic behaviour. There may also be exploration of the deeper schemata underlying this behaviour. Homework assignments may be used to gather data on how events influence thoughts and feelings, and to provide opportunities to practise different ways of interpreting weight- and eating-related events. Only once a working alliance has been achieved and the individual is motivated to at least consider change, can cognitive therapy begin.

Cognitive interventions may have multiple targets, including modifying inappropriate cognitions and developing autonomy. Emphasis may be placed on challenging perceptual/attitudinal distortions. While these may never change to perceptions of being thin, an awareness of distortions and an acceptance that they have some degree of exaggeration may help change the individual's willingness to eat. Autonomy may be encouraged by challenging negative cognitions and encouraging the individual to trust their own intuitions and feelings. **Cognitive challenges** encourage the individual to consider the high emotional cost of their behaviour, and help them to explore some of the more entrenched schemata that underpin this behaviour, such as the belief that body weight or shape can serve as the sole criterion for self-worth and that complete control of one's body is necessary. Participants in therapy may also be taught problem-solving techniques to help them deal with any crises that might occur more effectively.

Studies of CBT have shown mixed efficacy. A number of cohort studies following people treated with CBT-E have shown significant gains in weight over time in people with anorexia, particularly among younger participants (e.g. Dalle Grave et al. 2015). However, randomized controlled trials comparing this or very similar approaches with other psychological therapies have failed to find consistent evidence of its superiority. McIntosh et al. (2005), for example, compared the effectiveness of cognitive therapy, interpersonal therapy, and non-specific supportive clinical management. The latter was thought to be the baseline against which these active therapies were measured. However, it proved the most effective approach, with 56% of the people in this condition showing significant improvement, compared with 32% in the cognitive therapy condition and 10% of those in interpersonal therapy. The authors speculated that the CBT might have failed because the cognitive rigidity of the people with anorexia might make it difficult to achieve cognitive, and hence behavioural, change. This result was partially replicated by Zipfel et al. (2014), who compared three different approaches: 'optimized treatment as usual' (similar to that of McIntosh), focal dynamic psychotherapy, and CBT-E further enhanced by the addition of a range of more generic cognitive behavioural procedures including social skills training. No differences were found in the effectiveness of the interventions. More positively, Carter et al. (2009) found a year-long cognitive behavioural intervention to be more effective than usual care in preventing relapse in participants who had already achieved a criterion weight. By the end of the year, 64% of the comparison group had relapsed, while only 35% of the intervention condition had.

Family therapy approaches

A number of different family therapies have been used to treat anorexia, although all seek to change the power structure within the family by empowering parents, preventing alliances that cross generations, and reducing tensions and problems between parents. Note that this approach contrasts markedly with the cognitive behavioural interventions described above which encourage autonomy and personal control over eating.

One of the first family approaches to treating anorexia was reported by Minuchin et al. (1978; see Chapter 5). They reported their structural family therapy achieved an 85% success rate, although this has been viewed with some caution as it was based on a series of case reports with relatively young and 'intact' families rather than data from controlled trials. More recently, Russell et al. (1987) followed a similar therapeutic approach which focused on the underlying stresses within the family. The approach had three tasks. The first involved engaging the family in the therapy process. They termed the second part the refeeding phase. In this phase, the family was observed eating together to identify relationships, communication of support, and rules about food and eating. At this time, the 'identified patient' and their siblings were encouraged to align, in order to reinforce appropriate boundaries within the family. The final stage involved changes in the family system, including return of control of eating to parents, working to support cooperation between parents, and stopping alignments or collusion between one or other parent and the person with the eating disorder.

Behavioural family therapy (Robins et al. 1995) combines systemic and behavioural therapy approaches. The goals of therapy begin with restoration of weight. Strategies to achieve this include changing eating habits and cognitive therapy to minimize body image distortions, fear of fatness, and feelings of ineffectiveness. Family interaction patterns such as conflict avoidance, enmeshment, and over-protectiveness are also targeted. Therapy follows three phases. First, control of eating is taken away from the individual and given to the parents, to restore the family hierarchy. Parents are taught and encouraged to implement a behavioural weight-gain programme for their child, including making meals, regulating exercise, and establishing consequences for following or not following the plan. Once weight gain has been achieved, therapy moves to the second stage. This combines three elements:

1. Cognitive restructuring of distorted body image and unrealistic food beliefs
2. Working with the family to alter enmeshment, coalitions, and inappropriate family hierarchies (see Chapter 5)
3. Gradually giving control of eating to the person with the eating disorder.

Finally, the family may be taught problem-solving and communication skills. Robins et al. evaluated the effectiveness of their approach, comparing it with supportive individual therapy, in a group of female adolescents aged 12–19 years. At one-year follow-up, both forms of treatment had positive effects, although there were no between-group differences. Subsequently, Eisler et al. (2007) compared 'conjoint family therapy' with 'separated family therapy'. Both used the behavioural principles outlined above. However, in the conjoint therapy the therapists worked with the whole family together, while in the separated family intervention they worked with adolescent girls and their parents separately. Both interventions proved effective over a one-year-long period of treatment, achieving significant gains on measures of symptomatology such as bulimic symptoms, as well as on nutritional status and mood. Le Grange et al. (2016) also found whole family therapy to be less effective than a 'family' intervention working just with parents, at least in the short term; although both proved equally effective in the longer term. Importantly, though, Eisler et al. found that among families where there was significant maternal criticism towards the adolescent, the separated family intervention proved most effective. At 5-year follow-up there remained little difference between the groups, with 75% of their study population having no eating disorder at this time. These data are in accord with the findings of Perkins et al. (2005), who found that adolescent girls who did not want to involve their parents in their treatment for bulimia considered their mothers to be more blaming and to hold a more negative attitude towards them than those who wanted them to be involved. Accordingly, the choice of any intervention needs to take account of family dynamics.

Pharmacological interventions

Given the role of dopamine and serotonin in eating disorders, it should not be surprising that drugs involving these neurotransmitters have been used in the treatment of anorexia. Kaye et al. (2001b) reported an intervention in which women with anorexia were treated with either fluoxetine (an **SSRI**) or a **placebo** control. Of those on fluoxetine, 63% achieved a 'good' response as a result of gains in 'appropriate weight maintenance', obsessionality, 'core eating disorder symptoms', and mood. Only 16% of those in the placebo group achieved comparable gains. However, this positive finding may be rather optimistic, as Attia and Schroeder (2005) reviewed the evidence from all the controlled studies of the treatment of anorexia using antidepressants and **neuroleptics** then available, and found little evidence of benefit. While treatment with SSRIs may prove effective in the treatment of depression that may co-exist with anorexia, there is no evidence of consistent changes in 'core' anorexic symptoms (Claudino et al. 2006). Interestingly, antipsychotic medication may provide more, or at least comparable, benefits. Mondraty et al. (2005) found that anorexic individuals treated with an atypical antipsychotic (see Chapter 4) reported fewer ruminations than those treated with a **phenothiazine**. In addition, Bissada et al. (2008) reported that treatment with the atypical antipsychotic olanzapine, which includes weight gain among its side-effects, resulted in greater weight gain than a placebo intervention over a 10-week treatment period.

Research box 11

Le Grange, D., Hughes, E.K., Court, A. et al. (2016) Randomized clinical trial of parent-focused treatment and family-based treatment for adolescent anorexia nervosa, *Journal of the American Academy of Child and Adolescent Psychiatry*, 55: 683–92.

There have been relatively few trials of the effectiveness of family interventions targeting adolescents with a diagnosis of anorexia nervosa. These have had mixed results, but two have shown that separate parent and adolescent sessions may be equally as effective as those involving the whole family. This study examined this issue further, by comparing a family-based intervention (FBI) with a parent-focused intervention (PFI), in which the therapist actively worked with parents while the adolescent spent time being 'monitored' by a nurse.

Method

Participants

Participants were 107 referrals over a 4-year period to a specialist treatment clinic. They attended a one-day assessment clinic for diagnosis and treatment planning. Inclusion criteria were a DSM-IV/5 diagnosis of anorexia nervosa, age 12–18 years, and living with at least one parent. The weight criterion was being at or below the 90th or 95th percentile modified body mass index (mBMI) for adolescents depending on their height. Exclusion criteria included drug and alcohol dependence, risk of suicide, and current **psychotic** episode.

Assessments

Assessments were taken at baseline, end of therapy, and at 6- and 12-month follow-up. Key measures were:

- *Global Eating Disorder Examination (EDE)*: a standard interview focused on symptoms over the previous 4 weeks and which addresses: (i) restraint, (ii) eating concern, (iii) shape concern, and (iv) weight concern.
- *Weight*: taken wearing a surgical gown and 'after voiding'.

In addition, measures of a number of potential mediators of outcome included: the Child Depression Inventory, Yale-Brown Obsessive-Compulsive Scale, and Yale-Brown Eating Disorder Scale.

Interventions

Treatment in both conditions was manualized and conducted by trained therapists.

- *Family-based intervention (FBI)* involved three phases: (i) sessions 1–12, supported parents in their efforts to assist their child to gain weight, with a family meal in the second session; (ii) sessions 13–16, involved transitioning control over eating to the adolescent in a developmentally appropriate manner; and (iii) sessions 17–18, introduced adolescent developmental tasks once the eating disorder symptoms had largely abated. Weight was measured at each session.
- *Parent-focused intervention (PFI)* involved the adolescent meeting with a nurse prior to parents, when they were weighed and afforded brief supportive counselling. The focus and content of the parent sessions were the same as in FBI. However, they were conducted without any interaction with the adolescent or his or her siblings.

Results

At baseline, the mean percentile BMI was 81.9 (SD 6.1), the mean duration of symptoms was 10.5 months (SD 8.8), and the majority of participants were female (88%) and from intact families (63%). Table 1 reports the outcomes of the key outcomes at each assessment period.

The differences in remission rates at end of treatment and 6-month follow-up were significant (p = 0.016 and 0.05, respectively), but not at 12-month follow-up (p = 0.44). No differences emerged on any other primary outcome. At the end of treatment participants in the PFI condition were three times more likely to be in remission than those in the FBI condition (OR = 3.03; 95% CI = 1.23–7.46) and over twice as likely to be in remission at 6-month follow-up, although this difference was not significant.

Eighteen per cent of participants were hospitalized during treatment (FBI = 24%, PFI, 12%; NS, Fisher's exact test, p = 0.133). Fifteen per cent were hospitalized during follow-up (FBI = 20%, PFI, 11%; p = 0.271). Of the hospitalizations, 83% were for medical reasons.

Table 1 Changes on key outcomes over time

	End of treatment	6-month follow-up	12-month follow-up
Percent remission			
PFI	43	39	37
FBI	21	22	30
EDE Global, mean (SD)			
PFI	0.81 (1.22)	0.74 (1.01)	0.81 (1.13)
FBI	1.10 (1.32)	0.98 (1.28)	1.04 (1.24)
% mBMI, mean (SD)			
PFI	93.9 (10.4)	95.0 (11.4)	95.6 (10.0)
FBI	90.7 (8.7)	92.8 (9.9)	93.3 (9.7)

Further analyses of the EDE found no differences between conditions on the subscales of restraint, eating concerns, weight concerns or shape concerns. Nor were any differences found on any of the secondary measures.

Discussion

The two interventions proved equally effective in the long term. However, the PFI intervention achieved its results more quickly: an important finding given the distress and health risk associated with anorexia. Although the study had a relatively large sample size, it is possible that a larger sample may have led to the reporting of higher significance – although the failure to report **effect sizes** makes this difficult to assess. The relative benefits of parent-focused therapy are also valuable because this approach is potentially less therapeutically challenging and more likely to be achievable, without the specialist training involved in family therapy.

Interventions in bulimia

Cognitive behavioural therapy

In contrast to interventions in anorexia, those in bulimia are more structured and have a better prognosis. One of the pioneers of cognitive behavioural interventions in bulimia developed a three-stage approach (Fairburn 2008). The initial stage has two aims: first, to provide a rationale for the treatment, and second, to replace binge eating with a pattern of more regular eating. Eating is restricted to three planned meals a day, plus two or three planned snacks, none of which is followed by vomiting or other compensatory behaviours. This is not usually accompanied by weight gain. Indeed, reductions in the frequency of binge eating often result in weight loss. Distracting activities, such as having a bath or contacting friends, can be used to minimize the risk of bingeing. Once regular meals are established, the desire to vomit may reduce naturally. However, where this remains problematic, continued use of these inhibitory behaviours for an hour or so after eating may be necessary. Laxative and diuretic use should also be stopped at this time, with a phased withdrawal programme established for those who are unable to do so immediately. Knowledge that these strategies do not prevent food absorption aids this process. Towards the end of this phase, therapy sessions may involve both the **client** and key friends or relatives establishing an environment that will support behaviour change. This first stage may be sufficient to bring about therapeutic change, measured in term of both reductions in bulimic behaviour as well as related cognitions, as it has been found to achieve similar or even better outcomes than more complex interventions (Södersten et al. 2017).

Most cognitive behavioural interventions, however, progress to a second stage involving the using of both behavioural and cognitive procedures to counter concerns about shape and weight, and other cognitive distortions. Behavioural interventions may involve eating previously avoided types of food and, where necessary, increasing energy intake. This may be achieved by working up a hierarchy from relatively acceptable foods to those that initially invoke high levels of anxiety or urges to binge or purge. At the same time, participants are encouraged to identify negative assumptions about their shape and weight, and to find evidence in support of or against them using cognitive challenge techniques. Fairburn noted that many clients have a limited repertoire of such thoughts, triggered by a range of different circumstances. By repeatedly examining these thoughts and the circumstances that trigger them, their potency and automaticity gradually decline. Further behavioural hypothesis-testing may involve a gradual introduction of previously avoided and feared behaviours, including exposing body shape through wearing tight clothing, undressing at swimming baths, or even no longer undressing in the dark. The third stage involves maintenance of progress achieved in the first two stages and consideration of strategies to prevent relapse once therapy is terminated.

This approach is usually considered the treatment of choice for bulimia. Overall remission rates from this approach are about 50%, with up to 44% of successful participants relapsing in the year following treatment, and a similar percentage of those who make no gains during treatment subsequently achieving remission over this period (Södersten et al. 2017). One of the successful interventions involved remote treatment using 'internet-assisted cognitive behavioural therapy' (Ljotsson et al. 2007). Participants in the active intervention in this study were sent a book outlining Fairburn's treatment plan and were assigned homework related to each phase via email contact with a therapist over a 12-week period. They also had access to a private discussion forum involving other participants. Of those who completed the programme, 46% were no longer bingeing or purging after 12 weeks: a figure that reduced to 37% of those who started but did not complete. These gains were generally maintained up to 6 months follow-up.

Le Grange et al. (2007) reported outcomes of a family therapy intervention involving 20 sessions in which parents are first empowered to disrupt binge eating and control behaviours such as restrained eating and purging, and then hand back control over these behaviours to the adolescent. By the end of treatment,

39% of participants were no longer binge–purging, compared to 18% in the comparison group who received supportive psychotherapy. Schmidt et al. (2007) reported a direct comparison of an individual cognitive behavioural and family therapy intervention, finding that although the cognitive behavioural intervention proved superior at 6-month follow-up, there were no between-group differences at 1-year follow-up.

Case formulation

Ms F was a 23-year-old single woman living in Scotland. Her weight appeared normal, and according to her body mass index she was within the upper range of average for her height and age. She worked as a secretary for a local firm and lived with her parents. At school, she felt some awareness of and negativity towards her own physique – she considered herself to weigh a little heavier than ideal, but was not unduly worried by her appearance. However, she became more concerned over this when she and her long-term boyfriend split up, and he told her that he thought she was fat and this made her unattractive. She had had few previous boyfriends and found it difficult to develop such relationships as a consequence of shyness and low self-esteem. As a result, she had no history of more complimentary comments from boyfriends, and losing weight to become more attractive became a major goal in her life. She began to link having a boyfriend with losing weight, and withdrew from situations where she could potentially meet another boyfriend until she looked more attractive.

She initially tried to diet, but found it difficult to do this consistently and did not lose weight. So, she began to experiment with other ways of losing weight. She tried laxatives and found that she initially lost weight following their use, but then regained the weight over the next few days. She felt that she needed to take more extreme action and visited a website where she learned how to vomit effectively. She did not change her eating pattern (and may even have increased her food consumption), and still took meals with the family, even going out with them to a restaurant and eating a full meal with pudding. However, over the next month she began to visibly lose weight. This pleased her, but worried her family who considered her to be at an appropriate weight already, and were puzzled by her weight loss despite apparently eating normally. They also noted her absences from the room and trips to the toilet immediately following meals. After some detective work, her family recognized the reason for her weight loss, and confronted her about it. As a result of this, she agreed to stop the purging. However, she found this difficult to do, and continued to eat and purge albeit at a lower frequency than before. Further confrontations with her family led her to seek help from a specialist clinic.

Formulation

The formulation here is quite simple. She was engaging in purging behaviours in a drive to reduce her weight, make her (in her view) more attractive to men, and to bolster her self-esteem which was increasingly dependent on her losing weight. Any intervention needed to reduce her bulimic behaviour, shift her self-esteem from being weight-dependent, and to increase her self-esteem and confidence in general.

Intervention

Following the Fairburn model, the first stage of the intervention involved planning a regular eating programme – eating three meals a day, but avoiding large meals or bingeing. The aim was to eat the required number of calories to maintain her weight, and no more. The planned meals and calorie intake provided some reassurance to Ms F that she would not put on weight even if she did not purge. To help her cope with the anxieties that would inevitably follow eating without purging, she planned things to do following each meal, to distract away from bingeing. She wanted her family to be involved in helping her, so at home this involved such things as going for walks or playing card games with her parents in the half to one hour following meals. This approach proved successful, and she quickly reduced the degree to which she was eating and purging.

The second phase of the intervention involved modifying her dysfunctional beliefs about her body shape. This involved cognitive work, including discussion of societal understandings of attractiveness, questioning the validity of the previous boyfriend's statement about her weight, and reliance on thinness as a requirement within a relationship. At a broader level, she also explored her expectations of relationships and through this exploration to be less absolutist about them: to be willing to enter relationships with no expectation of longevity or success and to enjoy the relationship for what it was 'in the moment' and not to feel she had to compromise herself in doing so. On a behavioural level, she explored meeting new partners through going out dancing with friends and joining a dating agency. This led to her meeting a number of men, all of whom found her attractive, reinforcing her improved self-confidence and lack of dependence on weight control as a means of facilitating relationships.

Interpersonal psychotherapy

One other psychological approach appears to be particularly effective in the treatment of bulimia. **Interpersonal psychotherapy (IPT)** may be effective in the light of commonly reported interpersonal problems experienced by people with bulimia (Thompson-Brenner 2016) because it focuses on strategies for improving interpersonal relationships. Two studies have compared the approach with cognitive therapy. In one comparison, Fairburn et al. (1993) found it to be less effective than cognitive therapy in the short term. However, at one-year follow-up the differences between the two conditions were not significant, as a result of continued improvements among those who received IPT. Remission rates at this time were 46% for IPT and 39% for cognitive behavioural therapy. The authors speculated that these gains in the IPT condition resulted from an improvement in self-worth and relationships, which made weight and shape much less important to the individual. As the effects of IPT are more indirect than cognitive methods, they took longer to become apparent. A second comparison of the two approaches was undertaken by Agras et al. (2000), who reported a similar outcome. Cognitive therapy proved more effective than IPT at the end of a 20-week intervention, with 29% and 6% fully recovered, respectively. However, at one-year follow-up, although the cognitive therapy still appeared more successful, the differences between the groups were no longer significant (40% versus 27%).

Pharmacological interventions

A review by Ramacciotti et al. (2013) led them to conclude that SSRIs are success-ful in 'transiently' reducing binge eating. However, evidence of longer-term effec-tiveness was not strong, indicating that psychological alternatives may be better. Grilo et al. (2005) provided the most rigorous evaluation of this issue, comparing 16 weeks of treatment with an SSRI, a drug placebo, CBT plus placebo, and CBT plus SSRI (but not CBT alone). Their results were interesting in that on their key measure of remission (absence of binges for one month), CBT plus placebo proved the most effective intervention and SSRI was no more effective than pla-cebo (or even slightly less effective). Remission rates amongst those who com-pleted the treatments were: SSRI, 29%; placebo 30%; CBT plus SSRI, 55%; CBT plus placebo, 73%. Among those who dropped out, the SSRI proved even less effective, with remission rates of 22% for the SSRI, 26% for the placebo, 50% for CBT plus SSRI, and 61% CBT plus placebo. It seems in some cases treatment with SSRI can actually be counter-productive. However, SSRIs may prove a useful intervention among people who do not respond to cognitive behavioural interventions (Walsh et al. 2000).

12.3 Chapter summary

1. Anorexia is defined by the desire to achieve a body weight significantly below normal. This can be achieved in two ways: self-imposed starvation, or binge-ing and purging.
2. Anorexia has a relatively poor prognosis, with long-term mortality rates of up to 16% and complete 'recovery' in just over half of cases.
3. Bulimia has a better prognosis, with most people achieving something like normal eating patterns.
4. Cognitive models suggest that both conditions are driven by cognitions that prioritize control over one's eating and weight. The behaviour of people with each condition varies as a result of their abilities to control their responses to hunger. People who engage in type 1 anorexic behaviour are able to control their hunger; those who are bulimic occasionally give in to urges to eat and compensate by purging.
5. Psychoanalytic models of anorexia suggest that it forms a rejection of sexual instincts and risk of pregnancy.

6. Bruch suggested that anorexia arose out of chaotic parent–child interactions that leave the child confused about their own emotional and physical needs. They turn to their parents to provide feedback on their own feelings. At the time of adolescence, they seek but fail to achieve autonomy from their parents. As a response, they seek excessive control over their size and shape.

7. Socio-cultural models emphasize the role of social pressures in shaping young women's striving for thinness and the perfect body.

8. Family models suggest anorexia results from aberrant family dynamics. Minuchin, for example, suggested that the person with anorexia serves to maintain family cohesion as the family focuses on them and their needs, and ignores the dysfunctional relationship between their parents.

9. There appears to be a genetic risk for anorexia, possibly mediated through disorders of serotonin metabolism.

10. Interventions in anorexia usually involve two stages: first, weight gain to safe levels, and second, longer-term interventions involving cognitive behavioural therapy, family therapy, psychotherapy or drug therapy. The best intervention for each individual may depend on the specific factors that led to their problems, with each of the psychological approaches being of benefit to some. The long-term prognosis, however, is not good.

11. Cognitive behavioural interventions are acknowledged as the treatment of choice in bulimia, with most people making significant long-term gains. However, in some contexts, pharmacological therapy using SSRIs may be advantageous.

12.4 For discussion

1. Should we actively treat people with anorexia who are close to dying as a result of their restrained eating, or should we respect their desire not to eat whatever the consequences?

2. Anorexia is perhaps one of the most difficult psychological conditions to treat. Given the success of cognitive behavioural techniques in other conditions, why does anorexia remain so problematic?

3. Bulimic behaviour could be considered a highly functional way of controlling weight. If this is the case, should it be treated only where the affected individual is distressed by their way of controlling their weight?

12.5 Further reading

Douzenis, A. and Michopoulos, I. (2015) Involuntary admission: the case of anorexia nervosa, *International Journal of Law and Psychiatry*, 39: 31–35.

Fairburn, C. (2008) *Cognitive Behavior Therapy and Eating Disorders*, New York: Guilford Press.

Fisher, C.A., Skocic, S., Rutherford, K.A. et al. (2019) Family therapy approaches for anorexia nervosa, *Cochrane Database of Systematic Reviews*, 5: CD004780 [https://doi.org/10.1002/14651858.CD004780.pub4].

Hail, L. and Le Grange, D. (2018) Bulimia nervosa in adolescents: prevalence and treatment challenges, *Adolescent Health, Medicine and Therapeutics*, 9: 11–16.

NICE (2017) *Eating disorders: recognition and treatment*, NICE Guideline NG69, London: NICE [https://www.nice.org.uk/guidance/ng69].

Treasure, J. and Alexander, J. (2013) *Anorexia Nervosa: A Recovery Guide for Sufferers, Families and Friends*, London: Routledge.

13 Schizophrenia

Schizophrenia is one of the most controversial psychiatric diagnoses. Over time, debates have addressed whether a distinct state of schizophrenia actually exists, whether it results from genetic or environmental causes, and whether it should be treated using drug therapy, **electroconvulsive therapy (ECT)**, or more social or psychological approaches. They have also addressed whether this broad all-inclusive, some would say 'over-inclusive', title could be better considered in terms of its component elements. This chapter will address each of these issues, and after reading it, you should have an understanding of:

- The nature of schizophrenia
- Alternative understandings of the 'symptoms' of schizophrenia
- The possible causal role of genetic factors, the family, and psychosocial factors
- Neuronal and **neurotransmitter** models of the disorder
- Psychological models of the experiences of people diagnosed with schizophrenia
- Differing approaches to the treatment of schizophrenia and its constituent elements: **delusions** and **hallucinations**.

13.1 What is schizophrenia?

Originally identified by Kraepelin in 1883, and termed *dementia praecox*, the condition was considered to be a progressive and deteriorating condition, with no recovery. Later redefined some 25 years later by Bleueler as 'schizophrenia' (literally, split mind), it was then considered to involve ambivalence, disturbance of association and mood, and a preference for fantasy over reality. Now, schizophrenia is characterized by disorders of perception and thinking, the most obvious of which are:

- *Delusions*: strong and unshakeable beliefs including: (i) control over other people or being controlled by others; (ii) grandeur, being somehow special or famous; and (iii) reference, believing the behaviour of others relates directly to the individual.
- *Hallucinations*: anomalous perceptual experiences, which may affect all senses, but are most often auditory. They may appear in the voice of the individual or others, and can be malicious, commanding or benevolent.

The exact nature of schizophrenia remains hotly disputed. However, the consensus view is that it comprises a number of related disorders characterized by fundamental distortions of thinking and perception. Disturbances in thought processes are usually the most obvious symptom of schizophrenia. Conversations may lack coherence, jumping from topic to topic and idea to idea in an apparently incoherent manner. People with schizophrenia may use **neologisms** or make bizarre associations between words. They may feel that someone is putting thoughts into their mind and lose track of their conversation or thoughts, perhaps not completing sentences. They may have deluded and sometimes bizarre beliefs about themselves or others. These may include *delusions of control* (being able to control or being controlled by others), *delusions of grandeur* (believing they are rich, famous, talented), and *delusions of reference* (believing the behaviour of others is directly related to them: glances, looks, laughter, are all seen as being directed at the individual). People with schizophrenia may also experience hallucinations, the most frequent of which are auditory. Their content may vary from benign to persecutory. The emotions that such people experience are often described as *flattened*. That is, they experience a general lack of emotional responsiveness, although they may be prone to apparently inappropriate mood states such as anger or depression as a consequence of internal thoughts or hallucinations.

For a formal diagnosis of schizophrenia to be made, DSM-5 states that two or more symptoms should be present for a significant period of time over a one-month period, and at least one of them must be among the first three symptoms identified below:

- delusions
- hallucinations
- disorganized speech: frequent derailment or incoherence
- grossly disorganized or **catatonic behaviour**
- **negative symptoms**: diminished emotional expression or **avolition.**

In addition, the symptoms must result in significant impairment and the 'disturbance' should persist for at least 6 months, unless successfully treated. A second way of considering the symptoms is to divide them into **positive symptoms**, such as the *presence* of hallucinations or delusions, and negative symptoms denoted by the *absence* of faculties (e.g. Kirkpatrick et al. 2006). The latter include:

- *Blunted affect*: the limitation of an individual's ability to convey his or her emotions, causing diminished facial and emotional expressions; a flat voice, lack of eye contact, and blank or restricted facial expressions.

- *Alogia* or 'poverty of speech': a decrease in verbal output or verbal expressiveness, often limited to 'yes' and 'no' in response to questions.
- *Asociality*: a lack of involvement in social relationships or increased desire to spend time alone.
- *Avolition*: a marked lack of motivation to engage in social activities or meet goals, combined with a striking lack of concern for both minor and major matters, including eating and self-care.
- *Anhedonia*: an inability to experience pleasure in normally pleasurable activities.

A key problem with the **DSM** diagnostic criteria is that the same diagnosis can be given to individuals who present with very different experiences and problems. This contradicts the notion of a disorder that has one underlying mechanism: if this were the case, all people should present with the same cluster of symptoms. A related point is that different people with schizophrenia respond to different medications, including **neuroleptics**, lithium, and benzodiazepines. Others fail to respond to any of these medications. Together, these led Bentall to note, 'We are inevitably drawn to an important conclusion: "schizophrenia" appears to be a disease which has no particular symptoms, no particular course, and responds to no particular treatment' (1993: 227). On these grounds, he suggested that the diagnosis has no validity and that the concept of schizophrenia should be abandoned. Rather than attempting to explain multiple syndromes, he argued, future efforts should focus on explanations of particular behaviours or experiences: each of the various symptoms of 'schizophrenia' should be considered as a disorder in its own right, with differing underlying causes and treatments. A further issue of relevance here is that the experiences of people diagnosed with schizophrenia are not exclusive to them. Many people who do not come to the attention of the psychiatric services also hear voices. What distinguishes between them and people who seek help for their 'problem' appears to be differences in their responses to the voices and their ability to cope with them. Positive coping strategies include setting limits to the time spent listening to voices, talking back to them, and listening selectively to more positive voices (Romme and Escher 2000).

This diversity of opinion presents a challenge when writing about the disorder. Biological explanations tend to focus on the broad diagnosis of schizophrenia, while psychological explanations focus on more discrete explanations of hallucinations and delusions. Similarly, while most intervention studies have been conducted under the rubric of schizophrenia, a number have now specifically targeted the influence and emotional impact of delusional thinking. Reflecting these historical processes, some parts of this chapter will use the term schizophrenia. Elsewhere, the terms **psychosis**, hallucinations or delusions are preferred and used to describe the relevant phenomena.

About 1% of adults are diagnosed as having some form of schizophrenia (APA 2000). The **prevalence** of schizophrenia appears to be stable across countries, cultures, and over time, with onset typically occurring between the ages of 20 and 35 years. On average, women develop the condition 3–4 years later than men and show a second peak of onset around the menopause. The highest population rates of schizophrenia are among those in the lower socio-economic groups (Werner et al. 2007). It is an episodic condition with a poor prognosis. Of those people that have one episode, approximately half will experience a significant reduction in symptoms over the following 5 years. However, only a quarter are likely to maintain good social and vocational functioning, and only an eighth will meet the criteria for full recovery for 2 years or more (Robinson et al. 2004). Factors associated with a good prognosis include receiving appropriate treatment, an acute onset and short duration of the first episode, the presence of an identifiable stress trigger, a predominance of positive symptoms, good social support, no family history of schizophrenia, and having a job.

Personal experiences

The experiences of people diagnosed with schizophrenia vary markedly, as does the degree to which any experiences interfere with their life. Many people experience delusions over long periods without any significant impact. For others, the experience may be much more problematic. Two examples of this may be found in the experiences of Michael and David. Michael was a middle-aged man diagnosed with schizophrenia some years ago who was living a relatively normal life in a small flat in Cardiff. One of his delusional beliefs was that he is being attacked by lasers from an unknown, probably extra-terrestrial, source:

The lasers attack me. They aim for my head. I know when they are firing because I have pains when they hit me. They don't fire at me all the time. They come and go. I don't know what I have done to have them do this to me. But it's been going on for years. They usually hit me in the head, so I wear protection against it when they fire. I wrap metal foil over my head so it reflects the lasers away ... that way they can't get to me ... I think they are aliens that do this ... The last time they fired at me was Sunday morning. They woke me up – the lasers – with my head really hurting. I couldn't get out of bed because of the pain. I had to wear protection and take my time to get going because of the pain ... That was bad. Usually I can stop the lasers with the metal, but it can get through sometimes.

It is perhaps not coincidental that Michael had spent much of Saturday night drinking beer in a local pub.

A more acute and devastating set of delusional beliefs resulted in David being admitted to hospital as he was running naked down the middle of a city road proclaiming that he was the son of God come to save us from our sins. At the time he was brought into casualty he was proclaiming:

I am the messiah! I am David, David, the saviour ... I will save you from the sins you have committed that commit you to the heat of the hell not heaven of the Lord my God. You cannot hold me ... God is angry with you, the world, the whole round ... the devil will take you for your sins of holding me here ... the nine that follow will kill you for holding the son of God in your hall ... I have come to save the world ... you cannot hold me ... By the writings of Methuselah and the prophets and God and Jesus I am here. God speaks to me! Not you! And he is angry at the wickedness of the world and the work of the people and the things they have done ... the sins, things ... wings of angels will come for me to take me away from this hell.

13.2 Aetiology of schizophrenia

Genetic factors

Early studies (e.g. Kringlen 1993) reported concordance rates for schizophrenia in **monozygotic (MZ) twins** of between 30% and 40%, and in **dizygotic (DZ) twins** of between 10% and 15%, suggesting a partly genetically mediated risk for schizophrenia. Subsequently, Tienari et al. (2000) compared rates of schizophrenia in the adopted-away offspring of both mothers diagnosed with schizophrenia and those without the diagnosis. Risk for schizophrenia was four times greater among the children of the women diagnosed as having schizophrenia than among those of the comparison mothers: a total **incidence** of 8.1% versus 2.3%. However, this was not entirely due to genetic factors. Using data from the same study, Wahlberg et al. (2000) reported an interaction between genetic and environmental factors. Children of women diagnosed with schizophrenia who lived in households where there was good communication between family members were not at increased risk of schizophrenia. By contrast, the children of women diagnosed as having schizophrenia who were placed in families with evidence of communication deviance were at greater risk of developing schizophrenia than children with 'typical' mothers who were placed in such households. That is, the development of schizophrenia seemed to depend on both genetic risk *and* communication deviance within the adoptive family. Importantly, any communication deviance seemed to pre-date the adoption, and was not a consequence of the child's behaviour.

Together, these and other data have generally been seen by biological theorists as supporting a model in which genetic factors influence risk for schizophrenia but do not form the single causal agent. They form a vulnerability factor rather than a causal factor. The search for the location of genes that increase risk of schizophrenia, however, remains. Nevertheless, some candidate genes involved in the development of schizophrenia are emerging, including the *ERBB4* gene, responsible for dopamine regulation (Lu et al. 2010), and the *5-HTR2A* gene (Tee et al. 2010), which is involved in serotonin regulation.

Perhaps the gene that has received most attention is the *DISC1* (Disrupted in Schizophrenia 1) gene. Originally linked to schizophrenia in a Scottish family (Millar et al. 2000), alleles of the *DISC1* gene appear to influence neural growth and proliferation, and a number of processes including mitochondrial transport and cell-to-cell adhesion. They are expressed in brain regions known to be involved in schizophrenia, including the cerebral cortex and hippocampus, and are involved in neural development and brain maturation. They are highly

expressed during critical periods of brain development, particularly in the prenatal period and the onset of puberty, although they are active throughout life.
Although their mechanism is not fully understood, it appears that when some
gene alleles fail to work effectively, maturation of the brain, in key areas relevant
to schizophrenia, are disrupted. Variants of the *DISC1* gene have been linked to
reduced grey matter density and volume, abnormal hippocampal structure/func-
tion, and impaired memory, although even here the evidence is inconsistent
(Ma et al. 2018).

Biological mechanisms

Any genetic potential is likely mediated through inherited neurological mechanisms. The most widely accepted neurological model of schizophrenia involves
the dopamine systems (e.g. Gründer and Cumming 2016). The key feature of the
dopamine hypothesis is that the experiences of people diagnosed with schizophrenia result from either an excess of dopamine, or from the receptors at neuronal synapses being supersensitive to normal amounts of dopamine. Evidence
generally supports the latter, but either way this theory suggests that at least
some of the experiences of schizophrenia may result from excess activity in those
parts of the brain controlled by dopamine, including the limbic system, the brain
area A10, and links to the thalamus, hippocampus and frontal cortex, and the
substantia nigra. Early evidence of increased dopamine activity came from a
number of converging types of study including the effectiveness of **phenothiazine**
neuroleptic drugs (see Chapter 4), which block transmission of dopamine by preventing its uptake at the postsynaptic receptor site, and post-mortem evidence
showing marked increases in dopamine receptor sites in people with schizophrenia compared with 'normal' controls, suggesting a super-sensitivity to dopamine
(Lieberman et al. 1990).

A developmental extension of the model of schizophrenia provides an explanation of why symptoms frequently begin in adolescence and early adulthood and
change in nature over time – with the positive symptoms that are dominant in the
early stages subsequently being replaced by negative symptoms. According to
this model, the dopamine levels of the young child are generally unexceptional.
However, as a consequence of the normal levels of stress associated with adolescence or young adulthood, and possibly heightened social stress as a consequence
of their odd and asocial behaviour, vulnerable individuals may experience excess
dopamine release within the relevant neurological systems. As a consequence,
they experience a number of the positive symptoms, which may last many years.
However, as excessive dopaminergic activity is neurotoxic, this eventually causes
degeneration of the dopaminergic neurons, reduces dopamine activity, and
allows the emergence of negative and **disorganized symptoms**. Evidence for
this neuronal degeneration can be found in consistent findings of enlarged cerebral **ventricles** and decreased cortical volume especially in the temporal and
frontal lobes of people diagnosed with schizophrenia (Basso et al. 1998). The various brain areas affected include systems that influence attention, memory, and
mood (limbic system), planning and coordination (frontal and prefrontal lobe),
and acoustic and verbal memory (temporal lobes). Bleich-Cohen et al. (2009), for

example, found reduced functional processing in the amygdale and prefrontal cortex to be associated with a lack of sensitivity to bizarre facial expressions presented on a computer screen.

Although any behavioural evidence of these neurological changes may take time to become evident, damage may occur at a very early stage in the development of schizophrenia. Wood et al. (2005) compared hippocampal volumes of 79 young male subjects at ultra-high risk of schizophrenia with those of 49 healthy male volunteers. The high-risk participants had significantly smaller hippocampal volumes than the comparison group, a finding that provides at least tangential support for a dopamine–hippocampal damage association. Despite the increasing ability of the dopamine model to account for the changing symptoms of schizophrenia over time, however, dopamine is clearly not the only neurotransmitter involved. New-generation neuroleptics (see Chapter 4), for example, work on serotonin levels, while GABA and NMDA have also been implicated (e.g. Guo et al. 2009). However, their involvement is probably in addition to dopamine rather than as alternative mechanisms of schizophrenia.

A second set of risk factors linked to schizophrenia involve insult to the developing foetus. One route through which this may occur involves maternal viral infection. Brown and Derkits (2010) found maternal exposure to the flu virus during the first trimester of pregnancy was associated with a seven-fold increase in risk of a child subsequently being diagnosed with schizophrenia. Other viruses associated with increased risk of schizophrenia include rubella and herpes simplex. Stress during pregnancy may also increase risk, evident among children of mothers who have experienced a family death while pregnant, as well as more extended stressors such as invasion during the Second World War and the Israeli Six-Day War (e.g. Malaspina et al. 2008). The factor common to all these processes appears to be immune function activation. An excess of pro-inflammatory cytokines associated with inflammation can result in brain cell abnormalities associated with schizophrenia, and (in animal studies) a wide spectrum of behavioural abnormalities including impaired social interaction, increased (and occasionally decreased) anxiety, and increased impulsivity (Watanabe et al. 2010). These abnormalities may be the result of impaired neural development similar to that associated with the *DISC1* gene.

So far, this section has identified a number of factors that either increase risk of developing schizophrenia or explain the chronic degenerative changes associated with the condition. Given the episodic nature of the condition, these are likely to be psychological. However, one biochemical trigger may also be implicated. Amphetamines can cause transient **psychotic** experiences and precipitate relapse of an existing psychotic condition (Harro 2015). Even more problematic may be cannabis use. Reviewing the evidence, Ortiz-Medina et al. (2018) found consistent evidence that young heavy cannabis users were at double the risk of non-users of developing schizophrenia, and that higher dosages and earlier use were predictive of greater risk. Caspi et al. (2005) suggested that this risk may be largely specific to individuals with a particular genetic make-up (involving a functional polymorphism in the catechol-O-methyltransferase [*COMT*] gene): a contention that has largely been supported in subsequent studies (Misiak et al. 2018). A potential biochemical route through which cannabis exerts this influence has also been determined. The active metabolite of cannabis (delta-9 tetrahydrocannabinol) raises levels of cerebral dopamine and might precipitate psychosis. People with early experiences of schizophrenia may also take cannabis as a form of self-treatment to alleviate either negative experiences or depression (Peralta and Cuesta 1992), reversing the causal link.

Psychosocial factors

Developmental models identify some of the childhood stresses that increase vulnerability to schizophrenia, mediated through dopaminergic dysregulation. Not surprisingly, perhaps, childhood traumas such as sexual abuse or neglect are considered important risk factors. Varese et al. (2012), for example, reviewed the strong association between childhood abuse, whether physical or sexual, and schizophrenia. The prevalence of childhood sexual abuse among women and men diagnosed with schizophrenia or similar disorders was found to be between 22–46% and 22–39%, respectively: both rates are roughly double those in the wider population. The trauma is also likely to have begun at a relatively early age. Children diagnosed with schizophrenia are also more likely to have experienced parental hostility, to have run away from home, and to be placed in a children's home. Men who experienced parental abstinence and institutionalization during childhood are at higher than average risk of experiencing a range of experiences that include thought disorder, hallucinations, and delusions. There is also evidence of dopamine dysregulation in children and adults who experienced childhood trauma (Pruessner et al. 2004). In addition, the extent of damage to areas of adult brains, including to the hippocampus and prefrontal cortex, associated with excess dopamine activity appears to be related to the occurrence and severity of childhood sexual abuse (Egerton et al. 2016).

One of the first theories to consider a more subtle parental influence identified the mother–child relationship as a critical factor in schizophrenia. This psychoanalytic theory, developed by Fromm-Reichman (1948), suggested that schizophrenia is the outcome of being raised by a mother who appears warm and self-sacrificing, but is in reality self-centred, cold, and domineering: the *schizophrenogenic mother*. Fromm-Reichman suggested that the mixed signals that such a mother gives out confuse the child and make their world difficult to interpret, a process that eventually leads to chaotic behaviour and cognitions. A similar theory was proposed by Bateson et al. (1956). Their 'double-bind' theory suggested that some parents frequently deal with their children in contradictory and confusing ways. They may, for example, tell their children they love them in a tone of voice that implies the opposite, or ask them to do incompatible things: 'I think you should go out more often with your friends: please stay with me …'. Frequent exposure to these contradictory demands may confuse the child, and eventually prove so stressful that it results in the experience of schizophrenia. Both models have some logic, but they have little evidence in their support.

One family theory has proven more robust. A critical element in the family process seems to be the degree of family criticism that the individual experiences. According to this model, high levels of negative emotional expression, hostility or criticism may trigger a relapse in someone who has already had at least one episode of schizophrenia. The classic study of this phenomenon, now known as high negative expressed emotion (NEE), was that of Vaughn and Leff (1976) on readmission rates of people with schizophrenia discharged from the Maudsley Hospital during the 1970s. Their findings were dramatic: those who were discharged to high NEE households were much more likely to relapse than those whose home was rated low in NEE, particularly when they experienced this family environment for 35 hours or more a week. These findings have since been replicated in a number of countries and cultures (e.g. Weintraub et al. 2017).

The majority of studies have considered high NEE to be a trigger to relapse, though not to a first episode. As such, the high NEE environment is often thought to be a consequence of a family coping with an individual within it whose behaviour may be at odds with family values and processes. High NEE lies within a circle of causality, being both a response to 'difficult' or inexplicable behaviour and a contributor to its development. In keeping with this model, levels of NEE tend to be higher in families where odd behaviour is seen as wilful and under the control of the individual, and lower where it is attributed to an illness or an uncontrollable cause (Yang et al. 2004). Evidence that family processes may also trigger the initial onset of schizophrenia in vulnerable individuals can be found in Wahlberg and colleagues' (2000) study described earlier in the chapter. Also of note is that family processes may be moderated by a number of individual, cognitive, factors. Kéri and Kelemen (2009), for example, found that individuals with particularly poor attention and immediate memory experienced more 'unusual thoughts' and were the subject of more family criticism than those who had better attention and memory.

A psychobiological model

Combining the psychosocial and biological data suggests a possible stress–vulnerability model of schizophrenia involving three broad stages (Duncan et al. 1999):

- The first stage is one of disordered neuronal development resulting from genetic, natal or perinatal factors. These problems underlie subtle early cognitive, motor, and social impairments that constitute a *vulnerability* for schizophrenia.
- These deficiencies may lead to the second stage, which occurs in adolescence and early adulthood. At this time, stressful but normal human experiences result in increases in dopamine activity. As a consequence of this neuronal disorganization, dopaminergic neuronal systems become sensitized to existing levels of dopamine and become more reactive to them, resulting in the positive symptoms of schizophrenia. The greater the stress experienced, the greater the risk of dysregulation and onset of schizophrenia.
- If prolonged or recurrent, high levels of dopamine can lead to the degeneration of neurons, leading to structural damage, and the onset of negative symptoms.

Accordingly, the dysregulation that underpins schizophrenia may be a consequence of both biological factors that increase vulnerability and stress factors that trigger or exacerbate the condition. This model is consistent with findings that children who go on to develop schizophrenia have cognitive deficits including those related to **executive function** indicative of mild neural damage (e.g. Cannon et al. 2006). In addition, Poulton et al. (2000) found that 'quasi-psychotic phenomena' (including beliefs that people were reading their minds or spying on them) reported by young people were strong predictors of later psychosis. Accordingly, one can envisage a model in which these behaviours are both markers and contributors to risk if they trigger negative social responses, which contribute to additional stresses in childhood, and trigger the dopaminergic responses.

Stop and think ...

Schizophrenia is a devastating condition with significant impact on the individual, those close to them, and wider society in terms of the cost of care. If we can identify people at risk for schizophrenia as a consequence of their family history, genes or behavioural characteristics, are we duty bound to work with the families and schools of 'at-risk' children to try and prevent an initial psychotic episode thereby improving their quality of life and life chances? Or is this intrusive to the families, likely to lead to discrimination towards affected children and adolescents, and a significant use of resources that could be better targeted elsewhere?

Psychological models

Rather than attempt to identify factors that trigger 'episodes' of 'schizophrenia', psychological models of schizophrenia typically attempt to explain the processes that underlie each of the different experiences reported by people assigned the diagnosis.

Theory of mind

One of the most encompassing psychological models of schizophrenia was initially developed by Frith (e.g. Frith and Corcoran 1996). He proposed that our understanding of the social world around us depends on being able to interpret the causes of our own actions and the actions of other people. In social situations, we interpret others' verbal and non-verbal signals in order to try and understand what they are thinking, feeling, what they believe, what is real, and so on. In order to do so, theory of mind suggests we first of all need to understand our own cognitive processes, the way *we* interpret our world, and then translate this knowledge to understand the actions of others. A failure in this process makes it difficult to understand the social signals during any interaction and to understand the full meaning of any conversation: to understand the world we inhabit.

Frith suggested that a key deficit of people with schizophrenia is that they do not have a fully intact theory of mind. They cannot fully understand their own cognitive processes: in particular, they can have difficulties in monitoring their own intentions, leading to feelings of passivity and being out of control of their own actions. Other phenomena associated with this problem include the belief that thoughts are being placed in an individual's mind by others, and auditory hallucinations. In addition, affected individuals cannot understand the minds of other people, and therefore find it difficult to interpret what other people are thinking or feeling. This may lead to delusions of paranoia and reference. Finally, because such individuals find it difficult to interpret their world, they may become withdrawn and isolated in order to avoid any distress or confusion such attempts may engender.

The degree to which these problems exist varies across individuals. According to Frith, some people with a diagnosis of schizophrenia may have a complete inability to represent other people's mental states. In this, they may be similar to individuals who are autistic. Others, including those with paranoid delusions, have some understanding that other people have minds and motivations, but make significant errors due to an inaccurate or poorly developed theory of mind.

This theory has significant implications for a variety of processes involved in the symptoms of schizophrenia. It also provides a number of experimentally testable hypotheses. Such studies have attempted to identify how well people diagnosed with schizophrenia can understand other people's mental states, often through the use of analogue studies. These can involve quite complex cognitive tasks. One of the simpler methodologies has involved exploration of the understanding of jokes that involve deception, and therefore require an intact theory of mind to understand. In one such study, Marjoram et al. (2005) presented 20 people diagnosed with schizophrenia and 20 controls with 63 single-image cartoons. Thirty-one of these were considered to be 'theory of mind cartoons', in that understanding the joke required an attribution of ignorance, false belief or deception to one of its characters and, therefore, an analysis of their mental state. The other jokes were more slapstick in nature and subsequently did not require theory of mind capabilities for their correct interpretation. People with a diagnosis of schizophrenia showed less understanding of both types of jokes than the control group, as has been found elsewhere. In addition, they showed significantly less understanding of the theory of mind jokes than the slapstick cartoons, suggesting impairment in their theory of mind. Craig et al. (2004) used two tasks to measure theory of mind in people with paranoid delusions and healthy controls. The first assessed their ability to infer an individual's intentions based on hints within a short written passage; the second measured their ability to detect 'cognitive emotions' such as being embarrassed or pensive (which require inferences about other people's beliefs or intentions to fully understand) from photographs of faces showing only the eye region. People with a diagnosis of schizophrenia performed less well in both tasks.

A new generation of studies has not only found deficits of theory of mind in people with schizophrenia, but have begun to explore the neural substrates of these difficulties. Brüne et al. (2011), for example, recorded fMRI scans of people with a diagnosis of schizophrenia and 'healthy controls' while they were engaging in a task thought to trigger a 'theory of mind network'. The scans measured activity within a number of brain regions, including the prefrontal cortex and the cingulate cortex which are involved in distinguishing self from other, error monitoring and prediction, and in 'decoupling' hypothetical states from reality.

Levels of activation of this network were lower in people diagnosed with schizophrenia than in control participants. These findings have been replicated in a number of studies and can be considered relatively robust (see Jáni and Kašpárek 2018).

Hallucinations as a failure of attention

A number of explanations for hallucinations have been based on an early theory of attention and memory developed by Broadbent (1971). Early work suggested that people with schizophrenia were unable to filter out irrelevant and unwanted stimuli. They could not filter out, or decide, which were appropriate or inappropriate elements of their environment to attend to. As a consequence, they felt overwhelmed by sensory experiences and found it difficult to concentrate and respond to their environment appropriately. This approach was extended by Hemsley (1996), who considered many of the symptoms of schizophrenia to result from two key failures of processing:

- an impairment of the rapid and automatic assessment of sensory input
- a breakdown in relationship between stored memories and current sensory input.

Hemsley suggested that the focus of our attention within our sensory field is a consequence of our previous experience. We store in our memory what he referred to as 'regularities'; that is, information that determines our expectations or interpretations of any situation. This regulates our reactions in similar but novel situations. These processes occur rapidly and automatically and allow us to focus on what is important within our environment, and what is not. As a result of these stored memories, we know what to attend to when we go into a shop to buy a pair of shoes, when we play football, and so on. According to Hemsley, these automatic processes do not occur in people with schizophrenia, and the individual is unable to focus their attention appropriately. They attend to everything within their environment and become overwhelmed by sensory information. Three key problems arise from this sensory barrage:

- Hallucinations result from a failure to filter out redundant information and from giving all stimuli equal weight
- The individual's own thoughts cannot be distinguished from external stimuli, and can be perceived as an external voice
- Delusions occur when trying to impose meaning on a barrage of confusing internal and external stimuli.

This model explains the positive symptoms of schizophrenia. But Hemsley was also able to explain some of the negative symptoms. He suggested that symptoms such as social withdrawal, impoverished speech, and flat affect may arise either as a consequence of, or as a coping strategy with, this sensory overload.

Evidence for some of the key elements of the theory can be derived from a number of sources. One source of support stems from studies of people with speech hallucinations. There is consistent evidence that people with hallucinations have difficulty in identifying the spatial location of sounds and are less accurate than controls in determining the meaning of words when spoken against a background of white noise, despite being highly confident of the meaning they attach to such sounds. In one investigation of this phenomenon, Hoffman et al. (1999) examined the performance of three groups of people during a variety of tasks: individuals with a history of hallucinations, a diagnosis of schizophrenia but no history of hallucinations, and 'typical' controls. They took part in a masked speech tracking task with three levels of superimposed phonetic noise. Participants were asked to repeat the sentences they heard, as they heard them – to assess grammar-dependent verbal working memory. They also took part in a non-verbal tracking task to assess any differences in attention between the three groups. People with a history of hallucinations performed less well on the speech tracking task but were not impaired on the non-verbal tracking task. The authors took this to indicate that hallucinated voices in schizophrenia arise from disrupted speech perception and verbal working memory systems rather than from non-language cognitive or attentional deficits. Rossell and Boundy (2005) subsequently found that people who hallucinated were particularly poor at distinguishing words with an affective meaning, leaving them susceptible to misinterpreting emotionally laden words in ordinary life. More recently, evidence that people prone to hallucinations, and more likely to be distressed by them, are also more likely to be self-focused, provides tangential support for a model of biased attention (Úbeda-Gómez et al. 2015).

In a study of the neurological processes that may contribute to this phenomenon, McGuire et al. (1996) used positron emission tomography to measure the brain activity of people with a history of hallucinations, people with a diagnosis of schizophrenia with no such history, and 'typical' controls while they took part in a number of tasks. In the first condition, in which participants were asked to simply talk to themselves in their head, there were no differences in brain activity between the groups. However, when they were asked to imagine someone else talking in their head, people who had experienced hallucinations showed different brain activity from the other two groups. The 'hallucinations' group showed reduced activation in the left middle temporal gyrus and the rostral supplementary motor area regions, which were strongly activated in the other two groups. As this area is implicated in the monitoring of inner speech, they took this deficit to be a neurological substrate of the failure to identify the source of verbal information and for the hallucinations this group experienced.

A cognitive model of delusions

Perhaps the most common understanding of delusional beliefs is that they are qualitatively different from those held by 'ordinary people'. Bentall (e.g. Bentall and Fernyhough 2008) has argued that delusions are at the extreme end of a continuum of types of thought that runs from 'ordinary thoughts' to those that are bizarre and impossible, but all of which are the end-product of similar cognitive processes. Cognitions, including delusions, are seen as an interpretation of events, maybe even a rational attempt to make sense of anomalous circumstances. While the thought content may be out of the ordinary, the psychological processes underpinning it are not.

The model of persecutory beliefs developed by Bentall et al. (2001) drew on the humanistic concepts of the actual and ideal self. They suggested that many people with schizophrenia have a poor self-image and experience significant discrepancies between their actual- and ideal-self; that is, how they see themselves and how they would like to be. According to Bentall and colleagues, when discrepancies between actual- and ideal-self are activated by negative life events or other triggers, the individual tries to minimize this discrepancy by shifting this attribution onto others, as a form of psychological defence: 'I think I am OK, even though others don't'. It may be less distressing for the individual to think that others think poorly of them than to accept their own feelings of inadequacy.

Bentall and colleagues further suggested that the natural history of schizophrenia within the family can be explained by this model, as attributional styles may be learned from other family members, and parental criticism may precipitate relapse by triggering actual–ideal self-discrepancies. Developmental processes that may contribute to this attributional style implicate insecure attachment in childhood which continues into adulthood, combined with low self-esteem and difficulty in trusting others. Repeated experiences of victimization are likely to exacerbate negative self-esteem while provoking an externalizing explanatory style in which negative events are assumed to be caused by powers external to the self.

Evidence for this model has accrued since Bentall's original postulation, to the degree that Murphy et al. (2018) were able to conduct a **meta-analysis** of 27 relevant studies, and found evidence that people with persecutory delusions had a greater external attribution bias than general populations and people with psychosis but not experiencing delusions. In addition, paranoia severity was correlated with the degree of externalizing attribution bias. It should be noted, however, that the evidence is not unequivocal, with researchers such as Humphreys and Barrowclough (2006) failing to find evidence of this process specific to paranoid delusions, while Meehl et al. (2014) found that people with persecutory delusions showed a 'self-blaming' attribution style and were *more* likely to attribute negative events to themselves than others.

A trauma model of hallucinations

Romme and Escher (2000) began their exploration of the nature of hallucinations by considering them to be a normal response to traumatic events, particularly bereavement and sexual or physical assault. They considered that their function is to draw attention to emotional traumas that need resolving and to provide a defence against the emotional upset associated with them by placing them into the third person. This may be considered a form of dissociation similar to that involved in the processing of traumatic memories discussed in Chapter 9. The goal of therapy should therefore be to help people develop strategies to understand the meaning of the voices, not to rid them of their voices. This approach has received little empirical attention. However, one key element of their model is that many people hear voices. What distinguishes those who become 'patients' and those that do not is that the latter group perceive their voices as predominantly positive, are not alarmed by them, and feel in control of the experience (Powers et al. 2017)

In a review of data relevant to this model, Luhrmann et al. concluded that 'trauma sometimes plays a major role in hallucinations, sometimes a minor role, and sometimes no role at all' (2019: S24), a finding not dissimilar to that in many other mental health states. Nevertheless, Romme and Escher have had a significant impact on the normalization of the experiences of people with schizophrenia and supporting people who hear voices. The 'hearing voices network' (e.g. https://www.hearing-voices.org/), inspired by their work and supported by them, provides support to people with this type of experience. It started in the Netherlands in 1987 but now can be found worldwide. The aims of the network are:

- to raise awareness of voice hearing, visions, tactile sensations, and other sensory experiences
- to give people who have these experiences an opportunity to talk freely about this together
- to support anyone with these experiences seeking to understand, learn, and grow from them.

Support is provided through self-help groups, training sessions for health workers and the general public, an internet discussion site, and a telephone helpline.

13.2 Treatment of schizophrenia

Antipsychotic medication

Most people diagnosed with schizophrenia receive some form of medication, although dosages may be reduced or even discontinued during periods of remission. Chlorpromazine, haloperidol, and clozapine are three of the most commonly used drugs (see Chapter 4 for a review of their mode of action and effectiveness). Their most striking effect is one of sedation. They also have a direct effect on hallucinations and delusions, although their effectiveness varies markedly between individuals. Chlorpromazine and haloperidol seem to affect only the positive symptoms of schizophrenia. Clozapine, an atypical neuroleptic, is more successful in treating both positive and negative symptoms, and is often effective when other treatments fail (Essali et al. 2009).

Antipsychotic medication has been so successful in treating people with schizophrenia that their typical hospital stay during an acute episode has declined to less than 13 days, when formerly it was months, years, even a lifetime. Appropriate medication also lies at the heart of the relatively good levels of relapse (10% in the first year) reported earlier in the chapter, with a ten-fold increase in risk of relapse over a 2-year period if medication is not taken (Morken et al. 2008). Nevertheless, these antipsychotics appear to delay relapse rather than prevent it, and their use is not without problems. They have a variety of side-effects that frequently lead those receiving them to minimize or stop their use. Side-effects of chlorpromazine, for example, include a dryness of mouth and throat, drowsiness, visual disturbances, weight gain or loss, skin sensitivity to sunlight, constipation, and depression. More problematic, however, are what are known as **extrapyramidal symptoms**. These include the symptoms of Parkinsonism and tardive dyskinesia (see Chapter 4), which have been estimated to affect over a quarter of individuals who receive medium- to long-term neuroleptic treatment. Treatment by clozapine or other atypical neuroleptics does not carry this risk, but those who receive clozapine may be at risk of a condition known as **agranulocytosis**, which results in significant impairment of the immune system and can result in death. In addition, although **psychomotor** symptoms may not occur, people on clozapine experience more drowsiness, hypersalivation, and increases in temperature than those given conventional neuroleptics. Despite this, clozapine is the preferred medication (Essali et al. 2009).

Adherence to antipsychotic drug regimens can be as low as 25% among people living in the community (Donohoe et al. 2001). This does not seem to be associated with sociodemographic variables, severity of the disorder, or even the extent to which people experience extrapyramidal symptoms. Instead, low adherence seems to be related to attitudes towards medication, expectations of drug effectiveness, available social support, and the quality of the therapeutic alliance. Poor memory may contribute to accidental non-adherence.

Strategies to maximize adherence include education, developing a high-quality therapeutic alliance, the use of memory aids for those with a poor memory, and money! Financial incentives certainly are of benefit, with Moran and Priebe (2016) reporting increases in adherence from 68% to 88% following a year's incentive scheme, which gave participants between £75 and £735 over the year as rewards for receiving **depot injections** with a relatively long active therapeutic life. Regression analyses identified improved adherence, but not financial gain, to be predictive of improved quality of life during the scheme. One relatively new strategy is known as motivational interviewing (Miller and Rollnick 2013). This approach encourages the recipient to choose whether or not to take their medication as a result of a careful exploration of the costs and benefits to them of doing so. This gives them a degree of control over their treatment and maintains or improves the therapeutic alliance as the therapist is not seen as coercive. It also allows any misunderstandings about medication to be identified and corrected and seems to be more effective in encouraging drug use than direct attempts at persuasion (Coffey 1999). In one exploration of this approach, Kemp et al. (1998) compared motivational interviewing designed to increase adherence to medication with routine care following relapse. The group which received the motivational approach showed higher levels of adherence to the drug regimen and lower readmission rates over an 18-month period. This positive finding compares well against even quite sophisticated education programmes involving several sessions, which have not proven so effective (e.g. Byerly et al. 2005).

Psychological approaches

Psychoanalytic approaches

One of the first psychosocial treatments of schizophrenia was developed by Harry Stack Sullivan in the early part of the twentieth century. Sullivan (1953) considered schizophrenia to involve difficulties in living arising from problems in personal and social relationships, and that 'personality warps' were the lasting residue of earlier unsatisfactory personal experiences. His treatment approach involved examination of the individual's life history and the historical roots and current ramifications of their maladaptive interpersonal patterns, evident in their relationship with their doctor and in daily life. Characteristic difficulties were thought to include a basic mistrust of others, and a marked ambivalence in relationships, with swings between a longing for, and a terror of, close relationships. Resolution of this conflict through the psychotherapeutic process was thought to result in improvements in psychosis, and maturation of the patient and their non-psychotic personality. While Sullivan's interventions were important, as they encouraged the psychological treatment of people with schizophrenia, the approach has been found to be less effective than supportive therapy and although a few proponents are still advocating the use of **psychoanalysis** (Lucas 2003), it is not a recommended form of treatment in most healthcare systems.

Family interventions

The recognition that high NEE was contributing to relapse in schizophrenia resulted in a number of studies of family interventions targeted at its reduction. In one of the earliest of these, Leff and Vaughn (1985) randomly assigned people with schizophrenia who had at least 35 hours per week face-to-face contact with family members in a high NEE household to a family intervention or usual care condition. The intervention included a **psychoeducational programme** that focused on methods of reducing NEE within the household, family support, and the opportunity for family therapy. The programme was highly successful. Nine months after the end of therapy, 8% of the people in the treatment group had relapsed, in contrast to 50% of those in the comparison group. At 2-year follow-up, 40% of the treatment group and 78% of the control group had relapsed. A similar therapeutic approach was adopted by Falloon et al. (1982). Their intervention included education about the role of family stress in triggering episodes of schizophrenia and working with the family to develop family problem-solving skills. Their results were equally impressive. At 9-month follow-up, 5% of the people in families receiving treatment had relapsed, in contrast to 44% of those receiving standard medical treatment. At 2-year follow-up, relapse rates were 16% and 83%, respectively. Such is the success and proliferation of data following these seminal studies, Pharoah et al. (2010) was able to conclude that data from 53 family interventions showed a reduction in risk of relapse of about 50% when compared with standard medical care. They also noted that family interventions decreased the frequency of admissions to hospital, time spent in hospital, and improved compliance with medication regimens.

Cognitive behaviour therapy

Two forms of CBT are typically used with people with a diagnosis of schizophrenia. The first, **stress management**, involves working with individuals to help them cope with the stress leading to or associated with psychotic experiences. The second, known as belief modification, involves attempts to change the nature of delusional beliefs the individual may hold.

Stress management

Stress management approaches involve a detailed evaluation of the problems and experiences an individual is having, their triggers and consequences, and developing strategies to help cope with them. These include cognitive techniques such as distraction from intrusive thoughts or **cognitive challenge**, increasing or decreasing social activity as a means of distraction from intrusive thoughts or low mood, and using relaxation techniques.

This approach has proven successful in preventing or delaying individuals at high risk of developing schizophrenia moving into a first episode. McGorry et al. (2002), for example, randomized such individuals into either supportive psychotherapy focusing on social, work or family issues, or low-dose risperidone therapy combined with CBT. Each intervention lasted for 6 months. By the end of treatment, 36% of the people who received supportive psychotherapy progressed to first episode psychosis compared with 10% in the CBT–risperidone group. Short-term gains were also found following a purely cognitive intervention by Morrison et al. (2006), but at 3-year follow-up the intervention proved no more successful than usual care. Other studies have evaluated interventions intended to promote recovery following an acute episode of schizophrenia. In one such study, Tarrier et al. (2000) randomly assigned individuals to either drug therapy alone, or in combination with stress management or supportive counselling. The stress management intervention involved 20 sessions in 10 weeks, followed by four booster sessions over the following year. By the end of the first phase of treatment, those who received this intervention evidenced a greater improvement than those in the supportive counselling group, while people who received only drug therapy showed a slight deterioration. One-third of the people who received stress management achieved a 50% reduction in psychotic experiences; only 15% of the supportive counselling group achieved this level of benefit. Fifteen per cent of the stress management group and 7% of the supportive counselling condition were free of all positive symptoms. None of those in the drug therapy group achieved this criterion. One year later, there remained significant differences between the three groups, favouring those in the stress management condition. At 2-year follow-up, those who received only drug therapy had significantly more problems than those in the psychological treatment groups. However, the two psychological interventions proved equally effective.

Belief modification

More recently, psychological studies have begun to explore the impact of cognitive interventions focusing on changing the fundamental processes driving psychosis. Belief modification involves the use of verbal challenge and behavioural hypothesis-testing to counter delusional beliefs and/or hallucinations. Verbal challenge encourages the individual to view a delusional belief as just one of several possibilities. The person is not told that the belief is wrong but is asked to consider an alternative view provided by the therapist. New possibilities may then be tested in the 'real world' as appropriate. A similar process is used to challenge hallucinations, focusing on the patient's beliefs about their power, identity, and purpose. Behavioural hypothesis-testing involves challenging any thoughts in a more direct, behavioural way (see also discussion of these issues in Chapter 2).

This approach may be enhanced by additional components, including teaching general coping skills, motivational strategies for increasing adherence to medication, and CBT programmes and vocational support (e.g. Barton et al. 2009). In one study of this approach, Drury et al. (2000) reported the outcome of an intervention which involved both individual and group cognitive therapy in which participants learned to cope with delusions and hallucinations. In addition, they took part in a 6-month family psychoeducation programme and an activity programme including life-skills groups. The effects of this intervention were compared with those of an activity programme involving participants in sports, leisure, and social groups. The short- and mid-term impacts of the intervention were impressive. Those in the active therapeutic programme recovered more quickly following the relapse that brought them into therapy. At 9-month follow-up, 56% of the control group still had moderate or severe problems, compared with 5% of the intervention group. At 5-year follow-up, however, there was no evidence of any differences between the two groups as regards relapse rates or levels of positive symptoms. To achieve longer-term benefits, it may be necessary to introduce a second, perhaps less extensive, 'booster' intervention.

In a subsequent review, Health Quality Ontario (2018) examined the impact of this approach, focusing on interventions with between 16 sessions for first episode psychosis and 24 sessions for people who had relapsed or did not respond to pharmacological interventions. Participants in the studies they reviewed were typically receiving pharmacological intervention in both conditions. Summarizing the data, they noted that when compared with usual care, CBT programmes significantly improved overall psychotic symptoms, positive symptoms including hallucinations and delusions, and negative symptoms including blunted affect immediately following treatment. No significant gains were found on measures of social function, distress associated with psychosis, relapse or quality of life.

Research box 12

Morrison, A.P., Law, H., Carter, L. et al. (2018) Antipsychotic drugs versus cognitive behavioural therapy versus a combination of both in people with psychosis: a randomised controlled pilot and feasibility study, *Lancet Psychiatry*, 5: 411–23.

This is one of the few, and slightly controversial, studies directly comparing treatment with antipsychotics, CBT in unmedicated individuals, and a combination of the two. The contentious issue for the study is that it involved withholding what is a relatively 'standard' treatment with antipsychotics for those in the CBT-alone condition, and was therefore potentially unethical. The authors argue that the high levels of side-effects and poor adherence justify this manipulation.

Method

Participants

Eligible participants were over 15 years old, help-seeking, and met the ICD-10 criteria for schizophrenia, schizoaffective disorder or delusional disorder. Alternatively, they met the criteria for entry into a local psychosis service: on the Positive and Negative Syndrome Scale (PANSS) they scored >3 on the delusions or hallucinations items, or >4 on items measuring suspiciousness, persecution, and grandiosity. Exclusion criteria included being prescribed antipsychotic medication or receiving CBT with a qualified therapist within the past 3 months, or a score of >4 on the PANSS conceptual disorganization item.

Interventions

- *Cognitive behaviour therapy*: participants allocated to CBT received up to 26 sessions of cognitive therapy targeted at delusions and hallucinations (see more details in chapter). Up to four optional booster sessions were accessible over the following 6 months. Therapy sessions were usually offered weekly and delivered by qualified psychological therapists.
- *Pharmacological intervention*: antipsychotics were prescribed by the participants' responsible psychiatrist. They could switch antipsychotics, prescribe other necessary medication, and adjust doses as clinically indicated. Clinicians were encouraged to continue antipsychotic treatment for a minimum of 12 weeks, and preferably for at least 26 weeks.
- *Combined intervention*: participants received both forms of intervention.

Due to ethical concerns, participants assigned to either the CBT or pharmacological condition could be moved to the combined treatment group if their mental state declined during the study.

Measures

Measures were taken at baseline and at 6 weeks, 3 and 6 months, and one year.

- *Positive and Negative Syndrome Scale (PANSS)*: the total score of the PANSS, a semi-structured interview assessing dimensions of psychosis (delusions, hallucinations, suspiciousness, persecution, grandiosity, and conceptual disorganization).
- *Hospital Anxiety and Depression Scale (HADS)*: a well-validated (non-hospital-focused) measure of anxiety and depression, reported below as a combined measure of mood disturbance (HADS-total).
- *World Health Organization Quality of Life (WHOQoL)*: a quality-of-life measure.
- *Clinical Global Impressions (CGI)* of symptom severity and recovery. This comprises two 7-point clinician (CGI-C) and patient (CGI-P) completed scales providing an overall judgement of each domain. Reported here are the total scores.
- *Questionnaire about the Process of Recovery (QPR)*: a user-defined measure of recovery.

Results

Of 138 people screened for potential entry into the study, 75 were randomly assigned to each condition. Table 1 reports the means and standard deviations of key outcomes at baseline, close to end of therapy (week 12), and at 6- and 12-month follow-ups.

Table 1 Mean scores (and standard deviations) and relevant probability values on key outcomes over time

	Pharmacological	CBT	Combined	Significance
PANSS				
Baseline	70.13 (10.11)	70.35 (8.03)	70.76 (8.46	CBT vs.
24 weeks	60.81 (16.52)	63.74 (7.73)	58.40 (14.51)	Combined
6 months	61.09 (14.44)	60.50 (8.74)	53.77 (12.54)	$p = 0.019$
12 months	56.77 (14.10)	58.14 (11.68)	57.40 (13.58)	
QPR				
Baseline	38.71 (9.23)	40.13 (9.33)	41.8 (11.79)	All
24 weeks	44.86 (14.99)	47.81 (8.86)	52 (14.05)	comparisons
12 months	48.55 (14.73)	51.62 (9.25)	49.88 (11.04)	NS
HADS – total				
Baseline	41.05 (5.49)	37.54 (5.42)	36.36 (6.76)	All
24 weeks	35.55 (7.69)	35.36 (12.61)	30.37 (9.28)	comparisons
12 months	34.27 (9.08)	32.14 (6.96)	30.35 (6.98)	NS
WHOQoL				
Baseline	67.03 (14.99)	68.66 (13.41)	70.18 (15.41)	All
24 weeks	79.15 (20.95)	79.10 (14.03)	89.06 (18.87)	comparisons
12 months	81.36 (20.02)	83.81 (15.23)	82.93 (19.17)	NS
CGI-C				
Baseline	4.13 (0.74)	4.08 (0.63)	4.04 (0.68)	CBT versus
24 weeks	3.32 (1.17)	3.45 (0.91)	2.86 (1.06)	combined
12 months	3.23 (1.11)	3.38 (1.07)	3.00 (1.08)	$p = 0.026$
CGI-P				
Baseline	4.91 (0.97)	4.42 (0.99)	4.38 (1.54)	All
24 weeks	4.33 (1.56)	3.71 (1.23)	3.20 (1.54)	comparisons
12 months	3.91 (1.48)	3.50 (1.50)	3.94 (1.59)	NS

N.B. 6-month data was not available for some measures.

Discussion

This was a pilot study. That is, its intention was to determine the feasibility of the study design and the **effect size** of any between-group differences. This type of study forms a safety check, and should precede larger, more highly powered studies. However, the relatively few participants enrolled means that the study was somewhat underpowered and may have failed to identify significant differences between conditions that would be found in a larger trial. Nevertheless, the results are intriguing and suggest that while a combined intervention with both pharmacological and psychological interventions may be optimal, there is also some evidence that substituting psychological for pharmacological treatment may be a safe approach, with the resultant reduction in cost and also, more importantly, side-effects associated with medication over time.

Case formulation

John was a 23-year-old man who lived with three other people in a rented flat in a suburb of Birmingham. He had experienced problems in childhood as a consequence of both his parents' violence to each other and their neglect of their children. He had been moved from the family home, and away from his siblings, to a foster home as a consequence of these problems. He was quite happy in the foster home and school, and gained a number of A levels. However, after leaving home to go to college, he began a history of significant drug and alcohol use, and dropped out of college in his first year. Since then, he had had a number of short-term casual jobs, but nothing long term. He continued to be a heavy user of drugs including marijuana, amphetamines, and cocaine over a period of years. To sustain his drug use, he had engaged in petty crime and occasionally dealt drugs. He was known to the local police force, who had detained him on a number of occasions, although he had not been to prison. He was well known to the local probation officers.

John was admitted to a local hospital following the onset of an acute psychotic episode, which appeared to follow a break-up with a girlfriend of several weeks previously. His flatmates had noticed that his behaviour had become increasingly strange and withdrawn over a period of several weeks. He told them that he was hearing voices indicating that the police were after him and that they had put out a contract for him to be killed because of his history of crime and the way he had treated his girlfriend. He could hear the voices because they were being transmitted through the police radio system, which he was able to detect through radio receivers in his brain. He had locked himself in his room, closed the curtains, and was not eating. He felt frightened and believed that if he left the house, he would be found by the police, and either taken to prison or killed. In order to calm himself down he was using significant amounts of marijuana and alcohol. His flatmates' concern was such that they had contacted their family doctor, who had visited John in his flat. Under the guise of doing some tests to check out the reality of the changes to his brain and to try and sort them out, the doctor had persuaded John to be admitted to a local psychiatric hospital on a voluntary basis.

Once in hospital he was assessed by a psychiatrist and subsequently placed on antipsychotic medication. After a few weeks, although he felt calm and safe in hospital, he remained depressed and believed that the police were still 'after him'. He was therefore referred to a clinical psychologist in the hope that they could change his paranoid beliefs.

Formulation

John was a vulnerable individual as a consequence of his damaged upbringing, difficulties in engaging with others, and the stresses associated with relationships and use of non-prescription drugs. The incident appears to have been triggered by his breaking up a relationship with a woman he had been seeing for several months. He had not treated her well during the relationship and the break-up had been quite uncaring and disrespectful to her. According to Bentall et al. (2001), this may have evoked memories of his childhood and the pain he experienced at this time, making him feel guilty for his behaviour that was like that of his parents, from whom he received little respect or love. He differed significantly from an ideal self of being caring and cared for. This guilt led to ruminations and worry about how he had behaved, its implications for him, and the belief that he was a bad person. Exacerbated by the use of drugs, he had externalized these feelings of guilt and self-deprecation onto the police.

Intervention

The first stage of therapy involved a period during which John and his therapist simply talked about his experiences, in a process of gaining trust and gaining empathy. Evidence has shown this to be particularly important in the process of treating psychosis – too quick or too challenging, and the **client** is highly likely to disengage from therapy. After several sessions, during which the therapist identified and acknowledged (but not agreed with) several distorted beliefs and delusions, he began to gently probe their reality. The therapist did this by simply questioning whether or not John agreed with any of the negative beliefs about himself he believed the police to hold. This led to discussion of a number of negative beliefs about himself, his past, and the disappointment he felt with his life situation – without directly challenging his belief that the voices he heard were those of the police radio. Following this discussion (over a number of therapy sessions), the therapist began to gently question the foundations of some of John's beliefs: why would the police want to kill him for very minor offences? Would they do this with other people? Had they shown evidence of this attitude when he had previously been involved with the police? As a consequence of these discussions, John was able to question the likelihood of some of his beliefs being true, and became less disturbed by them. This allowed the therapist to move to a different approach: more direct challenges to his beliefs through the use of behavioural hypothesis-testing. One belief John held was that the police were watching him and would pick him up if he left the safety of the hospital ward. This was tested by encouraging John to walk out of the ward, first in the hospital grounds and then to local shops. He did so, with a degree of anxiety, but succeeded in doing so, and began to question further the strength of his paranoid beliefs, as they had not come true.

Over a period of several weeks of intensive therapy (meeting with his therapist twice a week), John was able to question and counter much of his paranoid ideation and delusions. This process was no doubt aided by him no longer taking non-prescription drugs and the use of antipsychotics. However, the positive outcome of these various processes was that John was able to leave hospital with the support of a social worker and **community mental health team**, and engage in longer-term processes of reducing his drug and alcohol use, dealing with unresolved issues from his childhood, and developing better relationships with friends and partners. But that is another story ...

13.4 Chapter summary

1. Schizophrenia is one of the most disabling of the mental health disorders.
2. DSM identifies four types of schizophrenia: disorganized, paranoid, catatonic, and residual.
3. An alternative classification system identifies two clusters of symptoms. Positive symptoms include hallucinations, delusions, and thought disorder, while negative symptoms are those related to a general lack of motivation.
4. Concerns over the nature of schizophrenia have led some to argue that the concept can no longer be considered valid. Instead, they argue that the various experiences of people diagnosed as having schizophrenia would be better considered as separate and unrelated factors.
5. There is no exclusive 'cause' of schizophrenia, although a number of factors have been implicated, including genetics and social and family stress.
6. The biological bases for schizophrenia include disruption of the dopamine system and neuronal degeneration, partly as a consequence of perinatal factors, partly due to excess dopamine.
7. Psychological models adopt a dimensional view of the disorder and attempt to understand the psychological processes that contribute to the experiences of people diagnosed with schizophrenia rather than to identify triggers to a 'condition' in which the individual differs categorically from the norm.
8. Theory of mind explanations of schizophrenia attribute the condition to an inability to monitor and understand one's own thought processes and those of others.
9. Cognitive explanations of delusions suggest they may form an attributional process, to help people cope with negative self-evaluations.
10. Cognitive models of hallucinations consider them to result from failures in attentional and filtering processes.
11. Treatment is largely with phenothiazines such as chlorpromazine and newer drugs including clozapine. These seem to delay rather than prevent the onset of further problems

12. Drug therapy may be significantly augmented by family therapy, particularly for those who live in a high NEE environment, which has been shown to profoundly alter the course of schizophrenia.
13. Cognitive behavioural techniques may also be of benefit for both the general treatment of schizophrenia, including relapse risk, and specific symptoms of delusions and hallucinations.

13.5 For discussion

1. Is the diagnosis of schizophrenia a valid one?
2. Should people with schizophrenia receive genetic or family counselling when planning a family?
3. Should family or cognitive therapy form the first-line treatment for schizophrenia, with drug therapy used only if this is unsuccessful?

13.6 Further reading

Bentall, R. (2001) *Madness Explained: Psychosis and Human Nature*, London: Penguin.
Cooke, A. (2017) *Understanding Psychosis and Schizophrenia*, Leicester: British Psychological Society [https://www.bps.org.uk/sites/www.bps.org.uk/files/Page%20-%20Files/Understanding%20Psychosis%20and%20Schizophrenia.pdf].
Insel, T. (2010) Rethinking schizophrenia, *Nature*, 468: 187–93.
NICE (2009) *Psychosis and schizophrenia: management*, Clinical Guideline CG82, London: NICE [https://www.nice.org.uk/guidance/cg82].
Torrey, E.F. (2019) *Surviving Schizophrenia: A Family Manual*, New York: Harper Perennial.

14 Developmental disorders

Chapter contents

This chapter looks at disorders within the diagnostic category of pervasive developmental difficulties: conditions which begin in childhood and are predictive of subsequent adult problems. First, the chapter considers the problems associated with disorders grouped under the broad category of learning difficulties. It then discusses the **aetiology** and treatment of more specific conditions: autism spectrum disorder and attention-deficit/hyperactivity disorder (ADHD). By the end of the chapter, you should have an understanding of:

- Definitions and some of the causes of learning difficulties
- Aspects of the social and psychological care of people with learning difficulties
- The biological and psychological bases of autism
- Treatment of autism and autistic behaviours
- Factors that contribute to ADHD
- Biological and psychological treatments of ADHD.

14.1 Learning difficulties

Learning difficulties is a broad term that encompasses a variety of conditions whose defining characteristic is a significant impairment of intellectual functioning. The terms used to describe people with this condition differ across the world and in time. In the UK, they have in the past been referred to as 'handicapped', 'subnormal' or 'retarded'. Now, all people with intellectual deficits, however profound, are referred to as having learning difficulties. The reasons for these changing terms are not trivial: they reflect attempts to minimize prejudice towards this group of people. In the USA, people with mild learning difficulties are referred to as having learning difficulties, while those with more profound deficits are still referred to as having mental retardation.

According to the British Psychological Society (2001), the first criterion for a diagnosis of having a learning disability is that its onset is before the age of 18 years, which excludes the effects of trauma or other neurological illness later in life. In addition, the individual must experience significant impairment in adaptive/ social functioning and score significantly below the norm on intelligence tests. The usual cut-off score for this diagnosis is between 70 and 75 on the standard IQ test: two standard deviations below the population mean of 100. This criterion is somewhat arbitrary, because as Webb and Whitaker (2012) noted, IQ tests in people with learning difficulties are prone to measurement error and IQ measures may tell little of how an individual engages and copes with the 'real world'. Nevertheless, using this criterion, about 1% of the population fall into this category (e.g. Zablotsky et al. 2017), which includes a range of differing abilities:

- *Mild learning difficulties*: includes about 85% of people with learning difficulties. As children, they may be superficially indistinguishable from children with normal IQs, although their school performance shows they have clear learning difficulties. As adults, they are likely to be able to hold down unskilled jobs, although they may need help with social and financial issues.
- *Moderate learning difficulties*: includes about 10% of people with learning difficulties. Within this group of people, learning difficulties are often combined with other neurological deficits, including problems with motor skills such as walking, holding implements, and so on. People in this group usually live independently within families or in group homes. Many have obvious brain damage and other pathologies.
- *Severe learning difficulties*: usually associated with genetically mediated physical abnormalities and limited sensorimotor control. Most people with severe learning difficulties live in institutions and require constant aid and supervision. As adults, they are typically lethargic and lack motivation. They may, nevertheless, communicate at a simple and concrete level.
- *Profound learning difficulties*: profound mental and physical problems mean that people with this degree of difficulty require total supervision and nursing care all their lives. They cannot communicate using language and cannot get around on their own.

Severe learning difficulties are more common among males than females. Mild learning difficulties are most common among males and those from economically deprived or adverse family backgrounds (Roeleveld et al. 1997). As the medical care of people with learning difficulties improves, the **prevalence** of older people with learning difficulties within society is increasing, at the same time as childhood prevalence is falling as a consequence of increased prenatal screening and better child healthcare.

Aetiology of learning difficulties

Only about 25% of cases of learning difficulty have an identified cause. These include:

- *Genetic conditions*: including Down syndrome and Fragile X syndrome
- *Infectious diseases*: including rubella, parental syphilis, and encephalitis
- *Environmental hazards*: including lead paint and exhaust fumes in leaded petrol
- *Antenatal events*: including parental infections (including rubella) and endocrine disorders such as hypothyroidism
- *Perinatal trauma*: including asphyxia during birth.

For many people, there is no known biological cause. This is unsurprising, as IQ and related abilities, like all other natural phenomena, follow a normal distribution within the population, with the exception of the so-called 'hump' within the lower end of the distribution that occurs as a consequence of biological causes (see Figure 14.1). This does not mean that poor performance on IQ tests is totally biologically determined. A significant number and type of psychosocial factors may impact on both IQ performance and skills of everyday life, particularly for people with mild-to-moderate learning difficulties. These include the quality of parental care and of teaching and expectations of teachers, as well as the wider social environment. A key issue for those experiencing childhood poverty may also be dietary restrictions that can influence the developing brain (see D'Angiulli et al. 2012).

Down syndrome

People affected by Down syndrome are short and stocky in stature, and have typical facial characteristics, including upward-slanting eyes, sparse, fine straight hair, and a large furrowed tongue which protrudes as the result of a small mouth. They may also have a number of other less obvious characteristics, including serious heart malformations. All people with this condition have some degree of learning difficulty. Autopsy reveals brain tissue very similar to that found in **Alzheimer's disease**.

Down syndrome occurs in about 1 in 500–600 live births and has been detected in about 3% of foetuses that spontaneously abort before 20 weeks' gestation. It occurs sporadically. People with the disorder are generally the children of parents without it, precluding an obvious genetic linkage. Because the risk of having a child with Down syndrome increases with the age of the mother, rising significantly in women giving birth over the age of 32 years, it was originally thought to

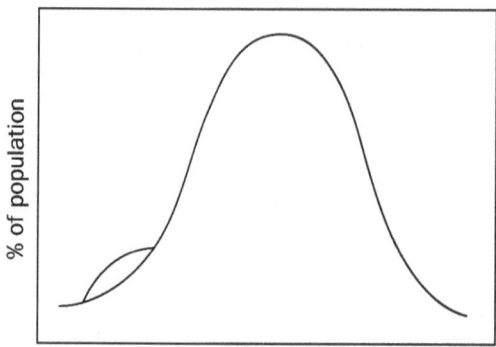

Figure 14.1 The genetic 'hump' within the distribution of IQ scores

be the result of an 'unfavourable' interaction between mother and foetus during pregnancy. However, it is now known to result from a chromosomal abnormality. People with Down syndrome have three, instead of two, **chromosomes**-21, leading to the more technical name of the disorder, trisomy-21.

This is the result of a process that occurs during the first few cell divisions that occur prior to fertilization. In trisomy-21, as the female egg cells duplicate, they fail to do so properly, and some sex cells receive two chromosomes-21; some receive none. If these eggs are fertilized by a normal sperm, the resultant cells contain either three or one chromosome-21. The latter is not a viable combination and the developing cells are aborted. However, in the case of trisomy-21, the embryo and then the foetus remain viable and survive. The age-related risk is thought to be the result of some kind of metabolic or physical damage accumulated by the egg cells while lying in the ovaries for decades before ovulating. Although Down syndrome is considered to be untreatable, some aspects of the syndrome may respond to medical treatment. Van Trotsenburg et al. (2005), for example, found that treatment with thyroxine immediately following birth may reduce the level of both motor and mental developmental delay during early childhood.

Fragile X syndrome

Fragile X syndrome affects approximately 1 in 1,000 male and 1 in 2,500 female births. This syndrome is caused by a defect within the *FMR-1* (Fragile X mental retardation-1) gene located on the X chromosome. In Fragile X syndrome, a small region of the gene undergoes repeated, unnecessary duplications of a number of amino acids that result in a longer gene. When the number of repeats is small (fewer than 200), the individual often has no signs of the disorder. Where there are a larger number of repeats, the learning difficulties associated with Fragile X syndrome are observed. In families that show evidence of Fragile X syndrome, both the number of repeats and the length of the chromosome increase with succeeding generations, with a proportional increase in the severity of symptoms.

Because of the X-linkage, the syndrome is seen more frequently in males than in females. This is because females typically have two X chromosomes, and males have one X and one Y chromosome. A female who inherits a chromosome carrying the Fragile X gene from either parent is likely to inherit a normal X chromosome from the other parent. This masks the presence of the Fragile X gene in a female. However, she may carry the gene and be capable of passing it on to her children. By contrast, because a male has only one X chromosome, if he inherits an affected X chromosome, he will inevitably inherit the condition. This simple genetic model does not always hold, however: about 20% of males who carry mutated forms of *FMR-1* are either unaffected or only mildly affected. In addition, a single copy of the Fragile X gene can be sufficient to cause the syndrome in some females. Why this happens is not understood.

Social interventions in learning difficulties

The lives of people with learning difficulties have been affected by socio-political factors as well as psychological and social interventions. One ideological movement, known as *normalization* (Wolfensberger 1972), has been particularly influential. This began in the 1960s in response to the poor institutional conditions in which many people with learning difficulties then lived in the USA. The movement called for people with learning difficulties to live a life as close to normal living conditions as possible, to have normal rhythms to their lives, and the means to establish and maintain behaviour as close to their cultural norms as possible. Under the rubric of *social role valorization* (Wolfensberger 1983), the movement subsequently called for the creation, support, and defence of valued social roles for people with learning difficulties. Its latest definition calls for the use of empirical knowledge to shape the roles of classes of individuals (in this case people with learning difficulties) through enhancement of their competencies and image so they are positively valued by society. These have led to five key aims of any service providing support for people with learning difficulties:

- *Community presence*: people with learning difficulties live in the community, in normal houses, not institutions. To avoid 'pockets' of disability, housing is distributed through the community.
- *Choice*: people with learning difficulties have the same choices of accommodation, care, and day-to-day routine that are available to the 'normal' population.
- *Competences*: the competences of people with learning difficulties are acknowledged and maximized.
- *Respect*: people with learning difficulties are afforded the respect due to all other people within the population.
- *Participation*: people with learning difficulties have equal rights of participation in society, including access to work, leisure facilities, political activities, and sexual relationships, as the rest of the population.

In the spirit of this integrated approach, children with learning difficulties are increasingly being taught in mainstream classes, and most adults with learning difficulties live in the community following the closure of large institutions. However, these changes fall short of the goals of normalization, and there is still work to do. Nearly two-thirds of British adults with learning difficulties, for example, continue to live with their family of birth: a significantly higher proportion than among the 'normal' population.

Schooling

Government policy within most Western countries is that all children should be educated in ordinary schools. Indeed, the UK government statutory guidance (Department for Education 2014) states that all children with learning difficulties (in their term, 'special education needs') must be accommodated within mainstream education and cannot be denied on the basis that their needs or disabilities are too great or complex. This right can be difficult at times to enact, with many children still denied it in practice (Independent Provider of Special Education Advice 2019). However, in order to refuse a child entry into a mainstream school, the local authority has to show evidence that the child or young person's presence would be incompatible with the 'efficient education of others' and that there are 'no reasonable steps' that can be taken to remove the incompatibility. This political and social policy is supported by the empirical evidence: educating children with learning difficulties in mainstream schools with additional support seems to be at least as effective as placing them in segregated 'special' schools. Buckley et al. (2007), for example, found gains in communication skills (including expressive language and literacy skills) among children with Down syndrome schooled in mainstream classrooms not found in those taught in specialist units.

Preparing for adulthood

The transition from school to adult life requires planning, as many people require some sort of social support in adulthood. Children leaving school are assessed and a care plan is drawn up, setting out how services will meet their continuing needs. Individual circumstances differ, but this process includes consideration of the following:

- *Future daytime activities*: including possible further education, supported employment, and attendance at day services
- *Living arrangements*: choices include remaining in the family home or moving to more independent living
- *Leisure opportunities*
- *Physical healthcare needs*.

Occupation and employment

Support in adulthood is usually provided through some form of day care or employment. In the UK, this has involved attendance at Adult Training Centres. In them, the individual takes part in a number of 'productive' activities, including simple contract work for which they receive a token 'wage', simple skills training, sports and arts and craft activities. These centres also provide day care for people with severe or complex disabilities.

More recently, significant effort has been given to placing people with learning difficulties into real working environments. One of the best models of this approach, known as the *supported employment model*, originated in the USA. It assumes that almost anyone can be employed if given sufficient support. It is colloquially known as a 'place, train, and maintain' model, because the process involves identifying a job suitable to the individual, training them to do the job effectively, and then supporting them in the job, with decreasing levels of support as appropriate. This can be effective in increasing integration into the workplace, and the development of increased adaptive skills, particularly where co-workers are prepared and receive appropriate training (Stephens et al. 2005).

Living away from institutions

Most adults with learning disabilities continue to live in their family of origin. Others may live independently in rented accommodation. A number of other options are available, each providing differing levels of support, including the following:

- *Registered care homes*: have up to 20 residents, though between 3 and 6 is more typical; 24-hour-a-day support is provided. All personal care and meals are provided.

- *Shared housing*: usually for groups of three or four people; levels of support vary from staff visiting once or twice a week to 24-hour-a-day support. Residents may do their own shopping, cooking, budgeting, and housework, with some support from staff.
- *Cluster of flats or bedsitters*: self-contained units, usually on a single site but occasionally dispersed across a neighbourhood. Support staff are available, but residents are more independent than in other settings.

Psychological interventions in learning difficulties

Psychological interventions for people with learning difficulties usually have one of two goals: either to teach people the skills necessary to maximize their abilities, or to reduce inappropriate behaviours. Both approaches are frequently based on the principles of **operant conditioning**, in which behaviour is shaped by a series of rewards and, less frequently, punishments. The remaining part of this section focuses on three interventions relevant to people with learning difficulties, starting with a programme aimed at preschool children. More programmes, developed for people with a combination of autism and learning difficulties, are described in the next section of the chapter.

Teaching skills

Most children with learning disabilities live in their family home. Preschool programmes provide opportunities for teaching age-dependent skills necessary for when the child starts to attend school. One of the most widely used systems through which this is provided is known as Portage (https://www.portage.org.uk/).

First established in the town of Portage, USA, this home-visiting service is now used in countries as far apart as India and Japan, as well as the USA, and is widely accessible in the UK (Russell 2007). The teaching process begins with assessment of the child's abilities. Therapists and parents then work together to develop a training programme that addresses six domains: infant stimulation, social development, communication speech and language, self-help, cognitive development, and motor development. Once the programme is designed, the parent works with the child on a planned programme of skills training, with weekly visits by health professionals who provide support and assess the child's progress. Parental interventions are facilitated by the provision of cards describing in detail how to teach 580 behaviours. Each card has a behavioural description of a skill (such as 'Mary will place 6 pieces in puzzle with verbal prompt'), suggested teaching materials, and the type of reinforcement to be used in its development. Despite its widespread use, there are relatively few formal evaluations of the approach. However, what evidence there is suggests it works. In a Chinese study, for example, Xiumei Liu et al. (2018) found significant gains on measures of gross and fine motor abilities, language, and social activity following a Portage programme that were not evident in a no-treatment control group.

Psychological methods can also be used to facilitate skills acquisition in adults. One frequently used approach involves the use of **self-instruction training** (Meichenbaum 1985) to either facilitate skills acquisition or lower anxiety levels associated with behaviours requiring sequencing or social skills. In these, the recipient is first talked through appropriate behaviours by the therapist using very specific and clear instructions, and then uses their own internal dialogue to do the same. This approach has been shown to be effective, even when treating an individual engaging in inappropriate sexual activity ('Think about prison. Walk away.'; Willner 2013). Outcomes studies are limited in number, partly because of the very individual strategies used in this type of intervention. Nevertheless, Corrigan (1991) was able to synthesize the outcomes of studies of this approach on measures of social skills of people with learning difficulties, **psychosis**, and offenders. People with learning difficulties gained significantly from the intervention. They performed best on measures of skill during role play and maintenance of skills over time. They were, however, less successful in transferring these skills to situations beyond the training setting; a common failing in this type of intervention, even in more intellectually able populations.

Coping with challenging behaviour

Between 10% and 15% of people with learning difficulties engage in challenging behaviours; that is, behaviours that transgress social rules, and usually involve aggression either towards themselves or others, destructive behaviours, or place the individual or others at risk of harm (e.g. Lowe et al. 2007). Episodes may re-occur over long periods of time, and are now considered to be operantly conditioned behaviours, through which people with restricted abilities try to achieve some degree of control over their environment and the people around them – for example, by attracting attention or getting someone to stop an unwanted action. Because each of the challenging behaviours differs in its causes, nature, and the type of intervention required, the effects of any intervention are not easily measured in randomized controlled trials. Indeed, Hassiotis and Hall (2008) found only four studies with more than four participants to include in their review of the area, and insufficient data to allow a **meta-analysis**. Nevertheless, a number of broad principles for reducing the frequency and severity of challenging behaviours have been developed. Emerson (1998), for example, identified the following three key intervention approaches, none of which involves punishing the individual.

Enrich the environment

Reinforcement theory suggests that the rate of behaviours maintained by positive reinforcement should reduce as the background level of reinforcement increases. Enriching environments by increasing social interaction or providing more things with which to engage and interest the individual should therefore reduce challenging behaviours. In one study of this approach, Golding et al. (2005) found an improvement in the challenging behaviours shown by a group of six men with mild-to-moderate learning difficulties when moved from an institution to a more enriched environment in a specialized community-based home. Following relocation, they found a significant increase in participants' domestic activity skills, a decrease in the occurrence of problem behaviours, and an increase in engagement and staff contact.

Reduce exposure to the triggers to challenging behaviour

One simple way in which challenging behaviour can be prevented is to minimize or obviate its triggers. Touchette et al. (1985), for example, identified that one woman's outbursts were associated with her attendance at pre-vocational and community living classes. Rescheduling them resulted in an almost total cessation in the frequency of her aggressive behaviour.

Teach or support alternative behaviours

Most challenging behaviour is considered to be functional; that is, it occurs in order to achieve a particular outcome. A key intervention, therefore, involves teaching people how to gain their desired outcome without engaging in challenging behaviour. To be effective, the new behaviour has to achieve exactly the same outcome as the original behaviour and be a more 'efficient' way of achieving this goal. An example of this approach was reported by Steege et al. (1990), who taught two young children with severe multiple disabilities to press a microswitch to activate a tape-recording of a request for a break from self-care activities, a process that led to marked reductions in self-injurious behaviour previously used to stop such activities.

Treating emotional problems

Psychological interventions to help people with learning difficulties to cope with emotional difficulties are perhaps less widely used than interventions used to address behavioural problems. Nevertheless, Nagel and Leiper (1999) found that 35% of their sample of clinical psychologists in the UK reported using CBT 'frequently' or 'very frequently'. Slightly fewer (31%) used humanistic approaches, while 17% reported using psychodynamic approaches with equal frequency. When used, CBT does appear to be of benefit, although the approach may need some simplification. Willner et al. (2013), for example, evaluated the impact of a simplified CBT approach to the treatment of anger. Compared to a no-treatment condition, participants in the CBT intervention reported fewer episodes of anger, which was validated by their key workers. This approach also appears to be of benefit when provided as a computer-assisted programme to help people with anxiety and depression (Cooney et al. 2017).

Case formulation

Mr R was a 27-year-old man with significant learning difficulties. As a child he lived at home, but as he got older his parents were unable to cope with his behaviour and were themselves ill, so he moved into a small residential home in his early teens. His behaviour in the home was generally unremarkable, and he developed good relationships with his fellow residents. However, he also experienced frequent and, at times, frightening episodes of anger and aggression towards residents and staff in the home. These were characterized at different times by screaming, shouting, banging his head, biting, becoming abusive and physically threatening. As he was a large man, these actions were very intimidating. As a result of these episodes, Mr R had been admitted to a local hospital for treatment on a number of occasions – each time following an aggressive outburst, and each time with the intention of preventing further episodes of this type of behaviour. Over the years, he had been given a number of medications (including **major tranquillizers** such as haloperidol), and taught basic anger management skills such as relaxation. He had also been on behavioural programmes that rewarded appropriate behaviour with, for example, social contact with staff, and punished inappropriate behaviours, which included being ignored by staff. These interventions had worked for short periods over the years, but their effects then faded, and his outbursts continued.

One reason for this episodic ebb and flow of his outbursts was that most of the interventions to reduce them had taken place in hospital, away from the residential home in which he lived. Accordingly, they influenced his behaviour while in hospital, but their effects did not generalize beyond this context. With this in mind, the staff in the home and a clinical psychologist attempted to develop an intervention to reduce his outbursts in the home.

Functional analysis

In contrast to self-management approaches, which require the individual concerned to deliberately change their behaviour, functional analysis aims to identify (and then change) external, environmental, factors that contribute to the triggering or maintenance of target behaviours. This process involves a period of naturalistic observation of the target behaviour, identifying when, where, and why it occurs and factors that contribute to it being maintained. This process is known as functional, or A-B-C, analysis in which A is the antecedent, B is the behaviour, and C is the consequence of the behaviour. In the case of Mr R, this process involved a psychology assistant spending time in the residential home observing Mr R through the day and keeping a diary of these issues. As key behaviours became evident – such as biting or shouting – the frequency of these specific events was recorded. In order to ensure a full understanding of the A-B-C process, the assistant worked at different times of the day to capture the full time-frame over which such incidents could occur. In addition to this diary keeping, staff in the home were asked their views about the causes and factors that maintained Mr R's behaviour and how they responded to it.

Formulation

The observation revealed a number of triggers to Mr R's behaviour. These included being teased by members of staff or other residents, and occasions on which Mr R was frustrated by waiting for things to happen: to be given food, staff attention, and so on. Conversations with staff members revealed that staff in the home responded very differently to Mr R's behaviour. Some tried to argue with him when he became angry, threatening sanctions, while others took a completely opposite approach of ignoring his outbursts. Some staff were consistent in their response; others responded differently depending on the context in which the behaviour occurred. Observation of incidents in the home suggested that his behaviour was worse and continued for longer if his outbursts were responded to with remonstrations or threats by staff or residents.

Intervention

Once the psychology team had completed their functional analysis and understood the causes and maintaining factors of Mr R's outbursts, they met with the home staff to develop a response to them. They planned a series of changes including avoiding triggers to the outbursts by ensuring that Mr R did not have long to wait for food, stopping any teasing, providing regular attention to him at appropriate times, and responding to any outbursts in a consistent manner: keeping a quiet and calm voice while talking to him, keeping a reasonable distance from him, and avoiding any appearance of confrontation. The staff team met at weekly intervals to share any problems they were experiencing or to suggest strategies they had found useful (within the overall behavioural programme). The assistant psychologist also continued to monitor the key target behaviours and to report back to these meetings how the intervention was progressing. The programme proved effective. After just one month, there was a marked reduction in the frequency of Mr R's outbursts. The inception of the programme resulted in a dramatic fall in the number of outbursts from two to three a day to two in the first week. This number fell to zero in the second week, and only one incident occurred in the third week. The programme could therefore be considered a success. The key to maintaining its success, of course, is that the staff continue their behavioural changes – and any new staff in the home learn to adopt their response style.

14.2 Autism spectrum disorder

Autism was first identified in 1943 and was differentiated from schizophrenia only in 1971. **DSM**-5 has shifted from considering autism as a distinct disorder, and now considers it to be a cluster of related deficits that range in severity from mild to severe: hence the new diagnostic label of autistic spectrum disorder (ASD). According to DSM-5, the characteristics of ASD are:

- Deficits in social communication and interaction across multiple contexts:
  - *Social-emotional reciprocity*: including reduced sharing of interests and emotions, and failure to initiate or respond to social interactions.
  - *Non-verbal communicative behaviours used for social interaction*: including abnormalities in eye contact and body language, deficits in understanding and the use of gestures, and lack of facial expressions.
  - *Developing, maintaining, and understanding relationships*: including failures to adjust behaviour to suit differing social contexts, sharing imaginative play, or in making friends, and the absence of interest in peers.

- Restricted, repetitive patterns of behaviour, interests or activities, as evidenced by at least two of the following:
  - Stereotyped or repetitive motor movements, use of objects, or speech (e.g. lining up toys, echolalia, idiosyncratic phrases).
  - Insistence on 'sameness', inflexible adherence to routines, or ritualized patterns of verbal and non-verbal behaviour (e.g. extreme distress at small environmental changes, difficulties with transitions, rigid thinking patterns, greeting rituals, need to travel on the same route and eat the same food every day).
  - Highly restricted, fixated interests that are abnormal in intensity or focus (e.g. strong attachment to or preoccupation with unusual objects, distress if separated from object of interest).
  - Exaggerated reactivity or indifference to sensory input, or unusual interests in sensory aspects of the environment (e.g. apparent indifference to pain/temperature, adverse response to particular sounds or textures, excessive smelling or touching of objects, fascination with lights or movement).

These deficits must be present in the early years but may not become evident until social demands exceed an individual's ability to cope with them. According to DSM, there are three levels of severity: (i) 'requiring support', (ii) 'requiring substantial support', and (iii) 'requiring very substantial support'. Some people with ASD are able to take an active part in society, with no deficits apparent to the casual observer, although they may have significant problems in establishing and maintaining relationships. About 80% of children with autism score less than 70 on intelligence tests, placing them in the learning disabilities range. These deficits are quite specific, and relate to abstract thought, symbolism, and sequential logic. Some people may have isolated skills that reflect great talent, including prodigious mathematical or memory skills, in a condition known as 'idiot savant'.

The latest DSM criteria have resulted in increased apparent rates of ASD, with the latest figures based on DSM-5 suggesting that among children, the prevalence of ASD is around 1.7%, with males four times more likely to be diagnosed than females (Baio et al. 2018). Of these children, 31% were found to have an IQ of less than 70, 25% were in the 'borderline' range (71–85), and 44% had scores in the average or above average range.

Core limitations of ASD

The core limitations associated with autism are social isolation, communication deficits, and obsessive-compulsive or ritual behaviours.

Social isolation

Many children with ASD act as if people have no special characteristics that distinguish them from inanimate objects. As babies, they do not respond to their mothers when being touched or fed and may reject attempts at cuddling by arching their back. By the age of 2 or 3 years, they may form a weak emotional bond with their parents. Few will initiate play with other children, and they are usually unresponsive to attempts by other children to engage them in play. Attempts at achieving eye contact are usually met with avoidance or movement away and carry no social message. By contrast, children may develop strong bonds with inanimate objects and carry them around with them if possible.

Communication deficits

About 50% of children with ASD never learn to speak. Those that do have some common abnormalities. One frequent speech characteristic is known as echolalia: the repetition of words or phrases spoken to the child immediately, hours or even days earlier. This is now thought to be an attempt at communication and may be associated with an event or stimulus. Repetition of the phrase, 'Do you want a sweet?', for example, may indicate a learned association between the phrase and being given a sweet. A second common characteristic is known as pronoun reversal, in which children refer to themselves in the third person. This may be associated with echolalia and reflect how they have heard others speak about them (e.g. 'How are you, Mary?' – 'She's here …'). This is highly resistant to change, even after intensive training programmes.

Obsessive-compulsive and ritualistic acts

Children with ASD rarely engage in symbolic play. More frequently, they engage in repetitive, **stereotypic**, and seemingly meaningless behaviour. These include ritualistic hand movements, such as flicking fingers across their face, or repetitive body movements, including rocking or walking on tip-toe. They may become upset if prevented from doing these behaviours or when minor elements of their daily routine are changed. Their play often has an obsessive flavour to it, lining up toys or constructing complex patterns with household objects.

Growing up

The prognosis of children with ASD is mixed. Those with learning difficulties often make a poor adjustment to adulthood, and most need some level of supervised care. By contrast, those without learning difficulties frequently go on to achieve an independent life, gain employment, and live independently. Some go on to make significant contributions in their lives. However, most continue to have markedly impaired social relationships and little understanding of the social and emotional aspects of life. For a powerful description of the feelings and development of a 'high functioning autistic' (her phrase), the story of Temple Grandin, a professor at Colorado State University (www.autism.org/temple-grandin-inside-asd/) provides fascinating insight. She describes, for example, how as a child being unable to speak was utterly frustrating. If an adult spoke to her she could understand every word they said, but could not respond. Working with a therapist, she learned to say 'bah' for ball with great stress by the age of 3. If pushed too hard by the therapist, she would throw a tantrum; if pushed too little, no progress was made: *'My mother and teachers wondered why I screamed. Screaming was the only way I could communicate …'*. Her description of the development of a 'squeezing machine' perhaps shows the paradox and constraints of her condition at their greatest. She reported, '*I wanted to feel the good feeling of being hugged, but when people hugged me the stimuli washed over me like a tidal wave ... I pulled away to avoid the all-engulfing tidal wave of stimulation. The stiffening up and flinching were like a wild animal pulling away*'. In response to this paradoxical urge to be held, but inability to cope with it, she built a 'squeezing machine': a device lined with foam rubber into which she could fit herself, and then 'hug' herself with control over the duration and amount of pressure she received.

Aetiology of autism

Genetic factors

Genetic studies of ASD are difficult to conduct as the condition is so rare, and there appears to be no one significant 'autism gene'. Nevertheless, the recurrence risk in siblings of affected children is approximately 2–8%, much higher than the prevalence in the general population but much lower than in single-gene diseases (Muhle et al. 2004), suggesting a moderate genetic influence on risk. Evidence is emerging from genetic studies of over 50 potential gene mutations linked to ASD, with a smaller number of genes likely to be the central influences. The exact mechanism of this influence is still to be determined, but it does appear that transmission of the genetic mutations may be through unaffected mothers, suggesting women may in some way be 'protected' against the influence of these mutations (Iossifov et al. 2015). Any genetic risk may also involve a number of related disorders, including attention-deficit/hyperactivity, developmental coordination, and tic disorders (Lichtenstein et al. 2010).

Biological mechanisms

The opioid theory

It has proved difficult to find a biochemical model of ASD. Perhaps the most widely advocated theory, the opioid theory, suggests the condition is the result of an early overload of the central nervous system by opioids. This is based on findings that certain behaviours found in autism, including stereotyped behaviour, can be artificially induced in animals following injection with opioid **agonists**. The excess opioids are thought to be the result of incompletely digested dietary gluten and/or casein found in barley, rye, oats, and milk products (Reichelt et al. 1991). These result from a lack of chemicals known as peptidases within the gut, which break down natural opioids found in these foodstuffs into innocuous metabolites. Unfortunately, what biological studies have been conducted have not always supported this theory. Neither Hunter et al. (2003) or Dettmer et al. (2007), for example, found any evidence of these opioid peptides in the urine of children with ASD.

Unfortunately, the opioid theory has also been linked to one of the most controversial research and public health issues in recent times. In the late 1990s, in a methodologically flawed study, Wakefield et al. (1998) examined 12 children referred to hospital with a normal developmental history followed by an apparently sudden loss of cognitive skills accompanied by a number of abdominal symptoms. Symptom onset was reported to have followed the measles, mumps, and rubella (MMR) vaccination in eight of the children; nine were diagnosed as having ASD. Each of these nine children was found to suffer from an inflammation of the bowel wall, known as lymphoid hyperplasia. Wakefield et al. suggested the MMR injection somehow resulted in a failure to break down dietary gluten and/or casein and, hence, triggered the onset of ASD. This finding, and the subsequent public reaction to MMR partly as a result of both mainstream and social media's fears in relation to vaccination (see, for example, https://vaccineresistancemovement.org/), sparked a widespread controversy and significant reductions in the uptake of the MMR vaccination.

Since that time a number of findings that significantly challenge the MMR–ASD link have been reported. Taylor et al. (1999), for example, examined trends in births and any subsequent registration of children with special needs and disabilities since 1979 in the UK. They noted a gradual increase in the numbers of children with ASD since that time, but no sudden increase coinciding with the introduction of the MMR vaccine, or any evidence of a cluster of children with developmental regression occurring within 2–4 months of MMR vaccination. In an even more clear-cut study, Honda et al. (2005) reviewed the rates of ASD diagnosed in the Kohuku area of Yokohama between 1988 and 2002. During that time, rates of MMR vaccinations fell dramatically (for reasons not related to the autism scare) and no MMR vaccines were administered from 1993 onwards. Nevertheless, rates of ASD rose throughout this period with the greatest increase beginning in the cohort of children born in 1993 – after the MMR vaccination was no longer given. These, and other data, led Demicheli et al. (2005) in their review of the evidence to suggest that exposure to MMR was unlikely to be associated with ASD or any other health condition.

So, why did so many people become convinced that MMR had caused their child to develop ASD? Perhaps the answer lies in the coincidence of timing between the MMR vaccine and the developmental history of the condition. About 600,000 children receive the MMR vaccine in any one year, most at the same age that ASD first becomes evident. It is possible that among these children, the identification of a small number of cases will coincide with vaccination. This apparent association could have been exaggerated by the highly selective way in which children were identified and assessed in the Wakefield study. In addition, it is possible that the link between receiving the MMR vaccine and the onset of symptoms made by parents may be inaccurate. It is usually difficult to identify the time of onset of symptoms of ASD, and most people search for a 'cause' of such problems. If parents were to attribute their child's problems to the vaccination, this may result in unconscious memory biases and inappropriate linkages of behaviour with the timing of the MMR vaccination.

An emerging alternative to the opioid theory, still incorporating the activity of the gut, suggests the gut microbiome may be implicated in ASD as well as a range of immune disorders. A number of reports looking at the intestinal flora of children with autism using stool samples have discovered differences between these samples and those of comparison children (e.g. Pulikkan et al. 2019) – however, the data again are very conflicting. All studies have been conducted on small numbers of children, and some have found no differences between children with

ASD and comparison children, and those that have found differences have found differences in different microbes. The idea that the biome affects mental health is still relatively recent, and the mechanisms appear to be related to inflammatory processes, but the link between the biome and ASD, while intriguing, has still to be fully established.

Another candidate for some of the problems associated with ASD is the dysregulation of serotonin both before and after birth. Reviewing the evidence, Whitaker-Azmitia (2005) suggested that in the early stages of development, when the blood–brain barrier is not yet fully formed, high levels of serotonin in the blood can enter the brain of genetically vulnerable foetuses and damage serotonin terminals during development. The loss of serotonergic nerve fibres persists throughout subsequent development and into adulthood (Chugani 2004), contributing to the symptoms of ASD. Although the evidence is mixed, studies comparing rates of ASD in the children of women both taking and who have discontinued SSRIs suggests the possibility that the continued use of these re-uptake inhibitors during pregnancy may increase risk for ASD, although this association may be more linked with the presence of a psychiatric disorder rather than SSRIs *per se* (Kaplan et al. 2017). Exactly where in the brain any damage may occur is also still not fully investigated, but animal studies suggest that the amygdala, a brain region involved in the fear-response, and the hypothalamus, involved in social memory and bonding, may be particularly vulnerable to damage. The anterior cingulated area of the brain, which is involved in face recognition, social, cognitive, and affective functions relevant to autism, may also be vulnerable to damage. It is noteworthy that the serotonin model may link to the biome. Enzymes in the biome are involved in the production of serotonin, and animal research has implicated dysregulation here as a contributor to the low levels of serotonin in ASD (Israelyan and Margolis 2019).

Psychological models

Early psychological theories of ASD focused on psychodynamic processes. Autistic behaviours were seen as a form of escape from environments that lacked warmth and care. Bettelheim (1967), for example, suggested that children who develop ASD have rejecting parents and are able to perceive their negative feelings. The infants learn that their actions have little or no impact on their parents' emotions or behaviour. They come to believe they have no power to influence the world, and so choose not to enter it. Instead, they build an 'empty fortress' against this pain and disappointment. Unfortunately, from Bettelheim's perspective, there is no evidence that the parents of children who develop ASD differ from those of children who develop normally. Cox et al. (1975), for example, found that the parents of children with ASD and those of children with problems in understanding speech did not differ in terms of emotional demonstrativeness, responsiveness to their children, or sociability.

A more biopsychosocial model can be found in the work of Koegel et al. (2001). They suggested that children who develop ASD lack motivation to engage with other people and, as a result, withdraw from social interactions. This may begin early in life as a result of neurological dysfunction. However, it can be exacerbated by carers' efforts to 'help' affected children by doing things for them regardless of their behaviour. Whatever the child does, they receive the same response from their environment. As a result of this, and because social interactions and communication are inherently difficult, they revert to early forms of communication such as crying or tantrums to get their needs met and avoid social interactions.

Treatment of autism

Pharmacological approaches

Given the hypothesized links between serotonin, opiates, and ASD, the primary pharmacological intervention would be expected to target these **neurotransmitters**. And indeed, a number of studies have investigated their effectiveness, though with less success than might be predicted. For example, summarizing the data from research trials on the use of SSRIs, Hurwitz et al. (2012) concluded that they may improve some symptoms, including irritability, hyperactivity, poor eye contact, and obsessive behaviours in the short term. However, they also place the individual at high risk of a number of adverse side-effects, including drowsiness and reduced activity levels, which may potentially obviate any therapeutic gains.

Opiate **antagonists**, such as naltrexone (see also Chapter 16), have been used with only modest effect. Perhaps the most consistent effect of naltrexone is a reduction in activity levels (Parikh et al. 2008). However, it neither proved beneficial in a behavioural programme conducted by Campbell et al. (1993), nor reduced self-injurious behaviour in a study reported by Willemsen-Swinkels et al. (1995). Indeed, in the latter study, treatment with naltrexone actually increased levels of stereotypic behaviour. As a consequence of these and related studies, Roy et al. (2015) concluded that naltrexone may be of benefit to some people with ASD as it may improve hyperactivity and restlessness, but it does not impact on the core symptoms of the disorder.

An alternative biological approach has been to reduce levels of dietary casein and gluten in order to reduce the extent to which opiates continue to be absorbed from the gut. Evidence of the effectiveness of this approach is also not convincing. Knivsberg et al. (1998), for example, reported on the outcomes of a group of 20 children who either received or did not receive this restricted diet for a period of one year. The authors claimed significant success, with improvements in the treated group relative to those who did not receive the diet on a combined measure of behaviour and communication. However, methodological weaknesses limit the robustness of their findings, and a number of small studies (e.g. Hyman et al. 2016) have subsequently found no consistent evidence of benefit, leading Piwowarczyk et al. (2018) to conclude that there is little evidence of a gluten-free diet being of benefit to people with ASD.

Finally, **neuroleptics**, which block the effects of dopamine (see Chapter 4) have also been used to treat some of the symptoms of ASD. The Research Units on Pediatric Psychopharmacology Autism Network (2005), for example, reported significant benefits arising from the use of risperidone in the treatment of severe tantrums, aggression, and/or self-injurious behaviour in a small group of adolescents, but as yet no study has found significant effects on the core ASD symptoms (Anagnostou 2018). To avoid the long-term adverse effects of neuroleptics, including tardive dyskinesia and Parkinsonism (see Chapter 4), the drugs may be used at relatively low dosage and episodically (5 days on, 2 days off) and still be effective.

Behavioural approaches

Many programmes to change behaviours associated with ASD have involved direct reinforcement of behaviours such as speech or pro-social behaviours. In these, the therapist/trainer typically provides a cue, usually a question or command, to evoke a specific response. This may be physically prompted if necessary, and performance of the behaviour is reinforced by a tangible reward such as a sweet: 'Look at me' – moves head to face therapist if necessary – reward with sweet.

One of the key researchers in this area is Ivar Lovaas, who developed a highly intensive operant programme for children. In his initial study (Lovaas 1987), therapy continued for much of the children's waking hours both at home and in school, for a period of 2 years. Children were rewarded for being less aggressive and more socially appropriate: talking, playing with other children, and so on. They were also punished, on occasion, for engaging in challenging behaviour. They were taught with their peers, not in special groups. This intensive intervention was compared with a similar treatment conducted for only 10 hours a week. The differences between the two groups were dramatic. By the end of the 2-year programme, the average IQ of the intervention group was 83 points, compared with 55 in the less intense intervention; 12 of the 19 children in the intensive intervention group had IQs at or above the norm, compared with 2 out of 40 in the less intensive intervention. These findings translated to school performance, with nine children in the intensive therapy group being accepted in the same age class as their peers; only one child in the less intensive therapy group achieved this. Four years later, the relative gains made by the children in the intensive therapy had been maintained. Unfortunately, these findings have been subject to significant critical debate as a result of the study's lack of methodological rigour, including non-random allocation to conditions and the use of differing measures across participants (Gresham and MacMillan 1998). Ospina and colleagues' (2008) take on these data, when combined with those of a less successful subsequent study conducted by Lovaas, was that while the approach did achieve some change on key measures, these were not clinically significant.

In an interesting development, Koegel et al. (2001) refined the operant approach by targeting a number of what they termed primary factors, which precede consequent or secondary factors: poor communication skills, for example, typically precede severe behaviour problems. In their Pivotal Response Treatment (PRT) approach, interventions to improve language and communication skills could, therefore, prevent the need for interventions to deal with disruptive behaviour. Koegel and colleagues argued for targeting a variety of pro-social behaviours that facilitate communication, including improving eye contact, head positioning, reducing stereotypical movements and unusual facial expressions, as well as encouraging children to initiate social interactions.

A second innovation was based on the idea that the goal of any behavioural programme should not just be to modify one particular behaviour, but to increase the individual's motivation to engage in a number of similar behaviours. A key element of their behavioural programmes, therefore, was to provide rewards for behaviours similar to the target one. An example of the difference between this and previous conditioning approaches was reported by Koegel et al. (1988). In this, the traditional operant approach reinforced specified phonetic sounds as they became increasingly word-like over time. For reinforcement to succeed, the child had to produce responses that were at least as good as their previous responses. This novel approach reinforced any attempts to verbalize, however accurate or inaccurate the noise made. In a direct comparison between the two approaches, Koegel et al. (1988) found the novel approach to result in more rapid gains in the use of appropriate speech and greater levels of pro-social behaviours than the traditional method.

A final innovation of their approach was to allow the child control over the reward they were given for engaging in the targeted behaviours. Perhaps the most extreme, and ultimately most rewarding, examples of this allowed the child to engage in stereotypical or ritualistic behaviours, which are intrinsically highly rewarding, as a reward for completion of other tasks. This strategy has been shown to reduce the **incidence** of aggressive tantrums and other 'off-task' behaviours and increase levels of engagement and initiation of peer social interactions (e.g. Koegel et al. 2013). The training is now in a form that can be conducted by parents as the key people interacting with the child, with some success on measures of child verbal communication and parent satisfaction (Bradshaw et al. 2017), and has now been successfully adapted to allow those who live far from areas of expertise to engage with the programme, with training provided via the internet (McGarry et al. 2020).

14.3 Attention-deficit/hyperactivity disorder

DSM-5 identifies three dimensions within attention-deficit/hyperactivity disorder (ADHD): problems of poor attention, hyperactive-impulsive behaviour, and a combination of the two. Most children with the disorder have both sets of problems. Criteria for each diagnosis are 'often' engaging in the behaviours outlined in Table 14.1 over a period of at least 6 months.

Table 14.1 Key features of the ADHD diagnostic categories

Inattention	Hyperactivity-impulsivity
• Has trouble maintaining attention on tasks or play activities	• Fidgets, taps hands or feet, or squirms in seat
• Fails to pay close attention to details or makes careless errors in schoolwork, work or other activities	• Runs around or climbs when it is not appropriate to do so (limited to feeling restless in adolescents/adults)
• Does not appear to listen when spoken to directly	• Appears driven or 'on the go'
• Fails to follow instructions or finish schoolwork, chores or workplace tasks	• Is unable to play or take part in leisure activities quietly
• Has trouble organizing tasks and activities	• Talks excessively
• Avoids, dislikes or is reluctant to do tasks that involve sustained mental effort	• Blurts out answers before questions are completed.
• Is easily distracted	• Interrupts or intrudes on others
• Is forgetful in daily activities	• Has trouble waiting turn
• Loses materials needed for tasks and activities: books, pencils, tools, toys, and so on	

The number of each criterion behaviour varies according to age. For those aged under 17 years, six or more inattention and hyperactivity criteria should be evident; for those aged 17 years and over, five or more should be present. In addition, problem behaviours need to have begun before the age of 12 years, be present in school, work and at home, and to significantly impair functioning. Many children with ADHD have difficulty in getting on with their peers and establishing friendships. They fail to recognize when their behaviour is annoying others and make significant social mistakes. They can usually understand such issues in hypothetical scenarios, but have trouble translating this understanding into the 'real world'. About 25% of children with ADHD have some form of learning difficulty, and many are placed in special education units as a consequence of their disruptive behaviour. Children with ADHD are more likely to drop out of school than those without the disorder.

An estimated 3–7% of children across the world could be diagnosed as having ADHD. A further 5% display difficulties that impact negatively on their life but are under the threshold for a diagnosis of ADHD (Sayal et al. 2018). Interestingly, rates across the US states vary between 3% and 6%, which has been taken to indicate differences in the diagnostic criteria being applied across educational systems (Fulton et al. 2009). Importantly, ADHD is not a uniquely American or Western problem. Kashala et al. (2005), for example, reported a prevalence of 6% among schoolchildren in the Democratic Republic of Congo.

Some, but not all, problems abate as the individual grows older. Of children identified with ADHD, 40% continue to have these problems in late adolescence, and about 10% have some level of symptoms in adulthood (Mannuzza and Klein 2000). Between 1% and 6% of adults meet the criteria for ADHD (Murphy and Barkley 1996). By this time, most people have learned to adapt to their symptoms and can hold down jobs, although adults diagnosed with ADHD tend to experience a number of negative outcomes, including difficulties in academic and workplace settings, relationship discord, and parenting issues, as well as more specific problems such as relatively poor driving performance. A suggestion that ADHD can begin in adulthood in the absence of any childhood problems has been recently posited, although Sibley and colleagues' (2018) longitudinal study suggests this may be erroneous with apparent adult-onset ADHD usually being the result of substance use in adulthood or missed early signs in adolescence.

Aetiology of ADHD

Biological mechanisms

The main characteristics of ADHD are thought to reflect problems with behavioural control and management. Impulsivity is not thought to result from an inability to attend but is the result of problems in **executive function**: a failure to decide when actions should be taken and how they should be executed (Tripp and Wickens 2009). This implicates dysfunction of the frontal lobe as central to the disorder, a hypothesis supported by consistent fMRI findings of hypoactivity within the frontal lobe and its links to other brain areas including the basal ganglia, thalamus, and parietal cortex among people with ADHD (e.g. Sharma and Couture 2014). The main neurotransmitter involved in ADHD seems to be dopamine. Data to support this hypothesis mainly stem from animal models and treatment studies that have found drugs that increase dopamine levels to be most effective in reducing or even eliminating the symptoms of ADHD. These include various types of amphetamines and indirect dopamine agonists. It seems paradoxical that an amphetamine could actually reduce levels of physical activity, but it appears to do so by increasing frontal activity and control over executive dysfunctions that underpin the behaviour. In fact, Sagvolden et al. (2005) suggested that dopamine dysregulation in three brain areas may lead to the key symptoms of ADHD:

- *Mesocortical system*: responsible for normal cognitive function within the frontal lobe. Dysregulation leads to deficiencies in attention and poor behavioural organization.
- *Mesolimbic system*: the reward pathway of the brain, linking (among other brain areas) the limbic and frontal lobes. Dysregulation leads to a shorter 'delay of reinforcement gradient' and deficient extinction of behaviour. That is, low levels of dopamine increase the salience of short-term rewards and reduce the ability to work towards longer-term rewards, leading to impulsiveness.
- *Nigrostriatal system*: dysregulation leads to clumsiness, and poor non-declarative, routine, habit learning.

A second, yet still important neurotransmitter involved in ADHD is norepinephrine. Evidence suggests there is lower than normal norepinephrine activity within the prefrontal cortex in ADHD, which may amplify responses to attended stimuli, and reduce responses to irrelevant stimuli (Sharma and Couture 2014).

Exploring the genetic contribution to the disorder, concordance between **monozygotic (MZ) twins** varies between 58% and 83%, versus 31% and 47% for **dizygotic (DZ) twins**, with heritability estimates for attention problems varying between 60% and 80% (Wender et al. 2001). Meta-analyses or pooled data analyses have supported associations between ADHD and polymorphisms in a number of genes that influence dopamine receptors and transporter processes (Thapar et al. 2005), as well as norepinephrine and serotonin transporter genes (Russell et al. 2005). However, a single gene increasing risk for ADHD has still to be identified, and risk is likely to be associated with a number of genes each contributing a small amount to the disorder (Neale et al. 2010).

Psychological explanations

As noted above, ADHD can be characterized not by hyperactivity, but by high levels of impulsivity – a failure to regulate responses to events. According to Barkley (1997), children with ADHD do things other children think of doing, but don't actually do. The urge to act is not inhibited. The first response to a situation is the response that is taken. In addition, children with ADHD are more emotionally responsive to events than most children. They are poor at controlling their feelings, and less able to tolerate negative emotions. Their emotions are driven by the moment and the object of their attention at that time. As a consequence, they have difficulties in maintaining goal-oriented behaviour, particularly when this is associated with some type of negative emotion. They have difficulty in sticking to a task in the expectation of future rewards or satisfaction on its completion. Schoolwork or other demanding and sometimes boring or frustrating tasks do not hold their attention and they move rapidly to other more immediately rewarding activities.

Barkley (1997) noted that as children grow older, they use an internal dialogue as a means of self-control. This internalized language develops at around the age of 3–4 years, the time that ADHD is often first identified. This is not coincidental: Barkley suggests that children with ADHD have disorganized internal speech, which contributes to their disorganized responses to external events. Barkley noted that children with ADHD often appear 'chatty', but their conversation usually deals with the present rather than the future: thoughts do not lead to planning and future expectations. This disorganization also means that children with ADHD have difficulties in dealing with abstract issues. They find it hard to explain things: they do not get to the point; they talk around it. Of interest is that while Barkley provided a psychological perspective on ADHD, he considered it to have a biological basis, and to be largely the result of biochemical and neurological factors. He described people with ADHD as 'biochemical outliers', acknowledging a dimensional view of their behaviour rather than a categorical one.

While Barkley's model is probably the most widely acknowledged psychological theory of ADHD, it is not without its critics. Sagvolden et al. (2005), for example, suggested the biochemical processes that underpin ADHD are more complicated than implied by the relatively simple model of Barkley. They also disagreed on the fundamental processes underpinning the condition. Barkley suggested ADHD involves a failure to inhibit urges to respond to the environment. Sagvolden and colleagues (e.g. Killeen et al. 2012) suggested a more complex process involving poor attention and behavioural organization, a failure to learn appropriate behavioural sequences, and a sensitivity to short-term reinforcers and lack of response to longer-term outcomes that rewards rapid, poorly thought-through responses to environmental stimuli. In support of this model, one study of the cognitive processes underpinning ADHD (Cornoldi et al. 2001) found that children with ADHD symptoms had working memory problems which led them to have difficulties suppressing information that initially had to be processed and subsequently excluded from memory, in order to perform a memory task effectively. The same research group (Sella et al. 2019) subsequently found that children with ADHD were less effective at identifying the best strategy through which to solve mathematical problems and were less accurate when using their strategy.

A biopsychosocial model

Bettelheim (1973) integrated biochemical models with social and psychological factors in a biopsychosocial model of ADHD. He suggested that ADHD develops when children with a biological predisposition to hyperactivity are raised in an environment with a strong authoritarian ethos or one where there is evident resentfulness at inappropriate behaviour. According to Bettelheim, if a child with a predisposition to hyperactivity is responded to with obvious frustration or impatience by their parents, they may feel unable to respond effectively to their parents' need for controlled behaviour and obedience. As both react to each other in negative ways, this may spiral into a continuous battle between child and parents, which spills over to other settings and eventually results in what may be termed ADHD.

Evidence of a role of family dynamics as a causal factor for ADHD, however, is not strong. Rey et al. (2000), for example, found an adverse family environment was associated with conduct disorder and oppositional defiant disorder, but was not associated with ADHD. That said, there does appear to be a link between disorganized attachment as a child and insecure attachment as an adult and ADHD; with ADHD-like behaviours used by the child as a means of gaining parental attention (Kissgen and Franke 2016). However, the data here are inconsistent, with one longitudinal study by Lifford et al. (2009) finding ADHD symptoms, particularly in boys, to trigger negative parental responses. It is possible some attention is better than no attention, but data such as these do not provide strong support for this hypothesis. Indeed, Sandberg (2005) suggested that ADHD is an adaptation to defective neurotransmission. The resulting behavioural style is usually maladaptive and not only increases vulnerability to adverse experiences, but also creates a context in which encountering adversity is more likely.

Treatment of ADHD

Pharmacological interventions

Perhaps the best-known pharmacological treatment of ADHD involves methylphenidate hydrochloride, better known as Ritalin. The combined results of studies investigating its efficacy suggest it achieves significant improvements in about 60% of those prescribed it, compared with about 10% of those prescribed **placebo** (Wender et al. 2001). The key benefit of Ritalin is that it moderates the symptoms of both inattention and hyperactivity, allowing the individual to focus more on educational, social, and family issues. Pelham et al. (1993), for example, compared an 8-week school-based behaviour modification programme combined with Ritalin and the same programme combined with placebo in the treatment of a group of 8-year-old boys with ADHD. The behavioural programme involved a points system with both rewards for appropriate behaviour and 'costs' for inappropriate classroom behaviours. Acquisition of a fixed number of points could be exchanged for a variety of items chosen by the child. The effect of the behavioural intervention combined with Ritalin was significantly greater than when it was combined with placebo on measures of both class behaviour and academic performance.

The benefits of Ritalin can be dramatic. Here, a teacher describes the impact of Ritalin on one child and his classmates:

He just came to us in Year 7, with a real history of paperwork behind him ... poor behaviour, learning difficulties. He came to the school in September. We thought he had ADHD because he was beyond control, reason. He couldn't stay seated – or wouldn't – he wandered round the classroom, started wandering about the school. He was a powerful lad, and just pushed people out of the way that tried to stop him. By the end of November he had been seen by the doctor. He was given a diagnosis of ADHD and prescribed Ritalin. He stayed at home a couple of days, because he was pretty zonked out on it. Then he came back to school. The change was instantaneous. He was a difficult child, and he still had behavioural problems ... but you could reason with him.

You could sit him down and talk to him. He decided he liked learning, as for the first time he could understand what he was being taught. He started reading ... which boosted his self-esteem ... lots of these kids with ADHD have low self-esteem as they fail in school ... Ritalin does allow them to access the curriculum. For the first time, they can concentrate on something and make progress. But when the medicine wears off you know about it. We start to give the mid-day dose at about a quarter to twelve. By this time, they [children with ADHD] have got more 'edgy', more loud. Lots of walking, winding people up: 'loud' is the predominant word ... Sometimes you think the poor kids don't have a chance. It's difficult at home – and they may trash their room. But you think sometimes it's a response to real problems they have with their parents. Some of them are like their child: they go from 'down here' to sky high in seconds. It's got to be bad for the kids.

In a Cochrane review of the relevant literature, Storebò et al. (2015) concluded that Ritalin had a consistent and significant positive benefit based on teacher reports of child behaviour and parental reports of quality of life. The authors also noted, more cautiously, that the studies on which these conclusions were based were generally methodologically weak. And although they found no increase in 'serious' adverse events, Ritalin was associated with an increased risk of non-serious events. Nevertheless, medical concerns in relation to Ritalin are not trivial, and include cardiac problems, loss of appetite, abdominal pain, weight loss, insomnia, and increased heart rate. Retardation of growth may also occur during prolonged therapy in children. Ritalin may also trigger **psychotic** symptoms, although the reportedly very high prevalence of psychotic symptoms (9%), including **hallucinations** and paranoia among 192 children treated with Ritalin for ADHD (Cherland and Fitzpatrick 1999), appears to have been rather exaggerated. An estimated prevalence of one case per 660 people prescribed the drug reported by Moran et al. (2019) appears more representative.

Many social problems with Ritalin result from its high level of prescribing. Some people believe it is over-prescribed, and used to control unruly or unwanted behaviour in the classroom, not just ADHD; an outcome, it has been argued, that has been orchestrated and facilitated by 'big Pharma' (see, for example, Schwarz 2016). Many schools in the USA, for example, have historically refused to accept 'difficult' children unless they are treated with Ritalin: a source of significant controversy. A final risk associated with Ritalin is its use as a drug of abuse, which is becoming increasingly common in the USA. As an amphetamine, it suppresses appetite, increases wakefulness, and produces an emotional high. When abused, tablets are either taken orally or crushed and snorted. Some abusers dissolve the tablets in water and inject the mixture, which can cause complications because insoluble fillers in the tablets can block small blood vessels. Students are also using Ritalin as a so-called 'smart drug' to improve exam performance.

Stop and think ...

ADHD provides a good example of the potential for 'difficult' or problematic behaviour to become a diagnosable 'disorder'. Once ascribed, this can then legitimize 'treatment' with medication, medicalizing what is essentially a behavioural problem. It also establishes a psychiatric 'label' which can follow an individual as they progress through the education and other systems, with a number of negative consequences, including not being accepted in some schools. But, of course, as discussed in the main text, appropriately targeted medication can be of benefit to some children and a diagnosis may trigger a range of supportive mechanisms. So, there are pros and cons to the use of any diagnostic label.

So, what are your views on this? How would you feel if one of your children was diagnosed with ADHD, prescribed medication, and how can we safeguard the process to be optimally beneficial to any child involved?

Other drug treatments are now emerging. The role of norepinephrine in ADHD has resulted in the development and use of a drug designed to increase levels of norepinephrine within the frontal lobe. Atomoxetine is a norepinephrine re-uptake inhibitor which may provide an alternative treatment to methylphenidate and is of similar therapeutic benefit. However, it also has more short-term side-effects, including anorexia, nausea, and vomiting, which are experienced by up to a third of those receiving the drug (Sharma and Couture 2014). Another form of treatment is provided by a drug known as modafinil. This psychostimulant has been used for treating excessive daytime sleepiness associated with **narcolepsy** and is now being used in ADHD. The mechanism of action of modafinil is unknown but, unlike other stimulants, the drug is highly selective for the central nervous system and has little effect on dopaminergic activity. Nevertheless, it appears effective in reducing the core symptoms of ADHD (S.M. Wang et al. 2017).

Working with children with ADHD

Training attention

The attention training tasks used to treat head injuries described in Chapter 15 can also be used to help children with ADHD. Semrud-Clikeman et al. (1999), for example, examined the effectiveness of the Attention Process Training Programme (Park et al. 1999: described in more detail in Chapter 15) combined with training in problem-solving in a school setting with children identified as having problems in attention and not completing work. As a result of the training programme, the children improved on the training tasks, completed more tasks in class, and their teachers reported that they seemed more attentive. Using materials specifically developed for young children, Kerns et al. (1999) reported improvements in a group of 7–11-year-old children following a similar attention training programme. By the end of the training period, participants achieved better scores on untrained cognitive tasks, academic performance, and teacher reports of impulsiveness.

Environmental manipulation

As many of the behaviours associated with ADHD are seen as immediate responses to the environment, one way in which they may be influenced is by environmental manipulation. The US Department of Education (2006) set out some clear guidelines, including the nature of the learning environment, to help teachers work with children with ADHD. These included:

- sit students with ADHD at the front of the class with their backs to the rest of the class to keep other students out of view
- surround students with ADHD with good role models
- avoid distracting stimuli
- produce a stimuli-reduced study area for teaching (which other children can access) to avoid isolation.

In addition to these environmental aspects, they considered a number of other factors, including guidelines for maintaining and enhancing self-esteem, responding to inappropriate behaviour, and the process of teaching, all of which contribute to best practice when teaching children with ADHD.

A different way of manipulating the environment, whether in school or the home, is to reward appropriate behaviours in an operant-conditioning-based intervention. This approach frequently involves a process known as a token economy, in which the child is rewarded for engaging in specific pre-specified behaviours with a token. Tokens can be collected and, when enough have been accrued, exchanged for a desired item. This approach has a number of variants, including charts on which stars are placed as a reward for appropriate behaviours and, again, exchanged for tangible rewards when enough are displayed. Although this type of intervention can be effective on its own, these procedures are frequently used in conjunction with treatment by some form of medication.

Token economies can provide a general set of rules and rewards for addressing key goals within a particular environment: one token for sitting in the chair quietly during a lesson, and so on. They may also be more personalized. In one study of this latter approach, Coelho et al. (2015) combined a cognitive behavioural and token economy intervention in the home. In the token economy, parents initially identified the ten most problematic problem behaviours at home, which became the focus of the intervention. Each problem behaviour was written on a card combined with a new, desirable behaviour or response. Over the course of the intervention, when an inappropriate behaviour occurred, parents reminded the child of the positive alternative response and provided a model of this. At the end of each week, the child was given a token for each appropriate behaviour in which they engaged. Over time, these could be exchanged for desired rewards including crayons and pencil cases. In addition, parents were taught to give praise for appropriate behaviours with the intention that this became a reinforcer of the behaviour independent of tokens. Over the course of the intervention, problematic behaviours decreased significantly in 7 of 11 categories measured: impulsiveness, hyperactivity, disorganization, disobeying rules and routines, poor self-care, low frustration tolerance, and antisocial behaviours. Measures of verbal/physical aggression, lack of initiative, and compulsive behaviours were unchanged (one further category, 'inattention', could not be assessed).

Other family approaches have adopted less behavioural, and perhaps more complex, strategies. Barkley et al. (2001), for example, compared the effectiveness of problem-solving communication training alone or following training in behavioural management skills in an attempt to minimize conflict within families. Problem-solving communication training involved a five-stage process through which the family combined to deal with problems: defining the problem, brainstorming potential solutions, negotiating and deciding within the family which solutions to implement, and then implementing the solution. The behavioural skills management involved parents learning to change triggers or responses to disruptive behaviour using operant procedures. The two interventions proved equally effective in those that completed them. However, three times as many people dropped out of training when the problem-solving approach was used alone than in the combined condition. Not all studies have shown benefit, however (see Bjornstad and Montgomery 2005), and given the evidence that family dynamics do not directly contribute to the development of ADHD, this approach may best be used when families are clearly experiencing stress and struggling to cope with a child's behaviour rather than as a standard approach given to all.

Research box 13

Bachmann, K., Lam, A.P., Sörös, P. et al. (2018) Effects of mindfulness and psychoeducation on working memory in adult ADHD: a randomised, controlled fMRI study, *Behaviour Research and Therapy*, 106: 47–56.

Impairments in working memory are central to the problems faced by individuals with ADHD. Mindfulness interventions have the potential to improve working memory, with evidence of improved attention, emotional regulation, and quality of life. The present study aimed to develop this research further by considering both experimental and neurological evidence of any changes following a mindfulness intervention in adults with ADHD. The latter evidence is likely to be manifest through functional changes in the frontoparietal networks and cingulate cortex and basal ganglia: the brain activity of the neural systems involved in working memory were monitored using fMRI.

Method

Participants

Participants were 40 adults (mean age 40 years; $n = 22$ women) being treated for ADHD in a large German university hospital or recruited via an advert on the centre's website. Inclusion criteria were age 18–65 years, a confirmed diagnosis of ADHD, and not on any medication or psychological treatment for at least 3 months. Exclusion criteria were evidence of psychosis, substance abuse or contraindications to MRI (e.g. metal implant, pregnancy). Twenty-nine participants were co-morbid for a range of other diagnoses, the most common of which was 'minor depressive disorder' ($n = 26$).

Interventions

Participants were randomly allocated to one of two conditions, each of which involved 8 weeks of contact between the study participants and therapists:

- *Mindfulness meditation (MM)*: this involved a programme of group psychotherapy, teaching a 'mindful mental attitude'. Participants completed a gradually increasing programme of group work and homework including daily seated meditation and exercises in everyday life, as well as focusing on how to manage ADHD problems using mindfulness techniques such as visualization.
- Group *psychoeducation (PE)*: this involved information on the causes, symptoms, and treatment options for ADHD in adulthood combined with the 'activation of [existing] organisational skills and stress management techniques' and mutual support from other group members.

Measures

- *fMRI – structural and functional*: images of the brain were acquired on a 3 T Siemens Magnetom Trio with a 12-channel head coil.
- *Working memory task*: fMRI images were acquired while participants performed a 'one-back letter task'. In this task, which followed two practice trials, participants were presented with two runs of 20 blocks of sequences of white letters on a black screen (visible through a projector and mirror) and instructed to indicate whether each letter matched or did not match the previous letter via a button press. In the case of two identical letters in a row (targets), participants pressed the right mouse button. Where there was no match, the left mouse button was pressed (non-targets).
- *Conners' Adult ADHD Rating Scales (CAARS) – self- and observer-rated*: measured ADHD symptom severity.

Results

The psychoeducational intervention was intended to form a placebo intervention allowing any between-group differences to be attributable to the specific effects of learning mindfulness. However, there was no evidence of this benefit on clinical measures of ADHD. Repeated-measures analysis of variance found all CAAR dimension scores to change significantly over time (at a minimum of $p < 0.02$), but no evidence of any time $\times$ condition interactions, suggesting the two interventions were equally effective (see Table 1). This pattern of results was replicated in the measures of task performance which found improvements over time ($p < 0.05$), but no effect of condition.

Table 1 Mean scores (and standard deviations) on key CAAR measures of ADHD symptomatology over time and across treatment conditions

	Baseline		Post-treatment	
	MM	**PE**	**MM**	**PE**
CAARS observer rating				
Inattention/ memory problems	18.71 (9.05)	17.58 (7.51)	16.29 (8.65)	15.53 (7.76)
Hyperactivity/ restlessness	14.10 (8.20)	17.68 (7.39)	12.48 (7.61)	13.21 (7.58)
Impulsivity/ emotional lability	13.86 (8.13)	13.11 (7.82)	11.62 (6.15)	9.47 (6.92)
CAARS self-rating				
Inattention/ memory problems	19.62 (7.54)	18.68 (6.58)	18.86 (8.18)	14.89 (6.26)
Hyperactivity/ restlessness	15.14 (7.53)	17.26 (8.25)	14.10 (7.85)	14.37 (6.47)
Impulsivity/ emotional lability	16.00 (8.33)	14.95 (9.55)	14.57 (7.67)	11.42 (6.75)
One-back performance				
Mean correct	61.29 (15.51)	57.13 (14.04)	70.05 (14.70)	64.55 (15.37)
% correct	54.55 (13.80)	50.85 (12.5)	62.35 (13.1)	57.45 (13.68)

The neurological measures, however, showed a more condition-specific effect. A two-sample paired t-test in each condition found no changes in neural activation in the psychoeducation group. However, the mindfulness participants evidenced higher activation in the left and right inferior parietal lobule, right posterior insula, and right precuneus following training in mindfulness (see Table 2).

Table 2 Brain areas showing significantly stronger activation after mindfulness training

Brain area	Hemisphere	x (mm)	y (mm)	z (mm)	Voxels	Max Z-value
Inferior parietal lobule	Left	−36	−64	46	354	3.58
Posterior insula	Right	36	−18	6	640	3.47
Inferior parietal lobule	Right	50	−26	22		3.20
Precuneus	Right	8	−60	30	319	3.25

Discussion

The study reports some intriguing findings. The interventions proved equally successful on both behavioural/clinical measures of ADHD and task performance, yet the neurological evidence suggests a more specific effect of mindfulness on the brain systems underpinning both task performance and behaviour. The authors provided a number of potential explanations for these findings, of which the strongest may be that the time-frame of the study did not permit any clinical changes driven by the altered neurological activation to be evident. It is also possible that the study was underpowered to detect such changes with any accuracy.

Working with adults who have ADHD

Self-management strategies

Adults with ADHD can be taught a number of self-management strategies to help them manage their attentional problems (Sohlberg and Mateer 2001). These include orienting procedures in which they regularly monitor their activities to ensure they focus on planned activities. An example of this approach may be the use of a watch that beeps every hour, reminding the individual to ask themselves, 'What am I currently doing? What was I doing before doing this? What am I supposed to do next?' An example of another orienting task, used with people who set off to drive somewhere and then forget their destination is, at the beginning of every trip, to routinely write down their destination, expected time of arrival, and the time at which it may be useful to ask for help if lost.

A second approach involves *pacing*. People with attention problems often experience fatigue or problems in maintaining concentration over extended periods of time. To combat this, they may benefit from pacing the demands they place upon themselves, by not setting too high standards of productivity and taking breaks at regular intervals. They can also be taught to monitor fatigue levels and take breaks at appropriate times rather than fighting through the fatigue and being unproductive. People with attention problems also find that they have difficulty in switching from one task to another. The *key ideas log* minimizes the problems associated with this by encouraging people with attention problems to quickly write down or voice-record ideas that spring to mind, so they do not disrupt their ongoing task. Ramsay (2010) contended that the very process of therapy may be of value to people with ADHD, because it involves what he termed, 'prolongation' – that is, a time of reflection, review of issues, and consideration of problem management, within therapy. Learning and practice of these skills regardless of the issue at hand is likely to be of benefit to people with ADHD. He also noted that CBT may also be used to challenge thoughts that perpetuate ADHD, including: 'I have plenty of time to do … I can do it later' or 'My reports are no good …', and can also act as prompts to some form of attention and behavioural activation: 'Can you commit to working on it for at least 5 minutes?'

Environmental strategies

A final intervention involves thinking through the impact that environmental factors have on attention and considering ways in which they can be modified to maximize cognitive performance (Sohlberg and Mateer 2001). Central to this approach is avoiding 'busy' or distracting environments and making use of 'quiet' environments when attention is required. This may involve, for example, shopping in quiet local shops rather than attempting to shop in bustling supermarkets. Further strategies may include minimizing the demands on attentional or organizational abilities by setting up standing orders to pay bills or labelling cupboards to ensure maximum organization. The use of 'Do not disturb' signs both at home and at work may also help minimize distraction from ongoing tasks. While these types of approaches would seem logical and likely to be effective, their highly individual nature has meant that their effectiveness has largely been explored through individual case reports rather than controlled trials (Sohlberg and Mateer 2001).

14.4 Chapter summary

1. About 3% of the UK population have learning difficulties.
2. Only about 25% of cases of learning difficulty have an identified cause. These causes include genetic conditions, infectious diseases, environmental hazards, and several perinatal factors.
3. Social factors contribute strongly to mild learning difficulties, less so to more severe problems.
4. Down syndrome and Fragile X syndrome are two common conditions resulting from differing genetic factors.
5. The principles of normalization and social role valorization ensure that people with learning difficulties achieve the same respect and rights as the rest of the population.
6. Care of people with learning difficulties includes both social and psychological interventions.

7. Psychological interventions are frequently based on operant conditioning approaches to skills learning or behavioural change, although cognitive behavioural interventions may also prove effective.

8. People with ASD have difficulties in three areas: social interaction, communication, and obsessive-compulsive or ritualistic acts.

9. When combined with learning difficulties, these may profoundly influence the outcome of affected individuals.

10. The opioid theory of autism suggests that the disorder results from an overdose of opioids as a result of a failure to metabolize gluten and casein from the gut. The MMR vaccine was thought to contribute to this problem – but is no longer seen as a cause of autism.

11. A newly emerging neurological factor appears to be damage to the brain due to high levels of serotonin before birth affecting key brain regions regulating behaviours affected by autism. A gut biome–brain interaction also appears important although any exact mechanisms are yet to be fully understood.

12. Bettelheim's psychodynamic model suggests that autism is an escape from an adverse family environment.

13. The biopsychosocial model of autism proposes that the disorder results from a combination of lack of motivation to engage in social interactions combined with a lack of appropriate responses from the environment.

14. Lovaas's controversial behavioural treatment has proven moderately effective in the treatment of autism. Koegel and colleagues have developed a more strategic approach to such interventions.

15. Pharmacological interventions have also been shown to reduce a limited number of negative behaviours.

16. An estimated 3–5% of children in the USA have ADHD.

17. ADHD seems to be driven by low levels of dopamine and serotonin and can be treated with drugs that increase these levels.

18. ADHD is driven by high levels of impulsivity, or lack of 'executive control'.

19. Barkley considered ADHD to reflect failures to control immediate impulses. By contrast, Sagvolden and colleagues considered the problem to reflect behavioural organization, an over-response to immediate reinforcers and a failure to learn routine behavioural sequences.

20. Family factors may also increase risk for ADHD, although relevant data are surprisingly sparse.

21. Treatment with Ritalin and atomoxetine has been shown to facilitate behavioural interventions and education in children and adults.

22. A variety of self-management programmes may be effective in treating adult ADHD.

14.5 For discussion

1. Do changes in technology and society help or hinder people with learning difficulties to cope with everyday living?
2. What are the implications for a family that has a child with a significant learning disorder?
3. What limits should there be to health professionals' responses to 'challenging behaviour'?
4. Given the range of experiences of people with ASD, from profound learning difficulties to the emotional and social difficulties identified by Grandin, how useful a label is this?
5. What are the implications for a family that has a child with ADH?
6. Should all families of children with ADHD be encouraged to take part in family therapy to minimize the negative impact of an adverse family environment?

14.6 Further reading

Fletcher, S. and Happé, F. (2019) *Autism: A New Introduction to Psychological Theory and Current Debate*, Abingdon: Routledge.

Grandin, T. and Panek, R. (2014) *The Autistic Brain*, London: Rider.

Haavik, J., Kuntsi, J., Larsson, H. et al. (2018) Live fast, die young? A review on the developmental trajectories of ADHD across the lifespan, *European Neuropsychopharmacology*, 28: 1059–88.

Jones, V. and Haydon-Laurelut, M. (eds.) (2019) *Working with People with Learning Disabilities: Systemic Approaches*, London: Red Globe Press.

Manos, M.J., Giuliano, K. and Geyer, E. (2017) ADHD: overdiagnosed and overtreated, or misdiagnosed and mistreated?, *Cleveland Clinic Journal of Medicine*, 84: 873–80.

Ratey, J.R. (2006) *Delivered from Distraction: Getting the Most Out of Life with Attention Deficit Disorder*, New York: Ballantine.

Reichow, B., Hume, K., Barton, E.E. et al. (2018) Early intensive behavioral intervention (EIBI) for young children with autism spectrum disorders (ASD), *Cochrane Database of Systematic Reviews*, 5: CD009260 [https://doi.org/10.1002/14651858.CD009260.pub3].

15 Neurological disorders

Chapter contents

Neurological disorders are the result of damage or degeneration of the brain following the onset of disease or trauma. This chapter focuses on the consequences of three types of disorder arising from two disease processes, **Alzheimer's disease** and multiple sclerosis (MS), as well as from head injury. In the case of Alzheimer's disease and MS, therapy is aimed at maintaining cognitive function and well-being in the face of a progressive deterioration of cognitive processes. Cognitive processes may be markedly impaired following head injury, but recover to some extent over time. Interventions here focus on maximizing the process of recovery and helping the individual cope with any residual cognitive deficits. By the end of the chapter, you should have an understanding of:

- The neurological processes that result in Alzheimer's disease and MS
- The psychological consequences of these diseases
- Interventions aimed at improving or maintaining both cognitive functioning and well-being as the diseases progress
- The immediate and long-term cognitive consequences of head injury
- Interventions used to maximize recovery following head injury.

15.1 Alzheimer's disease

Alzheimer's disease, now referred to as 'major or mild neurocognitive disorder due to Alzheimer's Disease' by **DSM**-5, is the most common type of dementia, affecting between 2% and 10% of those aged over 65 years, and at least 20% of those aged over 80 years (e.g. Fiest et al. 2016). Although generally a condition found in elderly people, this is not always the case. Indeed, Alois Alzheimer's first description of the condition in the early years of the twentieth century was of a middle-aged woman. The criteria for a diagnosis of Alzheimer's disease are quite complex:

- The diagnostic criteria for major or minor neurocognitive disorder are fulfilled: (i) memory impairment, (ii) impaired abstract thinking, (iii) impaired judgement, (iv) other disturbances of higher cortical function including aphasia, apraxia, and agnosia, (iv) personality change (either alteration or accentuation of pre-morbid traits), and (v) no change in consciousness.
- Insidious onset and gradual decline of cognitive function in one or more of the following domains for mild, or two or more domains for major, neurocognitive disorder: complex attention, **executive function**, learning and memory, language, perceptual-motor function, and social cognition (e.g. theory of mind, insight).
- The presence of Alzheimer's dementia genetic mutation based on family history or genetic testing.
- The following three indicators are present:
  o Decline in memory or learning, and one other cognitive domain evident over time
  o Steady cognitive decline, without periods of stability
  o No other psychological, neurological or medical problems responsible for cognitive decline.

More succinctly, DSM-IV-TR defined Alzheimer's disease as having the following characteristics (often summarized as the 4As):

- *Amnesia*: loss of memory
- *Aphasia*: language disturbance
- *Apraxia*: impaired ability to carry out motor activities despite intact motor function
- *Agnosia*: failure to recognize or identify objects despite intact sensory function

plus

- *Disturbance in executive functioning* (that is, planning, organizing, sequencing, abstracting).

Memory loss is progressive, with recent memories typically lost before remote ones, which are thought to be preserved as a consequence of rehearsal over life. However, as the disease progresses, even remote and emotionally charged memories are lost. Early forgetfulness becomes a pathologically poor memory for present events, daily routine, and even family members. Word-finding difficulties are common. In its final stages, Alzheimer's disease destroys the ability to communicate in any way.

In the early stages of Alzheimer's disease, levels of insight are high, and most people are aware of their deficits. However, as the disease progresses, insight is lost, all sense of self seems to vanish, and the individual becomes completely dependent on others for care. Suspiciousness, paranoia, and **delusions** are common. The individual may experience spontaneous changes in mood, including anger and irritability, as well as restlessness and agitation. Confusion is common, and may be worse at night when cues that may orient them in time and place are less obvious, and the oxygen supply to the brain is at its lowest. Although most healthcare services aim to maximize the independence of the individual and maintain them in their own home, there may come a time when they are hospitalized. By this time, they may be confused for much of the time, incontinent, and respond only vaguely to their environment.

The duration of Alzheimer's disease from time of diagnosis to death can be 20 years or more: the typical duration is between 4 and 8 years. Over this time the individual will progress through the following stages:

- *Questionable dementia*: the individual begins to behave 'oddly' and relatives suspect there is a problem
- *Mild dementia*: there is no question that there is a problem, but the affected individual can maintain independence
- *Moderate dementia*: help is required for routine tasks; 'problem' behaviours such as wandering or aggression may be evident
- *Severe dementia*: the individual becomes increasingly frail and eventually chair- or bed-bound.

The impact of Alzheimer's disease goes beyond the individual directly affected. Many elderly people (the preponderance of them women) care for people with dementia in their own home, often until the disease has progressed far. These carers typically experience significant stress (see Box 15.1). Molyneux et al. (2008), for example, reported that 21% of their sample of carers were clinically depressed, and that the higher the functional impairment of the person with Alzheimer's, the greater the risk and level of depression. This stress may spill over into the way they respond to the individual with dementia. Cooper et al. (2009), for example, found that 34% of carers reported abusing the person they were caring for 'at least sometimes' in the 3 months prior to their survey. Abuse was mainly verbal; only 1% reported physical abuse.

Box 15.1 Focus groups of people with mild-to-moderate dementia

One of my colleagues, Lucie Byrne, ran some focus groups exploring the factors that contributed to the quality of life of people with mild-to-moderate dementia. Below are some quotes taken from the focus groups, with people telling us what added to or detracted from their quality of life. The quotes are actually quite unremarkable, and could be made by virtually anyone of any age. Importantly, what the participants did not say was that their failing memory made their quality of life any worse, though some said that it might in the future. In fact, this became the theme related to this issue: however bad people's cognitive abilities were, they were always said not to be affecting their quality of life at the time, but that they might in the future. This is not to say that loss of memory is not an issue and concern for people with dementia – and some people may become profoundly depressed as a result of their failing abilities. But many other things contributed to their quality of life. This did not hinge only on their cognitive abilities.

Husband/wife/partner

- *Like I said, my husband is still there and so I'm all right.*
- *All I want is to be with my husband that I've been with practically since I left school.*
- *I think the majority would say if anything happens to the partner, there's nothing worse could happen, nothing worse could happen.*

Children/grandchildren

- *You got the love of a family and the grandchildren, like me.*
- *If I lost one of my children, I would be devastated.*

Family

- *Lack of friends or relations* [would make the quality of life worse].
- *I've got a good father and I had a good mother, but I'm afraid I've just lost my mum and dad, you know.*

Your friends

- *Lack of friends or relations, loneliness, all these things take away the quality of life.*
- *Friendship, that's very important, isn't it?*

Feeling happy

- *If you are happy, you are fair enough. Sometimes people are not happy and that must be awful.*

Feeling useful

- *If you could do a good turn for anybody, do it, that makes the quality of life, don't it?*
- *If you see a dirty cup there, what's stopping you picking it up and just giving it a swirl, helping that poor lady there? ... but people walk past ... and I like* [gestures angrily], *that's my way.*

Feeling content/satisfied

- *Well, I could say nothing* [could make the quality of life worse], *I'm quite contented as I am.*
- *Whatever I do, I am contented with.*

Feeling that you have had a good life

- *I'm an extremely lucky person, I think.*
- *I suppose you don't know me, but over the years I've really enjoyed my life.*

Aetiology of Alzheimer's disease

Neurological processes

Alzheimer's disease is the result of premature degeneration of brain systems. Degeneration is progressive, and over the course of the disease can be mapped against the geography of the brain affected. Problems typically initiate in the entorhinal cortex before proceeding to the hippocampus, and then gradually spread to other regions, particularly the cerebral cortex (Hedden and Gabrieli 2005). As the hippocampal neurons degenerate, short-term memory falters, as does the ability to perform routine tasks. As the disease spreads through the cerebral cortex, it begins to take away language.

The nature of the changes that occur appears to be both structural, including the development of beta-amyloid plaques and neurofibrillary tangles, and to involve a number of **neurotransmitters**. Beta-amyloid results from damage to amyloid precursor protein (APP), which lies within the neuron cell membranes. It is a member of a larger family of proteins which enclose cells and act as a barrier, to control which substances can enter and exit from them. Damage to APP results in the formation of beta-amyloid fragments, which may clump together to form amyloid plaques and cause neuronal death, perhaps because they form tiny channels in neuron membranes through which uncontrolled amounts of calcium can flow (Sinha et al. 2000). A second mechanism associated with APP proposed by Nikolaev et al. (2009) is that a 'fragment' of APP is involved in triggering the cell destruction associated with the neuronal pruning that occurs in the fast-growth phase of neurons during child development via a neuronal receptor called Death Receptor 6 (DR6). This process may be triggered for some reason in the ageing brain resulting in significant neuronal loss.

Neurofibrillary tangles comprise abnormal collections of twisted threads inside nerve cells. The chief component of these tangles is a protein called tau. In healthy individuals, tau binds and stabilizes the microtubules that carry nutrients and molecules from the bodies of the cells to the ends of the axon. In Alzheimer's disease, tau is changed chemically, and this altered tau twists the microfilaments around each other to form tangles. The resultant collapse of the transport system causes errors in communication between nerve cells and neuronal death (Luque and Jaffe 2009).

The most important neurotransmitter implicated in Alzheimer's disease is acetylcholine: levels decline moderately in normal ageing but drop by about 90% in people with Alzheimer's (Ferreira-Vieira et al. 2016). Acetylcholine is involved in memory formation and influences neuronal activity in the hippocampus and cerebral cortex. Other neurotransmitters may also be involved. Serotonin and norepinephrine levels are lower than normal in some people with Alzheimer's, which may contribute to sensory disturbances and aggressive behaviour (Zarros et al. 2005). They may also be linked to other psychological conditions associated with the early stages of Alzheimer's, including depression and anxiety.

Up to 50% of first-degree relatives of a person with Alzheimer's disease will develop the disorder (Korten et al. 1993). The presence of two *ApoE4* gene alleles, which are involved in lipid metabolism, may bring forward the onset of Alzheimer's by as much as 17 years (Robinson et al. 2017). However, this is found in only 40% of people who develop the disease, and many people who carry these alleles do not develop the condition. In addition, risk of Alzheimer's may be reduced by changing modifiable risk factors even in individuals at genetic risk due to *ApoE* variants (Schipper 2011). Mutations of three other genes have been identified as responsible for the rare early-onset familial form of the disease: amyloid precursor protein

(*APP*), presenilin 1 (*PSEN1*), and presenilin 2 (*PSEN2*), all of which are involved in the production and aggregation of toxic amyloid plaques. Mutations in these genes, however, account for less than 5% of the total number of cases of Alzheimer's disease (Rocchi et al. 2003). A cluster of other gene alleles have been implicated, are more frequently found in the general population, but also have significantly-less influence over risk of developing the disease (Robinson et al. 2017).

Modifiable risk factors

Risk for Alzheimer's disease is also determined in part by environmental factors, although their exact roles in its **aetiology** are not always fully understood. According to Livingston et al. (2017), nine potentially modifiable psychosocial factors explain around 35% of the risk for Alzheimer's:

- *Early life*: very low levels of education (none or primary school only)
- *Midlife*: hypertension, obesity, hearing loss
- *Later life*: smoking, depression, physical inactivity, social isolation, diabetes.

Some of these indicators may reflect underlying factors rather than being direct causes of Alzheimer's disease. Low levels of education, for example, may indicate low cognitive reserve, which enables individuals to compensate for at least some degree of neural degeneration. The mechanism linking hearing loss to Alzheimer's is unclear, but may involve either increased cognitive load on vulnerable brains, or an effect on social disengagement and depression. Findings show mid-life depression not to be a risk factor for Alzheimer's, but that later life depression is, have led to speculation that the depression is a consequence rather than cause of Alzheimer's disease. Nevertheless, plausible biological pathways including stress hormones and neural growth factors are influenced by depression (Ross et al. 2018). Other factors may contribute to high levels of cholesterol increasing risk for dementia as well as other cholesterol-related conditions such as coronary heart disease (Anstey et al. 2017).

One further and consistent risk factor appears to be a history of head injury, although surprisingly head injuries in which there is loss of consciousness do not appear to increase risk significantly (Li et al. 2017). Protective factors include high levels of physical activity, moderate levels of red wine, and a diet high in vitamins B6, B12, and folic acid. High levels of consumption of fatty fish may also be of benefit, probably because of its cholesterol-lowering effect. Huang et al. (2005) found that people who ate fatty fish at least twice a week were 41% less likely to develop Alzheimer's disease than those who ate it less than once a month. A number of medications may also be protective, including non-steroidal anti-inflammatory drugs and oestrogen replacement therapy in post-menopausal women.

Treatment of Alzheimer's disease

Pharmacological Interventions

If reductions in acetylcholine cause Alzheimer's disease, an increase in available acetylcholine may reverse its symptoms. Drugs that do so prevent its breakdown in the synaptic cleft by acetylcholinesterase and increase uptake in the postsynaptic receptor (see Chapter 4). An important group of drugs, known as acetylcholinesterase inhibitors, such as donepezil, generally achieve short-term cognitive improvements in individuals at early- and mid-stage Alzheimer's, although they delay rather than prevent cognitive decline, the effects are only modest, there are no improvements in quality of life or behavioural problems, and not all people respond to them (see Birks and Harvey 2018). Unfortunately, many people who take them also experience significant side-effects, most notably gastrointestinal tract disturbances, and up to 35% of participants in clinical trials have been withdrawn from medication for this reason (Rogers et al. 1998).

A different pharmacological approach involves attempts to block the production of beta-amyloid within the brain. In evaluating this approach, Sparks et al. (2005) compared the effectiveness of this type of drug (a statin) with that of a **placebo** intervention in people with mild-to-moderate Alzheimer's disease. At one-year follow-up, the active intervention proved superior to placebo, with people in this condition showing less disease progression. Whether these initial improvements will be maintained for longer periods is yet to be determined. Chu et al. (2018) estimated that statins may reduce the risk of developing Alzheimer's disease by around 25%, although the mechanism of this protection is not understood. Reflecting the difficulties of attempts to control the processes underpinning the disease, solanezumab, a drug that increases the clearance of beta-amyloid from the brain and prevent tangles, proved ineffective and placed participants at risk of cerebral swelling (Honig et al. 2018). Overall, effective long-term treatments for Alzheimer's have proved elusive, leading Briggs et al. (2016) to argue that we need to identify the markers of early disease to allow treatment much earlier than is now the norm, which may result in more effective interventions.

Psychological approaches

Most psychological interventions aim to maximize quality of life and functional ability as the disease progresses rather than 'cure' Alzheimer's, although there have been attempts to slow down progression through attempts to modify lipid metabolism and levels of amyloid and tau through exercise, albeit with little benefit (Frederiksen et al. 2018). Three more formal psychotherapeutic approaches are frequently used in its later stages.

Reality orientation

Reality orientation (RO; Holden and Woods 1995) involves providing confused elderly people with relevant information to help them maintain an accurate understanding of the world. There are two types of RO:

- *24-hour RO* involves establishing an environment with multiple cues to orient the individual in time, place, and person: large clocks and calendars, reminders of the name of an institution or ward, name badges, and so on. Social interactions with the person are also designed to provide relevant information ('Hello, Mr Jones. It's Tom here … It's really cold outside, like it usually is in January …'). Sentences are simple and specific, repeating information throughout the day and even within conversations.

- *Classroom RO* involves small groups of people meeting for between 30 and 60 minutes. Despite its name, these meetings are held in comfortable rooms, with easy chairs and a relaxed atmosphere. Attenders are matched according to ability, and sessions involve discussion and the provision of information, with memory triggered by multiple cues and modes of information: newspapers, pictures, talking, etc.

In their review of ten well-controlled trials of RO, Carrion et al. (2018) concluded that it achieved small but significant cognitive gains compared with no treatment or unstructured therapy, but that any gains following the cessation of therapy were soon dissipated and did not generalize to measures of daily functioning and use of language. Accordingly, RO may need to be a continuous form of intervention. It can also be combined with other treatments to maximize gains. For example, Onder et al. (2005) found that RO and donepezil contributed independently to cognitive gains made in a group of people with Alzheimer's disease.

Perhaps for reasons considered in the 'Stop and think' box below, more recent studies have evaluated a variant of RO, known as cognitive stimulation. A typical programme involves elements of reality orientation combined with less structured approaches to facilitating cognitive processing. A key difference between the two approaches is that cognitive stimulation places greater emphasis on information *processing* than the rote learning of RO. Thus, an activity known as 'faces' may ask group members 'Who looks the youngest?', 'What do these people have in common?', rather than 'Do you recognize these people?'. In a Cochrane review and **meta-analysis** of 16 studies of this approach, Woods et al. (2018) found it to have modest benefits, particularly when used in care homes: there was evidence of small but consistent improvements in quality of life, memory, and communication across a number of studies.

Stop and think ...

Whatever its outcome, RO can present difficulties for those trying to implement it, particularly when it may be necessary to remind people of distressing information. Many people with Alzheimer's, for example, forget about the death of a loved one, and in their confusion may start looking for them or demanding they come and see them. Proper adherence to RO involves a carer telling them that their loved one is dead. This can be devastating news and cause significant distress. Unfortunately, they may forget this information after a period of time and once more start looking for their loved one, requiring the carer to once more break the news of their loved one's death: a cycle that can be distressing for both the individual and carer. Is this fair and a reasonable way to treat people, or, in this case, is ignorance really bliss?

Validation therapy

As a consequence of the potentially problematic aspects of RO, Feil (1990) introduced a very different form of therapy. Validation therapy involves listening to the fears and concerns of the affected individual, taking time to fully understand their problems, and to 'validate' them by valuing what they have to say. These conversations can provide opportunities to identify and modify any false beliefs, but this is not a core element of this approach. The focus is on listening and responding to the emotional rather than the factual content of what is said.

In group therapy, small groups of individuals may engage in discussions designed to elicit 'universal' feelings of anger, separation or loss (Bleathman and Morton 1992). Feil suggested that by verbalizing memories and thoughts and having them validated by the group, the person gains a feeling of being accepted. This emphasis on the need to deal with unresolved conflicts has elements of psychodynamic therapy, while the therapeutic use of empathy and acceptance of the individual's personal view of the world provide a strong humanistic element. Evaluation of the effectiveness of this approach is largely anecdotal or based on uncontrolled case histories, although one small randomized controlled trial has been reported (Tondi et al. 2007). In this, older adults with dementia (of various kinds) were randomly allocated to either validation therapy or usual care. Those in the validation therapy experienced reductions in distress, agitation, apathy, and irritability. Whether validation therapy is better than other active interventions is not clear.

Reminiscence therapy

Reminiscence therapy is based on Erikson's (1980) developmental model in which life-review is considered to occur naturally towards the end of life. This review may be generally positive or negative, with a resultant outcome of **ego** integrity or despair. In individual therapy, the therapist aids the individual through this already occurring self-analysis in order to make it more conscious and efficient. There are three forms of reminiscence therapy (McMahon and Rhudick 1964). *Story-type reminiscence* involves remembering factual memories for pleasure. *Life-review* involves remembering and discussing memories, both good and bad, which come naturally to consciousness. Finally, *halo reminiscence* involves the repeated recollection of a particular situation involving guilt or despair. Life-review and halo reminiscence are thought to help resolve past conflicts. In group therapy, small groups typically review participants' lives through the use of prompts, including old photographs, television and radio broadcasts, and so on. As with validation therapy, there are few studies of the effectiveness of reminiscence therapy. Participants typically enjoy being part of reminiscence groups, and there are reports of small improvements in mood (Wang 2007) and increased self-esteem and life satisfaction (Lai et al. 2004) following group attendance. However, there is little evidence that it is more effective than other group activities, and some studies (e.g. Ito et al. 2007) have reported no benefit.

Helping the carers

Caring for people with Alzheimer's disease at home places enormous strain on the carers, who are usually elderly themselves and often in poor health (e.g. Gilhooly et al. 2016). Many benefit from some form of support and help. This can be provided by voluntary bodies such as the Alzheimer's Disease Society in the UK, and short periods during which the affected person stays in hospital to provide a break for the carer. They may also benefit from other, more formal interventions. In a meta-analysis of 44 studies designed to provide education and/or support to help carers cope more effectively with their stress, Thompson and Briggs (2000) concluded that group and individual interventions reduced both perceptions of burden and feelings of depression – although the effects across studies were varied and relatively modest. More recently, a review of the effect of mindfulness-based interventions for family carers found that there was some evidence of reductions in depressive symptoms and anxiety compared with controls, but any gains were marginal and inconsistent (Z. Liu et al. 2018). One interesting approach in this context has been to involve both carer and the person with dementia in a joint activity designed to enhance quality of life and potentially modify the course of the disease: exercise (Lamotte et al. 2017). As with the use of mindfulness, there are some encouraging signs that 'dyadic exercise interventions' may improve functional independence of the person with Alzheimer's and the perceived burden of their carer. However, the evidence is weak and needs further development.

A second way of helping carers cope is to provide them with strategies to help them manage the behaviour of their affected relative more effectively. In one such study, Gavrilova et al. (2009) examined the impact of a relatively brief intervention involving two sessions providing basic information about dementia, and two sessions developing personal strategies for coping with problem behaviours. Although measures of distress did not differ between those in the intervention group and a control condition at 6-month follow-up, those in the intervention group reported significantly less 'carer burden' (i.e. stress directly related to caring for the individual with dementia). More recently, Kales et al. (2018) identified carers as central to the management of behavioural and psychological symptoms in the main place of care: the home. Their model of care was adapted from their in-hospital system, and adopted a formulation-based approach, identifying specific problems and treating them as appropriate. This DICE model involved:

- *Describing the problematic behaviour*: this may vary from aggression to wandering, failure to remember routine tasks, and so on.
- *Investigating possible causes of the behaviour*: this approach may vary from simple assessment ('Why did he forget to do X?') to a more functional analysis ('What happens immediately before he loses his temper? How do I react to this? Does my reaction tend to reduce or increase his anger? What happens after?').
- *Creating a treatment plan*: based on the analysis of causes (changing possible triggers to the loss of temper, changing my reaction to his anger, and so on).
- *Evaluating the impact of the plan*: and maintaining or modifying as appropriate.

The pilot evaluation of this approach proved effective, with significant gains on measures of caregiver distress, as well as problematic behaviour frequency and severity compared with a **waiting list control** condition.

Case formulation

Mr F was a 74-year-old man, diagnosed with severe dementia, who was now living on a long-stay ward in a hospital in Southampton. He had held the rank of colonel in the army and had retired to the south coast with his wife, who was physically infirm. His children lived in northern England and had little contact with him. While living with his wife, he had become increasingly forgetful. Initially, this was attributed to his 'getting on', but it soon became evident that the problem was more severe. Over a period of a year, he began to forget the names of friends, became increasingly lost when away from their home, and lost any sense of time or order in his life. He even forgot the name of his wife, and on occasion did not recognize her, becoming aggressive and challenging the presence of this person in the room with him. His sleep–wake cycle was disrupted and he was often awake at night, when his confusion was worse. He became verbally aggressive when stopped doing things he wished to do such as leaving the house alone or driving their car, and his wife had to hide the house and car keys to avoid such confrontations. At these times he barked orders at her and expected her to do as he wished. She felt intimidated by his behaviour because she feared physical violence and was herself frail. He was admitted to hospital as a consequence of his confused and verbally aggressive behaviour. It took some weeks for him to adapt to his new environment, but the transition was eased by the regular visits made by his wife to see him. After a month of being in hospital, however, the ward staff were having increasing difficulties in dealing with his regular outbursts and verbally aggressive behaviour. They reported that these often occurred several times a day, and were quite frightening to some of the staff involved.

Assessment and formulation

In response to these episodes of aggressive behaviour, the ward staff asked the ward psychologist to conduct a functional analysis. In this, a psychology assistant observed Mr F's behaviour for a period of 2 weeks, noting down the antecedents, consequences, and nature of his aggressive behaviour at all times. Behaviour was observed at different times in the day: morning, evening, and during the night. It became clear that many of the incidents of aggressive behaviour were at times that Mr F went to the toilet – or should have gone. The antecedents to the outbursts were that Mr F would become agitated and start to wander around the ward. Staff would approach him to see why he was walking around the ward, an act that often increased his agitation. If they thought he was going to the toilet, they would take him there, and help him to take his trousers down. This provoked further anger and verbal aggression. If they did not spot that he was walking around the ward and intervene, he was frequently incontinent. His behaviour usually involved him becoming angry and verbally aggressive, demanding that he not be manhandled, and asking to be let out of the ward. The consequences were that Mr F remained agitated for some time after the incident and prone to further outbursts. Once he had been taken from the toilet to the patient seating area, staff generally ignored him.

From these observations, it was hypothesized that Mr F was not responding to early physical cues that he needed to urinate. As a consequence, he did not try to get to the toilet until his bladder was extremely full and he was desperate to go the toilet. His memory was poor, so he was unable to immediately remember the way to the toilet, which was some way from the patient seating area. His desperation led to some of his anger and agitation. In addition, he was unhappy about being helped to go to the toilet, wanting to do this himself, and expressed this anger towards whoever was trying to help him.

Intervention

Following the period of observation, the ward psychologist considered a number of solutions, each of which was relatively simple to initiate (at least in principle). The first involved preventing Mr F reaching the point of desperation before he tried to go the toilet. This could be achieved by instigating a regular series of prompts for him to go the toilet. Mr F could be asked by a designated member of the ward staff whether or not he wanted to go to the toilet on a regular basis throughout the day (every half to one hour). If he said he wanted to go, he would be reminded where the toilets were, but not taken there by a member of staff. If Mr F deviated from going to the toilet on any occasion, the same member of staff would remind him he was going to the toilet and accompany him to it. On a more general level, a coloured line could be painted on the (linoleum) floor between the toilet and the patient seating area. This should be the same colour as the toilets, and Mr F (and other patients with similar memory problems) could be reminded to follow the line to the toilets every time they were directed to them. It was hoped that by ensuring Mr F reached the toilet in plenty of time to sort himself out, help might not be needed. Accordingly, it might not be necessary for staff to help Mr F once at the toilet.

Thus the aims of the intervention were to: (i) increase the time available for Mr F to get to the toilet and obviate the stress and anger that were associated with his being desperate to urinate (and to avoid the risk of incontinence); (ii) provide cues to help Mr F get to the toilet without help; and (iii) minimize his embarrassment at being helped in the toilet by a member of the ward staff.

These intervention strategies were discussed with the ward staff who agreed to implement them. Accordingly, the staff modified their behaviour and the line was painted on the floor. The psychology assistant continued to monitor Mr F's behaviour for a further 2 weeks, and provided feedback to the ward staff and psychologist on any progress or problems they observed. Thankfully, the intervention progressed well. The staff explained to Mr F why they were regularly asking him if he wanted to go to the toilet. As he did not always remember why, they had to explain to him on a number of occasions. However, after a few days he stopped asking them why they were doing so. He also began to go to the toilet following the prompt. He had to be guided to the toilet on a number of occasions, but was always reminded that the coloured line on the floor led to the toilet – an association helped by the colour of the toilets being the same colour as the line. As a consequence, he was not only more likely to get to the toilet and avoid confrontation with staff, the frequency of his incontinence was also markedly reduced.

15.2 Neurocognitive disorder due to traumatic brain injury

As in Alzheimer's disease, a DSM diagnosis of neurocognitive disorder due to traumatic brain injury requires the individual to be experiencing the symptoms of major or minor neurological disorder. However, here, the cause is some degree of traumatic brain injury as a result of which the individual experienced one of more of: (i) loss of consciousness, (ii) post-traumatic amnesia, (iii) disorientation and confusion, and (iv) neurological signs including seizures, visual field deficits, and hemiparesis. These signs should be immediately present after the injury.

Closed head injury occurs when an individual is struck on the head with no resultant damage to the skull or specific brain injury. This type of trauma usually results in the whole brain shifting within the skull at the time of the incident, resulting in diffuse damage. About half of cases of closed head injury result from road traffic accidents. The second highest cause is falls, particularly among frail elderly people and young children. Violence accounts for a further 20% of cases, while sports injuries account for about 3%. Alcohol consumption also adds to the risk. People aged between 15 and 25 years are most at risk. In the UK, there are around 150 cases of closed head injury requiring hospitalization for every 100,000 people each year.

One simple index of the severity of injury is that of 'time to follow commands'; that is, the time after trauma it takes the head-injured person to be able to respond to simple commands. Mild head injury is indicated by a time to follow commands of less than one hour; for moderate head injury this time is between one hour and 13 days; for severe head injury it is 14 days or more. Between 30% and 50% of people will die as a result of severe head injury. About 10% will still be in a 'vegetative' (non-responsive) state 3 months after the trauma, decreasing to about 4% after 6 months, and 2–3% one year following injury. For those who survive their injury and recover consciousness, recovery follows a typical pattern. The first phase involves a period of acute confusion and disorientation during which they are unable to form and retain new memories: post-traumatic amnesia. The longer the period of amnesia, the poorer the long-term outcome (Willemse-van Son et al. 2007).

Following resolution of post-traumatic amnesia, the majority of people with moderate or severe head injuries experience significant physical, cognitive, and behavioural impairment, although younger and more intelligent people usually fare better than others due to their greater cognitive reserve (Steward et al. 2018). Most physical problems eventually resolve, although a minority of people continue to experience a wide range of symptoms including persistent muscle spasticity, impaired swallowing, and balance disturbances. About 5% of those with moderate-to-severe closed head injury develop epileptic seizures: this compares with 35–50% of people with penetrating head injuries. Risk for developing epilepsy continues to be higher than the population norm for as long as 5 years after the original trauma.

Cognitive and neurobehavioural deficits are the most common residual symptoms of closed head injury. Diffuse brain injury results in a typical pattern of cognitive deficits, including slowed cognitive speed, decreased attention and impaired memory, complex language skills and impaired 'executive function' (e.g. Malojcic et al. 2008; Schooler et al. 2008). The latter includes problems in working memory, problem-solving, monitoring performance, and organizing behaviour. Recovery is most marked in the first 6 months after injury, although recovery may continue more slowly for a further year. One month following injury, almost all people with moderate-to-severe injury have detectable cognitive impairments. Six months following injury, about 8% of those with moderate injury and 16% of those with severe injury will require hospital care as a result of cognitive disabilities. Ten per cent of people with a severe head injury will still require hospital care one year following the event, while around 70% will be considered 'functionally independent'; only about a quarter will ever return to work (e.g. Sveen et al. 2016). Of note in this context are the findings of van der Naalt et al. (2017), who found that 6-month recovery following mild brain injury was predicted by emotional distress and maladaptive coping following the trauma, and pre-injury mental health problems, as well as the severity of trauma.

Neurobehavioural symptoms experienced by people with head injuries include increased irritability, headaches, anxiety, difficulty concentrating, fatigue, restlessness, depression, and poorer quality of life and sleep (e.g. Ulvik et al. 2008). Around 10% of people with a traumatic brain injury go on to develop clinically diagnosed anxiety (Osborn et al. 2017) while rates of depression as high as 38% have been reported (Kreutzer et al. 2009). Features of long-term recovery include a lack of self-awareness, and a lack of understanding of the severity of any cognitive deficits (Bach and David 2006). Perhaps for this reason, relatives of people who have sustained a head injury frequently report more psychological changes than the affected individual, as well as high levels of depression (Rivera et al. 2007).

Research box 14

Mez, J., Daneshvar, D.H., Kiernan, P.T. et al. (2017) Clinicopathological evaluation of chronic traumatic encephalopathy in players of American football, *Journal of the American Medical Association*, 318: 360–70.

Followers of contact sport will be aware of the increasing concerns over the long-term consequences of minor repeated head trauma associated with direct contact with objects such as footballs, or aggressive tackles such as in rugby and American football. This is one study of this phenomenon, known as chronic traumatic encephalopathy (CTE), which has received significant scientific and social interest. It involves neuropathological assessment of the brains of over 200 US American football players donated to a medical donation programme on their deaths.

Method

Sample

The 202 brains examined in the study were drawn from donations to a 'brain bank' established by a range of institutions including Boston University and the Concussion Legacy Foundation. Next of kin of brain donors provided written informed consent for the examination. Inclusion criteria for the present study were: an American football player who died after the age of 35 years, with at least 2 years of college-level play, and with no need to have demonstrated any evidence of neurological symptoms during life.

Clinical evaluation

Personal history

Information about each individual was obtained from a range of sources, including online surveys and structured and semi-structured interviews with a range of informants. The interviewers were a behavioural neurologist, neuroscientist, and neuropsychologist. They obtained a detailed history, including a timeline of any cognitive, behavioural, mood, and motor symptoms. More formal assessment for the presence of a range of diagnosable disorders was also conducted. These included symptoms consistent with post-traumatic stress disorder, substance use disorder, and a range of neurological conditions including various forms of dementia and Parkinson disease. Finally, a range of personal history measures were taken including military and sporting history (such as type of sports played, age at first exposure), and evidence of traumatic brain injury including number of concussions.

Neurological assessment

This involved both measures of brain volume and macroscopic features associated with dementia, including tau and neurofibrillary tangles (see main text). These permitted the diagnosis of a range of dementias and motor neuron diseases to be made. In addition, the degree of CTE was classified into four levels of severity based on increasing levels of brain damage. Level 1 involved evidence of one or two isolated areas of brain damage;

level 2 involved lesions in the cerebral sulci in the frontal, temporal or parietal areas; level 3 involved involvement of areas including the amygdala and hypothalamus; level 4 included pervasive brain damage.

The clinical and neurological assessments were conducted blind, with the latter being reviewed by four neuropathologists.

Findings

The final sample comprised 202 deceased brain donors, with a median age of death of 66 years. The mean length of participation in football was 15.1 years. Some degree of CTE was diagnosed in 177 brains; 87% of the sample. Some degree of CTE was found in neither of 2 players that only played pre-high school, 3 of 14 (21%) who played in high school, 9 of 14 (64%) semi-professional players, and 110 of 111 (99%) National Football League (NFL) players. The most common cause of death amongst those with mild CTE was suicide (27%), with those having severe CTE being more likely to die from neurodegenerative disorders (47%).

The severity of CTE increased monotonically with the intensity of playing experience, and among those who experienced CTE it was progressive. Former high school players had mild pathology, while the majority of college (56%), semi-professional (56%), and professional (86%) players had severe pathology. Among participants with mild CTE pathology, 96% had evidence of behavioural and/or mood symptoms or both, 85% had cognitive symptoms, and 33% had signs of dementia. Among participants with severe CTE, 89% had behavioural and/or mood symptoms, 95% had cognitive symptoms, and 85% had signs of dementia.

Discussion

The alarming results indicated that virtually all former NFL players in their sample evidenced some degree of CTE, and this was frequently severe. The data on play were lacking in granularity, and it is not clear what factors within the experience of playing football contribute most to risk: duration of play, position, cumulative hits, and so on. However, that such a single indicator of risk appears to have such a powerful outcome is of concern. Despite these statistics, some caution needs to be applied. The sample was biased in that it was associated with participation in a brain donation programme with the potential of bias due to obvious pathology; thus the data cannot provide a measure of the absolute **prevalence** of neurological disorders within players of American football. Nevertheless, it provides a significant challenge for those involved in the game (and similar games such as rugby) on how to manage risk and the physical and mental health of its players.

Rehabilitation following head injury

A number of physical interventions have proved to be of benefit following head injury, including enhanced attention following treatment with methylphenidate (a drug used to treat ADHD; see Chapter 14) (Huang et al. 2016) and improvements in depression and executive function following repetitive transcranial magnetic stimulation (Lee and Kim 2018). However, the majority of interventions addressing the cognitive components of traumatic brain injury involve cognitive retraining and 'functional compensation'.

Coping with memory problems

A number of strategies can be used to improve memory, including memory drills, combining imagery with words to improve subsequent recall, and so on. Wilson (1989), for example, used a preview, question, read, state, and test (PQRST) model to improve encoding and recall of lists of words. This involved the participant examining the task, thinking about its requirements, and then reading a list of words over a number of trials both aloud and silently, before testing. The additional cognitive processing required in this approach was thought to enhance learning compared with simple repetition of lists of words. Unfortunately, memory gains made in such sessions frequently do not generalize beyond the specific memory task. In addition, as many people with head injuries underestimate their memory loss, attempts to implement such programmes are not always acceptable. These findings led Wilson (2005) to conclude that retraining memory is likely to have little impact on memory *per se*, but teaching people to cope with real-life memory problems (functional compensation), for example, through the use of memory aids, is potentially of more benefit. Memory aids may include use of a tape-recorder or handwritten notes, tablets, time reminders such as alarm clocks, phone calls or radio pagers, and the use of personal organizers or orientation boards within the home.

People with significant impairment may need lengthy training in the use of memory aids. Sohlberg et al. (2001), for example, recommended a three-stage process of training to use a memory notebook. The first stage involved systematic training in the contents and purpose of the notebook. This was reinforced by a question-and-answer approach ('What are the five sections of your notebook?'). During the application phase, individuals practised using the book through role play. Finally, participants used the notebook in their day-to-day lives. In one of their studies, it took one participant in their programme as long as 17 days to acquire the skills necessary to use the notebook. External memory aids can also be helpful in reminding the individual to do various tasks they otherwise may have forgotten to do. In a randomized controlled trial of this type of approach, Shum et al. (2011) evaluated a programme that had two components: (i) self-awareness training, which aimed to give participants insight into their memory problems (which can be significantly absent) and emphasized the need for compensatory behaviours; and (ii) the use of a diary or other organizational device and time management system within their existing daily regimens. This phase of the programme involved the participant learning the diary/organizer's structure and uses, developing and using a number of environmental cues to remind them to use it, learning basic note-taking skills to help them establish reminders to do things, and engaging with family and friends to support them in the use of these strategies. This second phase proved critical to the success of the programme.

Improving executive function

A second problem that people face following head injury is a decrement in problem-solving skills. Interventions designed to compensate for this have focused on breaking down problem-solving into specific stages. Levine et al. (2000) developed one such process, known as goal management training, This comprised a checklist of processes to follow when trying to solve problems: (i) stop – what am I doing, (ii) define the goal, (iii) list the steps, (iv) learn the steps, (v) check – am I doing what I planned. This strategy was then rehearsed during simulated tasks practised during therapy sessions and homework tasks. In-therapy practice involved a range of tasks and skills including clapping to words and inhibiting clapping to target words, decision-making, planning five activities within a 4-minute period, and mindfulness exercises. This approach has proven effective in a range of settings including US veterans with chronic traumatic brain injury who showed both improvements in cognitive functioning measured by performance of a 'complex functional task', and also in daily functioning, mood, and obtaining paid or voluntary employment (Novakovic-Agopian et al. 2019).

A number of standardized programmes have also been developed to remediate attention problems. The *Attention Process Training* (APT) programme of Park et al. (1999) did so by using a number of different strategies. Sustained attention was trained by exercises including attention tapes that required listening for target words or word/number sequences and pressing a buzzer when identified, listening to a paragraph and testing comprehension, and mental arithmetic exercises. Shifting attention was trained by exercises including tapes that required identification of one type of target word followed by identification of another. Tasks were presented in order of difficulty and repeated until the individual was able to cope effectively with the task demands. If necessary, the tasks were practised at home with the help of relatives as well as in the clinic. This type of approach has proven moderately effective, with most studies showing gains on psychometric measures of memory or attention following such interventions. Limited research has looked at 'real-world' improvements, however, and the effectiveness in these contexts is unclear (Michel and Mateer 2006).

Coping with negative emotions

Given the high levels of depression and suicide among people who have sustained a significant head injury, there is little doubt that many would benefit from some form of psychological or pharmacological intervention to help moderate their mood (e.g. Gómez-de-Regil et al. 2019). Such interventions should provide emotional support, explanations of the injury and its likely outcome, and help to achieve increased self-esteem by maximizing gains towards achievable goals, reduce denial, and increase the individual's ability to relate to family and society. The most widely used approach in this context is CBT, although other strategies have been used. Bell et al. (2005), for example, found that a series of telephone calls providing motivational strategies, counselling, and education for up to 9 months following discharge resulted in better outcomes on measures of functional status and well-being than standard care one year following discharge. Bradbury et al. (2008) found that a simplified cognitive behavioural approach, allowing for the memory and attentional problems of its recipients, delivered either by telephone or live in a group, depending on participant preferences, proved more successful in changing measures of well-being than an educational programme. Although trials of effectiveness are few in number, cognitive behavioural interventions have also proven successful in treating post-traumatic stress disorder and anxiety in people with traumatic brain injury (Soo and Tate 2007).

Helping the carers

Just as in Alzheimer's disease, people living with, and caring for, a person who has sustained a head injury may themselves experience significant stress and distress (Malec et al. 2017). While there is some evidence that strain on the family recedes as a consequence of improvements in cognitive deficits and health service input, there is a strong argument for the provision of services to help the family cope with the stress of caring for a person with a head injury. In their review of the relevant literature, Hart et al. (2019) identified a number of strategies that have been used to support carers in the USA. For mild traumatic brain injury, care usually involves education during acute care (often in the emergency treatment department) and is largely targeted at the affected individual. For more severe injuries, education tends to be provided later in care and involve families and caregivers. Interventions targeted at family members have involved education about injury, and skills training aimed at helping people cope with the behaviour of the injured person, including problem-solving solutions to difficult behaviours and problems (Rivera et al. 2008) and communication skills (Togher et al. 2013). Each has proved effective.

15.3 Multiple sclerosis

Multiple sclerosis (MS) is a neurological condition resulting from the destruction of the myelin sheath that surrounds all nerve cells within the brain and central nervous system. Sclerotic plaques develop where this destruction occurs, blocking or distorting the normal transmission of nerve impulses. As this may occur in any part of the brain or spinal cord, the symptoms they cause differ markedly across individuals, and include loss of limb function, loss of bowel and/or bladder control, blindness due to inflammation of the optic nerve, and cognitive impairment. Muscular spasticity is a common feature, particularly in the upper limbs; 95% of people with MS experience debilitating fatigue. This prevents any sustained physical activity in about 40% of people. Nearly half the people with MS consider this to be their most serious symptom (Rizzo et al. 2004). Between 30% and 50% of people with the condition require walking aids or a wheelchair for mobility.

The course of MS differs across individuals. Onset before the age of 15 years is rare; 20% of those who develop MS have a benign form of the disease in which symptoms show little or no progression after the initial attack. A few people experience malignant MS, resulting in a swift and relentless decline and significant disability or even death shortly after disease onset. Onset of this type of MS is usually after the age of 40 years. The majority of people have an episodic condition, with acute flare-ups followed by periods of remission. Each flare-up is usually followed by a failure to recover to previous levels of function, resulting in a slowly deteriorating condition. Death is usually due to complications of MS, including choking, pneumonia, and renal failure. Suicide rates are significantly higher among people with MS than in the general population (Brønnum-Hansen et al. 2005).

Susan provides a glimpse of what it feels like to have MS. At the time of our talk she was taking antidepressants for her depression and, as you will find, was having problems coming to terms with her disorder:

I developed MS about four years ago. It was odd to start with. I didn't think I had anything serious, although you do worry about symptoms you don't understand. It started when I had some problems with my sight. I couldn't see as well as I used to be able to – it came on suddenly so I didn't think it was age or anything normal. I think at the time I was also a bit more clumsy than I had been – nothing obvious, but I dropped things a bit more than before. Nothing really that you'd notice unless other things were happening as well. I went to my GP about my eyes and he sent me to see a neurologist. He tried to reassure me that there was nothing too badly wrong and that he wanted to check out a few symptoms. But I began to worry then ... you don't get sent on to see the hospital doctors unless there is anything really wrong with you. He suggested that he thought it might be MS, which was why he was not sending me to an eye specialist.

I got to see the neurologist pretty quickly and she ran a few tests over a few weeks – testing my muscle strength, coordination, scans and so on ... sticking needles into me at various times. The upshot of this was that I was diagnosed as having MS. My consultant told me and my husband together, and allowed us to ask questions about things. We also got to speak to a specialist nurse who has helped us over the years. She was able to take the time to tell us more than the doctor about what to expect and what support we could have. Although I think it was nice to hear the diagnosis from the doctor.

I must admit that I found it really hard to deal with things at the beginning – you don't know what to expect and perhaps you expect the worst. You hear all sorts of horror stories about people dying with MS and that. And no one can really reassure you that you won't have problems ... Over the last few years, I've got to know my body and seen things getting worse. But it happens gradually and a lot of the time there are no changes. So that is reassuring that things aren't going to collapse too quickly and I won't be left incontinent and unable to feed myself for a long time – hopefully not ever!

The worse thing is the tiredness and clumsiness. My eyes have actually got better, thank goodness. I use sticks to get around the house. Sometimes I can walk a little out of the house. Often I have to take the wheelchair. I just get exhausted too quickly, there isn't a lot of point trying to walk, because I cannot go far ...

I hate having MS. I used to take part in sports, go out, be lively. Now I can't do any of that. I'm tired ... down a lot of the time. I think the two often go together. My memory was never that good, but now it seems to be worse than ever. I can hold conversations, but keeping my concentration up for a long time is difficult. So, people find you difficult to deal with. I know my husband feels that way. He married a lively, sporty, slim woman ... now I'm lethargic, down, putting on weight because I eat and don't exercise – even though they tell me not to, so I can keep mobile and not develop skin problems. I don't go out very much because it's such a hassle in my wheelchair ... cities were not designed for people in wheelchairs ... and people don't like people in wheelchairs. You are ignored ... and just want to say, 'Hey, I'm here. I have a brain you know ...' I know this sounds sorry for myself. And sometimes I feel more positive. But I find living with uncertainty difficult. Will I have a bad day today? Will I have a flare-up – have to go to hospital, take mega-steroids, come out worse than when I went in? I guess you have to live for the day ... but it can be difficult.

Aetiology of multiple sclerosis

Genetic factors

The lifetime risk of developing MS for the general population is 1 in 800. This increases to 1 in 50 for the children of affected individuals and 1 in 20 for their siblings. However, increased concordance among family members may not exclusively indicate a genetic aetiology. Siblings who develop MS usually do so in the same calendar year rather than at the same age, indicating the possibility of common environmental factors impacting on risk for MS (Haines and Pericak-Vance 1999). Other evidence of genetic factors includes the markedly differing rates of the illness across the world (Rosati 2001). Multiple sclerosis is rare among a variety of groups including Uzbeks, Kazakhs, native Siberians, Chinese, Japanese, Africans, and New Zealand Maoris. Rates of MS in Sardinia, and among Parsis and Palestinians, are particularly high. Genes affecting immune processes (e.g. interleukin-2 and interleukin-7 receptor genes) are among around 15 gene alleles so far implicated in the condition (Tizaoui 2018).

Biological mechanisms

The aetiology of MS is still not fully understood, although the favoured hypotheses are that it is the result of errors in the immune system or a viral infection. One chemical within the immune system, gamma-interferon, is especially implicated in MS: high levels of gamma-interferon co-occur with high levels of MS activity. How gamma-interferon affects the disease process is not yet fully understood, but it is likely that it stimulates the immune system, through chemical messengers known as interleukins, to produce cytotoxic T cells, which are responsible for attacking and destroying diseased or damaged body cells. These cells can attack other cells directly and are usually able to discriminate between 'self' cells (those of the body) and 'non-self' cells (damaged or cancerous cells, or pathogens). In

MS, it seems to be that the activated cytotoxic T cells wrongly identify the myelin sheath of nerve cells within the brain and spinal column as 'non-self', and attempt to destroy it. Viral infections may act as a trigger to the production of gamma-interferon, hence the link between viral infections and MS.

Stress and MS

There is good evidence that stress can influence activity within the immune system. Given the role of the immune system in the aetiology of MS, it is therefore possible that stress may influence the onset and course of the condition. Evidence for the former was provided by Liu et al. (2009), who retrospectively found that the onset of MS was associated with high levels of negative life events, family problems, and a variety of negative emotions; all of which were higher than in a comparable group without MS. Longitudinal studies of the impact of stress on the progression of MS also indicate that stress may have a role in MS. In one such study, Mohr et al. (2000a) recorded various measures of stress and disease progression every 4 weeks for 28 to 100 weeks in a group of people with MS. They found that increases in personal conflict or disruption to routine typically preceded increases in disease activity. Similarly, Ackerman et al. (2002) found that 85% of the exacerbations in symptoms experienced by their cohort of women with MS were preceded by a period of stress, which typically occurred in the 2 weeks preceding the increase in symptoms. They estimated that participants were 13 times more likely to experience an exacerbation of their condition following an episode of stress than during periods of no stress. Of course, the exacerbation of symptoms may itself prove stressful. Schwartz et al. (1999), for example, found a bi-directional relationship between stress and MS: risk of disease progression increased as a consequence of stress, and increases in disease progression contributed to reported levels of stress – a vicious cycle between stress and disease progression. At a more fundamental level, Sorenson et al. (2013) found significantly higher levels of inflammation, measured by levels of cytokine production, among people with MS in response to day-to-day stress than among a control population.

Psychological sequelae of MS

Cognitive problems

As well as physical problems, people with MS frequently experience a number of cognitive deficits in memory, attention, conceptual reasoning, verbal fluency, and abstracting abilities. Nearly half of people with MS complain of some degree of cognitive impairment and memory problems, with deficits evident in around 20% of people even with relatively mild levels of MS (Patti et al. 2009). The latter do not follow a distinct progression, but usually involve problems in retrieval from long-term memory storage: short-term and recognition memory are seldom impaired. Speed of information processing is also slowed compared with people without the condition as a result of slowed neuronal activity (Manca et al. 2019). Visual and auditory attention may also be impaired. Perhaps because of the cognitive deterioration they experience, subjective reports of cognitive deficits may differ markedly from more objective measures (Christodoulou et al. 2005). Increasing cognitive deficits can be charted against progressive brain damage. In reviewing the relevant literature, Shi et al. (2014) noted that cortical demyelination correlates more strongly with cognitive deficits than visual, sensory, and motor symptoms. Cognitive reserve, measured by pre-diagnostic IQ or years in education, appears protective against the degenerative effects of MS (Benedict et al. 2010).

Emotional reactions

People with MS experience a variety of emotional responses. A review of 58 studies by Boeschoten et al. (2017), for example, showed that around 30% of people with MS are likely to be clinically depressed, while 22% will be clinically anxious. Such a high prevalence of depression is understandable given the nature of the disorder and has been associated with limited social support, inadequate coping and adjustment mechanisms, unpredictable disease course, loss of recreational activities, severe physical disability, and perceived physical incapacity (Ghaffar and Feinstein 2007). Suicide is a significant cause of mortality. Three per cent of people with MS take their own life, while up to 29% report suicidal ideation at some point in the course of their disorder (see Murphy et al. 2017). There is also evidence that disturbed affect may be a symptom as well as a consequence of MS. Depression can be the first sign of MS, preceding obvious neurocognitive symptoms by months or years (Feinstein et al. 2014). Proponents of the neurological model have suggested that this is the result of sclerotic plaques in brain areas, such as the limbic system, that mediate mood, prior to any obvious disorder to which the individual will react. An alternative biopsychosocial explanation could be that depression provides a trigger to the onset of MS (as may stress) rather than being an early indicator of its presence. In sharp contrast to the previous discussion, around 10% of people with MS experience periods of euphoria (Parvizi et al. 2001). This is found in people with advanced disease and is thought to be a consequence of scarring in the limbic system isolating it from frontal control. Steroids used to treat MS during acute flare-ups may also trigger such episodes. Finally, people with MS may experience significant bouts of anger, possibly as a consequence of neuronal damage (Nocentini et al. 2009).

Treatment of psychological problems associated with MS

Psychological interventions in MS have two primary foci: first, to help people manage the cognitive and other symptoms of MS, and second, to help people cope emotionally with the impact of the disease.

Coping with cognitive deficits

A number of studies have examined the impact of neurological rehabilitation techniques on cognitive abilities in MS, although the number of high-quality studies is limited (Goverover et al. 2018). Nevertheless, Goverover et al. identified several robust studies providing varying types of neurological training which achieved positive benefits on attentional and memory tasks. In the one study they considered to be 'grade I', Chiaravalloti et al. (2013) trained participants in the use of imagery as a way of facilitating learning over three phases: learning to visualize, applying visualization to facilitate learning new information, then transferring these skills to everyday life. Assessment involved formal memory tests and self-reports of memory in daily life. Compared with a placebo control condition, participants who received this training made gains on both types of measure. A second strong study found another sensory approach, the use of music, to enhance learning (Thaut et al. 2014). Attention training packages such as those used in head injury may also be of benefit.

Coping with emotional problems

A number of psychological interventions can be used to help people cope with the symptoms of MS. Ghielen et al. (2019), for example, conducted two meta-analyses of cognitive behavioural and mindfulness interventions in the treatment of psychological distress in people with MS. The first compared these interventions against treatment as usual; the second involved active treatment controls. Unsurprisingly, the differences in outcome were greater in the usual treatment control condition, but even when pitched against some form of active control, both interventions proved more beneficial. These interventions have proven equally effective in the treatment of MS-related fatigue (van den Akker et al. 2016).

Responding to the specific needs of this population, who may find it difficult to attend out-patient therapy appointments due to fatigue and poor mobility, Mohr et al. (2000b) examined the effectiveness of a cognitive behavioural programme for the treatment of depression delivered by telephone. The intervention lasted 8 weeks and involved a workbook with standardized assignments combined with telephone contacts. Assignments focused on identifying and modifying dysfunctional thoughts, increasing pleasant events, and developing strategies to manage fatigue. The latter included scheduling achievable amounts of exercise, scheduling breaks, and learning to identify physical cues to determine when to take breaks. The usual care control involved routine out-patient appointments. By the end of the intervention, participants in the cognitive behavioural programme reported lower levels of depression and were more likely to adhere to their interferon therapy than those in the normal care condition.

15.4 Chapter summary

1. Alzheimer's disease affects a significant proportion of elderly people.
2. It is characterized by a progressive process of cognitive and behavioural degeneration following a regular pattern as differing brain systems become involved.
3. The neurological processes underpinning the disorder appear to be neurofibrillary tangles and beta-amyloid plaques. Reduced levels of the neurotransmitter acetylcholine also appear to be implicated.
4. There is, as yet, no cure for Alzheimer's disease. In its early stages, interventions are aimed at maximizing cognitive abilities. As the illness progresses, interventions focus on minimizing cognitive load and maintaining independence.

5. Closed head injuries can result in profound and long-lasting cognitive deficits.
6. Psychological interventions in this population focus on cognitive retraining, although any gains often fail to generalize beyond the training context. Accordingly, many interventions incorporate the use of external aids to trigger routine behaviours as well as cognitive strategies for maintaining concentration.
7. Multiple sclerosis is a degenerative disease of varying course.
8. It impacts on both the cognitive and emotional life of people with the disease.
9. Stress may exacerbate or trigger the symptoms of MS.
10. Interventions for MS are therefore aimed at developing strategies for coping with both cognitive and emotional impairments. Both appear to be effective.

15.5 For discussion

1. Many frail and elderly people act as carers for people with Alzheimer's disease. How can their stress be minimized? How responsible should the state be for caring for such people, and when (if at all) should care begin?
2. Does cognitive retraining really provide meaningful benefit to people who have had a head injury, or are its effects too limited?
3. How can people with MS and their families be helped to cope effectively with their disease?

15.6 Further reading

Coetzer, R. (2010) *Anxiety and Mood Disorders following Traumatic Brain Injury: Clinical Assessment and Psychotherapy*, London: Routledge.

Gingold, J.N. (2011) *Facing the Cognitive Challenges of Multiple Sclerosis*, New York: Demos Medical Publishing.

Gómez-de-Regil, L., Estrella-Castillo, D.F. and Vega-Cauich, J. (2019) Psychological intervention in traumatic brain injury patients, *Behavioural Neurology* [https://doi.org/10.1155/2019/6937832].

Melunsky, N., Poland, F. and Moniz-Cook, E. (2016) Behavioural and psychological symptoms in dementia and the challenges for family carers: systematic review, *British Journal of Psychiatry*, 208: 429–34.

Rao, V. and Vaishnavi, S. (2016) *The Traumatized Brain: A Family Guide to Understanding Mood, Memory, and Behavior after Brain Injury*, Baltimore, MD: Johns Hopkins University Press.

Russell-Williams, J., Jaroudi, W., Perich, T. et al. (2018) Mindfulness and meditation: treating cognitive impairment and reducing stress in dementia, *Reviews in the Neurosciences*, 29: 791–804.

Zucchella, C., Sinforiani, E., Tamburin, S. et al. (2018) The multidisciplinary approach to Alzheimer's disease and dementia: a narrative review of non-pharmacological treatment, *Frontiers in Neurology*, 9: 1058 [https://doi.org/10.3389/fneur.2018.01058].

16 Addictions

Chapter contents

Ask someone to describe an addict, and they will usually give you a stereotypical description of someone addicted to 'hard' drugs such as heroin or cocaine. However, most chemical addictions are to legal drugs such as coffee, cigarettes, and alcohol. People may also be addicted to a variety of behaviours, including exercise or gambling. For these people, the neurochemical reaction to their behaviour is similar to that induced by drugs. After a brief introduction to drugs and drug dependence, this chapter considers the **aetiology**, implications, and treatment of four types of addiction: two to chemicals – alcohol and heroin, and two to behaviours – gambling and internet gaming. By the end of the chapter, you should have an understanding of:

- Why people take drugs, and the nature of dependence
- Factors leading to physical addiction (alcohol and opiate abuse) and psychological addiction (gambling and internet gaming disorders)
- The types of interventions used to treat each disorder, and their relative effectiveness.

16.1 Drugs and drug dependence

According to the WHO (2018b), 2.5% of the world population and 5.6% of those aged 15–16 years use cannabis, compared with 0.2% who use cocaine and 0.2% who take opiates (including heroin and the painkiller tramadol), amphetamines or prescription stimulants. Only 3% of the drug-using population injects. Despite their relatively low use, though, opioids cause the most harm; accounting for 76% of drug-related deaths. The rise in addiction to pharmaceutical opioids initially prescribed for pain in the USA, and now contributing to an epidemic of uncontrolled opioid use, has led to increased deaths from drug overdose there, with a 21% increase in death following overdose between 2015 and 2016.

With few exceptions, the quicker a drug's action, the more addictive it is. Cocaine, for example, was originally ingested by chewing coca leaves. This produced an increase in vigour and resistance to fatigue but little pleasure. More recently, it has been made into cocaine hydrochloride powder, which, when taken nasally, impacts on the brain within 4–10 minutes. Crack cocaine is a further refinement that allows it to be smoked and to impact on the brain in seconds. Each form of cocaine is thought to be increasingly addictive.

Problems arising from drug use defy simple categorization. They may be social, physical, legal, interpersonal or psychological. **DSM**-5 acknowledged these in its broad list of criteria involved in a diagnosis of substance misuse disorder:

- Taking the substance in larger amounts and/or over a longer period than intended
- Persistent attempts, or one or more unsuccessful efforts, to cut down or control use
- Significant amounts of time spent in activities necessary to obtain, use or recover from the effects of the substance
- Craving or strong urges to use the substance
- Recurring failures to fulfil major role obligations at work, school or home
- Continued use despite persistent or recurrent social or interpersonal problems associated with, or exacerbated by, use of the substance
- Important social, occupational or recreational activities given up or reduced
- Recurrent substance use in situations in which it is physically hazardous
- Substance use despite experiencing recurrent physical or psychological problems as a result of or exacerbated by the substance
- Tolerance, involving either:
  o significantly increased amounts of the substance required in order to achieve their desired effect
  o significantly reduced effect with continued use of the same amount
- Withdrawal, manifested by either:
  o the characteristic withdrawal syndrome for the substance
  o use of the same (or a closely related) substance to relieve or avoid these symptoms.

DSM-IV-TR identified two 'levels' of substance-related problems: *substance abuse*, involving hazardous use, social and interpersonal problems, neglecting major roles and legal problems; and *substance dependence*, which involves tolerance to the drug, needing more of it to achieve the desired experience, and withdrawal symptoms following stopping use of the drug. These various criteria have now been rolled into one diagnostic category, with severity based on the number of criteria met rather than the type of criteria.

16.2 Addiction: a common neurological pathway

The chapter considers addiction to a range of physical and psychological experiences including alcohol and heroin use, gambling and internet gaming. Despite their apparent differences, these experiences impact through a number of common neurological pathways and processes as well as more specific pathways associated with particular drug types:

Activation of the brain reward system

The immediate rewarding effects of addictive substances and experiences involve activation of the ventral tegmental area, which releases dopamine to the nucleus accumbens, the prefrontal cortex, amygdala, and septum, all of which are in what is often called the 'reward circuit', with the nucleus accumbens perhaps providing the focus of pleasure – leading to its label as the 'pleasure centre'. Cocaine, amphetamines, and nicotine directly increase dopamine activity within the system; opioids and alcohol do so indirectly by influencing activity within the neural opioid systems, which, in turn, influences dopaminergic activity within the reward circuit. Cannabinoids such as delta-9-tetrahydrocannabinol (THC) achieve dopaminergic release through their influence on the brain's endogenous cannabinoid system.

Anticipatory activation of the brain reward system

As experience with drugs or addictive behaviours increases, a conditioned response involving release of dopamine can be evoked in the presence of associated stimuli such as drug paraphernalia, bars or casinos. This establishes a process known as 'incentive salience', an urge to engage in behaviour that sustains that experience. Unfortunately, this may occur long after people have stopped taking a drug or engaging in addictive behaviours, forming a significant barrier to recovery.

Withdrawal effects

Over time, repeated use of drugs or engagement in addictive behaviours can adversely impact on the dopaminergic reward system, resulting in long-term reductions in the number of dopamine D2 receptors within the neurons of the reward circuit. The consequent decrease in the 'baseline' levels of dopaminergic activity results in a reduction in the sensitivity of the reward system, leading to an increase in drug use or addictive behaviour, as the individual strives to increase the pleasure associated with it and to prevent withdrawal effects. A second withdrawal process involves activation of stress **neurotransmitters**, including corticotrophin-releasing hormone and norepinephrine.

Pre-occupation/anticipation

Following cessation of drug or behavioural addictions, the individual may become pre-occupied with the focus on their addiction and begin to plan or actively resist re-engagement with them. The individual is caught in a 'go–stop' process. In this process, the frontal lobe is involved with planning the actions required to re-engage with the experience, with 'go' processes involving the pre-frontal cortex activating the nucleus accumbens and the pleasure circuit, leading to a powerful urge to repeat the addicted experience. Activation of the dorsal striatum may also trigger habitual behaviours, including those involved in seeking a 'high'. The 'stop' processes involve inhibition of these processes.

Along with these common neurological pathways, shared genetic factors may also influence risk for a range of addictions. Family studies reported by Kendler (e.g. Kendler et al. 2007), for example, found overlapping genetic risk for clusters of addictions including: (i) excess alcohol consumption, illicit drug use, and smoking, (ii) cannabis and cocaine use; and (iii) caffeine, alcohol, and nicotine consumption.

16.3 Alcohol abuse disorder

Acute intoxication can result in risk-taking or other behaviours that may damage the individual or others. Fifty per cent of deaths in single vehicle road accidents in Norway, for example, are associated with high levels of driver alcohol consumption (Christophersen and Gjerde 2014), while alcohol consumption has also been associated with an increased risk for violent crime, accidents at work, admissions for mental health problems, drownings, burns, and suicide. The influence on suicide is particularly dramatic. Borges et al. (2017), for example, identified a seven-fold increase in risk for attempted suicide amongst the acutely intoxicated, and a near trebling of risk among those with lower levels of alcohol consumption.

Chronic excess consumption can lead to a wider set of problems, including dependence on alcohol. The DSM criteria for what it terms alcohol abuse disorder (AAD) comprise specific examples of the wider criteria for substance abuse disorder; that is, simply swap the word 'alcohol' for 'substance' in the criteria outlined above. Around 9% of the population are likely to meet the criteria for AAD, with 5% being considered problem drinkers and 4% dependent on alcohol (Hasin and Grant 2015). However, the long-term dangers of alcohol abuse go significantly beyond problems of dependence, and include physical health problems such as cirrhosis of the liver, hypertension, and various cancers. They also include significant neurological problems. Wernicke's encephalopathy is caused by thiamine deficiencies common in heavy drinkers as a consequence of poor diet, and results from degenerative changes and small bleeds in the brain. Its symptoms include memory deficits, **ataxia**, and confusion. If not treated, it may progress to a more problematic disorder known as Korsakoff's syndrome. This irreversible condition affects about 5% of heavy drinkers and involves significant **retrograde amnesia** and **anterograde amnesia**. Anterograde memory deficits are usually the most marked problems, and individuals with the condition live a very 'minute-by-minute' existence, frequently **confabulating** in an effort to replace the memories they fail to sustain.

Alcohol abuse disorder is usually the end-point of a progression from social drinking to drinking at times of stress or difficulty, through to an increasing 'need' to drink to cope with social or psychological problems or prevent the onset of withdrawal symptoms. By this time, withdrawal results in a variety of symptoms, including tremor, nausea, sweating, and mood disturbance. Delirium tremens ('the DTs'), the most extreme element of withdrawal, usually begins within 3–4 days of abstinence and lasts between 2 and 3 days. It involves reductions in consciousness, impairment of memory, insomnia, and frightening auditory and/or visual **hallucinations**. Despite this apparently gradual process, drinking early in life is not necessarily predictive of subsequent dependence. Behrendt et al. (2008), for example, found that speed of transition from alcohol 'user' to alcohol 'dependence' was quickest among people who were older when they started to drink.

The story of Anne is typical of many people who drink to excess:

I first started drinking when I was 18. I was at college at the time – a part of the norm – drinking cider or lager at weekends. I met my first partner out drinking when I was about 22. We got into a crowd who were wine drinkers and so we started drinking more wine. He'd always been a heavy drinker – more than I ever did. And often as a result of his drinking he'd become quite violent towards me and arguments would follow after drinking. As a result of this, I began to drink more – to join him, to keep up. My violent marriage made me think about my childhood – which had been very unstable and unhappy for various reasons – and the more I brooded on that, the more I drank. I was drinking about two bottles of wine a night at this time. Drinking helped me cope with my marriage and memories of my childhood. It also made things in the relationship worse, of course.

By the time I was 28–29, the relationship had broken down, and my drinking fell a little – but not that much. Then one night, I was followed home by a man from a nightclub and sexually assaulted by him. My drinking escalated again. I felt I couldn't go out of the house. I was scared and felt trapped. I lost my job as a care worker with children and then I had nothing to keep me going, so I just drank through the day. I was drinking a couple of bottles of wine and perhaps a flagon of cider a day at this time. I did this for about 6 months or so, when I met my next partner, and I began to drink less. I managed to get another job. But the drinking was always there. I managed to get another job – as a healthcare assistant in an old people's home. I had a child – but things were never good in the relationship I suppose. For the last 20 years, things have pretty much been the same. I drink all the time – sometimes more, sometimes less. Drinking helps me forget my problems and go into oblivion – it blocks things out. And there's a lot to block out. I thought I had been an OK mother – perhaps not the best, but OK. But my son doesn't want to know me anymore. My partner has long gone. I've had jobs on and off over this time – that last one, about 8 years ago.

I feel guilty about my drinking. I've never really been there for my family – I've always been the drunk that doesn't fit in. I suppose if you are always drunk – quietly not loudly – you still can't do your best. Now, I stay in – I don't go out much. I'm ashamed when I go to the shops – people looking at me, talking about me. I feel they are looking at me – judging me. I don't feel good when I'm drunk, but I do feel in oblivion. I just sit there – or lie in bed all day. I'm drinking from the moment I get up – I have to control the tremors.

I want to stop drinking. I feel despair at the circle I'm caught up in – there's no way out. I try – I do all the right things from pouring the drink down the sink, going to the GP for help, and so on. But when I stop drinking I get violent stomach cramps. I shake. I get headaches. I feel paranoid, that people are talking about me. I can't cope with these withdrawals, so I end up drinking again.

Aetiology of alcohol abuse disorder

Biological factors

As well as its neural impact as described above, alcohol also enhances the action of GABA within the hypothalamus and sympathetic nervous system, helping calm mood and behaviour. As with the action of dopamine in the 'pleasure circuit', this results in a reduction in the natural production of GABA, with abstinence resulting in suboptimal levels of GABA, increased anxiety and agitation, and the onset of physical withdrawal symptoms. These are relieved by continued drinking or, in time, the body's resumption of normal levels of GABA.

Both family and biological studies indicate a genetic predisposition to alcohol problems. Prescott and Kendler (1999), for example, reported concordance for 'high lifetime alcohol consumption' of 47% in **monozygotic (MZ) twins** and 32% in **dizygotic (DZ) twins**. People with the 'at-risk' alleles of the *DRD2* and *CNR1* genes may be more sensitive to the effects of alcohol than those without it, and may be encouraged to initiate alcohol and other drug use because they find it easy to gain a 'high'. Conner et al. (2005), for example, found that male adolescents with a particular allele (A1) of the *DRD2* gene tried alcohol and became intoxicated more often than those without it. In addition, they were more likely to develop a smoking habit and experience a marijuana 'high'. This sensitivity to both cannabis and alcohol has also been found to co-exist in alleles of the *CNR1* gene (cannabinoid receptor 1; Marcos et al. 2012).

Socio-cultural factors

Alcohol is a socially sanctioned drug, and consumption is influenced by social and environmental factors. Initiating alcohol consumption is seen as one of the transitions from childhood to adulthood. The European School Survey Project on Alcohol and Other Drugs (ESPAD: http://www.espad.org/report/home), for example, found that around half of all European 15–16-year-old school students reported consuming alcohol in the month preceding the survey. The **prevalence** of drinking ranged from a low of 9% among Icelandic students to 66% or more in countries such as Austria, Denmark, and Greece. Consumption of alcohol by young people is associated with positive attitudes to its use, some of which are linked to family and peer attitudes and behaviours. Heavily drinking parents or parents with *laissez-faire* attitudes towards drinking, for example, may encourage early alcohol consumption (Murphy et al. 2016). Other social factors influence consumption once initiated. Round buying, for example, may increase consumption among young social drinkers. Life transitions, both good and bad, may also influence consumption. Developing relationships and families, or getting and maintaining a job, may inhibit consumption. Adverse life events may increase consumption, particularly among people who use alcohol as a means of coping with stress (Perreira and Sloan 2001).

Rates of drinking vary across cultural and social groups. Men are more likely to drink heavily than women. Blue-collar workers are more likely than white-collar workers to report problem drinking, as are workers with access to alcohol as part of their job. Among men, binge drinking is most frequent among the young, lower-income, and less-educated groups (Bloomfield et al. 2006). There is less evidence of such a social gradient among females. Levels of alcohol consumption may be particularly high in marginalized groups and groups under social pressure, such as the Native Americans in the USA (e.g. Hasin and Grant 2015).

Psychological factors

The path to problem drinking may be established early in life. The pleasurable effects of early drinking and its surrounding social gains may be positive reinforcers of consumption. Further down the pathway to dependence, a motivator to drink may be the negative reinforcement of avoidance of withdrawal symptoms. **Classical conditioning** may also occur as drinking becomes associated with particular cues or events, subsequent exposure to which may trigger episodes of drinking. These behavioural outcomes may be accompanied by a range of cognitive processes known as addictive beliefs (Beck et al. 2001). At the beginning of a history of alcohol use, positive beliefs such as 'It will be fun to get drunk' predominate. As the individual begins to rely on alcohol to counteract feelings of distress, relief-oriented thoughts ('I need a drink to get through the day') may take over. Addictive beliefs may also be accompanied by a wider set of negative core beliefs, including a negative view of oneself, one's circumstances and environment, which may contribute to depression or anxiety.

From a differing perspective, risk for alcohol dependency has been linked to early adversities such as rejection, neglect, and over-protection as a child: experiences that may translate into adulthood and foster the use of alcohol as a means of dampening feelings of (di)stress. Backer-Fulghum et al. (2012), for example, found adult-reported parental neglect as a child was associated with lower levels of self-esteem and the experience of higher levels of stress as adults, which in turn was linked to higher consumption of alcohol. Drinking may also be used as a means of coping with more immediate negative life events, although its ability to effectively achieve this is not clear. Bresin's (2019) review of the acute effects of alcohol following a range of stress-inducing experimental manipulations, for example, indicated only an inconsistent, small-to-modest reduction in stress associated with such tasks.

Interventions in excess alcohol consumption

The goals of therapy

A sharp divide can be found between the philosophy of treatment and the therapeutic goals set by different practitioners in relation to alcohol-associated problems.

Some consider what they term 'alcoholism' to be a biological disease, with the goal of any intervention being abstinence. Others argue that many people can learn to drink alcohol in moderation and appropriately, and this outcome should be the goal of therapy. Empirical data suggests that the degree of dependence on alcohol may be the best determinant. Unsurprisingly, perhaps, Miller et al. (1994) found that those with low alcohol dependency scores were likely to be successful on a programme of moderate drinking. Those with moderate-to-high scores benefited most from abstinence programmes, while those with low-to-moderate scores benefited equally from the two approaches.

Withdrawal

The initial treatment of people with alcohol dependence may involve a period of withdrawal. This may take 3–4 days and is usually aided by the use of sedatives such as diazepam, which moderate the severity of any withdrawal symptoms. Once they have withdrawn from alcohol, many people will receive one or more of the interventions described below.

Drug therapies

Some drugs deter consumption by causing the drinker to feel ill if they consume alcohol while taking them. The most commonly used drug of this type is disulfiram (Antabuse). It prevents alcohol being broken down further than its intermediate metabolite acetaldehyde. This accumulates in the body and, 15–20 minutes after consumption of alcohol, causes a number of symptoms, including flushing, headache, pounding in the head or chest, nausea, and occasional vomiting. Users may be given a test reaction to alcohol to alert them to the consequences of consumption. The benefits of disulfiram depend on its regular consumption. Where this is enforced, it appears an effective barrier to consumption. It is significantly less effective when taken voluntarily, an issue that has raised some ethical concerns (Brewer et al. 2017). Its use clearly follows a biological, abstinence model. However, some studies have evaluated the effectiveness of similar drugs in programmes that accept participants who may choose to drink on occasion. In these, it may be used as an occasional control to consumption, particularly when users feel they are losing control over their drinking (Sinclair 2001).

A second type of drug treatment, and one which does not carry the health risks of disulfiram, involves the use of opioid **agonists**, such as naltrexone, which reduce cravings. Such interventions, of course, encounter the same problems as those associated with Antabuse. If people want to drink, they simply stop taking the medication, although a version of the drug which is therapeutically effective for one month may prevent this. In one study of its effectiveness, O'Malley et al. (2007) found that people who were alcohol dependent were likely to remain abstinent for longer than people who received a **placebo** (41 versus 12 days). In addition, 70% of the treated group were considered 'responders' (that is, they had less than 2 days heavy drinking in any 28-day period) compared with 30% in the placebo-treated group. A final type of drug used to treat alcohol dependence reduces cravings through its action on GABA receptors. Boothby and Doering (2005) reviewed the evidence of effectiveness of one such drug, acamprosate, and found it to be of significant benefit. The percentage of patients who were completely abstinent across the studies they reviewed varied from 18% to 61%, compared with 4–45% taking a placebo.

In a review of the effectiveness of drugs in the treatment of alcohol problems, Goh and Morgan (2017) concluded that they are 'moderately efficacious with few safety concerns'; however, they also noted a reluctance among many doctors to prescribe them either on philosophical grounds or because of a lack of knowledge about or unfamiliarity with them. For example, despite being a recommended treatment in Australia, Morley et al. (2016) found that only 3% of people with alcohol dependence were prescribed such a drug.

Psychosocial interventions

Perhaps the best-known treatment for alcoholism is the 12-step programme of Alcoholics Anonymous (AA). It is premised on a belief that alcoholism is a physical, psychological, and spiritual illness that cannot be cured, but can be controlled by total abstinence from alcohol. The organization provides a strong social support network that encourages emotional expression and the admission of failure. Attendees at group meetings are encouraged to accept that they are powerless to control their drinking, to cease their struggle, and allow a 'higher power' to take control (Gorski 2008). The millions of attendees at AA meetings across the world attest to the potential benefits of this approach.

In a Cochrane review and **meta-analysis** of the relevant research, Kelly et al. (2020) analysed data from 27 studies comprising over 10,000 participants. They concluded that comparisons between the 12-step approach and interventions with different philosophical orientations, such as CBT, showed a 'manualized' version of the 12-step approach was consistently more effective on measures of continuous abstinence for up to 3 years following the beginning of treatment. On a less absolute measure of 'days abstinent', the 12-step programme appeared to be as effective as other interventions at one-year follow-up, and to perform better over more extended periods of time – presumably as a result of the continued access to support not found in most alternative programmes. Non-manualized versions of the intervention may be slightly less effective, but still as effective as other forms of intervention. Interestingly, Timko et al. (2000) found 64% of those who had gone through an AA programme reported maintaining a 'benign' drinking pattern at 3-year follow-up: an interesting finding not only because of the high success rate (albeit self-report) but because it appears that many people who went through this abstinence-based programme were actually drinking at relatively safe levels.

More time-limited programmes have adopted a number of approaches. Cognitive behavioural therapy typically involves training in skills to cope with day-to-day stresses, social skills, and strategies for preventing relapse (Magill and Ray 2009). Social skills training involves teaching interpersonal and assertive skills to help participants cope more effectively with stressful situations, to refuse drinks, and so on. In relapse prevention programmes, high-risk situations are identified, and the individual develops and rehearses strategies to manage them should they arise. These may include specific strategies to challenge addictive beliefs and to cope with cravings. These interventions may be combined with drug therapies. Feeney et al. (2002), for example, reported abstinence rates of 14% following a CBT relapse prevention programme, compared with 38% in a CBT plus acamprosate in a group of individuals considered to be at high risk of relapse. The combined intervention, however, was no more effective in improving psychological well-being and health status than CBT alone (Feeney et al. 2006).

Relapse is frequently associated with interpersonal problems and prevented by strong relationship cohesion. For this reason, some programmes involve the problem drinker's partner. O'Farrell and Fals-Stewart (2000), for example, described an intervention intended to increase communication and problem-solving skills of couples rather than just the problem drinker. Both the problem drinker and their partner learned strategies to reduce consumption, including the partner changing behaviours that might trigger alcohol use, finding new ways to discuss drinking and situations involving it, and new responses to their partner's drinking. A further strand of therapy focused on the type and quality of communication between the partners. In their review of the effectiveness of this approach, O'Farrell and Fals-Stewart concluded that it was consistently more effective than individual therapy on measures of alcohol consumption, abstinence, alcohol-related problems, and the quality of the relationship.

Finally, one widely used intervention has been developed as a single one-off interview designed to enhance the individual's motivation to change. Motivational interviewing (Miller and Rollnick 2013) is a non-confrontational approach in which the therapist encourages the drinker to explore both their reasons for drinking and the advantages (and disadvantages) associated with reducing their consumption. The aim is to trigger a state of dissonance in which the individual actively considers two sets of opposing beliefs: the 'good' and 'not so good' things about drinking. This may result in a rejection of the newly considered arguments, or (more positively) the adoption of new beliefs or behaviours, and increased motivation to reduce alcohol consumption. A longer-term, second, phase can involve problem-solving how to achieve change should the individual choose to do so. It has proven an effective intervention, particularly at times of potential change. Monti et al. (2016), for example, evaluated the effect of motivational interviewing among patients treated in the emergency department of two community hospitals in the US, focusing on unsafe sex practices and alcohol consumption. Compared to brief advice, the intervention had a positive effect on the number of heavy drinking days (an approximate 20% reduction), sex after drinking heavily, and 'condomless sex' up to 9 months following the intervention. A similar intervention provided by peers instead of health professionals also proved of benefit (Bazargan-Hejazi et al. 2005).

Project MATCH

Despite the differences in philosophy and strategies of the various treatment approaches, their effectiveness appears to be very similar. In order to tease out exactly which strategy is the best, Project MATCH, the largest ever alcohol treatment trial, involving over 1,500 participants (Project MATCH Research Group 1998), compared the effectiveness of a number of interventions, including motivational enhancement therapy (a longer-term version of motivational interviewing), CBT, and 12-step approaches. At one-year follow-up, 35% of all participants reported complete abstinence for the whole of the previous year; a further 25% reported having not having drunk heavily on more than 2 consecutive days in this time, a measure considered to reflect some degree of control over their alcohol consumption. At both 1-year and 3-year follow-up, there were no differences between the three intervention groups. The principal purpose of the study, however, was to determine which **clients** responded best to which treatments. The results were as follows:

- People who entered treatment with a high level of state/trait anger fared best in motivational enhancement therapy.
- Those whose social support systems favoured continued drinking rather than abstinence, who were highly dependent, and who had more severe mental health problems benefited most from the 12-step approach.
- People who were less dependent fared better if they received CBT.

So, it would appear that the best approach is likely the one chosen by the **client**.

Case formulation

Mr C was a 33-year-old married man with significant alcohol problems. At the time he was seen by a psychologist he was unemployed as a result of drunken behaviour and lack of discipline in a variety of jobs. He was experiencing financial problems as a result of his unemployment and continued expenditure on alcohol, as well as significant marital problems. He was seeking treatment because his partner of 8 years had threatened to leave the relationship if he continued to drink.

Long-term antecedents

Mr C had his first drink at the age of 14 years. His father and partner regularly drank around the house, and he was soon regularly accessing his father's alcohol at home, buying alcohol from the local off licence, or friends would buy it for him. By the age of 15, he was a regular drinker. He got high on alcohol, but was able to tolerate its effects rather more than the friends with whom he drank. He became a member of a group of young heavy drinkers on his local estate, with whom he regularly drank cheap alcohol, such as beer or strong cider. By the age of 18, he was drinking every day and night, drinking several pints of beer/cider as well as spirits (Jack Daniels, etc.). He had left school at 16, and had had a series of short-term manual jobs, losing each because of poor time-keeping and lack of commitment. He had a series of girlfriends, but no committed relationship and was prioritizing spending his money on alcohol to the exclusion of other things. He was also taking various other drugs and regularly smoking cannabis.

At the age of 25 his behaviour continued much as before. However, he then met a woman (in a bar) with whom he began a long-term relationship, moving in with her after 3 months. She had a job in a local hairdresser and was earning a modest but regular income. He was still drifting from job to job. In the first months of the relationship he reduced his alcohol consumption, made a significant attempt to get and hold down a longer-term job, and attempted to establish a good relationship with his new partner. He succeeded in doing so for a number of months, but gradually began to drink more, began to re-establish old relationships with his drinking friends, and eventually lost his job due to drinking alcohol while at work and previous irregular time-keeping. He then began to drink more in the day as well as during the evenings and nights. He tried to hide his consumption from his partner by drinking spirits in the day and hiding bottles around the house. However, he increasingly needed to drink during the day, starting when he woke up. His mood was becoming erratic and contributing to frequent highly verbally aggressive rows with his partner who was becoming increasingly frustrated by his drinking, lying about his drinking, the money (her money!) spent on his drinking, and their poor relationship.

Short-term antecedents

The trigger to his seeking help for his alcohol problems was a row with his partner, who moved back to her mother's flat saying she could no longer tolerate his drinking. He had told her that he would seek help for his drinking many times and had not done so. But in an attempt at one last reconciliation he agreed to seek help. He did so somewhat reluctantly and felt rather anxious and unsure of how much benefit it might prove. Nevertheless, he and his partner went to his local doctor and asked to be referred to the local alcohol treatment programme. Referral was delayed due to the waiting list of the services and he was eventually seen 3 months later. In this time, he tried to reduce his alcohol consumption, but had struggled to do so, and his partner (and now more accurately his ex-partner) was still living with her mother – although she had agreed to reconsider her decision if he were to change his drinking behaviour.

Formulation

Mr C was a fairly typical man with a drink problem, in that there was no one trigger to his drinking; rather, he had drifted over a period of years into heavy drinking. He found the process of drinking rewarding, as it made him feel good, and when he drank with his friends there was an added social bonding. Eventually, he also found that drinking relieved the discomfort of withdrawal symptoms and the low moods he experienced when not drinking. These immediate rewards became more powerful determinants of his behaviour than the longer-term and more incremental problems drinking was causing in the rest of his life.

Intervention

Mr C was drinking high volumes of alcohol when he first came to the service, so he underwent a home detoxification programme, overseen by a community psychiatric nurse. This involved him stopping drinking, while taking fairly high dosages of drugs designed to minimize any withdrawal effects, which also made him very sleepy. As a result, he was visited a number of times a day by the nurse, and over a period of 3 days the dosage of the drug was gradually reduced as did his withdrawal symptoms. Once he was detoxed, Mr C was seen by a drug and alcohol counsellor for psychological treatment.

The first phase of treatment involved a motivational interview, designed to identify and hopefully increase his motivation to change his drinking behaviour. This identified key motivators of his desire to change: his relationship with his partner, lack of success in having children and providing a stable background for them, and the lack of money to spend on other parts of his life. He wanted to succeed and to be seen to be succeeding very quickly so that he could reinstate his relationship with his estranged partner. He initially opted to aim for total alcohol abstinence, using Antabuse as a means of ensuring abstinence. He also wanted to involve his partner in any treatment programme so she would have confidence that he was improving. Accordingly, he was seen with his partner on four occasions, and on his own for a similar number. In the joint sessions, the counsellor addressed several issues particularly pertinent to the relationship, including issues related to intimacy and sexual matters as well as developing strategies to reduce the intensity and number of arguments they had been having – all of which were triggers to his drinking. They also negotiated a plan for coming to live back together. Mr C also developed strategies for coping with urges to drink and to prevent his relapse. These involved both strategies he could use on his own, including going to see his father or getting a buzz from involvement in other activities such as jogging (which he had begun following his withdrawal), and activities involving his partner, that could be as simple as watching TV together or talking. He initially avoided people he associated with drinking, although this was not easy as most of his friends were heavy drinkers. Over time, when he was confident he could resist a drink, he began to see some of them, but not in drinking contexts. Over time, he also developed strategies to engage in if he did have a drink, which included talking about this with his partner, ensuring regular use of Antabuse, re-invoking strategies of abstinence if he had begun to relax and not use them, and seeing his counsellor if necessary. He also was helped by a social worker to find a job, allowing some stability in his life.

16.4 Heroin use disorder

Opiates are a group of drugs derived from the opium poppy. The key derivatives, in order of strength and addictiveness, are opium, morphine, and heroin. Across the world, the most widely used form of the drug is heroin, although addiction to prescription opiates is now particularly problematic in the USA, with more people addicted to them than heroin (Center for Behavioral Health Statistics and Quality 2018) as a consequence of widespread over-prescription of synthetic opioid drugs such as fentanyl for medical conditions typically involving chronic pain. Many people transition to the use of heroin if they can no longer access their prescribed medication. Muhuri et al. (2013), for example, estimated that 80% of heroin users first misused prescription opioids.

Taking heroin results in profound feelings of warmth, relaxation, and euphoria. Worries, fears, and concerns are forgotten, and self-confidence increases. These effects last for between 4 and 6 hours, before the individual 'comes down' from the drug. Once dependent on the drug, withdrawal initially results in muscle pain, sweats, sneezes, and uncontrollable yawning. Within 36 hours, the symptoms become increasingly severe, and include uncontrollable muscle twitching, cramps, chills, sweating, and a high heart rate. The person is unable to sleep, vomits, and has diarrhoea. These symptoms are at their most acute for about 72 hours, gradually reducing over a period of between 5 and 10 days.

It is difficult to estimate heroin use within the general population. However, estimates in the US suggest the prevalence rose from 0.33% to 1.6% of the population between 2002 and 2013, and that for heroin use disorder from 0.21% to 0.69% (Martins et al. 2017). The prevalence of drug injectors (usually opiates but including amphetamines) across the countries of Europe is thought to lie somewhere between 0.26% of the population in Germany and 0.48% in Luxembourg (Kraus et al. 2003). Between the 1960s and the early 1990s, heroin was taken predominantly by intravenous injection. Now it is increasingly smoked, a practice known as 'chasing the dragon' and associated with an increased drug effect and perceived cost-effectiveness (Swift et al. 1999). Smyth et al. (2000) reported a 330% increase in the number of new attendees smoking heroin at Dublin drug clinics between 1991 and 1996. Chasers were more likely to be employed, younger, use fewer other drugs, to be more educated, and have a shorter history of use than people who injected. Cultural differences may also influence mode of consumption. Keen et al. (2014), for example, found that in Baltimore, 75% of black users smoked heroin, while 69% of white users injected.

Most heroin users use other drugs. Beswick et al. (2001) reported that 60% of their sample of attendees at a London clinic used crack cocaine, 58% used alcohol, 11% diazepam, 9% methadone, and 8% used cocaine powder at the same time as taking heroin. Rather more conservative polydrug use was reported by Bobashev et al. (2018), who found five clusters of drug use types in their US sample: people who (i) used heroin with alcohol and occasionally crack cocaine; (ii) used heroin and crack cocaine daily; (iii) used heroin daily and almost exclusively; (iv) used heroin and marijuana daily; and (v) were part-time drug users.

Stop and think ...

We tend to think of addictions as being highly rewarding experiences associated with drugs and behaviours such as gambling. But there is now evidence of addiction to a much more mundane and everyday stimulus: food! Some have argued that the neurological effects of eating, at least for some people, are identical to those more commonly associated with drug use or behaviours such as gambling.

This may lead to binge eating and even withdrawal symptoms in the short term, and obesity in the long term. Supporting evidence of this hypothesis can be found in early brain scanning studies, and also animal studies where controlled access to high sugar and/or high fat food can trigger compulsive eating. Countering such claims are arguments that any addictive substance within food has not been found, the lack of pleasure generally associated with binge eating, and more recent contrary evidence from neuroimaging studies. The concept of food addiction raises a number of questions. Does it exist? And more generally, where do the boundaries lie to the concept of an 'addiction'? If we enjoy and repeat a behaviour frequently, and feel sad if we can no longer engage in it, does this form an 'addiction'? If we can become addicted to such frequently encountered stimuli as food, should we consider binge watching of Netflix to be an 'addiction'? Or is this over-pathologizing ordinary behaviours?

Aetiology of heroin use

Biological factors

Opiates influence dopaminergic activity within the neural 'reward system'. In addition, they bind to the same receptor sites as endorphins and enkephalins, resulting in a state of well-being, as well as having a sedating effect. Both chemicals are found throughout the brain, although there are high concentrations in the midbrain, hypothalamus, and thalamus, as well as the spinal cord (Lingford-Hughes 2005). Also, regular heroin users evidence generalized dysfunctional connectivity throughout the brain, including the prefrontal cortex, amygdala, hippocampus, and corpus callosum. This may contribute to decreased self-control, impaired inhibitory function, as well as deficits in stress regulation in chronic heroin users (Liu et al. 2009).

Although environmental factors predominate in the development of drug addiction, there is some evidence of family transmission of a genetic vulnerability to drug abuse. Cadoret et al. (1995), for example, found that the adopted children of parents who abused alcohol were three times more likely to develop drug dependence than those from non-alcohol-dependent parents, suggesting the potential of a gene for an 'addictive personality' rather than one for opiate addiction in particular. As with addiction to alcohol, alleles of the *DRD2* dopamine gene may be involved in determining risk for opiate dependence, although somewhat confusingly, the gene may work in different ways in different phenotypes. Xu et al. (2004) found that the same alleles of the gene increased susceptibility to dependence in people of Chinese origin but were associated with a low risk of dependence in Caucasians. Other genes may also be involved, including those involved with serotonin (Saiz et al. 2009) and endorphin activity (Levran et al. 2008).

Socio-cultural factors

Only about 20% of individuals who initiate drug use do so with the primary goal of seeking pleasure (Nutt and Law 2000). Other reasons include self-medication, social pressure, and the search for 'meaning' or mystical experiences. Evidence of the use of heroin as a means of self-medication or as a means of reducing stress can be found in studies that show higher rates of heroin use among populations living in stressful environments or who have experienced stressful events. Perhaps the most dramatic evidence of this, and the ability to stop use following cessation of such stress, is the estimated 40% of American soldiers who used heroin during the Vietnam War, and the approximately 1% who continued to use it when back in the USA (Grinspoon and Bakalar 1986).

A second route to the use of heroin is as a progression from the use of other drugs, as users seek a greater 'high' than, or different experience from, those already achieved. Use can escalate to abuse, and then to dependence, involving increased tolerance of the drug, compulsive drug-taking and withdrawal symptoms if the drug is not taken regularly. Sharing needles is relatively common and may contain a social or ritual element. For many addicts, maintaining a drug habit can be expensive and beyond their financial resources, particularly where they find it difficult or choose not to hold down a job. As a result, use is often maintained by crime.

The 'addiction career' often involves cycles of cessation and relapse, often over many years. Between one-quarter and one-third of users will die of a drug-related cause, generally an overdose. An example of this history is afforded by Dai, a 29-year-old brought up in an economically marginalized council estate in South Wales. Here is the story of his drug-taking, its associated problems, and how it was at least partly maintained by the social world he inhabited:

I started smoking ciggies when I was 9 ... bunk off school – hang around with me mates – some of the older kids – just hang around all day – no worries – just wander the streets all day. Soon got into sniffing glue – did it for about a year, year and a half. Didn't start as a regular thing – every now and then – but did it most days after a while. Used to be one of us would have a bag and some glue. Gave us a buzz. Yeah! Move on to dope at about 12. Did it with my mates. Spend a day in someone's house shitless on dope. F***king good! Still smoke. Mellows me out. But then went on to speed. Took it about when I was 12 and something. Only took it at weekends, washed down with lager. Billy whiz ... keeps you going, going, going. Good for dancing ... After a while, taking the stuff everyday – starts getting expensive, so start lifting things, nicking, TWOCing [taking without consent: stealing cars]. Problems with the police – in front of the bench a few times. Got a fine, so have to nick again! Parents found out once got to police. Went ballistic when they found out. First time they knew I was taking drugs. Beaten shitless by my father. Grounded – not that that did much good. Old man's a hypocrite anyway – drinks loads, but dead against drugs. Anyway, tried loads of other shit after that – LSD, tabs [benzodiazepines], Temazies, E's, uppers, downers. Sixteen. Stoned out of my mind on dope, one of my mates asked if I wanted some smack. So I said, 'Yeah!' Anything for a buzz. He injected me. That did it. What a rush! I felt I was superman! I could do anything. That was it. Hooked. Stopped taking speed – smack was it.

Left school at 16. Parents knew I was taking smack. Took me to loads of docs, but didn't do anything. So, they washed their hands of me – didn't want to know – chucked me out. Crashed on my mates' floors for a while. Got a council house pretty quickly. Got chucked out pretty quickly too – didn't pay the rent! Not good at paying rent! Smack had me hooked. The more I used, the more money I needed. So, I got into breaking and entering – always getting caught. Fines, probation, then time in prison. But that didn't stop me taking the stuff. You can get anything you want inside if you know the right people. Went to prison for the first time just before my 18th birthday – 4 months for burglary.

Cut a long story short – been in and out of prison for the last 12 years. Had girl-friends. Lived with one woman for about 3 years. Got a daughter with her – see her sometimes, but not a lot. They don't come and see me when I'm inside ... Smack has a hold on me and I can't let go. My mates all take the stuff. I don't know anyone that doesn't use. So, I've nothing else. Did give up once. Went on a programme in prison. Came out clean – stayed clean for about 3 months. They put me up in a hostel when I came out – so I could stay away from my mates ... Stop using in the 'real world' ... But then I had to leave as they didn't have money to keep me there. So, I went back to my old haunts. Soon back to jacking up ...

Don't enjoy the dope now. I'm pissed with the routine – take drugs, steal, go to prison, take drugs ... Don't get the buzz from using. I've got to take it so it doesn't do my head in. I'm trying to get out of it – stop using. I'm on methadone [see p. 437], so I can stop taking the stuff. But they don't give enough ... still get withdrawals – heart pounding, sweats, cramps. So I'm still using – but less than I was – was using about three bags a day, now it's a bag, bag and a half. I'll try to get more methadone – try to keep off the smack altogether, but they don't like to give you too much.

Psychological factors

The psychological processes associated with opiate use are similar to those for all addictions. There is an **operant conditioning** process in which the individual is rewarded for taking the drug through the pleasurable effects and reductions in tension associated with its use, and then the avoidance of withdrawal symptoms. Classical conditioning triggers cravings for heroin when a user encounters conditions similar to its previous use. These conditioned responses may be both powerful and sustained over time. Meyer (1995), for example, reported that the sight of a needle may decrease the severity of withdrawal symptoms while coming off heroin. Conversely, cues conditioned to withdrawal may trigger its symptoms, even years after heroin use has been stopped. Cognitive factors are also involved in expectancies of both pleasure and, ultimately, fear of withdrawal.

A biopsychosocial model

Combining pharmacological and psychological processes within one model, the incentive sensitization theory of Robinson and Berridge (2008) contended that the most important psychological change associated with drug use is a 'sensitization' or hypersensitivity, at a neurological level, to what they termed the incentive motivational effects of drugs and drug-associated stimuli. Incentive sensitization involves a bias of attentional processing towards drug-associated stimuli and a pathological motivation for drugs (compulsive 'wanting'). When combined with impaired executive control over behaviour, incentive sensitization culminates in the core symptoms of addiction. As this is a partly (Pavlovian) conditioned process, this may be triggered in particular by contexts associated with previous drug use. Behavioural evidence of this sensitization can be found in drug addicts whose attention is biased to visual drug-associated cues at an overt and implicit level (Wiers and Stacy 2006). Neural evidence of sensitization can be found in studies that have shown repeated intermittent administration of amphetamines causes increased dopamine release in humans, even when a drug is given a year after the initial administration, while drug cues can also elicit a significant conditioned dopamine response even in the absence of the drug (Boileau et al. 2006).

Treatment of heroin use

Harm minimization

Harm minimization strategies do not attempt to 'treat' addiction. Instead, they reduce the harm associated with the continued use of drugs.

Opioid substitutes

Opioid substitute programmes typically provide a controlled amount of synthetic opioid, taken orally, to avoid withdrawal symptoms without the 'rush' associated with heroin. Drugs such as methadone and buprenorphine are intended to prevent the risks of needle-sharing, overdose, and withdrawal when individuals initially seek help: a time that may be particularly chaotic in their lives. They can be prescribed for periods of a year or more, during which time the recipient is expected to 'stabilize' their life and prepare for subsequent withdrawal from it. Users typically report daily to a registered provider (doctor, pharmacist, etc.) where they take medication under supervision. This maintains contact with support services and stops the medication being sold on the black market. About half of UK family doctors are providing methadone to opiate users at any one time (Strang et al. 2005).

This approach appears to be successful, although methadone is more effective than buprenorphine (Mattick et al. 2014). In the largest study of the use of methadone, the Drug Abuse Treatment Outcome Study (Hubbard et al. 1997) followed nearly 3,000 people receiving out-patient treatment. In the year following its prescription, the percentage of people using heroin weekly or daily fell from 90% to 30%. Reasons for continued use of heroin included perceptions of being maintained on too low a dose of methadone, an associated 'toxicity', the desire for the 'high' achieved with opiates, the strength of self-identity as an 'addict', and continued relationships with intravenous drug users (Avants et al. 1999). To address some of these issues, a more recent approach has involved the use of diacetylmorphine, essentially pure heroin; again, prescribed by doctors and accessed via pharmacists in an injectable form twice a day. Diacetylmorphine is less toxic than methadone, and achieves better adherence. In one study comparing the two approaches, Oviedo-Joekes et al. (2009) found that 88% of people receiving diacetylmorphine and 54% receiving methadone remained in treatment for a year.

Needle-exchange schemes

Needle-exchange schemes exchange old for new needles, preventing the need for sharing, and reducing risk of cross-infection of blood-borne viruses including HIV and hepatitis. First established in the Netherlands in 1983, this harm reduction approach has not been without controversy. In the US, for example, some right-wing and church groups claimed it maintained, or even encouraged, the use of drugs. As a result, needle-exchange schemes were banned in 33 US states, and federal law prevented their funding through the US government: a stance that changed in 2016, following a significant 'outbreak' of HIV infection in Indiana. Since then, central government has allocated funds to such schemes. This change was facilitated by empirical evidence that where syringes cannot legally be obtained elsewhere, needle-exchange programmes are effective in reducing the use of shared needles (Kerr et al. 2005), although their use can be far from optimal. Gindi et al. (2009), for example, reported users typically only made two visits to a Baltimore needle-exchange programme over a 12-month period.

Interventions to reduce/prevent use

Most of the interventions described below follow a period of withdrawal from heroin involving either a gradual reduction in drug use (typically involving an opiate substitute) or more acutely using drugs such as clonidine hydrochloride (Marsch et al. 2005) to minimize withdrawal symptoms over a period of around 3 days.

Drug therapies

Longer-term use of therapeutic drugs typically involves those that negate the effects of heroin. Naltrexone is an opiate **antagonist** that binds with opioid receptors in the brain and blocks the effect of opiates. If taken on a regular basis, it prevents the 'high' associated with opiates. Unfortunately, the majority of people offered this form of intervention choose to take it up, and many fail to take the drug regularly. Jarvis et al. (2018), for example, reported typical adherence of around 10% in routine care settings. Among highly motivated individuals who actually use naltrexone, outcomes are relatively good. It results in lower cravings for opiates, longer periods of abstinence, and greater improvements in psychosocial functioning than placebo. Abstinence rates as high as 64% have been found in well-supported and 'high coping' individuals at 18-month follow-up, although rates between 31% and 53% are more typical (Tucker and Ritter 2000). The effects of naltrexone may be added to by combining it with a benzodiazepine to reduce the insomnia and 'excitability' that may accompany its use (Stella et al. 2005).

Psychological approaches

Rewarding abstinence. Many people who take methadone also continue using opiates. In an attempt to address this, Gruber et al. (2000) investigated whether providing extrinsic rewards could increase attendance at methadone clinics and drug abstinence. Their incentives to attend counselling sessions included bus tokens and vouchers to be spent on activities or items agreed by their counsellor. Incentives for abstinence included free weekend recreational activities, lunches, a modest financial sum per week in vouchers, and help towards payment of rent. This approach was compared with a standard treatment approach in which individuals were encouraged to attend routine methadone clinics but were not rewarded for doing so. One month after entry, 61% of participants in the reward condition, compared with 17% of those in the standard treatment, were enrolled in treatment; the percentage achieving 30 days abstinence were 50% and 21%, respectively. Since then a number of similar studies have followed this basic approach with significant and consistent benefit (see Stitzer and Petry 2006).

Cognitive behavioural therapy. People who use heroin often lead chaotic lives and find it difficult to follow formal therapeutic programmes. Accordingly, interventions such as CBT are difficult to institute, drop-out levels are very high, and they struggle to be effective. Moore et al. (2016), for example, found participants who were dependent on opioid medications but not those who were primarily heroin users benefited from the addition of CBT to a buprenorphine treatment programme. More positively, Scherbaum et al. (2005) found a one-session group cognitive behavioural intervention to be as effective as its long-term equivalent. Although the authors found no immediate benefits following either approach, participants in the brief intervention were using fewer opiates than the standard treatment group 6 months following the intervention, suggesting that complex cognitive behavioural programmes may not be the treatment of choice.

16.5 Behavioural addictions

Gambling disorder

Most of us gamble at some time or other. However, for some, gambling can become addictive and as difficult to stop as recreational drugs. DSM-IV-TR considered gambling disorder to be a problem of impulse control, but it is now included within the category of substance-related and addictive disorders. Nevertheless, the DSM-5 criteria for gambling disorder differ from those of the other addictions so far considered. Their definition requires at least four of the following criteria to be experienced within one year:

- The need to gamble with more money to achieve the same levels of excitement
- Feeling restless or irritable when trying to reduce or stop gambling
- Repeated, unsuccessful attempts to reduce or stop gambling
- Frequent thoughts about gambling
- Gambling when depressed, guilty or anxious
- Trying to win back gambling losses: 'chasing the dragon'
- Lying to hide the extent of gambling
- Losing relationships, jobs or significant career opportunities as a result of gambling
- Becoming dependent on others for money to relieve gambling-related financial problems.

Gambling disorder is the endpoint of a progression through social, frequent, problem, and finally pathological gambling. The WHO estimated the prevalence of gambling disorder to lie between 0.1% and 6% of the population across different countries, with two to three times as many individuals experiencing less serious, 'subclinical' problems (Abbott 2017). In addition, it considered the degree of associated 'harm' to be substantially greater than that linked to drug dependence disorder: an estimated two-thirds of pathological gamblers, for example, have committed criminal offences in order to continue gambling (Turner et al. 2009). In addition, up to 30% of pathological gamblers may have alcohol-related problems. The relationship to alcohol is important, as some have taken it to suggest that both alcohol and gambling problems are indicative of a more general 'addictive' personality.

Aetiology of gambling disorder

Biological factors

A key driver of gambling is the 'buzz' of winning or coming close to winning, which is associated with dopamine release in the neural reward system (Zack and Poulos 2009) as well as increased norepinephrine. In social gamblers, these neurochemical processes typically occur while gambling. Among pathological gamblers, they occur while anticipating gambling or as a classically conditioned response to gambling-related stimuli. These effects are not trivial, and withdrawal from gambling may result in symptoms similar to, or even more severe than, those experienced in drug withdrawal. Cunningham-Williams et al. (2009) identified both physiological symptoms, particularly restlessness and irritability, and psychological symptoms such as depression, anger, and guilt as typifying symptoms experienced by around two-thirds of gamblers in withdrawal.

Family studies (e.g. Slutske et al. 2009) involving pairs of twins have found genetic factors to account for around 45% of the vulnerability to pathological gambling, with genes influencing dopamine, serotonin, opioid, and norepinephrine metabolism (e.g. *DRD2*, *TPH*, *ADRA2*) each contributing to risk (Hillemacher et al. 2016; Kim et al. 2019).

Research box 15

de Brito, A.M., de Almeida Pinto, M.G., Bronstein, G. et al. (2017) Topiramate combined with cognitive restructuring for the treatment of gambling disorder: a two-center, randomized, double-blind clinical trial, *Journal of Gambling Studies*, 33: 249–63.

The primary goal of this study was to evaluate the effectiveness of a drug, topiramate, which increases activation of GABA and blocks glutamate pathways, resulting in reduced dopamine release (presumably) in response to gambling-related cues and thus reduced cravings. It has previously been found to be effective in treating alcohol dependence and binge eating disorder.

Previous interventions with topiramate in problem gamblers have shown reductions in impulsiveness but no effects on craving or gambling. The study therefore combined topiramate with a cognitive behavioural intervention to determine whether such a combination would have more of an effect on gambling-related measures.

Method

This was a 12-week, placebo-controlled, double-blind randomized controlled trial of (i) a flexible dose of topiramate, dependent on the participant's response, combined with a four-session cognitive behavioural intervention versus (ii) placebo combined with the psychological intervention. Any between-group differences would therefore be attributable to the topiramate.

Participants

Thirty-eight participants were recruited (39 completers) through media adverts. Inclusion criteria were meeting four or more of the DSM-5 criteria for gambling disorder and having made a bet at least once a week in the previous 30 days. Exclusion criteria included women who might become pregnant, a history of drug dependence, a serious psychiatric disorder, or having received pharma- or psychological therapy in the previous 3 months. No differences on any measure were observed between the groups before the intervention. The mean age of participants was 48.2 years and 47% were female.

Treatment

- *Cognitive behavioural therapy (CBT)* for 4 weeks: week 1, raising awareness of gambling-related problems; week 2, motivational interview; week 3, identification and correction of gambling-related cognitive distortions; and week 4, developing strategies to cope with cravings and relapses.
- *Topiramate* involved doses titrated up to 300 mg per day over an 8-week period and maintained at this dosage for an additional month. Participants saw a doctor 'live' every 2 weeks, with telephone contact on the intervening weeks.

These were combined to form two conditions: CBT plus topiramate (CBT-T) and CBT plus placebo (CBT-P).

Measures

Key measures of gambling addiction were taken immediate before and after the intervention:

- *Gambling Symptom Assessment Scale (G-SAS)*: a single-dimension self-report scale assessing gambling-related craving, thoughts, and behaviours.

- *Yale Brown Obsessive Compulsive Scale adapted for Pathological Gambling (PG-YBOCS)*: a semi-structured interview providing an obsession score (craving and thoughts), a compulsion score (gambling-related distress), and a total (obsession-compulsion) score.
- *TFB interviews*: recollection time and money spent on gambling in the last 30 days.
- *Gambling Beliefs Questionnaire (GBQ)*: measures cognitive distortions about randomness and gambling superstitions. Note that higher scores indicate less distortion.

Results

Participants in both groups evidenced significant improvements over time on all outcome measures. However, analyses of variance identified significant group × time interactions favouring the CBT plus topiramate (CBT-T) condition. *Post-hoc* analyses found greater improvements on measures of craving (G-SAS), gambling-related obsessions and compulsions (PG-YBOCS), and time spent on gambling and cognitive distortions (GBQ). **Effect sizes** fell within the 'large' range.

Table 1 Means (and standard deviations) of key outcome measures

	CBT-T	CBT-P	Interaction *F*	*p*-value
G-SAS				
Pre-trial	25.8 (10.15)	19.9 (10.55)	6.434	0.02
Post-trial	7.9 (9.48)	13.0 (10.30)		
PG-YBOCS: Total				
Pre-trial	22.0 (6.07)	16.3 (6.83)	7.629	0.01
Post-trial	5.6 (7.31)	7.5 (6.89)		
PG-YBOCS: Obsessions				
Pre-trial	11.3 (3.37)	8.7 (3.29)	6.217	0.02
Post-trial	3.5 (4.27)	4.5 (4.05)		
PG-YBOCS: Compulsions				
Pre-trial	10.3 (3.49)	7.7 (3.77)	5.758	0.02
Post-trial	2.1 (3.11)	3.1 (3.08)		
TFB interview				
Time spent (hours)				
Pre-trial	45.9 (29.3)	26.6 (20.17)	8.704	0.007
Post-trial	3.5 (6.76)	9.5 (11.25)		
Money spent (dollars)				
Pre-trial	2558.55 (3450.33)	2714.98 (3340.38)	Wald = 3.94	0.05
Post-trial	133.48 (188.36)	682.40 (737.44)		
GBQ				
Pre-trial	84.2 (19.78)	94.1 (33.46)	10.569	0.003
Post-trial	121.7 (20.73)	104.7 (32.85)		

Discussion

Although the authors reported no significant differences at baseline on the key measures, there does appear to be consistent evidence that the CBT-P group was less problematic than the CBT-T group at baseline, which may have biased this group against higher therapeutic gains. From a methodological perspective, therefore, it might have been better to have conducted a simple one-way analysis of variance between conditions, with a covariate of the baseline score on each measure. This would have provided a slightly fairer comparison. Nevertheless, the data do seem to indicate a clear benefit from the addition of topiramate to CBT on all measures, including cognitive and behavioural outcomes. However, a key issue not addressed by the study is what happens after withdrawal from the medication. We know that many people on medication relapse at this point, and it is possible that any advantage conferred by the medication is lost at this point. Indeed, it is possible that if participants in the CBT-T condition saw changes as a consequence of receiving the drug, it could be that those that made changes without the drug (e.g. CBT-P) might have been more resilient when the drug was removed. The study provides interesting preliminary data, but longer-term follow-up is required before any strong conclusions can be drawn.

Socio-cultural factors

In general, ease of access to gambling opportunities seems to increase both social and problem gambling (Ladouceur et al. 1999). This effect may be particularly apparent for quick-win outcomes such as those associated with gaming machines (e.g. Lund 2009). The easy availability of online gambling is now increasingly problematic, with studies such as that of Columb and O'Gara (2018) finding this to be the most popular gambling activity, while Effertz et al. (2018) calculated the risks of becoming an addicted gambler when using online gambling websites to be significantly greater than the associated off-line gambling risk. Once in a gambling context, a number of factors may influence the extent of gambling. Ellery et al. (2005), for example, found drinking alcohol increased the time videopoker players spent gambling, the frequency with which they placed 'power bets', and the time played while losing money. However, many regular casino gamblers drink less while gambling than they usually do: a finding that led Dickerson and Baron (2000) to challenge the notion that gambling and alcohol consumption share a common genetic risk.

Psychological factors

High levels of impulsivity are a significant risk factor for pathological gambling. Vitaro et al. (1999), for example, investigated the predictive strength of four measures of impulsivity in 13–14-year-olds: teacher ratings, self-report and performance on a card-playing task, and a 'delay in gratification task'. Gambling was subsequently measured at the age of 17 years. Among the factors that predicted gambling were **perseveration** on the card-playing task and an inability to delay gratification. These findings were considered indicative of a tendency to respond excessively to positive outcomes, to require immediate reinforcement, and insensitivity to negative consequences, all characteristics of the pathological gambler.

Early models of gambling assumed that gambling was established and maintained by the intermittent reinforcement, both biological and economic, inherent in gambling. Losses would be sustained in the hope of later gains. Sharpe (2002) suggested that while these undoubtedly contribute to explanations of social gambling, they do not fully explain pathological gambling, where consistent and significant losses do not result in a cessation of gambling. Instead, Sharpe suggested that large pay-outs, and in particular a 'big win' early in a gambling career, establish and sustain pathological gambling. Evidence for this influence, though, is not strong. In their longitudinal study of young people transitioning into problem gambling adults, Edgerton et al. (2015) found this was not predictive of long-term gambling problems. Of the 11 indicators of potential risk in their study, the only reliable predictor was impulsivity.

More important may be cognitive events while gambling. Pro-gambling attitudes increase the likelihood of gambling (Oei and Raylu 2004) but do not sustain gambling once initiated. Other forms of cognitive self-talk may be important at this time. Sharpe (2002), for example, found that 75% of all game-related cognitions during gambling were irrational in nature and supportive of continued gambling. Such thoughts may disregard losses, involve inappropriate expectations of success, and even lead the individual to feel that they have some degree of control over their fate (e.g. Johansson et al. 2009). Within an episode of gambling, 'near wins' serve to maintain gambling, as they lead to over-estimation of how much the individual is actually winning and are viewed as 'exciting events' (Barton et al. 2017). Spada et al. (2015) examined the meta-cognitions surrounding gambling. In their study of gambling addicts, the goals of gambling were two-fold: relieving economic hardship and improving emotional state. Each episode of gambling was controlled by what they called start and stop signals. Start signals were ideas that gambling could solve their problems and the expectation that 'the time is right' for a win. Stop signals were running out of money.

Low mood or anxiety also appear to trigger gambling among pathological gamblers (Skokauskas and Satkeviciute 2007). The immersive nature and experience of 'flow' while playing slot machines, for example, may provide distance from emotional difficulties and escape from boredom and stress (Murch et al. 2017). **Dysphoric** mood before gambling may also result in more persistent gambling following losses. As a partial explanation of this phenomenon, Dickerson and Baron (2000) suggested that low mood may reduce perceptions of control over gambling and reduce attempts to curtail the activity even when losing.

These various findings each contributed to Sharpe's (2002) biopsychosocial model of gambling. She suggested that this may involve three early risk factors:

- a biological vulnerability involving the dopaminergic and serotonergic systems
- family attitudes that support gambling
- high levels of impulsivity.

These factors may lead to a number of gambling experiences as a relatively young individual, during which the individual becomes socialized into a gambling culture. A pattern of early wins may also reinforce gambling behaviours and distort beliefs about, and attitudes towards, gambling. Greater attention may be paid, for example, to success than failures. At the same time, the individual may become pleasantly physiologically aroused while gambling. All of these factors serve to maintain an interest. As a gambling career progresses, episodes may be triggered by hopes of avoiding stress, boredom or improving mood. Gambling is used to increase arousal and as a means of escape from reality. In the gambling context, cognitive biases and the arousal experienced serve to maintain the behaviour, whether winning or losing.

Treatment of pathological gambling

Pharmacological therapies

Given the multiple biochemical pathways that drive pathological gambling, several medications may be of benefit. Despite this, few controlled studies of their effectiveness have been conducted, and drop out from interventions tends to be significant (Kraus et al. 2020). The best candidate for treatment may be the opiate antagonist, naltrexone, although even this has had mixed results, with both better (Grant et al. 2008) and similar (Kovanen et al. 2016) effects compared with placebo. The latter study involved 'as needed' use of naltrexone rather than consistent dosage, which may have reduced its benefit.

Psychological therapies

Programmes such as the Gamblers Anonymous (GA) 12-step programme have achieved abstinence rates of around 8% over 1 year and 7% over 2 years (Stewart and Brown 1988). More formal 'therapeutic' interventions have reported one-year abstinence rates as high as 55%, although the optimum approach may be a combination of GA-type support combined with a formal therapeutic approach such as CBT (see Petry 2005). Cognitive behavioural interventions have certainly proved effective. Cowlishaw et al. (2012), for example, conducted a meta-analysis of 14 studies involving the use of cognitive therapies, including cognitive therapy, motivational interviewing, and imaginal desensitization. The authors found consistent evidence of short-term benefit. The longer-term outcomes were less clear as not all studies included follow-up assessments; however, those that did showed a continuing – albeit smaller – benefit.

In one such study, Ladouceur et al. (2001) randomly allocated pathological gamblers into cognitive therapy or a **waiting list control** group. The cognitive intervention had two elements. The first involved cognitive correction, in which participants' misconceptions on randomness were challenged. This involved both an educational component on the nature of randomness and the identification and challenge of erroneous cognitions made while gambling. This was achieved by tape-recording verbalizations ('… if I lose four times in a row, I will definitely win the next time …') made during a session of imaginal gambling followed by the therapist 'correcting' them within the therapy session. The second element involved training in relapse prevention, whereby participants identified high-risk situations and planned how to cope with them should they arise. The intervention was successful: 54% of participants in the cognitive intervention improved by at least 50% on a composite measure of recovery that included frequency of gambling and perceived control over gambling behaviour, compared with only 7% of the control group. Furthermore, 85% of participants in the treatment programme compared with only 14% in the control group achieved 50% improvements on at least three of the four measures. These gains were generally maintained at 6-month, 12-month, and 2-year follow-up (Ladouceur et al. 2003).

Interventions reported in clinical trials tend to be conducted by experts, following prescribed protocols, with selected participants – with the potential for exaggerated success rates compared with those likely to be achieved in the 'real world'. The study reported by Smith et al. (2018) is therefore especially interesting as it not only examined the impact of a 'gold standard' clinical trial of CBT for gambling disorder, it also compared data from the trial with that from routine provision of CBT in normal practice. Reassuringly, the majority of measures did not differ between the two, with around 60% of participants achieving the main outcome measure of the study: a significant reduction in the urge to gamble. Instead, the key determinant of outcome was the type of gambling the participants engaged in, with those who used poker gambling machines having a worse prognosis than those who bet on horses. One final study is also of particular interest. Petry et al. (2008) found a one-off motivational interview to be more effective in the short term, and equally effective in the longer term (9 months), than a more complex cognitive behavioural intervention. Complexity of intervention does not always equate with greater success, particularly for populations that are not strongly motivated to engage with any therapeutic programme.

(Internet) gaming disorder

It will probably come as no surprise that many internet users experience a range of compulsions to engage with the internet in differing ways. However, within this broad category of addictions one subcategory appears to be close to formal recognition within the DSM and has already been classified by its WHO equivalent – the International Classification of Diseases 11 (WHO 2018a). According to DSM-5, gaming disorder is likely to be accepted within its remit in the future, with criteria for the disorder potentially involving five or more of the following over a period of a year:

- Preoccupation with gaming
- Withdrawal symptoms when gaming is not possible
- The urge to spend more time gaming
- Repeated unsuccessful attempts to quit gaming
- Giving up, or loss of interest in, previously enjoyed activities due to gaming
- Continuing to game despite problems
- Deceiving others about the amount of time spent gaming
- Using gaming to relieve negative mood states
- Risking or losing a job or relationship due to gaming.

An estimated 2% of the overall population are likely to experience this problem, with higher rates in younger people, among whom a prevalence of as high as

10.8% has been reported in Taiwan (Ko et al. 2009). In their sample of 2,533 Italians aged 14–21 years, Poli and Agrimi (2012) found that 5% were moderately addicted and 0.79% were 'seriously' addicted to gaming. Many people experience problems for some time, with rates of continuing difficulties varying between 26% and 84% at 2-year follow-up (see Gentile et al. 2017). As the disorder continues, so too do social and family relationship problems. Scharkow et al. (2014), for example, found that the adolescents in their sample who remained addicted to gaming, experienced increased levels of depression and aggressive tendencies, and worsening academic performance and relationships with their parents.

Aetiology of gaming disorder

It should come as no surprise that vulnerable individuals experience some degree of compulsion or addiction related to game playing. Games are designed to provide an enjoyable way of spending time socializing with friends and distancing from daily concerns. Their design is deliberately engineered to provide a 'flow' (Csikszentmihalyi 1990) within an alternative world in which participants can gain a sense of control and lose sense of time and place, and they produce a neurological response involving increased dopaminergic activation of the reward network combined with reduced activity within the executive control system (Dong et al. 2015). Genetic analysis of gaming disorder is still in its infancy. However, it is already showing some surprising results. Park et al. (2018), for example, found no relationship with the genes controlling dopamine metabolism, as with other addictions, but did find a relationship with a gene allele involved in the stress response: the Corticotropin-Releasing Hormone Receptor 1.

Psychosocial risk factors for gaming disorder have not been explored in detail, but high levels of impulsivity and low social competence have been implicated (see Gentile et al. 2017). Rho et al. (2017) identified a number of predictors. Some, such as money spent on gaming, may have been manifestations of the disorder. However, a number appear more predictive. The strongest predictor was what they termed 'functional and dysfunctional impulsivity'; others included pursuit of desired appetitive goals, and anxiety. The social aspects of game playing both on- and offline appeared a particularly important predictor, while avoiding negative emotions associated with the 'real world' and gaining mastery and empowerment within the virtual world were also key motivators (Kuss and Griffiths 2012).

Several cognitive processes have also been identified as underpinning the disorder. It may be sustained as a consequence of a number of 'problematic' cognitions combined with behaviours which are maintained or magnified by the behaviour of those affected. King and Delfabbro (2014) consolidated a number of empirical findings to identify four cognitive underpinning dimensions:

- *Beliefs about game reward value and tangibility*: e.g. 'Rewards in video-games are as real to me as anything else in my life', 'I feel an emotional attachment to my avatar'.
- *Maladaptive and inflexible rules about gaming behaviour*: including sunk cost bias (I have invested too much time and effort in this game to leave') and procrastination/prioritization ('I will do other stuff later, I must finish the game now…').

- *Over-reliance on gaming to meet self-esteem needs*: e.g. 'I am good on the internet, but in the real world I am worthless', 'I would be a failure without my gaming', 'I have control over things on the internet'.
- *Gaming as a method of gaining social acceptance*: e.g. 'I can only relate to people in the online game', 'People who do not play video-games do not understand me', 'Other players admire and respect my gaming achievements'.

These may be added to by wider beliefs about the internet including feelings of safety in the online world and feeling unsafe off it.

Treatment of gaming disorder

Well-controlled studies of interventions to treat internet gaming disorder are lacking (King et al. 2017), with those that have been conducted typically foregoing control conditions, having small sample sizes, and other methodological weaknesses. Accordingly, although CBT appears to be of benefit, there is no definitive evidence as yet.

16.6 Chapter summary

1. Drug use is relatively common throughout most social groups, although some groups use more than others do.
2. Excess alcohol consumption results in a number of negative short-term social consequences, including risky or dangerous behaviours, and long-term health consequences, such as cirrhosis and Korsakoff 's syndrome.
3. Genetic factors may influence risk for high levels of alcohol consumption.
4. Alcohol influences mood through its impact on GABA and dopamine.
5. Social factors, including ease of access, peer influence, cost, and advertising, influence alcohol consumption.
6. Psychological explanations of drinking include operant and classical conditioning experiences and cognitions that support consumption.
7. Legal and social interventions impact on drinking levels throughout the population.
8. Treatment of alcohol-dependent individuals usually begins with a period of withdrawal.
9. Drugs such as disulfiram (Antabuse) can help maintain abstinence in highly motivated groups or where its use is compulsory.
10. Both the 12-step model, which advocates abstinence, and cognitive behavioural interventions that can support abstinence or controlled drinking appear equally effective in maintaining abstinence or appropriate drinking habits.
11. Couples therapy is particularly effective for people with drink problems.
12. Opiates exert their action via dopamine levels, endorphins and enkephalins.
13. Harm reduction strategies, including methadone maintenance and needle-exchange schemes, can be successful in reducing opiate use-related harm.
14. As with alcohol, behavioural therapy and social approaches can be effective in the treatment of opiate dependence: couples therapy may be the most effective intervention where appropriate.

15. Gambling results in similar neurochemical changes to those associated with drug use.
16. The biopsychosocial model implicates biological, family, psychological, and learning history factors in the aetiology of problem gambling.
17. Cognitive behavioural therapy, antidepressants, and opiate antagonists may prove effective in reducing gambling-related problems.

16.7 For discussion

1. Why might the various approaches to the treatment of alcohol-related problems differ little in their effectiveness?
2. Switzerland legalized opiate use in 2004. What are the costs and benefits of this approach for the individual and society?
3. Many people receiving treatment for addictions continue to engage in their addiction. Is this an acceptable behaviour within therapy?
4. Should access to gaming machines be controlled?
5. How should society regulate access to triggers to behavioural addictions such as online gambling, poker, and gaming? Or should it avoid legislation and control, allowing a 'free market' of choices?

16.8 Further reading

Chandler, C. and Andrews, A. (2018) *Addiction: A Biopsychosocial Perspective*, London: Sage.

Greenfield, D.N. (2018) Treatment considerations in internet and video game addiction: a qualitative discussion, *Child and Adolescent Psychiatric Clinics of North America*, 27: 327–44.

Nathan, P.E., Conrad, M. and Skinstad, A.H. (2016) History of the concept of addiction, *Annual Review of Clinical Psychology*, 12: 29–51.

Potenza, M.N., Balodis, I.M., Derevensky, J. et al. (2019) Gambling disorder, *Nature Reviews Disease Primers*, 5: 51 [https://doi.org/10.1038/s41572-019-0099-7].

Schüll, N. (2014) *Addiction by Design: Machine Gambling in Las Vegas*, Princeton, NJ: Princeton University Press.

Volkow, N.D., Jones, E.B., Einstein, E.B. et al. (2019) Prevention and treatment of opioid misuse and addiction: a review, *JAMA Psychiatry*, 76: 208–16.

Glossary

A

Aetiology explanations of the causes of disease

Agonist drug that increases the action of a neurotransmitter

Agranulocytosis condition in which the bone marrow fails to produce enough white blood cells called neutrophils. Leaves the individual prone to infection

Alexithymia a paucity of emotional experience and awareness, with an associated poverty of imagination and a tendency to focus upon the tangible and mundane

Alogia poverty of speech; literally, 'no words'

Alzheimer's disease the most common cause of dementia in old age

Antagonist drug that inhibits the action of a neurotransmitter

Anterograde amnesia lack of memory for events that occur after an episode that caused amnesia

Aphonia an inability to speak

Ataxia incoordination and unsteadiness as a result of the brain's failure to regulate posture and strength and direction of limb movement

Avolition lack of volition, or voluntary motivation

B

Behaviour therapy a form of therapy that targets behavioural change by altering the triggers or consequences of behaviour using operant or classical conditioning-based interventions

C

Catatonic behaviour type of behaviour observed in one form of schizophrenia; includes posturing, or 'waxy flexibility', mutism, and stupor

Catharsis reliving past repressed emotions in order to come to terms with past conflicts

Chromosome structures within a cell that contain genes

Classical conditioning the learned association between two co-occurring stimuli, such that a similar response is evoked by either

Client a term often used to denote an individual in therapy. In contrast to words such as patient or subject, it is used to indicate the helping, non-hierarchical nature of the therapeutic relationship between therapist and individual

Clinical supervision discussion and feedback on therapy by peers or experts intended to improve therapeutic formulation and treatment

Cognitive challenge the identification and disputation of maladaptive cognitions

Cognitive schema a consistent set of beliefs that influence mood and behaviour

Community mental health team a multidisciplinary team providing mental healthcare within the community, involving psychiatrists, community psychiatric nurses, psychologists, and other therapists

Confabulate to make up 'facts', usually to hide confusion or poor memory

D

Defence mechanism unconscious mental act that prevents the individual from psychological harm

Delusion a strongly held inappropriate belief; usually a belief that is normally considered impossible

Depot injection the injection of a slow-release drug that will provide a therapeutic dose for days or weeks

Disorganized symptoms (of schizophrenia) include confused thinking and speech and behaviour that does not make sense

DSM – the *Diagnostic and Statistical Manual* (now in its fifth edition, DSM-5: APA 2013) – US system of classification of mental health disorders

Dysphoric unhappy, but not sufficiently so to warrant a diagnosis of depression

Dizygotic (DZ) twins non-identical twins

E

Effect size provides a measure of the effect of an intervention; an effect size of 0.2 is considered a small effect, above 0.6 a large effect, and in between a moderate effect

Ego according to Freud, the part of the personality that operates under the reality principle and works to maximize gratification within the constraints of the 'real world'

Electroconvulsive therapy (ECT) treatment involving passing a brief electric current through the temporal lobe(s) as a treatment for depression and schizophrenia

Executive function neurological coordination of a number of complex processes, including speech, motor coordination, and behavioural planning

Extrapyramidal symptoms the symptoms that result from low levels of dopamine in the extrapyramidal regions of the brain, often as a result of long-term phenothiazine use. Includes Parkinsonism and tardive dyskinesia

F

Flattened mood lack of emotional response, either positive or negative, to events

G

Glucocorticoid a corticosteroid that has anti-inflammatory and immunosuppressive effects

H

Hallucination the experience of touch, visions or sounds in the absence of external stimuli

Heritability coefficient the degree to which individual differences are the result of genetic factors

Hyperalgesia abnormally increased pain sensation – a lowered pain threshold

Hyperventilation short rapid breaths that lead to low levels of carbon dioxide in the blood and physical sensations that include tingling in the arms, dizziness, and feelings of an inability to breathe

Hysterical disorder physical symptoms in the absence of physical pathology

I

Id according to Freud, the personality component driven by the basic instincts of sex and aggression

Ideas of reference the inappropriate belief that objects, events or people are of personal significance; for example, a person may think that a television programme he is watching is all about him. May reach sufficient intensity to constitute delusions

Incidence the frequency with which new cases of a condition arise within the population

Interpersonal psychotherapy a form of therapy focusing exclusively on changing interpersonal problems that contribute to mental health problems

L

Learned helplessness a belief that one has no control over events; results in a cessation of attempts at control

Lobotomy an early form of psychosurgery

M

Major tranquillizers see phenothiazines.

MAOI (monoamine oxidase inhibitor) a form of antidepressant, whose action is on the norepinephrine system.

Meta-analysis a statistical method of combining the data from several studies using similar measures that allows a more powerful analysis of the effect of the intervention than that provided by a single, relatively small study

Monozygotic (MZ) twins identical twins, with identical genetic structure

N

Narcolepsy a disorder characterized by sudden and uncontrollable, though often brief, attacks of deep sleep

Negative symptoms (of schizophrenia) an absence of activation, including apathy, lack of motivation or poverty of speech

Neologism a newly made-up word

Neuroleptics a broad class of drugs used to treat psychotic condition such as schizophrenia; otherwise known as major tranquillizers or phenothiazines

Neurotransmitter chemical involved in maintaining neuronal activity; transmits information across the synaptic cleft

O

Operant (Skinnerian) conditioning manipulation of behaviour through the use of reinforcement and punishment schedules

P

Perseveration inability to shift from a cognitive set, resulting in inappropriate repetitive behaviour, including speech

Pharmacotherapy treatment with drugs

Phenothiazines major tranquillizers used to treat schizophrenia, of which the best known is chlorpromazine; their action is usually on the dopaminergic system

Placebo an inactive condition (either pharmacological or psychological) against which active treatment trials are often evaluated. These allow the assessment of the general effects of receiving some form of attention or 'treatment'. Differences in outcomes between placebo and active intervention(s) are considered to show the specific effects of the therapy against which the placebo is compared

Polygenic caused by multiple genes

Positive symptoms (of schizophrenia) include hallucinations, delusions, disorganized speech, and positive thought disorder

Prevalence the frequency with which a particular condition is found within the population at any one time

Primary care basic or general healthcare focused on the point at which a patient ideally first seeks assistance from the medical care system

Psychoanalysis there are a number of different psychoanalytic therapies, most of which share a number of therapeutic goals, including gaining insight into the nature of the original trauma and bringing troubling material to consciousness so the individual can cope with it without the use of ego defence mechanisms.

Psychoeducational programme a treatment usually combining elements of education about a problem or means of coping with it with cognitive behavioural strategies of change

Psychomotor movements involving both mental and motor processes

Psychosis includes a number of mental health conditions, such as schizophrenia, each of which has the common symptom of a loss of contact with reality

Psychotherapist a generic term for someone who provides some form of therapy. In this book, it does not denote any particular therapeutic orientation, and may include therapists as diverse as cognitive and psychoanalytic in practice

Psychotic the presence of a mental health condition, such as schizophrenia, of which the main symptom is a loss of contact with reality

Psychotropic medication drugs used to treat mental health problems via their action on neurotransmitters

R

Retrograde amnesia lack of memory for events that occurred before an event that causes amnesia

S

Self-actualization described by the humanists as the experience of fulfilling one's potential for growth

Self-instruction training developed by Meichenbaum, involves the use of coping self-statements at times of stress

SNRIs (serotonin and norepinephrine re-uptake inhibitors) antidepressants thought to inhibit neuronal uptake of serotonin, norepinephrine and dopamine in the central nervous system.

Spillover a failure to separate work and home life, such that each intrudes on the other

SSRIs (selective serotonin re-uptake inhibitors) a form of antidepressant, whose action is on the serotonergic system

Stereotypic behaviours repetitive, non-spontaneous, apparently non-functional behaviours

Stress management a specialist cognitive behavioural intervention focusing on teaching people to cope with stress; includes the usual elements of this approach, such as relaxation, self-instruction, and cognitive challenge

Superego according to Freud, contains the individual's morals and societal values; the psychoanalytical equivalent of the conscience

T

Transference the unconscious transfer of experience from one interpersonal context to another – that is, the reliving of past interpersonal relationships in current situations, including therapies

Tricyclic a form of antidepressant whose action is on the serotonin and norepinephrine systems

V

Ventricle one of a system of four communicating cavities within the brain that are continuous with the central canal of the spinal cord

Vicarious learning learning the outcomes of behaviour or situations from observation of others

W

Waiting list control used in randomized controlled trials, it provides a group whose treatment is delayed, so comparisons can be made between treatment and no-treatment conditions without withholding treatment to some

Bibliography

Abbott, M. (2017) *The Epidemiology and Impact of Gambling Disorder and other Gambling-related Harm*, Geneva: WHO.

Abela, J.R.Z. and D'Alessandro, D.U. (2002) Beck's cognitive theory of depression: the diathesis-stress and causal mediation components, *British Journal of Clinical Psychology*, 41: 111–28.

Abela, J.R.Z. and Seligman, M.E.P. (2000) The hopelessness theory of depression: a test of the diathesis-stress component in the interpersonal and achievement domains, *Cognitive Therapy and Research*, 23: 361–78.

Abiodun, O.A. (1995) Pathways to mental health care in Nigeria, *Psychiatric Services*, 46: 823–26.

Abraham, H.C. (1956) Therapeutic and psychological approach to cases of unconsummated marriage, *British Medical Journal*, 1: 837–39.

Abramson, L.Y., Seligman, M.E. and Teasdale, J.D. (1978) Learned helplessness in humans: critique and reformulation, *Journal of Abnormal Psychology*, 87: 49–74.

Achtyes, E., Simmons, A., Skabeev, A. et al. (2018) Patient preferences concerning the efficacy and side-effect profile of schizophrenia medications: a survey of patients living with schizophrenia, *BMC Psychiatry*, 18: 292 [https://doi.org/10.1186/s12888-018-1856-y].

Ackerman, K.D., Heyman, R., Rabin, B.S. et al. (2002) Stressful life events precede exacerbations of multiple sclerosis, *Psychosomatic Medicine*, 64: 916–20.

Adamec, R., Bartoszyk, G.D. and Burton, P. (2004) Effects of systemic injections of Vilazodone, a selective serotonin reuptake inhibitor and serotonin 1A receptor agonist, on anxiety induced by predator stress in rats, *European Journal of Pharmacology*, 504: 65–77.

Adan, R.A. and Vink, T. (2001) Drug target discovery by pharmacogenetics: mutations in the melanocortin system and eating disorders, *European Neuropsychopharmacology*, 11: 483–90.

Adebowale, T.O. and Ogunlesi, A.O. (1999) Beliefs and knowledge about aetiology of mental illness among Nigerian psychiatric patients and their relatives, *African Journal of Medicine and Medical Science*, 28: 35–41.

Aghighi, A., Grigoryan, V.H. and Delavar, A. (2015) Psychological determinants of erectile dysfunction among middle-aged men, *International Journal of Impotence Research*, 27: 63–68.

Agras, W.S., Walsh, T., Fairburn, C.G. et al. (2000) A multicenter comparison of cognitive behavioral therapy and interpersonal psychotherapy for bulimia nervosa, *Archives of General Psychiatry*, 57: 459–66.

Ahern, J., Galea, S., Resnick, H. et al. (2002) Television images and psychological symptoms after the September 11 terrorist attacks, *Psychiatry*, 65: 289–300.

Ahmad, F., Quinn, T.J., Dawson, J. et al. (2008) A link between lunar phase and medically unexplained stroke symptoms: an unearthly influence?, *Journal of Psychosomatic Research*, 65: 131–33.

Alamy, S., Wei Zhang, Varia, I. et al. (2008) Escitalopram in specific phobia: results of a placebo-controlled pilot trial, *Journal of Psychopharmacology*, 22: 157–61.

Alcock, J., Maley, C.C. and Aktipis, C.A. (2014) Is eating behaviour manipulated by the gastrointestinal microbiota? Evolutionary pressures and potential mechanisms, *Bioessays*, 36: 940–49.

Allen, A., Hadley, S.J., Kaplan, A. et al. (2008) An open-label trial of venlafaxine in body dysmorphic disorder, *CNS Spectrum*, 13: 138–44.

Ali, J.S., Farrell, A.S., Alexander, A.C. et al. (2017) Race differences in depression vulnerability following Hurricane Katrina, *Psychological Trauma: Theory, Research, Practice and Policy*, 9: 317–24.

Amad, A., Thomas, P. and Perez-Rodriguez, M.M. (2015) Borderline personality disorder and oxytocin: review of clinical trials and future directions, *Current Pharmaceutical Design*, 21: 3311–16.

American Psychiatric Association (APA) (1987) *Diagnostic and Statistical Manual of Mental Disorders*, 3rd edition, text revision (DSM-III), Washington, DC: APA.

American Psychiatric Association (APA) (2000) *Diagnostic and Statistical Manual of Mental Disorders*, 4th edition, text revision (DSM-IV-TR), Washington, DC: APA.

American Psychiatric Association (2013) *Diagnostic and Statistical Manual of Mental Disorders*, 5th edition (DSM-5), Arlington, VA: American Psychiatric Publishing.

American Psychological Association (2008) *Report of the Task Force on Gender Identity and Gender Variance*. Washington, DC: American Psychological Association.

Anagnostopoulos, F. and Botse, T. (2016) Exploring the role of neuroticism and insecure attachment in health anxiety, safety-seeking behavior engagement, and medical services utilization: a study based on an extended interpersonal model of health anxiety, *SAGE Open* [https://doi.org/10.1177/2158244016653641].

Anagnostou, E. (2018) Clinical trials in autism spectrum disorder: evidence, challenges and future directions, *Current Opinion in Neurology*, 31: 119–25.

Anderson, A.B., Rosen, N.O., Price, L. et al. (2016) Associations between penetration cognitions, genital pain, and sexual well-being in women with provoked vestibulodynia, *Journal of Sexual Medicine*, 13: 444–52.

Anderson, I.M. (1998) SSRIs versus tricyclic antidepressants in depressed inpatients: a meta-analysis of efficacy and tolerability, *Depression and Anxiety*, 7 (suppl. 1): 11–17.

Anderson, K.E., Eberly, S., Marder, K.S. et al. (2019) The choice not to undergo genetic testing for Huntington disease: results from the PHAROS study, *Clinical Genetics*, 96: 28–34.

Anderson, M.C. and Hanslmayr, S. (2014) Neural mechanisms of motivated forgetting, *Trends in Cognitive Sciences*, 18: 279–92.

Anderson, R.N. and Smith, B.L. (2003) Deaths: leading causes for 2001, *National Vital Statistics Report*, 52: 1–86.

Andrews, B., Brewin, C.R., Rose, S. and Kirk, M.P. (2000) Predicting PTSD symptoms in victims of violent crime: the role of shame, anger, and childhood abuse, *Journal of Abnormal Psychology*, 109: 69–73.

Andrews, G., Stewart, G., Allen, R. et al. (1990) The genetics of six neurotic disorders: a twin study, *Journal of Affective Disorders*, 19: 23–29.

Anstey, K.J., Ashby-Mitchell, K. and Peters, R. (2017) Updating the evidence on the association between serum cholesterol and risk of late-life dementia: review and meta-analysis, *Journal of Alzheimer's Disease*, 56: 215–28.

Aouizerate, B., Pujol, H., Grabot, D. et al. (2003) Body dysmorphic disorder in a sample of cosmetic surgery applicants, *European Psychiatry*, 18: 365–68.

Apfel, B.A., Ross, J., Hlavin, J. et al. (2011) Hippocampal volume differences in Gulf War veterans with current versus lifetime posttraumatic stress disorder symptoms, *Biological Psychiatry*, 69: 541–48.

Appiah-Poku, J., Laugharne, R., Mensah, E. et al. (2004) Previous help sought by patients presenting to mental health services in Kumasi, Ghana, *Social Psychiatry and Psychiatric Epidemiology*, 39: 208–11.

Aragona, M., Onesti, E., Tomassini, V. et al. (2009) Psychopathological and cognitive effects of therapeutic cannabinoids in multiple sclerosis: a double-blind, placebo controlled, crossover study, *Clinical Neuropharmacology*, 32: 41–47.

Arcelus, J., Mitchell, A.J., Wales, J. et al. (2011) Mortality rates in patients with anorexia nervosa and other eating disorders: a meta-analysis of 36 studies, *Archives of General Psychiatry*, 68: 724–31.

Arch, J., Eifert, G.H., Davies, C. et al. (2012) Randomized clinical trial of cognitive behavioral therapy (CBT) versus acceptance and commitment therapy (ACT) for mixed anxiety disorders, *Journal of Consulting and Clinical Psychology*, 80: 750–65.

Arie, M., Apter, A., Orbach, I. et al. (2008) Autobiographical memory, interpersonal problem solving, and suicidal behavior in adolescent inpatients, *Comprehensive Psychiatry*, 49: 22–29.

Arntz, A., Klokman, J. and Sieswerda, S. (2005) An experimental test of the schema mode model of borderline personality disorder, *Journal of Behavior Therapy and Experimental Psychiatry*, 36: 226–39.

Ashok, A., Marques, T., Jauhar, S. et al. (2017) The dopamine hypothesis of bipolar affective disorder: the state of the art and implications for treatment, *Molecular Psychiatry*, 22: 666–79.

Ataoglu, A., Ozcetin, A., Icmeli, C. et al. (2003) Paradoxical therapy in conversion reaction, *Journal of Korean Medical Science*, 18: 581–84.

Attia, E. and Schroeder, L. (2005) Pharmacologic treatment of anorexia nervosa: where do we go from here?, *International Journal of Eating Disorders*, 37 (suppl.): S60–S63.

Aubry, T., Bourque, J., Goering, P. et al. (2019) A randomized controlled trial of the effectiveness of Housing First in a small Canadian city, *BMC Public Health*, 19: 1154 [https://doi.org/10.1186/s12889-019-7492-8].

Austen, B., Christodoulou, G. and Terry, J.E. (2002) Relation between cholesterol levels, statins and Alzheimer's disease in the human population, *Journal of Nutrition, Health and Aging*, 6: 377–82.

Avants, S.K., Margolin, A. and McKee, S. (1999) A path analysis of cognitive, affective, and behavioral predictors of treatment response in a methadone maintenance program, *Journal of Substance Abuse*, 11: 215–30.

Awad, A.D. and Vorungati, L.N. (1999) Quality of life and new antipsychotics in schizophrenia: are patients better off?, *International Journal of Social Psychiatry*, 45: 268–75.

Bacaltchuk, J., Hay, P. and Trefiglio, R. (2001) Antidepressants versus psychological treatments and their combination for bulimia nervosa, *Cochrane Database of Systematic Reviews*, 4: CD003385 [https://doi.org/10.1002/14651858.CD003385].

Bach, L.J. and David, A.S. (2006) Self-awareness after acquired and traumatic brain injury, *Neuropsychological Rehabilitation*, 16: 397–414.

Bachmann, K., Lam, A.P., Sörös, P. et al. (2018) Effects of mindfulness and psychoeducation on working memory in adult ADHD: a randomised, controlled fMRI study, *Behaviour Research and Therapy*, 106: 47–56.

Backer-Fulghum, L.M., Patock-Peckham, J.A., King, K.M. et al. (2012) The stress-response dampening hypothesis: how self-esteem and stress act as mechanisms between negative parental bonds and alcohol-related problems in emerging adulthood, *Addictive Behaviors*, 37: 477–84.

Baio, J., Wiggins, L., Christensen, D.L. et al. (2018) Prevalence of autism spectrum disorder among children aged 8 years – Autism and Developmental Disabilities Monitoring Network, 11 sites, United States, 2014, *MMWR Surveillance Summary*, 67 (6): 1–23 [https://www.cdc.gov/mmwr/volumes/67/ss/ss6706a1.htm].

Bancroft, J. (1999) Central inhibition of sexual response in the male: a theoretical perspective, *Neuroscience Biobehavioral Review*, 23: 763–84.

Bandelow, B., Krause, J., Wedekind, D. et al. (2005) Early traumatic life events, parental attitudes, family history, and birth risk factors in patients with borderline personality disorder and healthy controls, *Psychiatry Research*, 134: 169–79.

Bandelow, B., Späth, C., Tichauer, G.A. et al. (2002) Early traumatic life events, parental attitudes, family history, and birth risk factors in patients with panic disorder, *Comprehensive Psychiatry*, 43: 269–78.

Bandura, A. (1977) *Social Learning Theory*, Englewood Cliffs, NJ: Prentice-Hall.

Bandura, A. (1982) Self-efficacy mechanism in human agency, *American Psychologist*, 37: 122–47.

Bandura, A. (1999) A social cognitive theory of personality, in L. Pervin and O. John (eds.) *Handbook of Personality: Theory and Research*, 2nd edition, New York: Guilford Press.

Banerjee, T. and Banerjee, G. (1995) Determinants of help-seeking behaviour in cases of epilepsy attending a teaching hospital in India: an indigenous explanatory model, *International Journal of Social Psychiatry*, 41: 217–30.

Barbaree, H.E. (1990) Stimulus control of sexual arousal, in W.L. Marshall, D.R. Laws and H.E. Barbaree (eds.) *Handbook of Sexual Assault: Issues, Theories, and Treatment of the Offender*, New York: Plenum Press.

Barbaree, H.E. and Marshall, W.L. (1989) Erectile responses among heterosexual child molesters, father-daughter incest offenders and matched nonoffenders: five distinct age preference profiles, *Canadian Journal of Behavioural Science*, 21: 70–82.

Barbui, C., Hotopf, M., Freemantle, N. et al. (2000) Selective serotonin reuptake inhibitors versus tricyclic and heterocyclic antidepressants: comparison of drug adherence, *Cochrane Database of Systematic Reviews*, 4: CD002791 [https://doi.org/10.1002/14651858.CD002791].

Barkley, R.A. (1997) Behavioral inhibition, sustained attention and executive functions: constructing a unifying theory of ADHD, *Psychological Bulletin*, 121: 65–94.

Barkley, R.A., Edwards, G., Laneri, M. et al. (2001) The efficacy of problem solving communication training alone, behavior management training alone, and their combination for parent-adolescent conflict in teenagers with ADHD and ODD, *Journal of Consulting and Clinical Psychology*, 69: 926–41.

Barloon, T.J. and Noyes, R. (1997) Charles Darwin and panic disorder, *Journal of the American Medical Association*, 277: 138–41.

Barnes, A. (2008) Race and hospital diagnoses of schizophrenia and mood disorders, *Social Work*, 53: 77–83.

Barsky, A.J. and Ahern, D.K. (2004) Cognitive behavior therapy for hypochondriasis: a randomized controlled trial, *Journal of the American Medical Association*, 291: 1464–70.

Barsky, A.J., Ahern, D.K., Bailey, E.D. et al. (2001) Hypochondriacal patients' appraisal of health and physical risks, *American Journal of Psychiatry*, 158: 783–87.

Barth, J., Munder, T., Gerger, H. et al. (2013) Comparative efficacy of seven psychotherapeutic interventions for patients with depression, *PLoS: Medicine*, 10: e1001454 [https://doi.org/10.1371/journal.pmed.1001454].

Barton, G.R., Hodgekins, J., Mugford, M. et al. (2009) Cognitive behaviour therapy for improving social recovery in psychosis: cost-effectiveness analysis, *Schizophrenia Research*, 112: 158–63.

Barton, K.R., Yazdani, A., Ayer, N. et al. (2017) The effect of losses disguised as wins and near misses in electronic gaming machines: a systematic review, *Journal of Gambling Studies*, 33: 1241–60.

Bass, C. and Murphy, M. (1995) Somatoform and personality disorders: syndromal comorbidity and overlapping developmental pathways, *Journal of Psychosomatic Research*, 39: 405–27.

Bass, E. and Davis, L. (1988) *The Courage to Heal: A Guide for Women Survivors of Sexual Abuse*, New York: Harper & Row.

Basso, M.R., Nasrallah, H.A., Olson, S.C. et al. (1998) Neuropsychological correlates of negative, disorganized and psychotic symptoms in schizophrenia, *Schizophrenia Research*, 25: 99–111.

Batelaan, N.M., Van Balkom, A.J.L.M. and Stein, D.J. (2012) Evidence-based pharmacotherapy of panic disorder: an update, *International Journal of Neuropsychopharmacology*, 15: 403–15.

Bateson, G., Jackson, D.D., Haley, J. et al. (1956) Toward a theory of schizophrenia, *Behavioral Science*, 1: 251–64.

Batinić, B., Trajković, G., Duisin, D. et al. (2009) Life events and social support in a 1-year preceding panic disorder, *Psychiatria Danubina*, 21: 33–40.

Bauer, P.J. (2006) *Remembering the Time of Our Lives: Memory in Infancy and Beyond*, Mahwah, NJ: Erlbaum.

Baxter, A.J., Scott, K.M., Ferrari, A.J. et al. (2014) Challenging the myth of an 'epidemic' of common mental disorders: trends in the global prevalence of anxiety and depression between 1990 and 2010, *Depression and Anxiety*, 31: 506–16.

Bazargan-Hejazi, S., Bing, E., Bazargan, M. et al. (2005) Evaluation of a brief intervention in an innercity emergency department, *Annals of Emergency Medicine*, 46: 67–76.

Bechard, M., VanderLaan, D.P., Wood, H. et al. (2017) Psychosocial and psychological vulnerability in adolescents with gender dysphoria: a 'proof of principle' study, *Journal of Sex and Marital Therapy*, 43: 678–88.

Beck, A.T. (1976) Cognitive Therapy of Depression, in *Cognitive Therapy and the Emotional Disorders*, New York: Meridian.

Beck, A.T. (1997) Cognitive therapy: reflections, in J.K. Zeig (ed.) *The Evolution of Psychotherapy: The Third Conference*, New York: Brunner/Mazel.

Beck, A.T. (2008) The evolution of the cognitive model of depression and its neurobiological correlates, *American Journal of Psychiatry*, 165: 969–77.

Beck, A.T., Davis, D.D. and Freeman, A. (eds.) (2016) *Cognitive Therapy of Personality Disorders: A Guide for Clinicians*, New York: Guilford Press.

Beck, A.T., Freeman, A. and Associates (1990) *Cognitive Therapy of Personality Disorders*, New York: Guilford Press.

Beck, A.T., Rush, A.J., Shaw, B.F. and Emery, G. (1979) *Cognitive Therapy of Depression*, New York: Guilford Press.

Beck, A.T., Steer, R.A., Ball, R. et al. (1996) Comparison of Beck Depression Inventories – IA and – II in psychiatric outpatients, *Journal of Personality Assessment*, 67: 588–97.

Beck, A.T., Wright, F.D., Newman, C.F. et al. (2001) *Cognitive Therapy of Substance Abuse*, New York: Guilford Press.

Behrendt, S., Wittchen, H.-U., Hofler, M. et al. (2008) Risk and speed of transitions to first alcohol dependence symptoms in adolescents: a 10-year longitudinal community study in Germany, *Addiction*, 103: 1638–47.

Beidel, D.C. and Turner, S.M. (1986) A critique of the theoretical bases of cognitive-behavioral theories and therapy, *Clinical Psychology Review*, 6: 177–97.

Belbasis, L., Köhler, C.A., Stefanis, N. et al. (2018) Risk factors and peripheral biomarkers for schizophrenia spectrum disorders: an umbrella review of meta-analyses, *Acta Psychiatrica Scandinavica*, 137: 88–97.

Bell, K.R., Temkin, N.R. and Esselman, P.C. (2005) The effect of a scheduled telephone intervention on outcome after moderate to severe traumatic brain injury: a randomized trial, *Archives of Physical Medicine and Rehabilitation*, 86: 851–56.

Benbadis, S.R. and Allen Hauser, W. (2000) An estimate of the prevalence of psychogenic nonepileptic seizures, *Seizure*, 9: 280–81.

Benedict, R.H., Morrow, S.A., Weinstock Guttman, B. et al. (2010) Cognitive reserve moderates decline in information processing speed in multiple sclerosis patients, *Journal of the International Neuropsychological Society*, 16: 829–35.

Bennett, P., Conway, M. and Clatworthy, J. (2001a) Predicting post-traumatic symptoms in cardiac patients, *Heart and Lung*, 30: 458–65.

Bennett, P., Hunter, R., Johnston, S. et al. (2020) Covid-19: recording their stories provides emotional benefit to healthcare workers, *British Medical Journal*, 369: m2536 [https://doi.org/10.1136/bmj.m2536].

Bennett, P., Lowe, R. and Honey, K. (2002) Appraisals and emotions: a test of the consistency of reporting and their associations, *Cognition and Emotion*, 17: 511–20.

Bennett, P., Parsons, E., Brain, K. et al. (2010) Long-term cohort study of women at intermediate risk of familial breast cancer: experiences of living at risk, *Psycho-Oncology*, 19: 390–98.

Bennett, P., Williams, Y., Page, N. et al. (2001b) Associations between organizational and incident factors and emotional distress in emergency ambulance personnel, *British Journal of Clinical Psychology*, 12: 215–26.

Bennett, P., Williams, Y., Page, N. et al. (2004) Levels of mental health problems among UK emergency ambulance workers, *Emergency Medicine Journal*, 21: 235–36.

Bentall, R.P. (1993) Deconstructing the concept of 'schizophrenia', *Journal of Mental Health*, 2: 223–38.

Bentall, R.P., Corcoran, R., Howard, R. et al. (2001) Persecutory delusions: a review and theoretical integration, *Clinical Psychology Review*, 21: 1143–92.

Bentall, R.P. and Fernyhough, C. (2008) Social predictors of psychotic experiences: specificity and psychological mechanisms, *Schizophrenia Bulletin*, 34: 1012–20.

Beswick, T., Best, D., Rees, S. et al. (2001) Multiple drug use: patterns and practices of heroin and crack use in a population of opiate addicts in treatment, *Drug and Alcohol Review*, 20: 201–4.

Bettelheim, B. (1967) *The Empty Fortress*, New York: Free Press.

Bettelheim, B. (1973) Bringing up children, *Ladies Home Journal*, 90: 28.

Biederman, J., Petty, C., Faraone, S.V. et al. (2005) Childhood antecedents to panic disorder in referred and nonreferred adults, *Journal of Child and Adolescent Psychopharmacology*, 15: 549–61.

Bighelli, I., Castellazzi, M., Cipriani, A. et al. (2018) Antidepressants versus placebo for panic disorder in adults, *Cochrane Database of Systematic Reviews*, 4: CD010676 [https://doi.org/10.1002/14651858.CD010676.pub2].

Birbaumer, N., Veit, R., Lotze, M. et al. (2005) Deficient fear conditioning in psychopathy: a functional magnetic resonance imaging study, *Archives of General Psychiatry*, 62: 799–805.

Birks, J. (2006) Cholinesterase inhibitors for Alzheimer's disease, *Cochrane Database of Systematic Reviews*, 1: CD005593 [https://doi.org/10.1002/14651858.CD005593].

Birks, J.S. and Harvey, R.J. (2018) Donepezil for dementia due to Alzheimer's disease, *Cochrane Database of Systematic Reviews*, 6: CD001190 [https://doi.org/10.1002/14651858.CD001190.pub3].

Bishop, S.R., Lau, M., Shapiro, S. et al. (2004) Mindfulness: a proposed operational definition, *Clinical Psychology Science and Practice*, 11: 230–41.

Bissada, H., Tasca, G.A., Barber, A.M. et al. (2008) Olanzapine in the treatment of low body weight and obsessive thinking in women with anorexia nervosa: a randomized, double-blind, placebo-controlled trial, *American Journal of Psychiatry*, 165: 1281–88.

Bisson, J.I., Roberts, N.P., Andrew, M. et al. (2013) Psychological therapies for chronic post-traumatic stress disorder (PTSD) in adults, *Cochrane Database of Systematic Reviews*, 12: CD003388 [https://doi.org/10.1002/14651858.CD003388.pub4].

Bjornstad, G. and Montgomery, P. (2005) Family therapy for attention-deficit disorder or attention-deficit/hyperactivity disorder in children and adolescents, *Cochrane Database of Systematic Reviews*, 2: CD005042 [https://doi.org/10.1002/14651858.CD005042.pub2].

Black, D.W., Noyes, R., Jr., Goldstein, R.B. et al. (1992) A family study of obsessive-compulsive disorder, *Archives of General Psychiatry*, 49: 362–68.

Blanchard, R. (2010) The DSM diagnostic criteria for transvestic fetishism, *Archives of Sexual Behavior*, 39: 363–72.

Blaszczynski, A. (1995) Criminal offences in pathological gamblers, *Psychiatry, Psychology and Law*, 1: 129–38.

Blazer, D.G. and Wu, L.T. (2009) The epidemiology of substance use and disorders among middle aged and elderly community adults: national survey on drug use and health, *American Journal of Geriatric Psychiatry*, 17: 237–45.

Bleathman, C. and Morton, I. (1992) Validation therapy: extracts from 20 groups with dementia sufferers, *Journal of Advanced Nursing*, 17: 658–66.

Bleich-Cohen, M., Strous, R.D., Even, R. et al. (2009) Diminished neural sensitivity to irregular facial expression in first-episode schizophrenia, *Human Brain Mapping*, 30: 2606–16.

Bleuler, E. (1908) Die Prognose der Dementia praecox–Schizophreniegruppe, *Präger Medizinische Wochenschrift*, 16: 321–25.

Bloomfield, K., Grittner, U., Kramer, S. et al. (2006) Social inequalities in alcohol consumption and alcohol-related problems in the study countries of the EU concerted action 'Gender, Culture and Alcohol Problems: a Multi-national Study', *Alcohol and Alcoholism*, 41: i26–i36.

Blum, N., St. John, D., Pfohl, S. et al. (2008) Systems Training for Emotional Predictability and Problem Solving (STEPPS) for outpatients with borderline personality disorder: a randomized controlled trial and 1-year follow-up, *American Journal of Psychiatry*, 165: 468–78.

Bo, H.-X., Yang, Y. and Wang, Y. (2020) Posttraumatic stress symptoms and attitude toward crisis mental health services among clinically stable patients with COVID-19 in China, *Psychological Medicine* [https://doi.org/10.1017/S0033291720000999].

Bobashev, G., Tebbe, K., Peiper, N. et al. (2018) Polydrug use among heroin users in Cleveland, OH, *Drug and Alcohol Dependence*, 192: 80–87.

Boeschoten, R.E., Braamse, A.M.J., Beekman, A.T.F. et al. (2017) Prevalence of depression and anxiety in multiple sclerosis: a systematic review and meta-analysis, *Journal of the Neurological Sciences*, 372: 331–41.

Bogaerts, S., Vanheule, S. and Declerq, F. (2005) Recalled parental bonding, adult attachment style, and personality disorders in child molesters: a comparative study, *Journal of Forensic Psychiatry and Psychology*, 16: 445–58.

Boileau, I., Dagher, A., Leyton, M. et al. (2006) Modeling sensitization to stimulants in humans: an [11C]raclopride/positron emission tomography study in healthy men, *Archives of General Psychiatry*, 63: 1386–95.

Bonanno, R.A. and Hymel, S. (2013) Cyber bullying and internalizing difficulties: above and beyond the impact of traditional forms of bullying, *Journal of Youth and Adolescence*, 42: 685–97.

Borduin, C.M. (1999) Multisystemic treatment of criminality and violence in adolescents, *Journal of Consulting and Clinical Psychology*, 63: 569–78.

Borduin, C.M., Mann, B.J., Cone, L.T. et al. (1995) Multisystemic treatment of serious juvenile offenders: long-term prevention of criminality and violence, *Journal of Consulting and Clinical Psychology*, 63: 569–78.

Borges, G., Bagge, C.L., Cherpitel, C.J. et al. (2017) A meta-analysis of acute use of alcohol and the risk of suicide attempt, *Psychological Medicine*, 47: 949–57.

Bostock, S., Crosswell, A.D., Prather, A.A. et al. (2019) Mindfulness on-the-go: effects of a mindfulness meditation app on work stress and well-being, *Journal of Occupational Health Psychology*, 21: 127–38.

Boothby, L.A. and Doering, P.L. (2005) Acamprosate for the treatment of alcohol dependence, *Clinical Therapeutics*, 27: 695–714.

Bradbury, C.L., Christensen, B.K., Lau, M.A. et al. (2008) The efficacy of cognitive behavior therapy in the treatment of emotional distress after acquired brain injury, *Archives of Physical Medicine and Rehabilitation*, 89: S61–S68.

Bradshaw, J., Koegel, L.K. and Koegel, R.L. (2017) Improving functional language and social motivation with a parent-mediated intervention for toddlers with autism spectrum disorder, *Journal of Autism and Developmental Disorders*, 47: 2443–58.

Brand, B.L., Sar, V., Stavropoulos, P. et al. C. (2016) Separating fact from fiction: an empirical examination of six myths about dissociative identity disorder, *Harvard Review of Psychiatry*, 24: 257–70.

Brenneis, C.B. (2000) Evaluating the evidence: can we find authenticated recovered memory?, *Journal of the American Psychoanalytical Association*, 17: 61–77.

Bresin, K. (2019) A meta-analytic review of laboratory studies testing the alcohol stress response dampening hypothesis, *Psychology of Addictive Behaviors*, 33: 581–94.

Breton, J., Legrand, R., Akkerman, K. et al. (2016) Elevated plasma concentrations of bacterial ClpB protein in patients with eating disorders, *International Journal of Eating Disorders*, 49: 805–8.

Brewer, C., Streel, E. and Skinner, M. (2017) Supervised disulfiram's superior effectiveness in alcoholism treatment: ethical, methodological, and psychological aspects, *Alcohol and Alcoholism*, 52: 213–19.

Brewin, C.R. (2001) A cognitive neuroscience account of posttraumatic stress disorder and its treatment, *Behaviour Research and Therapy*, 39: 373–93.

Brewin, C.R. and Andrews, B. (1998) Recovered memories of trauma: phenomenology and cognitive mechanisms, *Clinical Psychology Review*, 18: 949–70.

Brewin, C.R. and Andrews, B. (2017) Creating memories for false autobiographical events in childhood: a systematic review, *Applied Cognitive Psychology*, 31: 2–23.

Brewis A.A. (2014) Stigma and the perpetuation of obesity, *Social Science and Medicine*, 118: 152–58.

Briggs, R., Kennelly, S.P. and O'Neill, D. (2016) Drug treatments in Alzheimer's disease, *Clinical Medicine (Lond.)*, 13: 247–53.

Briken, P., Hill, A. and Berner, W. (2003) Pharmacotherapy of paraphilias with long-acting agonists of luteinizing hormone-releasing hormone: a systematic review, *Journal of Clinical Psychiatry*, 64: 890–97.

British Psychological Society (BPS) (2001) *Learning Disability: Definitions and Contexts*, Leicester: BPS.

Broadbent, D.E. (1971) *Decision and Stress*, London: Academic Press.

Broft, A., Shingleton, R., Kaufman, J. et al. (2012) Striatal dopamine in bulimia nervosa: a PET imaging study, *International Journal of Eating Disorders*, 45: 648–56.

Bromberger, J.T., Schott, L.L., Matthews, K.A. et al. (2017) Childhood socioeconomic circumstances and depressive symptom burden across 15 years of follow-up during midlife: study of Women's Health Across the Nation (SWAN), *Archives of Women's Mental Health*, 20: 495–504.

Bronisch, T. and Wittchen, H.U. (1994) Suicidal ideation and suicide attempts: comorbidity with depression, anxiety disorders, and substance abuse disorder, *European Archives of Psychiatry and Clinical Neuroscience*, 244: 93–98.

Brønnum-Hansen, H., Stenager, E., Nylev Stenager, E. et al. (2005) Suicide among Danes with multiple sclerosis, *Journal of Neurology, Neurosurgery, and Psychiatry*, 76: 1457–59.

Brooks, S.K., Webster, R.K., Smith, L.E. et al. (2020) The psychological impact of quarantine and how to reduce it: rapid review of the evidence, *Lancet*, 395: 912–20.

Brown, A.S. and Derkits, E.J. (2010) Prenatal infection and schizophrenia: a review of epidemiologic and translational studies, *American Journal of Psychiatry*, 167: 261–80.

Brown, G.W., Birley, J.L.T. and Wing, J.K. (1972) The influence of family life on the course of schizophrenic disorders: a relocation, *British Journal of Psychiatry*, 121: 241–58.

Brown, R.F., Tennant, C.C., Sharrock, M. et al. (2006) Relationship between stress and relapse in multiple sclerosis: Part II. Direct and indirect relationships, *Multiple Sclerosis*, 12: 465–75.

Bruch, H. (1982) Anorexia nervosa: therapy and theory, *American Journal of Psychiatry*, 139: 1531–38.

Brüne, M. (2016) On the role of oxytocin in borderline personality disorder, *British Journal of Clinical Psychology*, 55: 287–304.

Brüne, M., Ozgürdal, S., Ansorge, N. et al. (2011) An fMRI study of 'theory of mind' in at-risk states of psychosis: comparison with manifest schizophrenia and healthy controls, *Neuroimage*, 55: 329–37.

Brunoni, A.R., Valiengo, L., Baccaro, A. et al. (2013) The sertraline vs. electrical current therapy for treating depression clinical study: results from a factorial, randomized, controlled trial, *Journal of the American Medical Association Psychiatry*, 70: 383–91.

Bucci, W. (1997) Symptoms and symbols: a multiple code theory of somatization, *Psychoanalytic Enquiry*, 2: 151–72.

Buckley, S., Bird, G., Sacks, B. et al. (2007) Mainstream or special education for teenagers with Down syndrome, in J.-A. Rondal and A. Rasore-Quartino (eds.) *Therapies and Rehabilitation in Down Syndrome*, Chichester: Wiley.

Buhlmann, U., Cook, L.M., Fama, J.M. et al. (2007) Perceived teasing experiences in body dysmorphic disorder, *Body Image*, 4: 381–85.

Buhlmann, U., Etcoff, N.L. and Wilhelm, S. (2006) Emotion recognition bias for contempt and anger in body dysmorphic disorder, *Journal of Psychiatric Research*, 40: 105–11.

Bulik, C.M., Blake, D. and Austin, J. (2019) Genetics of eating disorders: what the clinician needs to know, *Psychiatric Clinics of North America*, 42: 59–73.

Bulik, C.M., Prescott, C.A. and Kendler, K.S. (2001) Features of childhood sexual abuse and the development of psychiatric and substance use disorders, *British Journal of Psychiatry*, 179: 444–49.

Bulloch, A.G. and Patten, S.B. (2010) Non-adherence with psychotropic medications in the general population, *Social Psychiatry and Psychiatric Epidemiology*, 45: 47–56.

Burneo, J.G., Martin, R., Powell, T. et al. (2003) Teddy bears: an observational finding in patients with nonepileptic events, *Neurology*, 61: 714–15.

Burt, S.A. and Klump, K.L. (2014) Prosocial peer affiliation suppresses genetic influences on non-aggressive antisocial behaviors during childhood, *Psychological Medicine*, 44: 821–30.

Byeon, H. (2019) Developing a random forest classifier for predicting the depression and managing the health of caregivers supporting patients with Alzheimer's disease, *Technology and Health Care*, 27: 531–44.

Byerly, M.J., Fisher, R., Carmody, T. et al. (2005) A trial of compliance therapy in outpatients with schizophrenia or schizoaffective disorder, *Journal of Clinical Psychiatry*, 66: 997–1001.

Cadoret, R.J., Yates, G.A., Geyer, M.A. et al. (1995) Adoption study demonstrating two genetic pathways to drug abuse, *Archives of General Psychiatry*, 52: 45–52.

Calati, R. and Courtet, P. (2016) Is psychotherapy effective for reducing suicide attempt and non-suicidal self-injury rates? Meta-analysis and meta-regression of literature data, *Journal of Psychiatric Research*, 79: 8–20.

Calhoun, L.G. and Tedeschi, R.G. (1999) *Facilitating Posttraumatic Growth: A Clinician's Guide*, Mahwah, NJ: Erlbaum.

Campbell, M., Anderson, L.T., Small, A.M. et al. (1993) Naltrexone in autistic children: behavioral symptoms and attentional learning, *Journal of the American Academy of Child and Adolescent Psychiatry*, 32: 1283–91.

Campos, D., Bretón-López, J., Botella, C. et al. (2019) Efficacy of an internet-based exposure treatment for flying phobia (NO-FEAR Airlines) with and without therapist guidance: a randomized controlled trial, *BMC Psychiatry*, 19: 86 [https://doi.org/10.1186/s12888-019-2060-4].

Canivet, C., Bodin, T., Emmelin, M. et al. (2016) Precarious employment is a risk factor for poor mental health in young individuals in Sweden: a cohort study with multiple follow-ups, *BMC Public Health*, 16: 687 [https://doi.org/10.1186/s12889-016-3358-5].

Cannon, M., Moffitt, T.E., Caspi, A. et al. (2006) Neuropsychological performance at the age of 13 years and adult schizophreniform disorder: prospective birth cohort study, *British Journal of Psychiatry*, 189: 463–64.

Cao, J., Wei, J., Fritzsche, K. et al. (2019) Prevalence of DSM-5 somatic symptom disorder in Chinese outpatients from general hospital care, *General Hospital Psychiatry*, 62: 63–71.

Carney, T., Tait, D., Richardson, A. et al. (2008) Why (and when) clinicians compel treatment of anorexia nervosa patients, *European Eating Disorders Review*, 16: 199–206.

Carpenter, J.K., Andrews, L.A., Witcraft, S.M. et al. (2018) Cognitive behavioral therapy for anxiety and related disorders: a meta-analysis of randomized placebo-controlled trials, *Depression and Anxiety*, 35: 502–14.

Carr, A.T. (1974) Compulsive neurosis: a review of the literature, *Psychological Bulletin*, 81: 311–18.

Carrion, C., Folkvord, F., Anastasiadou, D. et al. (2018) Cognitive therapy for dementia patients: a systematic review, *Dementia and Geriatric Cognitive Disorders*, 46: 1–26.

Carter, J.C., McFarlane, T.L., Bewell, C. et al. (2009) Maintenance treatment for anorexia nervosa: a comparison of cognitive behavior therapy and treatment as usual, *International Journal of Eating Disorders*, 42: 202–7.

Cartwright-Hatton, S. and Wells, A. (1997) Beliefs about worry and intrusions: the Meta-Cognitions Questionnaire and its correlates, *Journal of Anxiety Disorders*, 11: 279–96.

Caslini, M., Bartoli, F., Crocamo, C. et al. (2016) Disentangling the association between child abuse and eating disorders: a systematic review and meta-analysis, *Psychosomatic Medicine*, 78: 79–90.

Caspi, A., Moffitt, T.E., Cannon, M. et al. (2005) Moderation of the effect of adolescent-onset cannabis use on adult psychosis by a functional polymorphism in the catechol-O-methyltransferase gene: longitudinal evidence of a gene × environment interaction, *Biological Psychiatry*, 57: 1117–27.

Cecil, C.A., Viding, E., Fearon, P. et al. (2017) Disentangling the mental health impact of childhood abuse and neglect, *Child Abuse and Neglect*, 63: 106–19.

Celada, P., Puig, M.V. and Artigas, F. (2013) Serotonin modulation of cortical neurons and networks, *Frontiers in Integrative Neuroscience*, 7: 25 [https://doi.org/10.3389/fnint.2013.00025].

Center for Behavioral Health Statistics and Quality (CBHSQ) (2018) *2017 National Survey on Drug Use and Health: Detailed Tables*, Rockville, MD: Substance Abuse and Mental Health Services Administration.

Cervenka, M.C., Lesser, R., Tran, T.T. et al. (2013) Does the teddy bear sign predict psychogenic nonepileptic seizures?, *Epilepsy and Behaviour*, 28: 217–20.

Chaix, B., Rosvall, M. and Merlo, J. (2007) Neighborhood socioeconomic deprivation and residential instability: effects on incidence of ischemic heart disease and survival after myocardial infarction, *Epidemiology*, 18: 104–11.

Chan, Y.Y., Lo, W.Y., Yang, S.N. et al. (2015) The benefit of combined acupuncture and antidepressant medication for depression: a systematic review and meta-analysis, *Journal of Affective Disorders*, 176: 106–17.

Chemtob, C., Roitblatt, H., Hamada, J. et al. (1988) A cognitive action theory of posttraumatic stress disorder, *Journal of Anxiety Disorders*, 2: 253–75.

Chen, J.A., Keller, S.M., Zoellner, L.A. et al. (2013) 'How will it help me?' Reasons underlying treatment preferences between sertraline and prolonged exposure in posttraumatic stress disorder, *Journal of Nervous and Mental Disease*, 201: 691–97.

Cherland, E. and Fitzpatrick, R. (1999) Psychotic side effects of psychostimulants: a 5-year review, *Canadian Journal of Psychiatry*, 44: 811–13.

Chew, K.K., Stuckey, B., Bremner, A. et al. (2008) Male erectile dysfunction: its prevalence in Western Australia and associated sociodemographic factors, *Journal of Sexual Medicine*, 5: 60–69.

Chiang, K.J., Tsai, J.C., Liu, D. et al. (2017) Efficacy of cognitive-behavioral therapy in patients with bipolar disorder: a meta-analysis of randomized controlled trials, *PloS One*, 12: e0176849 [https://doi.org/10.1371/journal.pone.0176849].

Chiang, Y.L., Yeh, S.S., Hsiao, C.C. et al. (1999) Treatment of a transvestic fetishist with cognitive-behavioral therapy and supportive psychotherapy: case report, *Changgeng Yi Xue Za Zhi*, 22: 299–312.

Chiaravalloti, N.D., Moore, N.B., Nikelshpur, O.M. et al. (2013) An RCT to treat learning impairment in multiple sclerosis: the MEMREHAB trial, *Neurology*, 81: 2066–72.

Children with ADHD (MTA) Cooperative Group (2018) Late-Onset ADHD reconsidered with comprehensive repeated assessments between ages 10 and 25, *American Journal of Psychiatry*, 175: 140–49.

Chorpita, B.F. and Barlow, D.H. (1998) The development of anxiety: the role of control in the early environment, *Psychological Bulletin*, 124: 3–21.

Chouinard, G. (2004) Issues in the clinical use of benzodiazepines: potency, withdrawal, and rebound, *Journal of Clinical Psychiatry*, 65 (suppl. 5): 7–12.

Christodoulou, C., Melville, P., Scherl, W.F. et al. (2005) Perceived cognitive dysfunction and observed neuropsychological performance: longitudinal relation in persons with multiple sclerosis, *Journal of the International Neuropsychological Society*, 11: 614–19.

Christophersen, A.S. and Gjerde, H. (2014) Prevalence of alcohol and drugs among car and van drivers killed in road accidents in Norway: an overview from 2001 to 2010, *Traffic Injury Prevention*, 15: 523–31.

Chu, C., Tseng, P., Stubbs, B. et al. (2018) Use of statins and the risk of dementia and mild cognitive impairment: a systematic review and meta-analysis, *Science Reports*, 8: 5804 [https://doi.org/10.1038/s41598-018-24248-8].

Chugani, D.C. (2004) Serotonin in autism and pediatric epilepsies, *Mental Retardation and Developmental Disabilities Research Reviews*, 10: 112–16.

Chung, W.C., De Vries, G.J. and Swaab, D.F. (2002) Sexual differentiation of the bed nucleus of the stria terminalis in humans may extend into adulthood, *Journal of Neuroscience*, 22: 1027–33.

Cladder-Micus, M.B., Speckens, A., Vrijsen, J.N. et al. (2018) Mindfulness-based cognitive therapy for patients with chronic, treatment-resistant depression: a pragmatic randomized controlled trial, *Depression and Anxiety*, 35: 914–24.

Clark, D.M. (1986) A cognitive approach to panic disorder, *Behaviour Research and Therapy*, 24: 461–70.

Clark, D.M., Canvin, L., Green, J. et al. (2018) Transparency about the outcomes of mental health services (IAPT approach): an analysis of public data, *Lancet*, 391: 679–86.

Clark, D.M., Salkovskis, P.M., Gelder, M. et al. (1988) Tests of a cognitive model of panic, in I. Hand and U. Wittchen (eds.) *Panic and Phobias*, vol. 2, Berlin: Springer.

Clark, D.M., Salkovskis, P.M., Hackmann, A. et al. (1994) A comparison of cognitive therapy, applied relaxation and imipramine in the treatment of panic disorder, *British Journal of Psychiatry*, 164: 759–69.

Clark, T.C., Lucassen, M.F., Bullen, P. et al. (2014) The health and well-being of transgender high school students: results from the New Zealand adolescent health survey (Youth'12), *Journal of Adolescent Health*, 55: 93–99.

Clarke, D.M., Piterman, L., Byrne, C.J. et al. (2008) Somatic symptoms, hypochondriasis and psychological distress: a study of somatisation in Australian general practice, *Medical Journal of Australia*, 189: 560–64.

Claudino, A.M., Silva de Lima, M., Hay, P.P.J. et al. (2006) Antidepressants for anorexia nervosa, *Cochrane Database of Systematic Reviews*, 1: CD004365 [https://doi.org/10.1002/14651858.CD004365.pub2].

Cleckley, H. (1941) *The Mask of Sanity: An Attempt to Reinterpret the So-Called Psychopathic Personality*, St. Louis, MO: C.V. Mosby.

Clemente, A.S., Diniz, B.S., Nicolato, R. et al. (2015) Bipolar disorder prevalence: a systematic review and meta-analysis of the literature, *Revista Brasileira de Psiquiatria*, 37: 155–61.

Cluxton-Keller, F. and Bruce, M.L. (2018) Clinical effectiveness of family therapeutic interventions in the prevention and treatment of perinatal depression: a systematic review and meta-analysis, *PLoS One*, 13: e0198730 [https://doi.org/10.1371/journal.pone.0198730].

Coelho, H.F., Canter, P.H. and Ernst, E. (2007) Mindfulness-based cognitive therapy: evaluating current evidence and informing future research, *Journal of Consulting and Clinical Psychology*, 75: 1000–5.

Coelho, L.F., Barbosa, D.L., Rizzutti, S. et al. (2015) Use of cognitive behavioral therapy and token economy to alleviate dysfunctional behavior in children with attention-deficit hyperactivity disorder, *Frontiers in Psychiatry*, 6: 167 [https://doi.org/10.3389/fpsyt.2015.00167].

Coffey, M. (1999) Psychosis and medication: strategies for improving adherence, *British Journal of Nursing*, 8: 225–30.

Cohen, L.J., McGeoch, P.G., Gans, S.W. et al. (2002) Childhood sexual history of 20 male pedophiles vs. 24 male healthy control subjects, *Journal of Nervous and Mental Diseases*, 190: 757–66.

Coid, J., Yang, M., Tyrer, P. et al. (2006) Prevalence and correlates of personality disorder in Great Britain, *British Journal of Psychiatry*, 188: 423–31.

Coles, J., Lee, A., Taft, A. et al. (2015) Childhood sexual abuse and its association with adult physical and mental health: results from a national cohort of young Australian women, *Journal of Interpersonal Violence*, 30: 1929–44.

Columb, D. and O'Gara, C. (2018) A national survey of online gambling behaviours, *Irish Journal of Psychological Medicine*, 35: 311–19.

Conner, B.T., Noble, E.P., Berman, S.M. et al. (2005) DRD2 genotypes and substance use in adolescent children of alcoholics, *Drug and Alcohol Dependency*, 79: 379–87.

Conway, K., Compton, W., Stinson, F. et al. (2006) Lifetime comorbidity of DSM-IV mood and anxiety disorders and specific drug use disorder: results from the National Epidemiologic Survey on Alcohol and Related Conditions, *Journal of Clinical Psychiatry*, 67: 247–57.

Coolidge, F.L., Thede, L.L. and Young, S.E. (2002) The heritability of gender identity disorder in a child and adolescent twin sample, *Behavioral Genetics*, 32: 251–57.

Cooney, P., Jackman, C., Coyle, D. et al. (2017) Computerised cognitive-behavioural therapy for adults with intellectual disability: randomised controlled trial, *British Journal of Psychiatry*, 211: 95–102.

Cooper, C., Selwood, A., Blanchard, M. et al. (2009) Abuse of people with dementia by family carers: representative cross sectional survey, *British Medical Journal*, 338: b115 [https://doi.org/10.1136/bmj.b155].

Cornoldi, C., Marzocchi, G.M., Belotti, M. et al. (2001) Working memory interference control deficit in children referred by teachers for ADHD symptoms, *Neuropsychology, Development, and Cognition, section C: Child Neuropsychology*, 7: 230–40.

Cororve, M.B. and Gleaves, D.H. (2001) Body dysmorphic disorder: a review of conceptualizations, assessment, and treatment strategies, *Clinical Psychology Review*, 6: 949–70.

Corrigan, P.W. (1991) Social skills training in adult psychiatric populations: a meta-analysis, *Journal of Behavior Therapy and Experimental Psychiatry*, 22: 203–10.

Costa, P.T. and McCrae, R.R. (1992) The five-factor model of personality and its relevance to personality disorders, *Journal of Personality Disorders*, 6: 343–59.

Costa, R., Dunsford, M., Skagerberg, E. et al. (2015) Psychological support, puberty suppression, and psychosocial functioning in adolescents with gender dysphoria, *Journal of Sexual Medicine*, 12: 2206–14.

Cowlishaw, S., Merkouris, S., Dowling, N. et al. (2012) Psychological therapies for pathological and problem gambling, *Cochrane Database of Systematic Reviews*, 11: CD008937 [https://doi.org/10.1002/14651858.CD008937.pub2].

Cox, A., Rutter, M., Newman, S. et al. (1975) A comparative study of infantile autism and specific developmental language disorders. 2: Parental characteristics, *British Journal of Psychiatry*, 126: 146–59.

Craddock, N. and Jones, I. (1999) Genetics of bipolar disorder, *Journal of Medical Ethics*, 36: 585–94.

Craig, J.S., Hatton, C., Craig, F.B. et al. (2004) Persecutory beliefs, attributions and theory of mind: comparison of patients with paranoid delusions, Asperger's syndrome and healthy controls, *Schizophrenia Research*, 69: 29–33.

Craig, T.K., Bialas, I., Hodson, S. et al. (2004) Intergenerational transmission of somatization behaviour. 2: Observations of joint attention and bids for attention, *Psychological Medicine*, 34: 199–209.

Craig, T.K., Boardman, A.P., Mills, K. et al. (1993) The South London Somatization Study. I: Longitudinal course and the influence of early life experiences, *British Journal of Psychiatry*, 163: 579–88.

Craig, T.K., Cox, A.D. and Klein, K. (2002) Intergenerational transmission of somatization behaviour: a study of chronic somatizers and their children, *Psychological Medicine*, 32: 805–16.

Crawford, L.L., Holloway, K.S. and Domjan, M. (1993) The nature of sexual reinforcement, *Journal of Experimental Analysis of Behaviour*, 60: 55–66.

Creed, E. and Barsky, A. (2004) Systematic review of the epidemiology of somatisation disorder and hypochondriasis, *Journal of Psychosomatic Research*, 56: 391–408.

Crimlisk, H.L., Bhatia, K., Cope, H. et al. (1998) Slater revisited: 6 year follow up study of patients with medically unexplained motor symptoms, *British Medical Journal*, 316: 582–86.

Cristea, I.A., Gentili, C., Cotet, C.D. et al. (2017) Efficacy of psychotherapies for borderline personality disorder: a systematic review and meta-analysis, *JAMA Psychiatry*, 74: 319–28.

Crits-Christoph, P., Newman, M.G., Rickels, K. et al. (2011) Combined medication and cognitive therapy for generalized anxiety disorder, *Journal of Anxiety Disorders*, 25: 1087–94.

Cross, D., Shaw, T., Epstein, M. et al. (2018) Impact of the Friendly Schools whole-school intervention on transition to secondary school and adolescent bullying behavior, *European Journal of Education*, 53: 495–513.

Csikszentmihalyi, M. (1990) *Flow: The Psychology of Optimal Experience*, New York: Harper & Row.

Cui, Y. and Zheng, Y. (2016) A meta-analysis on the efficacy and safety of St. John's wort extract in depression therapy in comparison with selective serotonin reuptake inhibitors in adults, *Neuropsychiatric Disease and Treatment*, 12: 1715–23.

Cuijpers, P., Reijnders, M. and Huibers, M. (2019) The role of common factors in psychotherapy outcomes, *Annual Review of Clinical Psychology*, 15: 207–31.

Cunningham-Williams, R.M., Gattis, M.N., Dore, P.M. et al. (2009) Towards DSM-V: considering other withdrawal-like symptoms of pathological gambling disorder, *International Journal of Methods in Psychiatric Research*, 18: 13–22.

Dabbs, C., Watkins, E.Y., Fink, D.S. et al. (2014) Opiate-related dependence/abuse and PTSD exposure among the active-component U.S. military, 2001 to 2008, *Military Medicine*, 179: 885–90.

Dakanalis, A., Gaudio, S., Serino, S. et al. (2016) Body-image distortion in anorexia nervosa, *Nature Reviews Disease Primers*, 2: 16026 [https://doi.org/10.1038/nrdp.2016.26].

Dalenberg, C.J., Brand, B.L., Gleaves, D.H. et al. (2012) Evaluation of the evidence for the trauma and fantasy models of dissociation, *Psychological Bulletin*, 138: 550–88.

Dalle Grave, R., Calugi, S., Sartirana, M. et al. (2015) Transdiagnostic cognitive behaviour therapy for adolescents with an eating disorder who are not underweight, *Behaviour Research and Therapy*, 73: 79–82.

D'Angiulli, A., Lipina, S.J. and Olesinska, A. (2012) Explicit and implicit issues in the developmental cognitive neuroscience of social inequality, *Frontiers in Human Neuroscience*, 6: 254 [https://doi.org/10.3389/fnhum.2012.00254].

Dargis, M., Newman, J. and Koenigs, M. (2016) Clarifying the link between childhood abuse history and psychopathic traits in adult criminal offenders, *Personality Disorders: Theory, Research, and Treatment*, 7: 221–28.

Daros, A.R., Zakzanis, K.K. and Ruocco, A.C. (2013) Facial emotion recognition in borderline personality disorder, *Psychological Medicine*, 43: 1953–63.

Davey, G.C.L. (1997) A conditioning model of phobias, in G.C.L. Davey (ed.) *Phobias: A Handbook of Theory, Research and Treatment*, Chichester: Wiley.

Davidson, K. (2000) *Cognitive Therapy for Personality Disorders*, Oxford: Butterworth-Heinemann.

Davidson, K.M., Tyrer, P., Tata, P. et al. (2008) Cognitive behaviour therapy for violent men with antisocial personality disorder in the community: an exploratory randomized controlled trial, *Psychological Medicine*, 39: 569–77.

Davies, J. (2013) *Cracked: Why Psychiatry is Doing More Harm than Good*, London: Icon Books.

Davies, M.N., Verdi, S., Burri, A. et al. (2015) Generalised anxiety disorder – a twin study of genetic architecture, genome-wide association and differential gene expression, *PLoS One*, 10: e0134865 [https://doi.org/10.1371/journal.pone.0134865].

Davis, T. E., III, Ollendick, T.H. and Öst, L.-G. (2019) One-session treatment of specific phobias in children: recent developments and a systematic review, *Annual Review of Clinical Psychology*, 15: 233–56.

Davoodi, E., Wen, A., Dobson, K.S. et al. (2018) Early maladaptive schemas in depression and somatization disorder, *Journal of Affective Disorders*, 235: 82–89.

Day, J.C., Bentall, R.P., Roberts, C. et al. (2005) Attitudes toward antipsychotic medication: the impact of clinical variables and relationships with health professionals, *Archives of General Psychiatry*, 62: 717–24.

Dayan, P. and Huys, Q.J.M. (2008) Serotonin, inhibition, and negative mood, *PLoS Computational Biology*, 4: e4 [https://doi.org/10.1371/journal.pcbi.0040004].

Deblinger, E., Pollio, E. and Dorsey, S. (2016) Applying trauma-focused cognitive-behavioral therapy in group format, *Child Maltreatment*, 21: 59–73.

de Brito, A.M., de Almeida Pinto, M.G., Bronstein, G. et al. (2017) Topiramate combined with cognitive restructuring for the treatment of gambling disorder: a two-center, randomized, double-blind clinical trial, *Journal of Gambling Studies*, 33: 249–63.

Decety, J., Chen, C., Harenski, C. et al. (2013) An fMRI study of affective perspective taking in individuals with psychopathy: imagining another in pain does not evoke empathy, *Frontiers in Human Neuroscience*, 7: 489 [https://doi.org/10.3389/fnhum.2013.00489].

DeFife, J.A., Drill, R., Nakash, O. et al. (2010) Agreement between clinician and patient ratings of adaptive functioning and developmental history, *American Journal of Psychiatry*, 167: 1472–78.

de Jonge, P., Wardenaar, K.J., Lim, C. et al. (2018) The cross-national structure of mental disorders: results from the World Mental Health Surveys, *Psychological Medicine*, 48: 2073–84.

De la Fuente, J.M., Goldman, S., Stanus, E. et al. (1997) Brain glucose metabolism in borderline personality disorder, *Journal of Psychiatric Research*, 31: 531–41.

Demicheli, V., Jefferson, T., Rivetti, A. et al. (2005) Vaccines for measles, mumps and rubella in children, *Cochrane Database of Systematic Reviews*, 5: CD004407 [https://doi.org/10.1002/14651858.CD004407.pub2].

Demyttenaere, K., Van Ganse, E., Gregoirre, J. et al. (1998) Compliance in depressed patients treated with fluoxetine or amitriptyline. Belgian Compliance Study Group, *International Clinical Psychopharmacology*, 13: 11–17.

Department for Education (2014) *Special Educational Needs and Disability Code of Practice: 0 to 25 Years*, London: HMSO.

Depue, B.E., Curran, T. and Banich, M.T. (2007) Prefrontal regions orchestrate suppression of emotional memories via a two-phase process, *Science*, 317: 215–19.

DeRubeis, R.J., Gelfand, L.A., Tang, T.Z. et al. (1999) Medications versus cognitive behavior therapy for severely depressed outpatients: mega-analysis of four randomized comparisons, *American Journal of Psychiatry*, 156: 1007–13.

Dettmer, K., Hanna, D., Whetstone, P. et al. (2007) Autism and urinary exogenous neuropeptides: development of an on-line SPE-HPLC-tandem mass spectrometry method to test the opioid excess theory, *Analytical and Bioanalytical Chemistry*, 388: 1643–51.

Deveney, C.M. and Deldin, P.J. (2006) A preliminary investigation of cognitive flexibility for emotional information in major depressive disorder and non-psychiatric controls, *Emotion*, 6: 429–37.

De Venter, M., Van Den Eede, F., Pattyn, T. et al. (2017) Impact of childhood trauma on the course of panic disorder, *European Psychiatry*, 41: S69 [https://doi.org/10.1016/j.eurpsy.2017.01.223].

Dhawan, S. and Marshall, W.L. (1996) Sexual abuse histories of sexual offenders, *Sexual Abuse: A Journal of Research and Treatment*, 8: 7–15.

Dhillon, S., Yang, L.P. and Curran, M.P. (2008) Bupropion: a review of its use in the management of major depressive disorder, *Drugs*, 68: 653–89.

Dias-Amaral, A. and Marques-Pinto, A. (2018) Female genito-pelvic pain/penetration disorder: review of the related factors and overall approach, *Revista Brasileira de Ginecologia e Obstetrícia*, 40: 787–93.

Dickerson, M. and Baron, E. (2000) Contemporary issues and future directions for research into pathological gambling, *Addiction*, 95: 1145–59.

Didie, E.R., Menard, W., Stern, A.P. et al. (2008) Occupational functioning and impairment in adults with body dysmorphic disorder, *Comprehensive Psychiatry*, 49: 561–69.

Didie, E.R., Tortolani, C.C. and Pope, C. (2006) Childhood abuse and neglect in body dysmorphic disorder, *Child Abuse and Neglect*, 30: 1105–15.

di Giacomo, E., Krausz, M., Colmegna, F. et al. (2018) Estimating the risk of attempted suicide among sexual minority youths: a systematic review and meta-analysis, *JAMA Pediatrics*, 172: 1145–52.

Distel, M.A., Trull, T.J., Derom, C.A. et al. (2008) Heritability of borderline personality disorder features is similar across three countries, *Psychological Medicine*, 38: 1219–29.

Docter, R.F. and Prince, V. (1997) Transvestism: a survey of 1032 crossdressers, *Archives of Sexual Behavior*, 26: 589–605.

Dodds, T.J. (2017) Prescribed benzodiazepines and suicide risk: a review of the literature. *Primary Care Companion for CNS Disorders*, 19: 16r02037 [https://doi.org/10.4088/PCC.16r02037].

Dollard, J. and Miller, N.E. (1950) *Personality and Psychotherapy*, New York: McGraw-Hill.

Dong, G., Lin, X., Hu, Y. et al. (2015) Imbalanced functional link between executive control network and reward network explain the online-game seeking behaviors in Internet gaming disorder, *Scientific Reports*, 5: 9197 [https://doi.org/10.1038/srep09197].

Dong, N., Nezgovorova, V., Hong, K. et al. (2019) Pharmacotherapy in body dysmorphic disorder: relapse prevention and novel treatments, *Expert Opinion on Pharmacotherapy*, 20: 1211–19.

Dong, X., Beck, T. and Simon, M.A. (2010) The associations of gender, depression and elder mistreatment in a community-dwelling Chinese population: the modifying effect of social support, *Archives of Gerontology and Geriatrics*, 50: 202–8.

Donohoe, G., Owens, N., O'Donnell, C. et al. (2001) Predictors of compliance with neuroleptic medication among inpatients with schizophrenia: a discriminant function analysis, *European Psychiatry*, 16: 293–98.

Drury, V., Birchwood, M. and Cochrane, R. (2000) Cognitive therapy and recovery from acute psychosis: a controlled trial. 3: Five-year follow-up, *British Journal of Psychiatry*, 177: 8–14.

Dugas, M.J., Marchand, A., Ladouceur, R. et al. (2005) Further validation of a cognitive behavioral model of generalized anxiety disorder: diagnostic and symptom specificity, *Journal of Anxiety Disorders*, 19: 329–43.

Dumais, A., Lesage, A.D., Alda, M. et al. (2005) Risk factors for suicide completion in major depression: a case-control study of impulsive and aggressive behaviors in men, *American Journal of Psychiatry*, 162: 2116–24.

Duncan, G.E., Sheitman, B.B. and Lieberman, J.A. (1999) An integrated view of pathophysiological models of schizophrenia, *Brain Research Reviews*, 29: 250–64.

Duncan, L.E., Ratanatharathorn, A., Aiello, A. et al. (2018) Largest GWAS of PTSD ($N = 20\,070$) yields genetic overlap with schizophrenia and sex differences in heritability, *Molecular Psychiatry*, 23: 666–73.

Duncan, R. and Oto, M. (2008) Predictors of antecedent factors in psychogenic nonepileptic attacks: multivariate analysis, *Neurology*, 71: 1000–5.

Durham, R.C., Murphy, T., Allan, T. et al. (1994) Cognitive therapy, analytic psychotherapy and anxiety management training for generalised anxiety disorder, *British Journal of Psychiatry*, 16: 315–23.

Durkheim, E. ([1897] 1951) *Suicide*, New York: Free Press.

Durwood, L., McLaughlin, K.A. and Olson, K.R. (2017) Mental health and self-worth in socially transitioned transgender youth, *Journal of the American Academy of Child and Adolescent Psychiatry*, 56: 116–23.

Dworkin, E.R., Ullman, S.E., Stappenbeck, C. et al. (2018) Proximal relationships between social support and PTSD symptom severity: a daily diary study of sexual assault survivors, *Depression and Anxiety*, 35: 43–49.

Dyck, M., Habel, U., Slodczyk, J. et al. (2009) Negative bias in fast emotion discrimination in borderline personality disorder, *Psychological Medicine*, 39: 855–64.

Dyrbye, L.N., Shanafelt, T.D., Werner, L. et al. (2017) The impact of a required longitudinal stress management and resilience training course for first-year medical students, *Journal of General Internal Medicine*, 32: 1309–14.

Eamon, M.K. and Mulder, C. (2005) Predicting antisocial behavior among Latino young adolescents: an ecological systems analysis, *American Journal of Orthopsychiatry*, 75: 117–27.

Eastman, C.I., Gallo, L.C., Lahmeyer, H.W. et al. (1993) The circadian rhythm of temperature during light treatment for winter depression, *Biological Psychiatry*, 34: 210–20.

Eaton, W., Bienvenue, O.J. and Miloyan, B. (2018) Specific phobias, *Lancet Psychiatry*, 5: 678–86.

Ebert, A. and Dyck, M.J. (2004) The experience of mental death: the core feature of complex posttraumatic stress disorder, *Clinical Psychology Review*, 24: 617–35.

Eddy, J.M. and Chamberlain, P. (2000) Family management and deviant peer associations as mediators of the impact of treatment condition on youth antisocial behavior, *Journal of Consulting and Clinical Psychology*, 68: 857–63.

Eddy, K.T., Dorer, D.J., Franko, D.L. et al. (2008) Diagnostic crossover in anorexia nervosa and bulimia nervosa: implications for DSM-V, *American Journal of Psychiatry*, 165: 245–50.

Edgerton, J.D., Melnyk, T.S. and Roberts, L.W. (2015) Problem gambling and the youth-to-adulthood transition: assessing problem gambling severity trajectories in a sample of young adults, *Journal of Gambling Studies*, 31: 1463–85.

Effertz, T., Bischof, A., Rumpf, H.J. et al. (2018) The effect of online gambling on gambling problems and resulting economic health costs in Germany, *European Journal of Health Economics*, 19: 967–78.

Egerton, A., Valmaggia, L.R., Howes, O.D. et al. (2016) Adversity in childhood linked to elevated striatal dopamine function in adulthood, *Schizophrenia Research*, 176: 171–76.

Eguchi, H., Tsutsumi, A., Inoue, A. et al. (2018) Association of workplace social capital with psychological distress: results from a longitudinal multilevel analysis of the J-HOPE Study, *BMJ Open*, 8: e022569 [https://doi.org/10.1136/bmjopen-2018-022569].

Ehsan, A., Klaas, H.S., Bastianen, A. et al. (2019) Social capital and health: a systematic review of systematic reviews, *SSM Population Health*, 8: 100425 [https://doi.org/10.1016/j.ssmph.2019.100425].

Eisler, I., Simic, M., Russell, G.F.M. et al. (2007) A randomized controlled trial of two forms of family therapy in adolescent anorexia nervosa: a five-year follow-up, *Journal of Child Psychology and Psychiatry*, 48: 552–60.

Eke, A.W., Helmus, M. and Seto, M.C. (2019) A validation study of the Child Pornography Offender Risk Tool, *Sexual Abuse*, 32: 456–76.

Elkin, I., Shea, T., Watkins, J.T. et al. (1989) National Institute of Mental Health Treatment of Depression Collaborative Research Program: general effectiveness of treatments, *Archives of General Psychiatry*, 46: 971–82.

Elkins, G., Rajab, M.H. and Marcus, J. (2005) Complementary and alternative medicine use by psychiatric inpatients, *Psychological Reports*, 96: 163–66.

Ellery, M., Stewart, S.H. and Loba, P. (2005) Alcohol's effects on video lottery terminal (VLT) play among probable pathological and non-pathological gamblers, *Journal of Gambling Studies*, 21: 299–324.

Ellis, A. (1977) The basic clinical theory of rational-emotive therapy, in A. Ellis and R. Grieger (eds.) *Handbook of Rational-Emotive Therapy*, New York: Springer.

Elzinga, B.M., Phaf, R.H., Ardon, A.M. et al. (2003) Directed forgetting between, but not within, dissociative personality states, *Journal of Abnormal Psychology*, 112: 237–43.

Emerson, E. (1998) Working with people with challenging behaviour, in E. Emerson, C. Hatton, J. Bromley et al. (eds.) *Clinical Psychology and People with Intellectual Disabilities*, Chichester: Wiley.

Emmelkamp, P.M., Benner, A., Kuipers, A. et al. (2006) Comparison of brief dynamic and cognitive-behavioural therapies in avoidant personality disorder, *British Journal of Psychiatry*, 189: 60–64.

Enander J., Andersson E., Mataix-Cols, D. et al. (2016) Therapist guided internet based cognitive behavioural therapy for body dysmorphic disorder: single blind randomised controlled trial, *British Medical Journal*, 352: i241 [https://doi.org/10.1136/bmj.i241].

English, D., Lambert, S.F., Evans, M.K. et al. (2014) Neighborhood racial composition, racial discrimination, and depressive symptoms in African Americans, *American Journal of Community Psychology*, 54: 219–28.

Erikson, E. (1980) *Growth and Crisis of the Healthy Personality: Identity and the Life Cycle*, New York: W.W. Norton.

Escobar, J.I., Gara, M.I., Diaz-Martinez, A.M. et al. (2007) Effectiveness of a time-limited cognitive behavior therapy-type intervention among primary care patients with medically unexplained symptoms, *Annals of Family Medicine*, 5: 328–35.

Essali, A., Al-Haj Haasan, N., Li, C. et al. (2009) Clozapine versus typical neuroleptic medication for schizophrenia, *Cochrane Database of Systematic Reviews*, 1: CD000059 [https://doi.org/10.1002/14651858.CD000059.pub2].

Fagan, P.J., Wise, T.N., Schmidt, C.W., Jr. et al. (2002) Pedophilia, *Journal of the American Medical Association*, 288: 2458–65.

Fahlen, T. (1995) Personality traits in social phobia. II: Changes during drug treatment, *Journal of Clinical Psychiatry*, 56: 569–73.

Fairburn, C.G. (2008) *Cognitive Behaviour Therapy and Eating Disorders*, New York: Guilford Press.

Fairburn, C.G., Cooper, Z. and Shafran, R. (2003) Cognitive behaviour therapy for eating disorders: a 'transdiagnostic' theory and treatment, *Behaviour Research and Therapy*, 41: 509–28.

Fairburn, C.G., Jones, R., Peveler, R.C. et al. (1993) Psychotherapy and bulimia nervosa: the longer-term effects of interpersonal psychotherapy, behaviour therapy and cognitive behaviour therapy, *Archives of General Psychiatry*, 50: 419–28.

Fallon, B.A., Petkova, E., Skritskaya, N. et al. (2008) A double-masked, placebo-controlled study of fluoxetine for hypochondriasis, *Journal of Clinical Psychopharmacology*, 28: 638–45.

Fallon, J. (2014) *The Psychopath Inside: A Neuroscientist's Personal Journey into the Dark Side of the Brain*, New York: Current.

Fallon, P.E., Fallon, E., Harris, B.S. et al. (2014) Prevalence of body dissatisfaction among a United States adult sample, *Eating Behaviors*, 15: 151–58.

Falloon, I.R., Boyd, J.L., McGill, C.W. et al. (1982) Family management in the prevention of exacerbations of schizophrenia: a controlled study, *New England Journal of Medicine*, 306: 1437–40.

Fardouly, J. and Vartanian, L.R. (2015) Negative comparisons about one's appearance mediate the relationship between Facebook usage and body image concerns, *Body Image*, 12: 82–88.

Farrington, D.P., Ttofi, M.M. and Piquero, A.R. (2016) Risk, promotive, and protective factors in youth offending: results from the Cambridge study in delinquent development, *Journal of Criminal Justice*, 45: 63–70.

Favarelli, C., Salvatori, S., Galassi, F. et al. (1997) Epidemiology of somatoform disorders: a community survey in Florence, *Social Psychiatry and Psychiatric Epidemiology*, 32: 24–29.

Feeney, G.F., Connor, J.P., Young, R. et al. (2006) Is acamprosate use in alcohol dependence treatment reflected in improved subjective health status outcomes beyond cognitive behavioural therapy alone?, *Journal of Addictive Diseases*, 25: 49–58.

Feeney, G.F., Young, R.M., Connor, J.P. et al. (2002) Cognitive behavioural therapy combined with the relapse-prevention medication acamprosate: are short-term treatment outcomes for alcohol dependence improved?, *Australian and New Zealand Journal of Psychiatry*, 36: 622–28.

Feil, N. (1990) Validation therapy helps staff reach confused patients, *Nursing*, 16– 33–34.

Feinstein, A., Magalhaes, S., Richard, J. et al. (2014) The link between multiple sclerosis and depression, *Neurology*, 10: 507–17.

Feiring, C., Taska, L. and Lewis, M. (2002) Adjustment following sexual abuse discovery: the role of shame and attributional style, *Developmental Psychology*, 38: 79–92.

Feldman-Summers, S. and Pope, K.S. (1994) The experience of 'forgetting' childhood abuse: a national survey of psychologists, *Journal of Consulting and Clinical Psychology*, 62: 636–39.

Feliu, M., Edwards, C.L., Sudhakar, S. et al. (2008) Neuropsychological effects and attitudes in patients following electroconvulsive therapy, *Neuropsychiatric Diseases and Treatment*, 4: 613–17.

Felner, R.D., Brand, S., Adan, A.M. et al. (1993) Restructuring the ecology of the school as an approach to prevention during school transitions: longitudinal follow-ups and extensions of the School Transitional Environment Project (STEP), *Prevention in Human Services*, 10: 103–9.

Fergusson, D., Doucette, S., Glass, K.C. et al. (2005) Association between suicide attempts and selective serotonin reuptake inhibitors: systematic review of randomised controlled trials, *British Medical Journal*, 330: 396–99.

Ferreira-Vieira, T.H., Guimaraes, I.M., Silva, F.R. et al. (2016) Alzheimer's disease: targeting the cholinergic system, *Current Neuropharmacology*, 14: 101–15.

Fiest, K.M., Roberts, J.I., Maxwell, C.J. et al. (2016) The prevalence and incidence of dementia due to Alzheimer's disease: a systematic review and meta-analysis, *Canadian Journal of Neurological Sciences*, 43: S51–S82.

Fink, P., Hansen, M.S. and Oxhoj, M.-L. (2004) The prevalence of somatoform disorders among internal medical inpatients, *Journal of Psychosomatic Research*, 56: 413–18.

Finkelhor, D. (1984) *Child Sexual Abuse: New Theory and Research*, New York: Free Press.

First, M.B., Williams, J.B., Karg, R.S. et al. (2016) *Structured Clinical Interview for DSM-5 Disorders – Clinician Version SCID-5-CV*, Arlington, VA: American Psychiatric Publishing.

Fisher, C.A., Skocic, S., Rutherford, K.A. et al. (2019) Family therapy approaches for anorexia nervosa, *Cochrane Database of Systematic Reviews*, 5: CD004780 [https://doi.org/10.1002/14651858.CD004780.pub4].

FitzGerald, C. and Hurst, S. (2017) Implicit bias in healthcare professionals: a systematic review, *BMC Medical Ethics*, 18: 19 [https://doi.org/10.1186/s12910-017-0179-8].

Fitzsimons, E., Goodman, A. and Smith, J.P. (2017) Poverty dynamics and parental mental health: determinants of childhood mental health in the UK, *Social Science and Medicine*, 175: 43–51.

Flook, L., Goldberg, S.B., Pinger, L. et al. (2015) Promoting prosocial behavior and self-regulatory skills in preschool children through a mindfulness-based kindness curriculum, *Developmental Psychology*, 51: 44–51.

Foa, E.B. and Kozak, M.J. (1986) Emotional processing of fear: exposure to corrective information, *Psychological Bulletin*, 99: 20–35.

Foreman, M., Hare, L., York, K. et al. (2019) Genetic link between gender dysphoria and sex hormone signaling, *Journal of Clinical Endocrinology and Metabolism*, 104: 390–96.

Forneris, C.A., Nussbaumer-Streit, B., Morgan, L.C. et al. (2019) Psychological therapies for preventing seasonal affective disorder, *Cochrane Database of Systematic Reviews*, 5: CD011270 [https://doi.org/10.1002/14651858.CD011270.pub3].

Fosse, R. and Read, J. (2013) Electroconvulsive treatment: hypotheses about mechanisms of action, *Frontiers in Psychiatry*, 4: 94 [https://doi.org/10.3389/fpsyt.2013.00094].

Frederiksen, K.S., Gjerum, L., Waldemar, G. et al. (2018) Effects of physical exercise on Alzheimer's disease biomarkers: a systematic review of intervention studies, *Journal of Alzheimer's Disease*, 61: 359–72.

Freud, S. (1900) *The Interpretation of Dreams*, New York: Wiley.

Freud, S. (1906) Analysis of a phobia in a five-year-old boy, in *The Standard Edition of the Complete Psychological Works*, vol. 10 (ed. and trans. J. Strachey), London: Hogarth Press.

Freud, S. (1914) On narcissism: an introduction, in *The Standard Edition of the Complete Psychological Works*, vol. 14 (ed. and trans. J. Strachey), London: Hogarth Press.

Freud, S. ([1917] 1957) Mourning and melancholia, in *The Standard Edition of the Complete Psychological Works*, vol. 14 (ed. and trans. J. Strachey), London: Hogarth Press.

Freud, S. ([1920] 1990) *Beyond the Pleasure Principle*, New York: W.W. Norton.

Freud, S. (1922) *Introductory Lectures on Psychoanalysis*, London: George Allen & Unwin.

Freud, S. and Breuer, J. (2004) *Studies in Hysteria* (trans. N. Luckhurst), London: Penguin.

Freyd, J.J. (1996) *Betrayal Trauma: The Logic of Forgetting Childhood Abuse*, Cambridge, MA: Harvard University Press.

Frith, C.D. and Corcoran, R. (1996) Exploring 'theory of mind' in people with schizophrenia, *Psychological Medicine*, 26: 521–30.

Fromm-Reichman, F. (1948) Notes on the development of treatment of schizophrenia by psychoanalytic psychotherapy, *Psychiatry*, 11: 263–73.

Fukunishi, I. (1997) Alexithymic characteristics of bulimia nervosa in diabetes mellitus with end-stage renal disease, *Psychological Reports*, 81: 627–33.

Fulton, B.D., Scheffler, R.M., Hinshaw, S.P. et al. (2009) National variation of ADHD diagnostic prevalence and medication use: health care providers and education policies, *Psychiatric Services*, 60: 1075–83.

Gadsby, S. (2017) Distorted body representations in anorexia nervosa, *Consciousness and Cognition*, 51: 17–33.

Gagné, G.G., Furman, M.J., Carpenter, L.L. et al. (2000) Efficacy of continuation ECT and antidepressant drugs compared to long-term antidepressants alone in depressed patients, *American Journal of Psychiatry*, 157: 1960–69.

Galatzer-Levy, I.R. and Bryant, R.A. (2013) 636,120 ways to have posttraumatic stress disorder, *Perspectives on Psychological Science*, 8: 651–62.

Galea, S., Vlahov, D., Resnick, H. et al. (2003) Trends of probable post-traumatic stress disorder in New York City after the September 11 terrorist attacks, *American Journal of Epidemiology*, 158: 514–24.

Galla, B.M., O'Reilly, G.A., Kitil, M.J. et al. (2015) Community-based mindfulness program for disease prevention and health promotion: targeting stress reduction, *American Journal of Health Promotion*, 30: 36–41.

Gannon, T., Terrier, R. and Leader, T. (2012) Ward and Siegert's Pathways Model of child sexual offending: a cluster analysis evaluation, *Psychology, Crime and Law*, 18: 129–53.

Gannon, T., Ward, T. and Polaschek, D. (2004) Child sexual offenders, in M. Connolly (ed.) *Violence in Society: New Zealand Perspectives*, Christchurch: Te Awatea Press.

Garbazza, C. and Benedetti, F. (2018) Genetic factors affecting seasonality, mood, and the circadian clock, *Frontiers in Endocrinology*, 9: 481 [https://doi.org/10.3389/fendo.2018.00481].

Garcia, R. (2017) Neurobiology of fear and specific phobias, *Learning and Memory*, 24: 462–71.

García-Vega, E., Camero, A., Fernández, M. et al. (2018) Suicidal ideation and suicide attempts in persons with gender dysphoria, *Psicothema*, 30: 283–88.

Garner, D.M. and Bemis, K.M. (1985) Cognitive therapy for anorexia nervosa, in D.M. Garner and P.E. Garfinkel (eds.) *Handbook of Psychotherapy for Anorexia Nervosa and Bulimia*, New York: Guilford Press.

Garrouste-Orgeas, M., Flahault, C., Vinatier, I. et al. (2019) Effect of an ICU diary on posttraumatic stress disorder symptoms among patients receiving mechanical ventilation: a randomized clinical trial, *Journal of the American Medical Association*, 322: 229–39.

Gava, I., Barbui, C., Aguglia, E. et al. (2007) Psychological treatments versus treatment as usual for obsessive compulsive disorder (OCD), *Cochrane Database of Systematic Reviews*, 2: CD005333 [https://doi.org/10.1002/14651858.CD005333.pub2].

Gavrilova, S.I., Ferri, C.P., Mikhaylova, N. et al. (2009) Helping carers to care – the 10/66 dementia research group's randomized control trial of a caregiver intervention in Russia, *International Journal of Geriatric Psychiatry*, 24: 347–54.

Gelso, C. (2014) A tripartite model of the therapeutic relationship: theory, research, and practice, *Psychotherapy Research*, 24: 117–31.

Gentile, D.A., Bailey, K., Bavelier, D. et al. (2017) Internet gaming disorder in children and adolescents, *Pediatrics*, 140: S81–S85.

Gentile, M.G., Manna, G.M., Ciceri, R. et al. (2008) Efficacy of inpatient treatment in severely malnourished anorexia nervosa patients, *Eating and Weight Disorders*, 13: 191–97.

George, M.P., Garrison, G.M., Merten, Z. et al. (2018) Impact of personality disorder cluster on depression outcomes within collaborative care management model of care, *Journal of Primary Care and Community Health*, 9: 2150132718776877 [https://doi.org/10.1177/2150132718776877].

Geraerts, E., Lindsay, D.S., Merckelbach, H. et al. (2009) Cognitive mechanisms underlying recovered-memory experiences of childhood sexual abuse, *Psychological Science*, 20: 92–97.

Ghaffar, O. and Feinstein, A. (2007) The neuropsychiatry of multiple sclerosis: a review, *Current Opinion in Psychiatry*, 20: 278–85.

Ghielen, I., Rutten, S., Boeschoten, R.E. et al. (2019) The effects of cognitive behavioral and mindfulness-based therapies on psychological distress in patients with multiple sclerosis, Parkinson's disease and Huntington's disease: two meta-analyses, *Journal of Psychosomatic Research*, 122: 43–51.

Gibb, B.E., Alloy, L.B., Abramson, L.Y. et al. (2001) History of childhood maltreatment, negative cognitive styles, and episodes of depression in adulthood, *Cognitive Therapy and Research*, 25: 425–46.

Giesen-Bloo, J., van Dyck, R., Spinhoven, P. et al. (2006) Outpatient psychotherapy for borderline personality disorder: randomized trial of schema-focused therapy vs. transference-focused psychotherapy, *Archives of General Psychiatry*, 63: 649–58.

Gilhooly, K.J., Gilhooly, M.L., Sullivan, M.P. et al. (2016) A meta-review of stress, coping and interventions in dementia and dementia caregiving, *BMC Geriatrics*, 16: 106 [https://doi.org/10.1186/s12877-016-0280-8].

Gillespie, K., Duffy, M., Hackmann, A. et al. (2002) Community based cognitive therapy in the treatment of post-traumatic stress disorder following the Omagh bomb, *Behaviour Research and Therapy*, 40: 345–57.

Gillespie, N.A., Zhu, G., Heath, A.C. et al. (2000) The genetic aetiology of somatic distress, *Psychological Medicine*, 30: 1051–61.

Gillman, P.K. (2007) Tricyclic antidepressant pharmacology and therapeutic drug interactions updated, *British Journal of Pharmacology*, 151: 737–48.

Gindi, R.M., Rucker, M.G., Serio-Chapman, C.E. et al. (2009) Utilization patterns and correlates of retention among clients of the needle exchange program in Baltimore, Maryland, *Drug and Alcohol Dependence*, 103: 93–98.

Gladue, B.A. (1985) Neuroendocrine response to estrogen and sexual orientation, *Science*, 230: 960–61.

Gleaves, D.H. (1996) The sociocognitive model of dissociative identity disorder: a reexamination of the evidence, *Psychological Bulletin*, 120: 42–59.

Gleaves, D.H., May, M.C. and Cardena, E. (2001) An examination of the diagnostic validity of dissociative identity disorder, *Clinical Psychology Review*, 21: 577–608.

Goh, E.T. and Morgan, M.Y. (2017) Review article: Pharmacotherapy for alcohol dependence – the why, the what and the wherefore, *Alimentary Pharmacology and Therapeutics*, 45: 865–82.

Golding, L., Emerson, E. and Thornton, A. (2005) An evaluation of specialized community-based residential supports for people with challenging behaviour, *Journal of Intellectual Disability*, 9: 145–54.

Goldman, M.S. (1999a) Expectancy operation: cognitive and neural models and architectures, in I. Kirsch (ed.) *Expectancy, Experience, and Behavior*, Washington, DC: APA Books.

Goldman, M.S. (1999b) Risk for substance abuse: memory as a common etiological pathway, *Psychological Science*, 10: 196–98.

Goldstein, I., Lue, T.F., Padma-Nathan, H. et al. (1998) Oral sildenafil in the treatment of erectile dysfunction: Sildenafil Study Group, *New England Journal of Medicine*, 338: 1397–404.

Goldstein, L., Chalder, T., Chigwedere, C. et al. (2010) Cognitive-behavioral therapy for psychogenic nonepileptic seizures: a pilot RCT, *Neurology*, 74: 1986–94.

Gómez-de-Regil, L., Estrella-Castillo, D.F. and Vega-Cauich, J. (2019) Psychological intervention in traumatic brain injury patients, *Behavioural Neurology*, 2019: 6937832 [https://doi.org/10.1155/2019/6937832].

González-Sanguino, C., Ausin, B., Castellanos, M.A. et al. (2020) Mental health consequences during the initial stage of the 2020 Coronavirus pandemic (COVID-19) in Spain, *Brain, Behavior, and Immunity*, 87: 172–76.

Gooding, P. and Tarrier, N. (2009) A systematic review and meta-analysis of cognitive-behavioural interventions to reduce problem gambling: hedging our bets?, *Behaviour Research and Therapy*, 47: 592–607.

Goodman, G.S., Ghetti, S., Quas, J.A. et al. (2003) A prospective study of memory for abuse: new findings relevant to the repressed memory debate, *Psychological Science*, 14: 113–18.

Goodwin, R.D. (2003) The prevalence of panic attacks in the United States: 1980 to 1995, *Journal of Clinical Epidemiology*, 56: 914–16.

Goodyear-Smith, F.A., Laidlaw, T.M. and Large, R.G. (1997) Memory recovery and repression: what is the evidence?, *Health Care Analysis*, 5: 99–111.

Gorski, T.T. (2008) *Understanding the Twelve Steps*, New York: Prentice-Hall/Parkside.

Gould, K.L., Coventry, W.L., Olson, R.K et al. (2018) Gene–environment interactions in ADHD: the roles of SES and chaos, *Journal of Abnormal Child Psychology*, 46: 251–63.

Goverover, Y., Chiaravalloti, N.D., O'Brien, A.R. et al. (2018) Evidenced-based cognitive rehabilitation for persons with multiple sclerosis: an updated review of the literature from 2007 to 2016, *Archives of Physical Medicine and Rehabilitation*, 99: 390–407.

Grant, B.F., Chou, S.P., Goldstein, R.B. et al. (2008) Prevalence, correlates, disability, and comorbidity of DSM-IV borderline personality disorder: results from the Wave 2 National Epidemiologic Survey on Alcohol and Related Conditions, *Journal of Clinical Psychiatry*, 69: 533–45.

Grant, B.F., Stinson, F.S., Hasin, D.S. et al. (2005) Prevalence, correlates, and comorbidity of bipolar I disorder and axis I and II disorders: results from the National Epidemiologic Survey on Alcohol and Related Conditions, *Journal of Clinical Psychiatry*, 66: 1205–15.

Gray, J.A. (1983) A theory of anxiety: the role of the limbic system, *Encephale*, 9 (suppl. 2): 161B–66B.

Green, R. and Blanchard, R. (1995) Gender identity disorders, in H.I. Kaplan and B.J. Sadock (eds.) *Comprehensive Textbook of Psychiatry*, Baltimore, MD: Williams & Wilkins.

Greeven, A., van Balkom, A.J., Visser, S. et al. (2007) Cognitive behavior therapy and paroxetine in the treatment of hypochondriasis: a randomized controlled trial, *American Journal of Psychiatry*, 164: 91–99.

Greist, J.H., Bandelow, B., Hollander, E. et al. (2003) Long-term treatment of obsessive-compulsive disorder in adults, *CNS Spectrums*, 8: 7–16.

Gresham, F.M. and MacMillan, D.L. (1998) Early intervention project: can its claims be substantiated and its effects replicated?, *Journal of Autism and Developmental Disorders*, 28: 5–13.

Grilo, C.M., Masheb, R.M. and Wilson, G.T. (2005) Efficacy of cognitive behavioral therapy and fluoxetine for the treatment of binge eating disorder: a randomized double-blind placebo-controlled comparison, *Biological Psychiatry*, 57: 301–9.

Grilo, C.M., Pagano, M.E., Skodol, A.E. et al. (2007) Natural course of bulimia nervosa and of eating disorder not otherwise specified: 5-year prospective study of remissions, relapses, and the effects of personality disorder psychopathology, *Journal of Clinical Psychiatry*, 68: 738–46.

Grimland, M., Apter, A. and Kerkhof, A. (2006) The phenomenon of suicide bombing: a review of psychological and nonpsychological factors, *Crisis*, 27: 107–18.

Grinspoon, L. and Bakalar, J.B. (1986) Can drugs be used to enhance the psychotherapeutic process?, *American Journal of Psychotherapy*, 40: 393–404.

Gruber, K., Chutuape, M.A. and Stitzer, M.L. (2000) Reinforcement-based intensive outpatient treatment for inner city opiate abusers: a short-term evaluation, *Drug and Alcohol Dependence*, 57: 211–23.

Gründer, G. and Cumming, P. (2016) The dopamine hypothesis of schizophrenia: current status, in T. Abel and T. Nickl-Jockschat (eds.) *The Neurobiology of Schizophrenia*, San Diego, CA: Academic Press.

Grupp, F., Moro, M.R., Nater, U.M. et al. (2018) 'It's that route that makes us sick': exploring lay beliefs about causes of post-traumatic stress disorder among sub-Saharan African asylum seekers in Germany, *Frontiers in Psychiatry*, 9: 628 [https://doi.org/10.3389/fpsyt.2018.00628].

Grzywacz, J.G., Almeida, D.M., Neupert, S.D. et al. (2004) Socioeconomic status and health: a micro level analysis of exposure and vulnerability to daily stressors, *Journal of Health and Social Behavior*, 45: 1–16.

Gude, T. and Vaglum, P. (2001) One-year follow-up of patients with cluster C personality disorders: a prospective study comparing patients with 'pure' and comorbid conditions within cluster C, and 'pure' C with 'pure' cluster A or B conditions, *Journal of Personality Disorders*, 15: 216–28.

Gunderson, J.G., Zanarini, M.C., Choi-Kain, L.W. et al. (2011) Family study of borderline personality disorder and its sectors of psychopathology, *Archives of General Psychiatry*, 68: 753–62.

Gunn, J., Robertson, G., Dell, S. et al. (1978) *Psychiatric Aspects of Imprisonment*, London: Academic Press.

Gunnell, D., Bennewith, O., Kapur, N. et al. (2012) The use of the internet by people who die by suicide in England: a cross sectional study, *Journal of Affective Disorders*, 141: 480–83.

Guo, X., Hamilton, P.J., Reish, N.J. et al. (2009) Reduced expression of the NMDA receptor-interacting protein SynGAP causes behavioral abnormalities that model symptoms of schizophrenia, *Neuropsychopharmacology*, 34: 1659–72.

Gupta, M.A. and Johnson, A.M. (2000) Nonweight-related body image concerns among female eating-disordered patients and nonclinical controls: some preliminary observations, *International Journal of Eating Disorders*, 27: 304–9.

Guthrie, E. (1996) Psychotherapy for somatisation disorders, *Current Opinion in Psychiatry*, 9: 182–87.

Haddad, P. and Anderson, I. (2007) Recognising and managing antidepressant discontinuation symptoms, *Advances in Psychiatric Treatment*, 13: 447–57.

Haines, J.L. and Pericak-Vance, M.A. (1999) Genetics of multiple sclerosis, in A.N. Theofilopoulos (ed.) *Genes and Genetics of Autoimmunity*, Current Directions in Autoimmunology vol. 1, Basel: Karger.

Halliburton, M. (2005) 'Just some spirits': the erosion of spirit possession and the rise of 'tension' in South India, *Medical Anthropology*, 24: 111–44.

Ham, P., Waters, D.B. and Oliver, M.N. (2005) Treatment of panic disorder, *American Family Physician*, 71: 733–39.

Hankin, B.L., Fraley, R.C., Lahey, B.B. et al. (2005) Is depression best viewed as a continuum or discrete category? A taxometric analysis of childhood and adolescent depression in a population-based sample, *Journal of Abnormal Psychology*, 114: 96–110.

Hansen, B., Vogel, P.A., Stiles, T.C. et al. (2007) Influence of co-morbid generalized anxiety disorder, panic disorder and personality disorders on the outcome of cognitive behavioural treatment of obsessive-compulsive disorder, *Cognitive Behaviour Therapy*, 36: 145–55.

Haraldsen, I.R., Opjordsmoen, S., Egeland, T. et al. (2003) Sex-sensitive cognitive performance in untreated patients with early onset gender identity disorder, *Psychoneuroendocrinology*, 28: 906–15.

Hare, R.D. (1991) *The Hare Psychopathy Checklist-Revised (PCL-R)*, Toronto: Multi-Health Systems.

Hare, R.D., Clark, D., Grann, M. et al. (2000) Psychopathy and the predictive utility of the PCL-R: an international perspective, *Behavioural Sciences and the Law*, 18: 623–45.

Harrison, A., Fernández de la Cruz, L., Enander, J. et al. (2016) Cognitive-behavioral therapy for body dysmorphic disorder: a systematic review and meta-analysis of randomized controlled trials, *Clinical Psychology Review*, 48: 43–51.

Harrison, P.J., Geddes, J.R. and Tunbridge, E.M. (2018) The emerging neurobiology of bipolar disorder, *Trends in Neurosciences*, 41: 18–30.

Harro, J. (2015) Neuropsychiatric adverse effects of amphetamine and methamphetamine, *International Review of Neurobiology*, 120: 179–204.

Harrow, M., Grossman, L.S., Jobe, T.H. and Herbener, E.S. (2005) Do patients with schizophrenia ever show periods of recovery? A 15-year multi-follow-up study, *Schizophrenia Bulletin*, 31: 723–34.

Hart, T., Driver, S., Sander, A. et al. (2019) Traumatic brain injury education for adult patients and families: a scoping review, *Brain Injury*, 32: 1295–306.

Hartmann, A.S., Cordes, M., Hirschfeld, G. et al. (2019) Affect and worry during a checking episode: a comparison of individuals with symptoms of obsessive-compulsive disorder, anorexia nervosa, bulimia nervosa, body dysmorphic disorder, illness anxiety disorder, and panic disorder, *Psychiatry Research*, 272: 349–58.

Hartnett, D., Carr, A., Hamilton, E. et al. (2017) The effectiveness of functional family therapy for adolescent behavioral and substance misuse problems: a meta-analysis, *Family Process*, 56: 607–19.

Harvey, A., Watkins, E., Mansell, W. et al. (2004) *Cognitive Behavioural Processes Across Psychological Disorders: A Transtheoretical Approach to Research and Treatment*, Oxford: Oxford University Press.

Hasin, D.S. and Grant, B.F. (2015) The National Epidemiologic Survey on Alcohol and Related Conditions (NESARC) Waves 1 and 2: review and summary of findings, *Social Psychiatry and Psychiatric Epidemiology*, 50: 1609–40.

Hassiotis, A.A. and Hall, I. (2008) Behavioural and cognitive-behavioural interventions for outwardly-directed aggressive behaviour in people with learning disabilities, *Cochrane Database of Systematic Reviews*, 3: CD003406 [https://doi.org/10.1002/14651858.CD003406.pub3].

Hawker, D.M., Durkin, J. and Hawker, D.S. (2011) To debrief or not to debrief our heroes: that is the question, *Clinical Psychology and Psychotherapy*, 18: 453–63.

Haworth-Hoeppner, S. (2000) The critical shapes of body image: the role of culture and family in the production of eating disorders, *Journal of Marriage and the Family*, 62: 212–27.

Hawton, K., Catalan, J. and Fagg, J. (1992) Sex therapy for erectile dysfunction: characteristics of couples, treatment outcome and prognostic factors, *Archives of Sexual Behavior*, 21: 161–75.

Hayes, S.C., Luoma, J.B., Bond, F.W. et al. (2006) Acceptance and commitment therapy: model, processes and outcomes, *Behaviour Research and Therapy*, 44: 1–25.

Hayes, S.C., Strosahl, K.D., Bunting, K. et al. (2004) What is acceptance and commitment therapy?, in S.C. Hayes and K.D. Strosahl (eds.) *A Practical Guide to Acceptance and Commitment Therapy*, New York: Springer.

Health Quality Ontario (2017) Psychotherapy for major depressive disorder and generalized anxiety disorder: a health technology assessment, *Ontario Health Technology Assessment Series*, 17: 1–167.

Health Quality Ontario (2018) Cognitive behavioural therapy for psychosis: a health technology assessment, *Ontario Health Technology Assessment Series*, 18: 1–141.

Hedden, T. and Gabrieli, J.D. (2005) Healthy and pathological processes in adult development: new evidence from neuroimaging of the aging brain, *Current Opinion in Neurology*, 18: 740–47.

Hedman E., Axelsson E., Andersson E. et al. (2016) Exposure-based cognitive-behavioural therapy via the internet and as bibliotherapy for somatic symptom disorder and illness anxiety disorder: randomised controlled trial, *British Journal of Psychiatry*, 209: 407–13.

Hellawell, S.J. and Brewin, C.R. (2004) A comparison of flashbacks and ordinary autobiographical memories of trauma: content and language, *Behaviour Research and Therapy*, 42: 1–12.

Hellström, K., Fellenius, J. and Öst, L.-G. (1996) One versus five sessions of applied tension in the treatment of blood phobia, *Behaviour Research and Therapy*, 34: 101–12.

Hemsley, D.R. (1996) Schizophrenia: a cognitive model and its implications for psychological intervention, *Behavior Modification*, 20: 139–69.

Hendin, H. (1992) The psychodynamics of suicide, *International Review of Psychiatry*, 4: 157–67.

Henggeler, S.W., Melton, G.B. and Smith, L.A. (1992) Family preservation using multisystemic therapy: an effective alternative to incarcerating serious juvenile offenders, *Journal of Consulting and Clinical Psychology*, 60: 953–61.

Henry, D.B., Tolan, P.H. and Gorman-Smith, D. (2001) Longitudinal family and peer group effects on violence and nonviolent delinquency, *Journal of Clinical Child and Adolescent Psychology*, 30: 172–86.

Herrera-Guzmán, I., Gudayol-Ferré, E., Herrera-Guzmán, D. et al. (2009) Effects of selective serotonin reuptake and dual serotonergic-noradrenergic reuptake treatments on memory and mental processing speed in patients with major depressive disorder, *Journal of Psychiatric Research*, 43: 855–63.

Hettema, J.M., Neale, M.C. and Kendler, K.S. (2001a) A review and meta-analysis of the genetic epidemiology of anxiety disorders, *American Journal of Psychiatry*, 158: 1568–78.

Hettema, J.M., Prescott, C.A. and Kendler, K.S. (2001b) A population-based twin study of generalized anxiety disorder in men and women, *Journal of Nervous and Mental Disorders*, 189: 413–20.

Hilker, R., Helenius, D., Fagerlund, B. et al. (2018) Heritability of schizophrenia and schizophrenia spectrum based on the nationwide Danish Twin Register, *Biological Psychiatry*, 83: 492–98.

Hillemacher, T., Frieling, H., Buchholz, V. et al. (2016) Dopamine-receptor 2 gene-methylation and gambling behavior in relation to impulsivity, *Psychiatry Research*, 239: 154–55.

Hiller, W., Rief, W. and Brähler, E. (2006) Somatization in the population: from mild bodily misperceptions to disabling symptoms, *Social Psychiatry and Psychiatric Epidemiology*, 41: 704–12.

Hirschfeld, R.M.A. (1999) Efficacy of SSRIs and newer antidepressants in severe depression: comparison with TCAs, *Journal of Clinical Psychiatry*, 60: 326–35.

Hirschtritt, M.E., Bloch, M.H. and Mathews, C.A. (2017) Obsessive-compulsive disorder: advances in diagnosis and treatment, *Journal of the American Medical Association*, 317: 1358–67.

Hodges, S. and Marks, M. (1998) Cognitive characteristics of seasonal affective disorder: a preliminary investigation, *Journal of Affective Disorders*, 50: 59–64.

Hoffman, R.E., Rapaport, J., Mazure, C.M. et al. (1999) Selective speech perception alterations in schizophrenic patients reporting hallucinated 'voices', *American Journal of Psychiatry*, 156: 393–99.

Hofmann, S.G. (2008) Cognitive processes during fear acquisition and extinction in animals and humans: implications for exposure therapy of anxiety disorders, *Clinical Psychology Review*, 28: 199–210.

Hoge, E.A., Tamrakar, S.M., Christian, K.M. et al. (2006) Cross-cultural differences in somatic presentation in patients with generalized anxiety disorder, *Journal of Nervous and Mental Disease*, 194: 962–66.

Holden, U.P. and Woods, R.T. (1995) *Positive Approaches to Dementia Care*, Oxford: Churchill Livingstone.

Hollander, E., Tracy, K.A., Swann, A.C. et al. (2003) Divalproex in the treatment of impulsive aggression: efficacy in cluster B personality disorders, *Neuropsychopharmacology*, 28: 1186–97.

Hollon, S.D., DeRubeis, R.J., Shelton, R.C. et al. (2005) Prevention of relapse following cognitive therapy vs. medications in moderate to severe depression, *Archives of General Psychiatry*, 62: 417–22.

Holmes, S. (2000) Treatment of male sexual dysfunction, *British Medical Bulletin*, 56: 798–808.

Home Office (2019) *Drug Misuse: Findings from the 2018/19 Crime Survey for England and Wales. Statistical Bulletin: 21/19*, London: National Statistics.

Honda, H., Shimizu, Y. and Rutter, M. (2005) No effect of MMR withdrawal on the incidence of autism: a total population study, *Journal of Child Psychology and Psychiatry*, 46: 72–79.

Honig, L.S., Vellas, B., Woodward, M. et al. (2018) Trial of solanezumab for mild dementia due to Alzheimer's disease, *New England Journal of Medicine*, 378: 321–30.

Horndasch, S., Heinrich, H., Kratz, O. et al. (2015) Perception and evaluation of women's bodies in adolescents and adults with anorexia nervosa, *European Archives of Psychiatry and Clinical Neuroscience*, 265: 677–87.

Horowitz, M.J. (1986) Stress-response syndromes: a review of posttraumatic and adjustment disorders, *Hospital and Community Psychiatry*, 37: 241–49.

Hoshiai, M., Matsumoto, Y., Sato, T. et al. (2010) Psychiatric comorbidity among patients with gender identity disorder, *Psychiatry and Clinical Neurosciences*, 64: 514–19.

Hoven, C.W., Duarte, C.S., Lucas, C.P. et al. (2005) Psychopathology among New York City public school children 6 months after September 11, *Archives of General Psychiatry*, 62: 545–52.

Huang, B., Grant, B.F., Dawson, D.A. et al. (2006) Race-ethnicity and the prevalence and co-occurrence of Diagnostic and Statistical Manual of Mental Disorders, fourth edition, alcohol and drug use disorders and axis I and II disorders: United States, 2001 to 2002, *Comprehensive Psychiatry*, 4: 252–57.

Huang, C.H., Huang, C.C., Sun, C.K. et al. (2016) Methylphenidate on cognitive improvement in patients with traumatic brain injury: a meta-analysis, *Current Neuropharmacology*, 14: 272–81.

Huang, T.L., Zandi, P.P., Tucker, K.L. et al. (2005) Benefits of fatty fish on dementia risk are stronger for those without APOE epsilon4, *Neurology*, 65: 1409–14.

Huang, X., Lei, Z., Li, X.P. et al. (2009) Response of sodium pump to ouabain challenge in human glioblastoma cells in culture, *World Journal of Biological Psychiatry*, 10: 884–92.

Huang, Y. and Zhao, N. (2020) Generalized anxiety disorder, depressive symptoms and sleep quality during COVID-19 outbreak in China: a web-based cross-sectional survey, *Psychiatry Research*, 288 [https://doi.org/10.1016/j.psychres.2020.112954].

Hubbard, R.L., Craddock, S.G., Flynn, P.M. et al. (1997) Overview of 1-year follow-up outcomes in the Drug Abuse Treatment Outcome Study (DATOS), *Psychological Addiction and Behavior*, 4: 1303–10.

Huhn, M., Nikolakopoulou, A., Schneider-Thoma, J. et al. (2019) Comparative efficacy and tolerability of 32 oral antipsychotics for the acute treatment of adults with multi-episode schizophrenia: a systematic review and network meta-analysis, *Lancet*, 394: 939–51.

Hulshoff Pol, H.E., Cohen-Kettenis, P.T., Van Haren, N.E. et al. (2006) Changing your sex changes your brain: influences of testosterone and estrogen on adult human brain structure, *European Journal of Endocrinology*, 155: S107–S114.

Humphreys, L. and Barrowclough, C. (2006) Attributional style, defensive functioning and persecutory delusions: symptom-specific or general coping strategy?, *British Journal of Clinical Psychology*, 45: 231–46.

Hunter, E. (1997) Memory loss for childhood sexual abuse: distinguishing between encoding and retrieval factors, in D. Read and D.S. Lindsay (eds.) *Recollections of Trauma: Scientific Research and Clinical Practice*, New York: Plenum Press.

Hunter, L.C., O'Hare, A., Herron, W.J. et al. (2003) Opioid peptides and dipeptidyl peptidase in autism, *Developmental Medicine and Child Neurology*, 45: 121–28.

Hurwitz, R., Blackmore, R., Hazell, P. et al. (2012) Tricyclic antidepressants for autism spectrum disorders (ASD) in children and adolescents, *Cochrane Database of Systematic Reviews*, 3: CD008372 [https://doi.org/10.1002/14651858.CD008372.pub2].

Hyman, I.E., Husband, T.H. and Billings, F.J. (1995) False memories of childhood experiences, *Applied Cognitive Psychology*, 9: 181–97.

Hyman, S.L., Stewart, P.A., Foley, J. et al. (2016) The gluten-free/casein-free diet: a double-blind challenge trial in children with autism, *Journal of Autism and Developmental Disorders*, 46: 205–20.

Independent Provider of Special Education Advice (IPSEA) (2019) Saffron Walden: IPSEA [https://www.ipsea.org.uk/the-right-to-a-mainstream-education].

International Society for the Study of Trauma and Dissociation (2011) Guidelines for treating dissociative identity disorder in adults, third revision, *Journal of Trauma and Dissociation*, 12: 115–87.

Iossifov, I., Levy, D., Allen, J. et al. (2015) Low load for disruptive mutations in autism genes and their biased transmission, *Proceedings of the National Academy of Sciences USA*, 112: E5600–E5607.

Israelyan, N. and Margolis, K.G. (2019) Serotonin as a link between the gut-brain-microbiome axis in autism spectrum disorders, *Pharmacological Research*, 140: 115–20.

Ito, T., Meguro, K., Akanuma, K. et al. (2007) A randomized controlled trial of the group reminiscence approach in patients with vascular dementia, *Dementia and Geriatric Cognitive Disorders*, 24: 48–54.

Jackson, P. (2012) Re E (Medical treatment: Anorexia) (Rev 1) [2012] EWCOP 1639 (15 June 2012) [https://www.bailii.org/ew/cases/EWHC/COP/2012/1639.html].

Jacob, C., Domschke, K., Gajewska, A. et al. (2010) Genetics of panic disorder: focus on association studies and therapeutic perspectives, *Expert Review of Neurotherapeutics*, 10: 1273–84.

Jacobi, F., Wittchen, H.-U., Holting, C. et al. (2004) Prevalence, co-morbidity and correlates of mental disorders in the general population: results from the German Health Interview and Examination Survey (GHS), *Psychological Medicine*, 34: 597–611.

Jacobs, M.J., Roesch, S., Wonderlich, S.A. et al. (2009) Anorexia nervosa trios: behavioral profiles of individuals with anorexia nervosa and their parents, *Psychological Medicine*, 39: 451–61.

Jacobson, N.S. and Hollon, S.D. (1996) Cognitive-behavior therapy versus pharmacotherapy: now that the jury's returned its verdict, it's time to present the rest of the evidence, *Journal of Consulting and Clinical Psychology*, 64: 74–80.

Jaffe, S.R., Moffitt, T.E., Caspi, A. et al. (2002) Differences in early childhood risk factors for juvenile-onset and adult-onset depression, *Archives of General Psychiatry*, 59: 215–22.

Jagielska, G. and Kacperska, I. (2017) Outcome, comorbidity and prognosis in anorexia nervosa, *Psychiatria Polska*, 51: 205–18.

Jáni, M. and Kašpárek, T. (2018) Emotion recognition and theory of mind in schizophrenia: a meta-analysis of neuroimaging studies, *World Journal of Biological Psychiatry*, 19: S86–S96.

Janssen, P.L. (1985) Psychodynamic study of male potency disorders: an overview, *Psychotherapy and Psychosomatics*, 44: 6–17.

Jarvis, B.P., Holtyn, A.F, Subramaniam, S. et al. (2018) Extended-release injectable naltrexone for opioid use disorder: a systematic review, *Addiction*, 113: 1188–209.

Jáuregui-Garrido, B. and Jáuregui-Lobera, I. (2012) Sudden death in eating disorders, *Vascular Health and Risk Management*, 8: 91–98.

Jenike, M.A. (1998) Neurosurgical treatment of obsessive-compulsive disorder, *British Medical Journal*, 163: s75–s90.

Jenike, M.A., Ballantine, H.T., Martuza, R.L. et al. (1991) Cingulotomy for refractory obsessive-compulsive disorder: a long-term follow-up of 33 patients, *Archives of General Psychiatry*, 48: 548–55.

Jiang, C., Mitran, A., Miniño, A. et al. (2015) Racial and gender disparities in suicide among young adults aged 18–24: United States, 2009–2013, *CDC: Health E-Stat*, Hyattsville, MD: Centers for Disease Control and Prevention [https://www.cdc.gov/nchs/data/hestat/suicide/racial_and_gender_2009_2013.pdf].

Jin, D.C., Cao, H.L., Xu, M.Q. et al. (2016) Regulation of the serotonin transporter in the pathogenesis of irritable bowel syndrome, *World Journal of Gastroenterology*, 22: 8137–48.

Jin, X., Jin, Y., Zhou, S. et al. (2018) Attentional biases toward body images in males at high risk of muscle dysmorphia, *PeerJ*, 6: e4273 [https://doi.org/10.7717/peerj.4273].

Johansson, A., Grant, J.E., Kim, S.W. et al. (2009) Risk factors for problematic gambling: a critical literature review, *Journal of Gambling Studies*, 25: 67–92.

Johnson, R.A., Albright, D.L., Marzolf, J.R. et al. (2018) Effects of therapeutic horseback riding on post-traumatic stress disorder in military veterans, *Military Medical Research*, 5: 3 [https://doi.org/10.1186/s40779-018-0149-6].

Johnson, S.L. (2005) Mania and dysregulation in goal pursuit, *Clinical Psychology Review*, 25: 241–62.

Johnson, S.L., Meyer, B., Winett, C. et al. (2000) Social support and self-esteem predict changes in bipolar depression but not mania, *Journal of Affective Disorders*, 58: 79–86.

Johnstone, L. (2003) A shocking treatment?, *The Psychologist*, 16: 236–39.

Jones, A.T., O'Connell, N.K. and David, A.S. (2020) Epidemiology of functional stroke mimic patients systematic review and meta-analysis, *European Journal of Neurology*, 27: 18–26.

Jónsdóttir, H., Friis S., Horne, R. et al. (2008) Beliefs about medications: measurement and relationship to adherence in patients with severe mental disorders, *Acta Psychiatrica Scandinavica*, 118: 78–84.

Joseph, S., Williams, R. and Yule, W. (1995) Psychosocial perspectives on posttraumatic stress, *Clinical Psychology Review*, 15: 515–44.

Joy, E., Kussman, A. and Nattiv, A. (2016) 2016 update on eating disorders in athletes: a comprehensive narrative review with a focus on clinical assessment and management, *British Journal of Sports Medicine*, 50: 154–62.

Joyce, S., Shand, F., Tighe, J. et al. (2018) Road to resilience: a systematic review and meta-analysis of resilience training programmes and interventions, *BMJ Open*, 8: e017858 [https://doi.org/10.1136/bmjopen-2017-017858].

Judge, C., O'Donovan, C., Callaghan, G. et al. (2014) Gender dysphoria – prevalence and co-morbidities in an Irish adult population, *Frontiers in Endocrinology*, 5: 87 [https://doi.org/10.3389/fendo.2014.00087].

Jung, C.G. ([1912] 1956) *Symbols of Transformation*, New York: Bollingen, no. 5 (original edition published in 1912 as *The Psychology of the Unconscious*).

Kabat-Zinn, J. (1990) *The Full Catastrophe Living: Using the Wisdom of Your Body and Mind to Face Stress, Pain, and Illness*, New York: Delacorte.

Kaewpradub, N., Kiatrungrit, K., Hongsanguansri, S. et al. (2017) Association among internet usage, body image, and eating behaviors of secondary school students, *Shanghai Archives of Psychiatry*, 29: 208–17.

Kales, H.C., Gitlin, L.N., Stanislawski, B. et al. (2018) Effect of the WeCareAdvisor™ on family caregiver outcomes in dementia: a pilot randomized controlled trial, *BMC Geriatrics*, 18: 113 [https://doi.org/10.1186/s12877-018-0801-8].

Kaltiala-Heino, R., Bergman, H., Työläjärvi, M. et al. (2018) Gender dysphoria in adolescence: current perspectives, *Adolescent Health, Medicine and Therapeutics*, 9: 31–41.

Kam, C.-M., Greenberg, M.T. and Kusche, C.A. (2004) Sustained effects of the PATHS curriculum on the social and psychological adjustment of children in special education, *Journal of Emotional and Behavioral Disorders*, 12: 66–78.

Kamphuis, J.H., Emmelkamp, P.M. and Bartak, A. (2003) Individual differences in posttraumatic stress following post-intimate stalking: stalking severity and psychosocial variables, *British Journal of Clinical Psychology*, 42: 145–56.

Kanno, M., Matsumoto, M., Togashi, H. et al. (2003) Effects of repetitive transcranial magnetic stimulation on behavioral and neurochemical changes in rats during an elevated plus-maze test, *Journal of Neurological Sciences*, 211: 5–14.

Kaplan, Y.C., Keskin-Arslan, E., Acar, S. et al. (2017) Maternal SSRI discontinuation, use, psychiatric disorder and the risk of autism in children: a meta-analysis of cohort studies, *British Journal of Clinical Pharmacology*, 83: 2798–806.

Kappelmann, N., Lewis, G., Dantzer, R. et al. (2018) Antidepressant activity of anti-cytokine treatment: a systematic review and meta-analysis of clinical trials of chronic inflammatory conditions, *Molecular Psychiatry*, 23: 335–43.

Karasz, A. (2005) Cultural differences in conceptual models of depression, *Social Science and Medicine*, 60: 1625–35.

Kashala, E., Tylleskar, T., Elgen, I. et al. (2005) Attention deficit and hyperactivity disorder among school children in Kinshasa, Democratic Republic of Congo, *African Health Sciences*, 5: 172–81.

Kasper, S. and Resinger, E. (2001) Panic disorder: the place of benzodiazepines and selective serotonin reuptake inhibitors, *European Neuropsychopharmacology*, 11: 307–21.

Katan, M. (1953) Mania and the pleasure principle, in P. Greenacre (ed.) *Affective Disorders*, New York: International Universities Press.

Kaye, W.H., Frank, G.K., Meltzer, C.C. et al. (2001a) Altered serotonin 2A receptor activity in women who have recovered from bulimia nervosa, *American Journal of Psychiatry*, 158: 1152–55.

Kaye, W.H., Fudge, J.L. and Paulus, M. (2009) New insights into symptoms and neurocircuit function of anorexia nervosa, *Nature Reviews Neuroscience*, 10: 573–84.

Kaye, W.H., Gwirtsman, H.E., Brewerton, T.D. et al. (1991) Altered serotonin activity in anorexia nervosa after long-term weight restoration: does elevated cerebrospinal fluid 5-hydroxyindoleacetic acid level correlate with rigid and obsessive behaviour?, *Archives of General Psychiatry*, 48: 556–62.

Kaye, W.H., Nagata, T., Weltzin, T.E. et al. (2001b) Double-blind placebo-controlled administration of fluoxetine in restricting- and restricting-purging-type anorexia nervosa, *Biological Psychiatry*, 49: 644–52.

Kaye, W.H. and Weltzin, T.E. (1991) Serotonin activity in anorexia and bulimia nervosa: relationship to the modulation of feeding and mood, *Journal of Clinical Psychiatry*, 52 (suppl.): 41–48.

Keating, L., Tasca, G.A. and Bissada, H. (2015) Pre treatment attachment anxiety predicts change in depressive symptoms in women who complete day hospital treatment for anorexia and bulimia nervosa, *Psychology and Psychotherapy*, 88: 54–70.

Keck, P.E., Jr., McIntyre, R.S. and Shelton, R.C. (2007) Bipolar depression: best practices for the outpatient, *CNS Spectrum*, 12 (suppl. 20): 1–14.

Keel, P.K., Klump, K.L., Miller, K.B. et al. (2005) Shared transmission of eating disorders and anxiety disorders, *International Journal of Eating Disorders*, 38: 99–105.

Keen, L., II, Khan, M., Clifford, L. et al. (2014) Injection and non-injection drug use and infectious disease in Baltimore City: differences by race, *Addictive Behaviors*, 39: 1325–28.

Keijsers, G.P., Schaap, C.P. and Hoogduin, C.A. (2000) The impact of interpersonal patient and therapist behavior on outcome in cognitive-behavioral therapy: a review of empirical studies, *Behavior Modification*, 24: 264–97.

Kellett, S. (2005) The treatment of dissociative identity disorder with cognitive analytic therapy: experimental evidence of sudden gains, *Journal of Trauma and Dissociation*, 6: 55–81.

Kellogg, S. and Young, J. (2006) Schema therapy for borderline personality disorder, *Journal of Clinical Psychology*, 62: 445–58.

Kells, M. and Kelly-Weeder, S. (2016) Nasogastric tube feeding for individuals with anorexia nervosa: an integrative review, *Journal of the American Psychiatric Nurses Association*, 22: 449–68.

Kelly, J.F., Humphreys, K. and Ferri, M. (2020) Alcoholics Anonymous and other 12-step programs for alcohol use disorder, *Cochrane Database of Systematic Reviews*, 3: CD012880 [https://doi.org/10.1002/14651858.CD012880.pub2].

Kemp, R., Kirov, G., Everitt, B. et al. (1998) Randomised controlled trial of compliance therapy: 18-month follow-up, *British Journal of Psychiatry*, 172: 413–19.

Kendler, K.S., Myers, J. and Prescott, C.A. (2007) Specificity of genetic and environmental risk factors for symptoms of cannabis, cocaine, alcohol, caffeine, and nicotine dependence, *Archives of General Psychiatry*, 64: 1313–20.

Kendler, K.S., Neale, M.C., Kessler, R.C. et al. (1993) Panic disorder in women: a population-based twin study, *Psychological Medicine*, 40: 397–406.

Kéri, S. and Kelemen, O. (2009) The role of attention and immediate memory in vulnerability to interpersonal criticism during family transactions in schizophrenia, *British Journal of Clinical Psychology*, 48: 21–29.

Kernberg, O.F. (1985) *Borderline Conditions and Pathological Narcissism*, Northvale, NJ: Jason Aronson.

Kerns, A., Eso, K., Thomson, J. et al. (1999) Investigation of a direct intervention for improving attention in young children with ADHD, *Developmental Neuropsychology*, 16: 273–95.

Kerr, T., Tyndall, M., Li, K. et al. (2005) Sager injection facility use and syringe sharing in injection drug users, *Lancet*, 366: 316–18.

Kessing, L.V., Søndergård, L., Kvist, K. et al. (2007) Adherence to lithium in naturalistic settings: results from a nationwide pharmacoepidemiological study, *Bipolar Disorders*, 9: 730–36.

Kessler, A., Sollie, S., Challacombe, B. et al. (2019) The global prevalence of erectile dysfunction: a review, *British Journal of Urology International*, 124: 587–99.

Kessler, R.C., McGonagle, K.A., Zhao, S. et al. (1994) Lifetime and 12-month prevalence of DSM-III-R psychiatric disorders in the United States: results from the National Comorbidity Survey, *Archives of General Psychiatry*, 5: 8–19.

Ketcher, D., Trettevik, R., Vadaparampil, S.T. et al. (2020) Caring for a spouse with advanced cancer: similarities and differences for male and female caregivers, *Journal of Behavioral Medicine*, 43: 817–28.

Key, B.L., Rowa, K., Bieling, P. et al. (2017) Mindfulness-based cognitive therapy as an augmentation treatment for obsessive-compulsive disorder, *Clinical Psychology and Psychotherapy*, 24: 1109–20.

Khan, S., Amjad, A. and Rowland, D. (2019) Potential for long-term benefit of cognitive behavioral therapy as an adjunct treatment for men with erectile dysfunction, *Journal of Sexual Medicine*, 16: 300–6.

Kiehl, K.A., Smith, A.M., Hare, R.D. et al. (2001) Limbic abnormalities in affective processing by criminal psychopaths as revealed by functional magnetic resonance imaging, *Biological Psychiatry*, 50: 677–84.

Killeen, P.R., Tannock, R. and Sagvolden, T. (2012) The four causes of ADHD: a framework, *Current Topics in Behavioral Neurosciences*, 9: 391–425.

Kilpatrick D.G., Resnick H.S., Milanak, M.E. et al. (2013) National estimates of exposure to traumatic events and PTSD prevalence using DSM-IV and DSM-5 criteria, *Journal of Traumatic Stress*, 26: 537–47.

Kim, K.M., Choi, S.W., Kim, D. et al. (2019) Associations among the opioid receptor gene (OPRM1) A118G polymorphism, psychiatric symptoms, and quantitative EEG in Korean males with gambling disorder: a pilot study, *Journal of Behavioral Addictions*, 8: 463–70.

Kim, Y.K. and Park, S.C. (2019) Classification of psychiatric disorders, *Advances in Experimental Medicine and Biology*, 1192: 17–25.

King, D.L. and Delfabbro, P.H. (2014) The cognitive psychology of internet gaming disorder, *Clinical Psychology Review*, 34: 298–308.

King, D.L., Delfabbro, P.H., Wu, A. et al. (2017) Treatment of internet gaming disorder: an international systematic review and CONSORT evaluation, *Clinical Psychology Review*, 54: 123–33.

Kiosses, D.N., Alexopoulos, G.S., Hajcak, G. et al. (2018) Cognitive Reappraisal Intervention for Suicide Prevention (CRISP) for middle-aged and older adults hospitalized for suicidality, *American Journal of Geriatric Psychiatry*, 26: 494–503.

Kirkpatrick, B., Fenton. W.S., Carpenter, W.T. et al. (2006) The NIMH-MATRICS consensus statement on negative symptoms, *Schizophrenia Bulletin*, 32: 214–19.

Kirmayer, L.J., Groleau, D., Looper, K.J. et al. (2004) Explaining medically unexplained symptoms, *Canadian Journal of Psychiatry*, 49: 663–72.

Kissgen, R. and Franke, S. (2016) An attachment research perspective on ADHD (English translation), *Klinik, Diagnostik, Therapie und Rehabilitation*, 30: 63–68.

Kleiman, S.C., Watson, H.J., Bulik-Sullivan, E.C. et al. (2015) The intestinal microbiota in acute anorexia nervosa and during renourishment: relationship to depression, anxiety, and eating disorder psychopathology, *Psychosomatic Medicine*, 77: 969–81.

Klein, M. (1927) The psychological principles of infant analysis, *International Journal of Psychoanalysis*, 8: 25–37.

Kleindienst, N., Engel, R.R. and Greil, W. (2005) Psychosocial and demographic factors associated with response to prophylactic lithium: a systematic review for bipolar disorders, *Psychological Medicine*, 35: 1685–94.

Kleinman, A.M. (1977) Depression, somatization and the 'new cross-cultural psychiatry', *Social Science and Medicine*, 11: 3–10.

Kleinstäuber, M., Witthöft, M., Steffanowski, A. et al. (2014) Pharmacological interventions for somatoform disorders in adults, *Cochrane Database of Systematic Reviews*, 11: CD010628 [https://doi.org/10.1002/14651858.CD010628.pub2].

Klucken, T., Schweckendiek, J., Merz, C.J. et al. (2009) Neural activations of the acquisition of conditioned sexual arousal: effects of contingency awareness and sex, *Journal of Sexual Medicine*, 6: 3071–85.

Klump, K.L., Miller, K.B., Keel, P.K. et al. (2001) Genetic and environmental influences on anorexia nervosa syndromes in a population-based twin sample, *Psychological Medicine*, 31: 737–40.

Knivsberg, A.M., Reichelt, K.L., Hien, T. et al. (1998) Parents' observations after one year of dietary intervention for children with autistic syndromes, in P. Shattock and G. Linfoot (eds.) *Psychobiology of Autism: Current Research and Practice*, Sunderland: Autism Research Unit, 13–24.

Ko, C.H., Yen, J.Y., Chen, C.S. et al. (2009) Predictive values of psychiatric symptoms for internet addiction in adolescents: a 2-year prospective study, *Archives of Pediatric and Adolescent Medicine*, 163: 937–43.

Koegel, R., Kim, S., Koegel, L. et al. (2013) Improving socialization for high school students with ASD by using their preferred interests, *Journal of Autism and Developmental Disorders*, 43: 2121–34.

Koegel, R.L., Koegel, L.K. and McNerney, E.K. (2001) Pivotal areas in intervention for autism, *Journal of Clinical Child Psychology*, 30: 19–32.

Koegel, R.L., O'Dell, M.C. and Dunlap, G. (1988) Producing speech use in nonverbal autistic children by reinforcing attempts, *Journal of Autism and Developmental Disorders*, 18: 525–38.

Koenen, K.C., Amstadter, A.B., Ruggiero, K.J. et al. (2009) RGS2 and generalized anxiety disorder in an epidemiologic sample of hurricane-exposed adults, *Depression and Anxiety*, 26: 309–15.

Kontis, D. and Theochari, E. (2012) Dopamine in anorexia nervosa: a systematic review, *Behavioural Pharmacology*, 23: 496–515.

Koran, L.M., Abujaoude, E., Large, M.D. et al. (2008) The prevalence of body dysmorphic disorder in the United States adult population, *CNS Spectrum*, 13: 316–22.

Korten, A.E., Jorm, A.F., Henderson, A.S. et al. (1993) Assessing the risk of Alzheimer's disease in first-degree relatives of Alzheimer's disease cases, *Psychological Medicine*, 23: 915–23.

Kovanen, L., Basnet, S., Castrén, S. et al. (2016) A randomised, double-blind, placebo-controlled trial of as-needed naltrexone in the treatment of pathological gambling, *European Addiction Research*, 22: 70–79.

Kraepelin, E. ([1883] 1981) *Clinical Psychiatry* (trans. A.R. Diefendorf), Delmar, NY: Scholar's Facsimiles and Reprints.

Krasucki, C., Howard, R. and Mann, A. (1998) The relationship between anxiety disorders and age, *International Journal of Geriatric Psychiatry*, 13: 79–99.

Kraus, L., Augustan, R., Frischer, M. et al. (2003) Estimating prevalence of problem drug use at national level in countries of the European Union and Norway, *Addiction*, 98: 471–85.

Kraus, S.W., Etuk, R. and Potenza, M.N. (2020) Current pharmacotherapy for gambling disorder: a systematic review, *Expert Opinion on Pharmacotherapy*, 21: 287–96.

Krautwurst, S., Gerlach, A.L. and Witthöft, M. (2016) Interoception in pathological health anxiety, *Journal of Abnormal Psychology*, 125: 1179–84.

Krebs, G., Fernández de la Cruz, L., Monzani, B. et al. (2017) Long-term outcomes of cognitive-behavioral therapy for adolescent body dysmorphic disorder, *Behavior Therapy*, 48: 462–73.

Kreutzer, J.S., Seel, R.T. and Gourley, E. (2009) The prevalence and symptom rates of depression after traumatic brain injury: a comprehensive examination, *Brain Injury*, 15: 563–76.

Kringlen, E. (1993) Genes and environment in mental illness: perspectives and ideas for future research, *Acta Psychiatrica Scandinavica*, 370: 79–84.

Kripke, D.F., Nievergelt, C.M., Joo, E. et al. (2009) Circadian polymorphisms associated with affective disorders, *Journal of Circadian Rhythms*, 7: 2 [https://doi.org/10.1186/1740-3391-7-2].

Kronsell, A., Nordenskjöld, A. and Tiger, M. (2019) Less memory complaints with reduced stimulus dose during electroconvulsive therapy for depression, *Journal of Affective Disorders*, 259: 296–301.

Kruijver, F.P., Zhou, J.N., Pool, C.W. et al. (2000) Male-to-female transsexuals have female neuron numbers in a limbic nucleus, *Journal of Clinical Endocrinology and Metabolism*, 85: 2034–41.

Krupp, L.B., Christodoulou, C., Melville, P. et al. (2004) Donepezil improved memory in multiple sclerosis in a randomized clinical trial, *Neurology*, 63: 1579–85.

Kuhn, A., Bodmer, C., Stadlmayr, W. et al. (2008) Quality of life 15 years after sex reassignment surgery for transsexualism, *Fertility and Sterility*, 92: 1685–89.

Kulacaoglu, F. and Kose, S. (2018) Borderline personality disorder (BPD): in the midst of vulnerability, chaos, and awe, *Brain Sciences*, 8: 201 [https://doi.org/10.3390/brainsci8110201].

Kulka, R.A., Schlenger, W.E., Fairbank, J.A. et al. (1990) *Trauma and the Vietnam War Generation: Report of Findings from the National Vietnam Veterans Readjustment Study*, New York: Brunner/Mazel.

Külz, A.K., Landmann, S., Cludius, B. et al. (2019) Mindfulness-based cognitive therapy (MBCT) in patients with obsessive-compulsive disorder (OCD) and residual symptoms after cognitive behavioral therapy (CBT): a randomized controlled trial, *European Archives of Psychiatry and Clinical Neuroscience*, 269: 223–33.

Kurlansik, S.L. and Maffei, M.S. (2016) Somatic symptom disorder, *American Family Physician*, 93: 49–54.

Kuss, D.J. and Griffiths, M.D. (2012) Internet gaming addiction: a systematic review of empirical research, *International Journal of Mental Health and Addiction*, 10: 278–96.

Kuyken, W., Warren, F.C., Taylor, R.S. et al. (2016) Efficacy of mindfulness-based cognitive therapy in prevention of depressive relapse: an individual patient data meta-analysis from randomized trials, *JAMA Psychiatry*, 73: 565–74.

Laakso, M.P., Vaurio, O., Koivisto, E. et al. (2001) Psychopathy and the posterior hippocampus, *Behavioural Brain Research*, 118: 187–93.

Ladouceur, R., Jacques, C., Ferland, F. et al. (1999) Prevalence of problem gambling: a replication study 7 years later, *Canadian Journal of Psychiatry*, 44: 802–4.

Ladouceur, R., Sylvain, C., Boutin, C. et al. (2001) Cognitive treatment of pathological gambling, *Journal of Nervous and Mental Disease*, 189: 774–80.

Ladouceur, R., Sylvain, C., Boutin, C. et al. (2003) Group therapy for pathological gamblers: a cognitive approach, *Behavioural Research and Therapy*, 41: 87–96.

LaFrance, W.C., Jr., Baird, G.L., Barry, J.J. et al. (2014) Multicenter pilot treatment trial for psychogenic nonepileptic seizures: a randomized clinical trial, *JAMA Psychiatry*, 71: 997–1005.

Lahaie, M.A., Amsel, R., Khalife, S. et al. (2014) Can fear, pain, and muscle tension discriminate vaginismus from dyspareunia/provoked vestibulodynia? Implications for the new DSM-5 diagnosis of genito-pelvic pain/penetration disorder, *Archives of Sexual Behavior*, 44: 1537–50.

Lai, C.K., Chi, I. and Kayser-Jones, J. (2004) A randomized controlled trial of a specific reminiscence approach to promote the well-being of nursing home residents with dementia, *International Psychogeriatrics*, 16: 33–49.

Lai, D.W. (2004) Impact of culture on depressive symptoms of elderly Chinese immigrants, *Canadian Journal of Psychiatry*, 49: 820–27.

Lam, D., Ancelin, M.L., Ritchie, K. et al. (2018) Genotype-dependent associations between serotonin transporter gene (SLC6A4) DNA methylation and late-life depression, *BMC Psychiatry*, 18: 282 [https://doi.org/10.1186/s12888-018-1850-4].

Lam, D.H., Hayward, P., Watkins, E.R. et al. (2005) Relapse prevention in patients with bipolar disorder: cognitive therapy outcome after 2 years, *American Journal of Psychiatry*, 162: 324–29.

Lam, D.H., Watkins, E.R., Hayward, P. et al. (2003) A randomized controlled study of cognitive therapy for relapse prevention for bipolar affective disorder, *Archives of General Psychiatry*, 60: 145–52.

Lam, R.W., Lönn, S.L. and Despiégel, N. (2010) Escitalopram versus serotonin noradrenaline reuptake inhibitors as second step treatment for patients with major depressive disorder: a pooled analysis, *International Clinical Psychopharmacology*, 25: 199–203.

Lambert, M.J. and Ogles, B.M. (2014) Common factors: post hoc explanation or empirically based therapy approach?, *Psychotherapy*, 51: 500–4.

Lamotte, G., Shah, R.C., Lazarov, O. et al. (2017) Exercise training for persons with Alzheimer's disease and caregivers: a review of dyadic exercise interventions, *Journal of Motor Behavior*, 49: 365–77.

Laney, C. and Loftus, E.F. (2005) Traumatic memories are not necessarily accurate memories, *Canadian Journal of Psychiatry*, 50: 823–28.

Långström, N., Babchishin, K.M., Fazel, S. et al. (2015) Sexual offending runs in families: a 37-year nationwide study, *International Journal of Epidemiology*, 44: 713–20.

Långström, N., Enebrink, P., Laurén, E.-M. et al. (2013) Preventing sexual abusers of children from reoffending: systematic review of medical and psychological interventions, *British Medical Journal*, 347: f4630 [https://doi.org/10.1136/bmj.f4630].

Långström, N. and Zucker, K.J. (2005) Transvestic fetishism in the general population: prevalence and correlates, *Journal of Sexual and Marital Therapy*, 31: 87–95.

Lantz, E.L., Gaspar, M.E., DiTore, R. et al. (2018) Conceptualizing body dissatisfaction in eating disorders within a self-discrepancy framework: a review of evidence, *Eating and Weight Disorders*, 23: 275–91.

Larochelle, S., Diguer, L., Laverdière, O. (2011) Predictors of psychological treatment noncompletion among sexual offenders, *Clinical Psychology Review*, 31: 554–62.

Larsson, H., Tuvblad, C., Rijsdijk, F.V. et al. (2007) A common genetic factor explains the association between psychopathic personality and antisocial behavior, *Psychological Medicine*, 37: 15–26.

Lavender, J.M. and Mitchell, J.E. (2015) Eating disorders and their relationship to impulsivity, *Current Treatment Options in Psychiatry*, 2: 394–401.

Laws, D.R. and Marshall, W.L. (1991) Masturbatory reconditioning with sexual deviates: an evaluative review, *Advances in Behavior Research and Therapy*, 13: 13–25.

Lecerof, S.S., Stafström, M., Westerling, R. et al. (2016) Does social capital protect mental health among migrants in Sweden?, *Health Promotion International*, 31: 644–52.

Lee, C.S. and Dik, B.J. (2017) Associations among stress, gender, sources of social support, and health in emerging adults, *Stress and Health*, 33: 378–88.

Lee, R., Kavoussi, R.J. and Coccaro, E.F. (2008) Placebo-controlled, randomized trial of fluoxetine in the treatment of aggression in male intimate partner abusers, *International Clinical Psychopharmacology*, 23: 337–41.

Lee, S.A. and Kim, M.K. (2018) Effect of low frequency repetitive transcranial magnetic stimulation on depression and cognition of patients with traumatic brain injury: a randomized controlled trial, *Medical Science Monitor*, 24: 8789–94.

Lefaucheur, J.P., Aleman, A., Baeken, C. et al. (2020) Evidence-based guidelines on the therapeutic use of repetitive transcranial magnetic stimulation (rTMS): an update (2014–2018), *Clinical Neurophysiology*, 131: 474–528.

Leff, J. and Vaughn, C. (1985) *Expressed Emotions in Families: Its Significance for Mental Illness*, New York: Guilford Press.

Legrand, L.N., Keyes, M., McGue, M. et al. (2008) Rural environments reduce the genetic influence on adolescent substance use and rule-breaking behavior, *Psychological Medicine*, 38: 1341–50.

Le Grange, D., Crosby, R.D., Rathouz, P.J. et al. (2007) A randomized controlled comparison of family-based treatment and supportive psychotherapy for adolescent bulimia nervosa, *Archives of General Psychiatry*, 64: 1049–56.

Le Grange, D., Hughes, E.K., Court, A. et al. (2016) Randomized clinical trial of parent-focused treatment and family-based treatment for adolescent anorexia nervosa, *Journal of the American Academy of Child and Adolescent Psychiatry*, 55: 683–92.

Lengua, L.J., Long, A.C., Smith, K.I. et al. (2005) Pre-attack symptomatology and temperament as predictors of children's responses to the September 11 terrorist attacks, *Journal of Child Psychology and Psychiatry*, 46: 631–45.

Lenox, R.H., McNamara, R.F., Papke, R.L. et al. (1998) Neurobiology of lithium: an update, *Journal of Clinical Psychiatry*, 59 (suppl. 6): 37–47.

Leuzinger-Bohleber, M., Hautzinger, M., Fiedler, G. et al. (2019) Outcome of psychoanalytic and cognitive-behavioural long-term therapy with chronically depressed patients: a controlled trial with preferential and randomized allocation, *Canadian Journal of Psychiatry*, 64: 47–58.

Levin, H.S. (1993) Neurobehavioral sequelae of closed head injury, in P.R. Cooper (ed.) *Head Injury*, Baltimore, MD: Williams & Wilkins.

Levine, B., Robertson, I.H., Clare, L. et al. (2000) Rehabilitation of executive functioning: an experimental-clinical validation of goal management training, *Journal of the International Neuropsychological Society*, 6: 299–312.

Levinson, H. (2011) The strange and curious history of lobotomy, *BBC News Magazine*, 8 November [https://www.bbc.co.uk/news/magazine-15629160].

Levinson, C.A., Zerwas, S.C., Brosof, L.C. et al. (2019) Associations between dimensions of anorexia nervosa and obsessive-compulsive disorder: an examination of personality and psychological factors in patients with anorexia nervosa, *European Eating Disorders Review*, 27: 161–72.

Levran, O., Londono, D., O'Hara, K. et al. (2008) Genetic susceptibility to heroin addiction: a candidate gene association study, *Genes, Brain, and Behavior*, 7: 720–29.

Lewinsohn, P.M., Youngren, M.A. and Grosscup, S.J. (1979) Reinforcement and depression, in A. Depue (ed.) *The Psychobiology of the Depressive Disorders*, New York: Academic Press.

Lewy, A.J., Bauer, V.K. and Cutler, N.L. (1998) Morning vs. evening light treatment of patients with winter depression, *Archives of General Psychiatry*, 55: 890–96.

Lewy, A.J., Lefler, B.J., Emens, J.S. et al. (2006) The circadian basis of winter depression, *Proceedings of the National Academy of Sciences USA*, 103: 7414–19.

Li, Y., Li, Y., Li, X. et al. (2017) Head injury as a risk factor for dementia and Alzheimer's disease: a systematic review and meta-analysis of 32 observational studies, *PloS One*, 12: e0169650 [https://doi.org/10.1371/journal.pone.0169650].

Liao, Y.C., Chou, C.Y., Chang, C.T. et al. (2017) Qi deficiency is associated with depression in chronic hemodialysis patients, *Complementary Therapies in Medicine*, 30: 102–6.

Lichtenstein, P., Carlström, E., Råstam, M. et al. (2010) The genetics of autism spectrum disorders and related neuropsychiatric disorders in childhood, *American Journal of Psychiatry*, 167: 1357–63.

Liddle, P., Carpenter, W.T. and Crow, T. (1994) Syndromes of schizophrenia: classic literature, *British Journal of Psychiatry*, 165: 721–27.

Lieberman, J.A., Kinon, B.J. and Loebel, A.D. (1990) Dopaminergic mechanisms in idiopathic and drug-induced psychoses, *Schizophrenia Bulletin*, 16: 97–109.

Lifford, K.J., Harold, G.T. and Thapar, A. (2009) Parent-child hostility and child ADHD symptoms: a genetically sensitive and longitudinal analysis, *Journal of Child Psychology and Psychiatry*, 50: 1468–76.

Lim, G.Y., Tam, W.W., Lu, Y. et al. (2018) Prevalence of depression in the community from 30 countries between 1994 and 2014, *Science Reports*, 8: 2861 [https://doi.org/10.1038/s41598-018-21243-x].

Lin, W., Gong, L., Xia, M. et al. (2018) Prevalence of posttraumatic stress disorder among road traffic accident survivors: a PRISMA-compliant meta-analysis, *Medicine*, 97: e9693 [https://doi.org/10.1097/MD.0000000000009693].

Linde, K., Treml, J., Steinig, J. et al. (2017) Grief interventions for people bereaved by suicide: a systematic review, *PloS One*, 12: e0179496 [https://doi.org/10.1371/journal.pone.0179496].

Linehan, M.M. (1993) *Cognitive Behavioral Treatment of Borderline Personality Disorder*, New York: Guilford Press.

Linehan, M.M., Comtois, K.A., Murray, A.M. et al. (2006) Two-year randomized controlled trial and follow-up of dialectical behavior therapy vs. therapy by experts for suicidal behaviors and borderline personality disorder, *Archives of General Psychiatry*, 63: 757–66.

Linehan, M.M., Korslund, K.E., Harned, M.S. et al. (2015) Dialectical behavior therapy for high suicide risk in individuals with borderline personality disorder: a randomized clinical trial and component analysis, *JAMA Psychiatry*, 72: 475–82.

Linehan, M.M., McDavid, J.D., Brown, M.Z. et al. (2008) Olanzapine plus dialectical behavior therapy for women with high irritability who meet criteria for borderline personality disorder: a double-blind, placebo-controlled pilot study, *Journal of Clinical Psychiatry*, 69: 999–1005.

Lingford-Hughes, A. (2005) Human brain imaging and substance abuse, *Current Opinion in Pharmacology*, 5: 42–46.

Lisanby, S.H., Maddox, J.H., Prudic, J. et al. (2000) The effects of electroconvulsive therapy on memory of autobiographical and public events, *Archives of General Psychiatry*, 57: 581–90.

Liu, S.K., Fitzgerald, P.B., Daigle, M. et al. (2009) The relationship between cortical inhibition, antipsychotic treatment, and the symptoms of schizophrenia, *Biological Psychiatry*, 65: 503–9.

Liu, X., Wang, X.M., Ge, J.J. et al. (2018) Effects of the portage early education program on Chinese children with global developmental delay, *Medicine*, 97: e12202 [https://doi.org/10.1097/MD.0000000000012202].

Liu, Z., Sun, Y.Y. and Zhong, B.L. (2018) Mindfulness-based stress reduction for family carers of people with dementia, *Cochrane Database of Systematic Reviews*, 8: CD012791 [https://doi.org/10.1002/14651858.CD012791.pub2].

Livingston, G., Sommerlad, A., Orgeta, V. et al. (2017) Dementia prevention, intervention, and care, *Lancet*, 390: 2673–734.

Ljotsson, B., Lundin, C., Mitsell, K. et al. (2007) Remote treatment of bulimia nervosa and binge eating disorder: a randomized trial of Internet-assisted cognitive behavioural therapy, *Behaviour Research and Therapy*, 45: 649–61.

Lloyd-Evans, D. and Johnson, S. (2014) *Crisis resolution teams – how are they performing*, Shoreham-by-Sea: Mental Health Today [https://www.mentalhealthtoday.co.uk/crisis-resolution-teams-how-are-they-performing; accessed November 2019].

Lock, J., Le Grange, D., Agras, W.S. et al. (2010) Randomized clinical trial comparing family-based treatment with adolescent-focused individual therapy for adolescents with anorexia nervosa, *Archives of General Psychiatry*, 67: 1025–32.

Loebel, J.P., Loebel, J.S., Dager, S.R. et al. (1991) Anticipation of nursing home placement may be a precipitant of suicide among the elderly, *Journal of the American Geriatric Society*, 39: 407–8.

Loewe, B., Zipfel, S., Buchholz, C. et al. (2001) Long-term outcome of anorexia nervosa in a prospective 21-year follow-up study, *Psychological Medicine*, 31: 881–90.

Loftus, E.F. and Coan, D. (1998) The construction of childhood memories, in D. Peters (ed.) *The Child Witness in Context: Cognitive, Social, and Legal Perspectives*, New York: Kluwer.

Loftus, E.F. and Davis, D. (2006) Recovered memories, *Annual Review of Clinical Psychology*, 2: 469–98.

Loftus, E.F. and Ketcham, K. (1994) *The Myth of Repressed Memory*, New York: St. Martin's Press.

Lopez, V.A. and Emmer, E.T. (2002) Influences of beliefs and values on male adolescents' decision to commit violent offenses, *Psychology of Men and Masculinity*, 3: 28–40.

Lopresti, A.L. and Drummond, P.D. (2014) Saffron (*Crocus sativus*) for depression: a systematic review of clinical studies and examination of underlying antidepressant mechanisms of action, *Human Psychopharmacology: Clinical and Experimental*, 29: 517–27.

Lorant, V., Deliège, D., Eaton, W. et al. (2003) Socioeconomic inequalities in depression: a meta-analysis, *American Journal of Epidemiology*, 157: 98–112.

Lotrich, F.E. (2015) Inflammatory cytokine-associated depression, *Brain Research*, 1617: 113–25.

Lovaas, O.I. (1987) Behavioral treatment and normal educational and intellectual functioning in young autistic children, *Journal of Consulting and Clinical Psychology*, 55: 3–9.

Lowe, K., Allen, D., Jones, E. et al. (2007) Challenging behaviours: prevalence and topographies, *Journal of Intellectual Disability Research*, 51: 625–36.

Lu, C.L., Wang, Y.C., Chen, J.Y. et al. (2010) Support for the involvement of the *ERBB4* gene in schizophrenia: a genetic association analysis, *Neuroscience Letters*, 481: 120–25.

Lucas, R. (2003) The relationship between psychoanalysis and schizophrenia, *International Journal of Psychoanalysis*, 84: 3–15.

Ludwig, L., Pasman, J.A., Nicholson, T. et al. (2018) Stressful life events and maltreatment in conversion (functional neurological) disorder: systematic review and meta-analysis of case-control studies, *Lancet Psychiatry*, 5: 307–20.

Luhrmann, T.M., Alderson-Day, B., Bell, V. et al. (2019) Beyond trauma: a multiple pathways approach to auditory hallucinations in clinical and nonclinical populations, *Schizophrenia Bulletin*, 45: S24–S31.

Lund, C. and Cois, A. (2018) Simultaneous social causation and social drift: longitudinal analysis of depression and poverty in South Africa, *Journal of Affective Disorders*, 229: 396–402.

Lund, I. (2009) Gambling behaviour and the prevalence of gambling problems in adult EGM gamblers when EGMs are banned: a natural experiment, *Journal of Gambling Studies*, 25: 215–25.

Luque, F.A. and Jaffe, S.L. (2009) The molecular and cellular pathogenesis of dementia of the Alzheimer's type: an overview, *International Review of Neurobiology*, 84: 151–65.

Lynam, D.R., Caspi, A., Moffitt, T.E. et al. (2005) Adolescent psychopathy and the big five: results from two samples, *Journal of Abnormal Child Psychology*, 33: 431–43.

Lynn, S.J., Lilienfeld, S.O., Merckelbach, H. et al. (2014) The trauma model of dissociation: inconvenient truths and stubborn fictions. Comment on Dalenberg et al. (2012), *Psychological Bulletin*, 140: 896–910.

Lyon, H.M., Startup, M. and Bentall, R.P. (1999) Social cognition and the manic defense: attributions, selective attention, and self-schema in bipolar affective disorder, *Journal of Abnormal Psychology*, 108: 273–82.

Lyon-Caen, O., Jouvent, R., Hauser, S. et al. (1986) Cognitive function in recent onset demyelinating diseases, *Archives of Neurology*, 43: 1138–41.

Ma, J.H., Sun, X.Y., Guo, T.J. et al. (2018) Association on DISC1 SNPs with schizophrenia risk: a meta-analysis, *Psychiatry Research*, 270: 306–9.

MacMillan, H.L., Fleming, J.E., Streiner, D.L. et al. (2001) Childhood abuse and lifetime psychopathology in a community sample, *American Journal of Psychiatry*, 58: 1878–83.

Maes, S., Verhoeven, C., Kittel, F. et al. (1998) Effects of the Brabantia-project, a Dutch wellness-health programme at the worksite, *American Journal of Public Health*, 88: 1037–41.

Magill, M. and Ray, L.A. (2009) Cognitive-behavioral treatment with adult alcohol and illicit drug users: a meta-analysis of randomized controlled trials, *Journal of Studies on Alcohol and Drugs*, 70: 516–27.

Magnusson, A. and Partonen, T. (2005) The diagnosis, symptomatology, and epidemiology of seasonal affective disorder, *CNS Spectrum*, 10: 625–34.

Magnusson, A. and Partonen, T. (2010) Prevalence, in T. Partonen and S.R Pandi-Perumal (eds.) *Seasonal Affective Disorder: Practice and Research*, 2nd edition, New York: Oxford University Press.

Mahmood, T. and Silverstone, T. (2001) Serotonin and bipolar disorder, *Journal of Affective Disorders*, 66: 1–11.

Maia, T.V., Cooney, R.E. and Peterson, B.S. (2008) The neural bases of obsessive-compulsive disorder in children and adults, *Development and Psychopathology*, 20: 1251–83.

Maibom, H.L. (2014) To treat a psychopath, *Theoretical Medicine and Bioethics*, 35: 31–42.

Malaspina, C., Corcoran, K.R., Kleinhaus, M.C. et al. (2008) Acute maternal stress in pregnancy and schizophrenia in offspring: a cohort prospective study, *BMC Psychiatry*, 8: 71 [https://doi.org/10.1186/1471-244X-8-71].

Malec, J.F., Van Houtven, C.H., Tanielian, T. et al. (2017) Impact of TBI on caregivers of veterans with TBI: burden and interventions, *Brain Injury*, 31: 1235–45.

Malesky, L.A., Jr. and Ennis, L. (2004) Supportive distortions: an analysis of posts on a pedophile internet message board, *Journal of Addictions and Offender Counseling*, 24: 92–100.

Malik, M., Bilal, F., Kazmi, S. et al. (2010) Depression and anxiety in dissociative (conversion) disorder patients at a tertiary care psychiatric facility, *Rawal Medical Journal*, 35: 224–26.

Malizia, A.L. (2000) Neurosurgery for psychiatric disorders, in M.G. Gelder, J.J. Lopez-Ibor, Jr. and N.C. Andreasen (eds.) *New Oxford Textbook of Psychiatry*, Oxford: Oxford University Press.

Malojcic, B., Mubrin, Z., Coric, B. et al. (2008) Consequences of mild traumatic brain injury on information processing assessed with attention and short-term memory tasks, *Journal of Neurotrauma*, 25: 30–37.

Manca, R., Mitolo, M., Stabile, M.R. et al. (2019) Multiple brain networks support processing speed abilities of patients with multiple sclerosis, *Postgraduate Medicine*, 131: 523–32.

Mann, J.J. and Michel, C.A. (2016) Prevention of firearm suicide in the United States: what works and what is possible, *American Journal of Psychiatry*, 173: 969–79.

Mannuzza, S. and Klein, R.G. (2000) Long-term prognosis in attention-deficit/hyperactivity disorder, *Child and Adolescent Psychiatric Clinics of North America*, 9: 711–26.

Marcos, M., Pastor, I., de la Calle, C. et al. (2012) Cannabinoid receptor 1 gene is associated with alcohol dependence, *Alcoholism, Clinical and Experimental Research*, 36: 267–71.

Marcus, D.K., Gurley, J.R., Marchi, M.M. et al. (2006) Cognitive and perceptual variables in hypochondriasis and health anxiety: a systematic review, *Clinical Psychology Review*, 27: 127–39.

Marjoram, D., Tansley, H., Miller, P. et al. (2005) A Theory of Mind investigation into the appreciation of visual jokes in schizophrenia, *BMC Psychiatry*, 5: 12 [https://doi.org/10.1186/1471-244X-5-12].

Marks, I. (1977) Phobias and obsessions: clinical phenomena in search of laboratory models, in J.D. Maser and M.E.P. Seligman (eds.) *Psychopathology: Experimental Models*, San Francisco, CA: Freeman.

Marks, I., Gelder, M. and Bancroft, J. (1970) Sexual deviants two years after electric shock aversion, *British Journal of Psychiatry*, 117: 173–85.

Marks, I., Green, R. and Mataix-Cols, D. (2000) Adult gender identity disorder can remit, *Comprehensive Psychiatry*, 41: 273–75.

Marks, I., Lovell, K., Noshirvani, H. et al. (1996) Treatment of post-traumatic stress disorder by exposure and/or cognition restructuring, *Archives of General Psychiatry*, 55: 317–25.

Marques, J.K., Wiederanders, M., Day, D.M. et al. (2005) Effects of a relapse prevention program on sexual recidivism: final results from California's sex offender treatment and evaluation project (SOTEP), *Sexual Abuse*, 17: 79–107.

Marsch, L.A., Bickel, W.K., Badger, G.J. et al. (2005) Comparison of pharmacological treatments for opioid-dependent adolescents: a randomized controlled trial, *Archives of General Psychiatry*, 62: 1157–64.

Marshall, J.C., Halligan, P.W., Fink, G.R. et al. (1997) The functional anatomy of a hysterical paralysis, *Cognition*, 64: B1–B8.

Martins, S.S., Sarvet, A., Santaella-Tenorio, J. et al. (2017) Changes in US lifetime heroin use and heroin use disorder: prevalence from the 2001–2002 to 2012–2013 National Epidemiologic Survey on Alcohol and Related Conditions, *JAMA Psychiatry*, 74: 445–55.

Maslow, A.H. (1970) *Motivation and Personality*, New York: Harper & Row.

Mason, K.E., Baker, E., Blakely, T. et al. (2013) Housing affordability and mental health: does the relationship differ for renters and home purchasers?, *Social Science and Medicine*, 94: 91–97.

Masters, W.H. and Johnson, V.E. (1970) *Human Sexual Inadequacy*, Boston, MA: Little, Brown.

Matthews, K.A., Räikkönen, K., Gallo, L. et al. (2008) Association between socioeconomic status and metabolic syndrome in women: testing the reserve capacity model, *Health Psychology*, 27: 576–83.

Mattick, R.P., Breen, C., Kimber, J. et al. (2014) Buprenorphine maintenance versus placebo or methadone maintenance for opioid dependence, *Cochrane Database of Systematic Reviews*, 2: CD002207 [https://doi.org/10.1002/14651858.CD002207.pub4].

Maunder, R.G., Hunter, J.J., Atkinson, L. et al. (2017) An attachment-based model of the relationship between childhood adversity and somatization in children and adults, *Journal of Psychosomatic Medicine*, 79: 506–513.

Mayou, R., Bryant, B. and Ehlers, A. (2001) Prediction of psychological outcomes one year after a motor vehicle accident, *American Journal of Psychiatry*, 158: 1231–38.

McConaghy, N., Blaszczynski, A. and Frankova, A. (1991) Comparison of imaginal desensitization with other behavioural treatments of pathological gambling: a two to nine year follow-up, *British Journal of Psychiatry*, 159: 390–93.

McCormick, R. (2017) Does access to green space impact the mental well-being of children: a systematic review, *Journal of Pediatric Nursing*, 37: 3–7.

McGarry, E., Vernon, T. and Baktha, A. (2020) Brief report: A pilot online Pivotal Response Treatment training program for parents of toddlers with autism spectrum disorder, *Journal of Autism and Developmental Disorders*, 50: 3424–31.

McGorry, P.D., Yung, A.R., Phillips, L.J. et al. (2002) Randomized controlled trial of interventions designed to reduce the risk of progression to first-episode psychosis in a clinical sample with subthreshold symptoms, *Archives of General Psychiatry*, 59: 921–28.

McGuffin, P., Katz, R., Watkins, S. et al. (1996) A hospital-based twin register of the heritability of DSM-IV unipolar depression, *Archives of General Psychiatry*, 53: 129–36.

McGuire, P.K., Silbersweig, D.A., Wright, I. et al. (1996) The neural correlates of inner speech and auditory verbal imagery in schizophrenia: relationship to auditory verbal hallucinations, *British Journal of Psychiatry*, 169: 148–59.

McIntosh, V.W., Jordan, J., Carter, F.A. et al. (2005) Three psychotherapies for anorexia nervosa: a randomized, controlled trial, *American Journal of Psychiatry*, 162: 741–47.

McKay, R., Langdon, R. and Coltheart, M. (2005) Paranoia, persecutory delusions and attributional biases, *Psychiatry Research*, 136: 233–45.

McLaughlin, K.A., Kubzansky, L.D., Dunn, E.C. et al. (2010) Childhood social environment, emotional reactivity to stress, and mood and anxiety disorders across the life course, *Depression and Anxiety*, 27: 1087–94.

McLean, P.D., Whittal, M.L., Thordarson, D.S. et al. (2001) Cognitive versus behavior therapy in the group treatment of obsessive-compulsive disorder, *Journal of Consulting and Clinical Psychology*, 69: 205–14.

McMahon, A. and Rhudick, P. (1964) Reminiscing, *Archives of General Psychiatry*, 10: 292–98.

McManus, F., Surawy, C., Muse, K. et al. (2012) A randomized clinical trial of mindfulness-based cognitive therapy versus unrestricted services for health anxiety (hypochondriasis), *Journal of Consulting and Clinical Psychology*, 80: 817–28.

McManus, S., Bebbington, P., Jenkins, R. et al. (eds.) (2016) *Mental Health and Wellbeing in England: Adult Psychiatric Morbidity Survey 2014*, Leeds: NHS Digital.

McNally, R.J. (2012) Searching for repressed memory, in R.F. Belli (ed.) *True and False Recovered Memories: Toward a Reconciliation of the Debate*, Nebraska Symposium on Motivation vol. 58, Dordrecht: Springer.

McNally, R.J., Lasko, N.B., Clancy, S.A. et al. (2004) Psychophysiological responding during script-driven imagery in people reporting abduction by space aliens, *Psychological Science*, 15: 493–97.

Meana, M., Fertel, E. and Maykut, C. (2017) Treating genital pain associated with sexual intercourse, in Z.D. Peterson (ed.) *The Wiley Handbook of Sex Therapy*, Chichester: Wiley-Blackwell.

Meehl, P.E. (1990) Towards an integrated theory of schizotaxia, schizotypy, and schizophrenia, *Journal of Personality Disorders*, 4: 1–99.

Meehl, S., Landsberg, M.W., Schmidt, A.C. et al. (2014) Why do bad things happen to me? Attributional style, depressed mood, and persecutory delusions in patients with schizophrenia, *Schizophrenia Bulletin*, 40: 1338–46.

Meesters, Y., Beersma, D.G., Bouhuys, A.L. et al. (1999) Prophylactic treatment of seasonal affective disorder (SAD) by using light visors: bright white or infrared light?, *Biological Psychiatry*, 46: 239–46.

Meichenbaum, D. (1985) *Stress Inoculation Training*, New York: Pergamon Press.

Meier, S.M. and Deckert, J. (2019) Genetics of anxiety disorders, *Current Psychiatry Reports*, 21: 16 [https://doi.org/10.1007/s11920-019-1002-7].

Melchior, M., Caspi, A., Milne, B.J. et al. (2007) Work stress precipitates depression and anxiety in young, working women and men, *Psychological Medicine*, 37: 1119–29.

Mendez, M.F., Chow, T., Ringman, J. et al. (2000) Pedophilia and temporal lobe disturbances, *Journal of Neuropsychiatry and Clinical Neuroscience*, 12: 71–76.

Meng, F.Q., Han, H.Y., Luo, J. et al. (2019) Efficacy of cognitive behavioural therapy with medication for patients with obsessive-compulsive disorder: a multicentre randomised controlled trial in China, *Journal of Affective Disorders*, 253: 184–92.

Mental Health Foundation (MHF) (2016) *Fundamental Facts about Mental Health*, London: MHF.

Mental Health Foundation (MHF) (2019) *Black, Asian and Minority Ethnic (BAME) communities*, London: MHF [https://www.mentalhealth.org.uk/a-to-z/b/black-asian-and-minority-ethnic-bame-communities].

Merckelbach, H. and de Jong, P.J. (1999) Evolutionary models of phobias, in G.C.L. Davey (ed.) *Phobias: A Handbook of Theory, Research, and Treatment*, Chichester: Wiley.

Merskey, H. (1995) *The Analysis of Hysteria: Understanding Conversion and Dissociation*, 2nd edition, London: Gaskell.

Mews, A., Di Bella, L. and Purver, M. (2017) *Impact Evaluation of the Prison-based Core Sex Offender Treatment Programme*, London: Ministry of Justice.

Meyer, R.E. (1995) Biology of psychoactive substance dependence disorders: opiates, cocaine, ethanol, in A.F. Schatzberg and C.B. Nemeroff (eds.) *The American Psychiatric Press Handbook of Psychopharmacology*, Washington, DC: American Psychiatric Press.

Mez, J., Daneshvar, D.H., Kiernan, P.T. et al. (2017) Clinicopathological evaluation of chronic traumatic encephalopathy in players of American football, *Journal of the American Medical Association*, 318: 360–70.

Michel, J.A. and Mateer, C.A. (2006) Attention rehabilitation following stroke and traumatic brain injury: a review, *Europa Medicophysica*, 42: 59–67.

Mihailides, S., Devilly, G.J. and Ward, T. (2004) Implicit cognitive distortions and sexual offending, *Sexual Abuse: A Journal of Research and Treatment*, 16: 333–50.

Miklowitz, D.J., Simponeau, T.L., George, E.L. et al. (2003) Family-focused treatment of bipolar disorder: year effects of a psychoeducational program in conjunction with pharmacotherapy, *Biological Psychiatry*, 48: 582–92.

Mikton, C. and Grounds, A. (2007) Cross-cultural clinical judgment bias in personality disorder diagnosis by forensic psychiatrists in the UK: a case vignette study, *Journal of Personality Disorders*, 21 (4): 400–17.

Millar, J.K., Wilson-Annan, J.C., Anderson, S. et al. (2000) Disruption of two novel genes by a translocation co-segregating with schizophrenia, *Human Molecular Genetics*, 9: 1415–23.

Miller, E. (1999) Conversion hysteria: is it a viable concept?, in P. Halligan (ed.) *Conversion Hysteria: Towards a Neuropsychological Account*, Hove: Psychology Press.

Miller, W.R. and Rollnick, S. (2013) *Motivational Interviewing: Preparing People for Change*, 3rd edition, New York: Guilford Press.

Miller, W.R., Zweben, A., DiClemete, C.C. et al. (1994) *Motivational Enhancement Therapy Manual*, Rockville, MD: National Institute on Alcohol Abuse and Alcoholism.

Miltz, A., Lampe, F., McCormack, S. et al. (2019) Prevalence and correlates of depressive symptoms among gay, bisexual and other men who have sex with men in the PROUD randomised clinical trial of HIV pre-exposure prophylaxis, *BMJ Open*, 9: e031085 [https://doi.org/10.1136/bmjopen-2019-031085].

MIND (2018) *Neurosurgery for Mental Disorder (NMD)*, London: MIND [https://www.mind.org.uk/information-support/drugs-and-treatments/neurosurgery-for-mental-disorder-nmd/about-nmd/#.XhhFB3d2vnM].

Minden, S.L. and Schiffer, R.B. (1990) Affective disorders in multiple sclerosis: review and recommendations for clinical research, *Archives of Neurology*, 47: 98–104.

Minuchin, S., Rosman, B. and Baker, L. (1978) *Psychosomatic Families: Anorexia Nervosa in Context*, Cambridge, MA: Harvard University Press.

Miranda, J. and Gross, J.J. (1997) Cognitive vulnerability depression, and the mood-state dependent hypothesis: is it out of sight out of mind?, *Cognition and Emotion*, 11: 585–605.

Misiak, B., Stramecki, F., Gawęda, Ł. et al. (2018) Interactions between variation in candidate genes and environmental factors in the etiology of schizophrenia and bipolar disorder: a systematic review, *Molecular Neurobiology*, 55: 5075–100.

Mistretta, E.G., Davis, M.C., Temkit, M. et al. (2018) Resilience training for work-related stress among health care workers: results of a randomized clinical trial comparing in-person and smartphone-delivered interventions, *Journal of Occupational and Environmental Medicine*, 60: 559–68.

Mitte, K., Noack, P., Steil, R. and Hautzinger, M. (2005) A meta-analytic review of the efficacy of drug treatment in generalized anxiety disorder, *Journal of Clinical Psychopharmacology*, 25: 141–50.

Moene, F.C., Spinhoven, P., Hoogduin, K.A. et al. (2003) A randomized controlled clinical trial of a hypnosis-based treatment for patients with conversion disorder, motor type, *International Journal of Clinical and Experimental Hypnosis*, 51: 29–50.

Mogg, K., Baldwin, D.S., Brodrick, P. et al. (2004) Effect of short-term SSRI treatment on cognitive bias in generalised anxiety disorder, *Psychopharmacology*, 176: 466–70.

Mohr, D.C., Goodkin, D.E., Bacchetti, P. et al. (2000a) Psychological stress and the subsequent appearance of new brain MRI lesions in MS, *Neurology*, 55: 55–61.

Mohr, D.C., Likosky, W., Bertagnolli, A. et al. (2000b) Telephone-administered cognitive-behavioral therapy for the treatment of depressive symptoms in multiple sclerosis, *Journal of Consulting and Clinical Psychology*, 68: 356–61.

Mokros, A. and Banse, R. (2019) The 'Dunkelfeld' Project for self-identified pedophiles: a reappraisal of its effectiveness, *Journal of Sexual Medicine*, 16: 609–13.

Molyneux, G.J., McCarthy, G.M., McEniff, S. et al. (2008) Prevalence and predictors of carer burden and depression in carers of patients referred to an old age psychiatric service, *International Psychogeriatrics*, 20: 1193–202.

Mondraty, N., Birmingham, C.L., Touyz, S. et al. (2005) Randomized controlled trial of olanzapine in the treatment of cognitions in anorexia nervosa, *Australasian Psychiatry*, 13: 72–75.

Montgomery, S.A., Dufour, H., Brion, S. et al. (1993) Guidelines for treatment of depressive illness with antidepressants, *Journal of Psychopharmacology*, 7: 19–23.

Monti, P.M., Mastroleo, N.R., Barnett, N.P. et al. (2016) Brief motivational intervention to reduce alcohol and HIV/sexual risk behavior in emergency department patients: a randomized controlled trial, *Journal of Consulting and Clinical Psychology*, 84: 580–91.

Moore, B.A., Fiellin, D.A., Cutter, C.J. et al. (2016) Cognitive behavioral therapy improves treatment outcomes for prescription opioid users in primary care buprenorphine treatment, *Journal of Substance Abuse Treatment*, 71: 54–57.

Moran, K. and Priebe, S. (2016) Better quality of life in patients offered financial incentives for taking anti-psychotic medication: linked to improved adherence or more money?, *Quality of Life Research*, 25: 1897–902.

Moran, L.V., Ongur, D., Hsu, J. et al. (2019) Psychosis with methylphenidate or amphetamine in patients with ADHD, *New England Journal of Medicine*, 380: 1128–38.

Morey, L.C. and Hopwood, C.J. (2019) Expert preferences for categorical, dimensional, and mixed/hybrid approaches to personality disorder diagnosis, *Journal of Personality Disorders* [https://doi.org/10.1521/pedi_2019_33_398].

Morey, R.A., Gold, A.L., LaBar, K.S. et al. (2012) Amygdala volume changes in posttraumatic stress disorder in a large case-controlled veterans group, *Archives of General Psychiatry*, 69: 1169–78.

Morimoto, T., Hashimoto, K., Yasumatsu, H. et al. (2002) Neuropharmacological profile of a novel potential atypical antipsychotic drug Y-931 (8-fluoro-12-(4-methylpiperazin-1-yl)-6H-[1]benzothieno[2,3-b][1,5] benzodiazepine maleate), *Neuropsychopharmacology*, 26: 456–67.

Morken, G., Widen, J.H. and Grawe, R.W. (2008) Non-adherence to antipsychotic medication, relapse and rehospitalisation in recent-onset schizophrenia, *BMC Psychiatry*, 8: 32 [https://doi.org/10.1186/1471-244X-8-32].

Morley, K.C., Logge, W., Pearson, S.A. et al. (2016) National trends in alcohol pharmacotherapy: findings from an Australian claims database, *Drug and Alcohol Dependence*, 166: 254–57.

Morrison, A.P., French, P., Parker, S. et al. (2006) Three-year follow-up of a randomized controlled trial of cognitive therapy for the prevention of psychosis in people at ultrahigh risk, *Schizophrenia Bulletin*, 33: 682–87.

Morrison, A.P., Law, H., Carter, L. et al. (2018) Antipsychotic drugs versus cognitive behavioural therapy versus a combination of both in people with psychosis: a randomised controlled pilot and feasibility study, *Lancet Psychiatry*, 5: 411–23.

Morton, J., Andrews, B., Bekerian, D. et al. (1995) *Recovered Memories*, Leicester: British Psychological Society.

Mostert, J.P., Koch, M.W., Heerings, M. et al. (2008) Therapeutic potential of fluoxetine in neurological disorders, *CNS Neuroscience and Therapeutics*, 14: 153–64.

Mowrer, O.H. (1947) On the dual nature of learning: a reinterpretation of 'conditioning' and 'problem solving', *Harvard Education Review*, 17: 102–48.

Moul, C., Dobson-Stone, C., Brennan, J. et al. (2013) An exploration of the serotonin system in antisocial boys with high levels of callous-unemotional traits, *PloS One*, 8: e56619 [https://doi.org/10.1371/journal.pone.0056619].

Muhle, R., Trentacoste, S.V. and Rapin, I. (2004) The genetics of autism, *Pediatrics*, 113: e472–e486.

Muhuri, P.K., Gfroerer, J.C. and Davies, M.C. (2013) Associations of nonmedical pain reliever use and initiation of heroin use in the United States, *CBHSQ Data Review*, August [https://www.samhsa.gov/data/sites/default/files/DR006/DR006/nonmedical-pain-reliever-use-2013.htm].

Mulle, J.G., Sharp, W.G. and Cubells, J.F. (2013) The gut microbiome: a new frontier in autism research, *Current Psychiatry Reports*, 15: 337 [https://doi.org/10.1007/s11920-012-0337-0].

Murad, M.H., Elamin, M.B., Garcia, M.Z. et al. (2010) Hormonal therapy and sex reassignment: a systematic review and meta-analysis of quality of life and psychosocial outcomes, *Clinical Endocrinology*, 72: 214–31.

Murch, W.S., Chu, S.W.M. and Clark, L. (2017) Measuring the slot machine zone with attentional dual tasks and respiratory sinus arrhythmia, *Psychology of Addictive Behaviors*, 31: 375–84.

Muris, P., de Jongh, A., Merckelbach, H. et al. (1998) Thought suppression in phobic and nonphobic dental patients, *Anxiety, Stress and Coping*, 11: 275–87.

Murphy, E., O'Sullivan, I., O'Donovan, D. et al. (2016) The association between parental attitudes and alcohol consumption and adolescent alcohol consumption in Southern Ireland: a cross-sectional study, *BMC Public Health*, 16: 821 [https://doi.org/10.1186/s12889-016-3504-0].

Murphy, K. and Barkley, R.A. (1996) Attention deficit hyperactivity disorder in adults: comorbidities and adaptive impairments, *Comprehensive Psychiatry*, 37: 393–401.

Murphy, P., Bentall, R.P., Freeman, D. et al. (2018) The paranoia as defence model of persecutory delusions: a systematic review and meta-analysis, *Lancet Psychiatry*, 5: 913–29.

Murphy, R., O'Donoghue, S., Counihan, T. et al. (2017) Neuropsychiatric syndromes of multiple sclerosis, *Journal of Neurology, Neurosurgery and Psychiatry*, 88: 697–708.

Murray, J.B. (2000) Psychological profiles of pedophiles and child molesters, *Journal of Psychology*, 134: 211–24.

Murray, L., Creswell, C. and Cooper, P.J. (2009) The development of anxiety disorders in childhood: an integrative review, *Psychological Medicine*, 39: 1413–23.

Murray, L., De Rosnay, M., Pearson, J. et al. (2008) Intergenerational transmission of social anxiety: the role of social referencing processes in infancy, *Child Development*, 79: 1049–64.

Myers, S.G. and Wells, A. (2005) Obsessive-compulsive symptoms: the contribution of metacognitions and responsibility, *Journal of Anxiety Disorders*, 19: 806–17.

Myhr, G., Sookman, D. and Pinard, G. (2004) Attachment security and parental bonding in adults with obsessive-compulsive disorder: a comparison with depressed out-patients and healthy controls, *Acta Psychiatrica Scandinavica*, 109: 447–56.

Myles, N., Large, M., Myles, H. et al. (2017) Australia's economic transition, unemployment, suicide and mental health needs, *Australia and New Zealand Journal of Psychiatry*, 51: 119–23.

Nagel, B. and Leiper, R. (1999) A national survey of psychotherapy with people with learning disabilities, *Clinical Psychology Forum*, 129: 14–18.

National Health Service (NHS) (undated) *Adult Improving Access to Psychological Therapies Programme* [https://www.england.nhs.uk/mental-health/adults/iapt/; accessed 20 November 2019].

National Institutes of Health (NIH) (1985) Electroconvulsive therapy, *NIH Consensus Statement Online*, 5: 1–23.

Neale, B.M., Medland, S., Ripke, P. et al. (2010) Case-control genome-wide association study of attention-deficit/hyperactivity disorder, *Journal of the American Academy of Child and Adolescent Psychiatry*, 49: 906–20.

Neto, D., Lambaz, R., Aguiar, P. et al. (2008) Effectiveness of sequential combined treatment in comparison with treatment as usual in preventing relapse in alcohol dependence, *Alcohol and Alcoholism*, 43: 661–68.

Neumeister, A., Praschak-Rieder, N., Hesselmann, B. et al. (1997) Rapid tryptophan depletion in drug-free depressed patients with seasonal affective disorder, *American Journal of Psychiatry*, 154: 1153–55.

New, A.S., Buchsbaum, M.S., Hazlett, E.A. et al. (2004) Fluoxetine increases relative metabolic rate in prefrontal cortex in impulsive aggression, *Psychopharmacology*, 176: 451–58.

Newby, J.M. and McElroy, E. (2019) The impact of internet-delivered cognitive behavioural therapy for health anxiety on cyberchondria, *Journal of Anxiety Disorders*, 69: 102150 [https://doi.org/10.1016/j.janxdis.2019.102150].

Newby, J.M., Smith, J.M., Uppal, S. et al. (2018) Internet-based cognitive behavioral therapy versus psychoeducation control for illness anxiety disorder and somatic symptom disorder: a randomized controlled trial, *Journal of Consulting and Clinical Psychology*, 86: 89–98.

Newcomb, M.D. (1985) The role of perceived relative parent personality in the development of heterosexuals, homosexuals, and transvestites, *Archives of Sexual Behavior*, 14: 147–64.

Newman, C.F., Leahy, R.L., Beck, A.T. et al. (2002) *Bipolar Disorder: A Cognitive Therapy Approach*, Washington, DC: American Psychological Association.

Newton-Howes, G., Tyrer, P., Anagnostakis, K. et al. (2010) The prevalence of personality disorder, its comorbidity with mental state disorders, and its clinical significance in community mental health teams, *Social Psychiatry and Psychiatric Epidemiology*, 45: 453–60.

NICE (2009a) *Guidance on the use of electroconvulsive therapy*, Technology Appraisal Guidance TA59, London: NICE [https://www.nice.org.uk/guidance/ta59].

NICE (2009b) *Depression in adults: recognition and management*, Clinical Guideline CG90, London: NICE [https://www.nice.org.uk/guidance/cg90].

Nicholson, T.R., Aybek, S., Craig, T. et al. (2016) Life events and escape in conversion disorder, *Psychological Medicine*, 46: 2617–26.

Nielsen, G., Stone, J., Matthews, A. et al. (2015) Physiotherapy for functional motor disorders: a consensus recommendation, *Journal of Neurology, Neurosurgery, and Psychiatry*, 86: 1113–19.

Nigg, J.T. and Goldsmith, H.H. (1994) Genetics of personality disorders: perspectives from personality and psychopathology research, *Psychological Bulletin*, 115: 346–80.

Nikolaev, A., McLaughlin, T., O'Leary, D.D. et al. (2009) APP binds DR6 to trigger axon pruning and neuron death via distinct caspases, *Nature*, 457: 981–89.

Niolu, C., Barone, Y., Bianciardi, E. et al. (2015) Predictors of poor adherence to treatment in inpatients with bipolar and psychotic spectrum disorders, *Rivista Di Psichiatria*, 50: 285–94.

Noblitt, J.R. and Perskin, P.S. (2000) *Cult and Ritual Abuse: Its History, Anthropology, and Recent Discovery in Contemporary America*, Westport, CT: Praeger.

Nobre, P.J. and Pinto-Gouveia, J. (2008) Cognitive and emotional predictors of female sexual dysfunctions: preliminary findings, *Journal of Sex and Marital Therapy*, 34: 325–42.

Nocentini, U., Tedeschi, G., Migliaccio, R. et al. (2009) An exploration of anger phenomenology in multiple sclerosis, *European Journal of Neurology*, 16: 1312–17.

Nock, M.K. and Kazdin, A.E. (2005) Randomized controlled trial of a brief intervention for increasing participation in parent management training, *Journal of Consulting and Clinical Psychology*, 73: 872–79.

Noh, H.J., Tang, R., Flannick, J. et al. (2017) Integrating evolutionary and regulatory information with a multispecies approach implicates genes and pathways in obsessive-compulsive disorder, *Nature Communications*, 8: 774 [https://doi.org/10.1038/s41467-017-00831-x].

Noh, S., Kaspar, V., Wickrama, K.A. (2007) Overt and subtle racial discrimination and mental health: preliminary findings for Korean immigrants, *American Journal of Public Health*, 97: 1269–74.

Nordahl, H.M., Borkovec, T.D., Hagen, R. et al. (2018) Metacognitive therapy versus cognitive-behavioural therapy in adults with generalised anxiety disorder, *BJPsych Open*, 4: 393–400 [https://doi.org/10.1192/bjo.2018.54].

Nordahl, H.M. and Stiles, T.C. (1997) Perceptions of parental bonding in patients with various personality disorders, lifetime depressive disorders, and healthy controls, *Journal of Personality Disorders*, 11: 391–402.

Nordentoft, M., Mortensen, P.B. and Pedersen, C.B. (2011) Absolute risk of suicide after first hospital contact in mental disorder, *Archives of General Psychiatry*, 68: 1058–64.

Novakovic-Agopian, T., Kornblith, E., Abrams, G. et al. (2019) Long-term effects of executive function training among veterans with chronic TBI, *Brain Injury*, 33: 1513–21.

Noyes, R., Stuart, S.P., Langbehn, D.R. et al. (2003) Test of an interpersonal model of hypochondriasis, *Psychosomatic Medicine*, 65: 292–300.

Nugent, A.C., Milham, M.P., Bain, E.E. et al. (2006) Cortical abnormalities in bipolar disorder investigated with MRI and voxel-based morphometry, *Neuroimage*, 30: 485–97.

Nutt, D.J. and Law, F.D. (2000) Pharmacological and psychological aspects of drugs of abuse, in M.G. Gelder, J.J. Lopez-Ibor, Jr. and N.C. Andreasen (eds.) *New Oxford Textbook of Psychiatry*, Oxford: Oxford University Press.

Oakley, D.A. (1999) Hypnosis and conversion hysteria: a unifying model, in P. Halligan and A.S. David (eds.) *Conversion Hysteria: Towards a Neuropsychological Account*, Hove: Psychology Press.

O'Donoghue, B., Lyne, J.P., Fanning, F. et al. (2014) Social class mobility in first episode psychosis and the association with depression, hopelessness and suicidality, *Schizophrenia Research*, 157: 8–11.

O'Donovan, M.C. and Owen, M.J. (2016) The implications of the shared genetics of psychiatric disorders, *Nature Medicine*, 22: 1214–19.

Oei, T.P. and Raylu, N. (2004) Familial influence on offspring gambling: a cognitive mechanism for transmission of gambling behavior in families, *Psychological Medicine*, 34: 1279–88.

O'Farrell, T.J. and Fals-Stewart, W. (2000) Behavioral couples therapy for alcoholism and drug abuse, *Journal of Drug Abuse Treatment*, 18: 51–54.

Öhman, A. and Mineka, S. (2001) Fears, phobias, and preparedness: toward an evolved module of fear and fear learning, *Psychological Review*, 108: 483–522.

Oke, S. and Kanigsberg, E. (1991) Occupational therapy in the treatment of individuals with multiple personality disorder, *Canadian Journal of Occupational Therapy*, 58: 234–40.

Okechukwu, C.A., El Ayadi, A.M., Tamers, S.L. et al. (2012) Household food insufficiency, financial strain, work–family spillover, and depressive symptoms in the working class: the Work, Family, and Health Network study, *American Journal of Public Health*, 102: 126–33.

Okur Güney, Z.E., Sattel, H., Witthöft, M. et al. (2019) Emotion regulation in patients with somatic symptom and related disorders: a systematic review, *PLoS One*, 14: e0217277 [https://doi.org/10.1371/journal.pone.0217277].

Olaya, B., Moneta, M.V., Miret, M. et al. (2018) Epidemiology of panic attacks, panic disorder and the moderating role of age: results from a population-based study, *Journal of Affective Disorders*, 241: 627–33.

Oldershaw, A., Lavender, T., Sallis, H. et al. (2015) Emotion generation and regulation in anorexia nervosa: a systematic review and meta-analysis of self-report data, *Clinical Psychology Review*, 39: 83–95.

Ollendick, T.H. and Davis, T.E., III (2013) One-session treatment for specific phobias: a review of Öst's single-session exposure with children and adolescents, *Cognitive Behaviour Therapy*, 42: 275–83.

Oltedal, L., Bartsch, H., Sørhaug, O.J. et al. (2017) The Global ECT-MRI Research Collaboration (GEMRIC): establishing a multi-site investigation of the neural mechanisms underlying response to electroconvulsive therapy, *Neuroimage Clinical*, 14: 422–32.

O'Malley, S., Garbutt, J., Gastfriend, D. et al. (2007) Efficacy of extended-release naltrexone in alcohol-dependent patients who are abstinent before treatment, *Journal of Clinical Psychopharmacology*, 27: 507–12.

Onder, G., Zanetti, O., Giacobini, E. et al. (2005) Reality orientation therapy combined with cholinesterase inhibitors in Alzheimer's disease: randomised controlled trial, *British Journal of Psychiatry*, 187: 450–55.

Ong, A., Fuller-Rowell, T. and Burrow, A. (2009) Racial discrimination and the stress process, *Journal of Personality and Social Psychology*, 96: 1259–71.

Oppenheimer, R., Howells, K., Palmer, R.L. et al. (1985) Adverse sexual experience in childhood and clinical eating disorders: a preliminary description, *Journal of Psychiatric Research*, 19: 357–61.

Ortiz-Medina, M.B., Perea, M., Torales, J. et al. (2018) Cannabis consumption and psychosis or schizophrenia development, *International Journal of Social Psychiatry*, 64: 690–704.

Osborn, A.J., Mathias, J.L., Fairweather-Schmidt, A.K. et al. (2017) Anxiety and comorbid depression following traumatic brain injury in a community-based sample of young, middle-aged and older adults, *Journal of Affective Disorders*, 213: 214–21.

Osman, S., Cooper, M., Hackmann, A. et al. (2004) Spontaneously occurring images and early memories in people with body dysmorphic disorder, *Memory*, 12: 428–36.

Ospina, M.B., Krebs Seida, J., Clark, B. et al. (2008) Behavioural and developmental interventions for autism spectrum disorder: a clinical systematic review, *PloS One*, 3: e3755 [https://doi.org/10.1371/journal.pone.0003755].

Ost, J., Easton, S., Hope, L. et al. (2017) Latent variables underlying the memory beliefs of chartered clinical psychologists, hypnotherapists, and undergraduates, *Memory*, 25: 57–68.

Öst, L.-G. (2014) The efficacy of acceptance and commitment therapy: an updated systematic review and meta-analysis. *Behaviour Research and Therapy*, 61: 105–21.

Öst, L.G. and Hellström, K. (1997) Blood-injury-injection phobia, in G.C.L. Davey (ed.) *Phobias: A Handbook of Theory, Research & Treatment*, New York: Wiley.

Otgaar, H., Howe, M.L., Patihis, L. et al. (2019) The return of the repressed: the persistent and problematic claims of long-forgotten trauma, *Perspectives on Psychological Science*, 14: 1072–95.

Ovesey, L. and Person, E. (1973) Gender identity and sexual pathology in men: a psychodynamic analysis of heterosexuality, transsexualism, and transvestism, *Journal of the American Academy of Psychoanalysis*, 1: 53–72.

Oviedo-Joekes, E., Brissette, S., Marsh, D. et al. (2009) Diacetylmorphine versus methadone for the treatment of opioid addiction, *New England Journal of Medicine*, 361: 777–86.

Ovuga, E., Oyok, T.O. and Moro, E.B. (2008) Post traumatic stress disorder among former child soldiers attending a rehabilitative service and primary school education in northern Uganda, *African Health Sciences*, 8: 136–41.

Owen, M., Liddell, M. and McGuffin, P. (1994) Alzheimer's disease, *British Medical Journal*, 308: 672–73.

Pacchiarotti, I., Bond, D.J., Baldessarini, R.J. et al. (2013) The International Society for Bipolar Disorders (ISBD) task force report on antidepressant use in bipolar disorders, *American Journal of Psychiatry*, 170: 1249–62.

Pappa, S., Ntella, V., Giannakas, T. et al. (2020) Prevalence of depression, anxiety, and insomnia among healthcare workers during the COVID-19 pandemic: a systematic review and meta-analysis, *Brain, Behavior, and Immunity*, 88: 901–7.

Parikh, M.S., Kolevzon, A. and Hollander, E. (2008) Psychopharmacology of aggression in children and adolescents with autism: a critical review of efficacy and tolerability, *Journal of Child and Adolescent Psychopharmacology*, 18: 157–78.

Paris, J. (1996) Antisocial personality disorder: a biopsychosocial model, *Canadian Journal of Psychiatry*, 41: 75–80.

Paris, J. (2008) Clinical trials of treatment for personality disorders, *Psychiatric Clinics of North America*, 31: 517–26.

Paris, J. and Zweig-Frank, H. (2001) A 27-year follow-up of patients with borderline personality disorder, *Comprehensive Psychiatry*, 42: 482–87.

Park, J., Sung, J.Y., Kim, D.K. et al. (2018) Genetic association of human Corticotropin-Releasing Hormone Receptor 1 (CRHR1) with internet gaming addiction in Korean male adolescents, *BMC Psychiatry*, 18: 396 [https://doi.org/10.1186/s12888-018-1974-6].

Park, N.W., Proulx, G.B. and Towers, W.M. (1999) Evaluation of the Attention Process Training programme, *Neuropsychological Rehabilitation*, 9: 135–54.

Parnas, J., Cannon, T., Schulsinger, F. and Mednick, S.A. (1995) Early predictors of onset and course of schizophrenia: results from the Copenhagen High-Risk Study, in H. Häfner and W.F. Gattaz (eds.) *Search for the Causes of Schizophrenia*, vol. 3, Berlin: Springer.

Partonen, T. and Lonnqvist, J. (1998) Seasonal affective disorder, *Lancet*, 352: 1369–74.

Parvizi, J., Anderson, S.W., Martin, C.O. et al. (2001) Pathological laughter and crying: a link to the cerebellum, *Brain*, 124: 1708–19.

Patel, V., Musara, T., Butau, T. et al. (1995) Concepts of mental illness and medical pluralism in Harare, *Psychological Medicine*, 25: 485–93.

Patihis, L. and Pendergrast, M. (2019) Reports of recovered memories of abuse in therapy in a large age-representative U.S. national sample: therapy type and decade comparisons, *Clinical Psychological Science*, 7: 3–21.

Patti, F., Armato, M., Trojano, M. et al. (2009) Cognitive impairment and its relation with disease measures in mildly disabled patients with relapsing-remitting multiple sclerosis: baseline results from the Cognitive Impairment in Multiple Sclerosis (COGIMUS) study, *Multiple Sclerosis*, 15: 779–88.

Pavlov, I.P. ([1927] 1960) *Conditioned Reflexes* (ed. and trans. G.V. Anrep), New York: Dover.

Pehek, E.A., Nocjar, C., Roth, B.L. et al. (2006) Evidence for the preferential involvement of 5-HT2A serotonin receptors in stress- and drug-induced dopamine release in the rat medial prefrontal cortex, *Neuropsychopharmacology*, 31: 265–77.

Pelham, W.E., Carlson, C., Sams, S.E. et al. (1993) Separate and combined effects of methylphenidate and behavior modification on boys with attention deficit/hyperactivity in the classroom, *Journal of Consulting and Clinical Psychology*, 61: 506–15.

Peralta, V. and Cuesta, M.J. (1992) Influence of cannabis abuse on schizophrenic psychopathology, *Acta Psychiatrica Scandinavica*, 85: 127–30.

Perkins, S., Schmidt, U., Eisler, I. et al. (2005) Why do adolescents with bulimia nervosa choose not to involve their parents in treatment?, *European Child and Adolescent Psychiatry*, 14: 376–85.

Perreira, K.M. and Sloan, F. (2001) Life events and alcohol consumption among mature adults: a longitudinal analysis, *Journal of Studies on Alcohol*, 62: 501–8.

Petras, H., Kellam, S.G., Brown, C.H. et al. (2008) Developmental epidemiological courses leading to antisocial personality disorder and violent and criminal behavior: effects by young adulthood of a universal preventive intervention in first- and second-grade classrooms, *Drug and Alcohol Dependence*, 95: S45–S59.

Petry, N.M. (2005) Gamblers Anonymous and cognitive-behavioral therapies for pathological gamblers, *Journal of Gambling Studies*, 21: 27–33.

Petry, N.M., Weinstock, J., Ledgerwood, D.M. et al. (2008) A randomized trial for brief interventions for problem and pathological gamblers, *Journal of Consulting and Clinical Psychology*, 76: 318–28.

Pevalin, D.J., Reeves, A., Baker, E. et al. (2017) The impact of persistent poor housing conditions on mental health: a longitudinal population-based study, *Preventive Medicine*, 105: 304–10.

Pharoah, F., Mari, J., Rathbone, J. et al. (2010) Family intervention for schizophrenia, *Cochrane Database of Systematic Reviews*, 12: CD000088 [https://doi.org/10.1002/14651858.CD000088. pub3].

Phillipou, A., Castle, D.J. and Rossell, S.L. (2019) Direct comparisons of anorexia nervosa and body dysmorphic disorder: a systematic review, *Psychiatry Research*, 274: 129–37.

Phillips, K.A. (1996) *The Broken Mirror*, New York: Oxford University Press.

Phillips, K.A. (2004) Psychosis in body dysmorphic disorder, *Journal of Psychiatric Research*, 38: 63–72.

Phillips, K.A., Keshaviah, A., Dougherty, D. et al. (2016) Pharmacotherapy relapse prevention in body dysmorphic disorder: a double-blind placebo-controlled trial, *American Journal of Psychiatry*, 173: 887–95.

Phillips, K.A., Menard, W., Fay, C. et al. (2006a) Gender similarities and differences in 200 individuals with body dysmorphic disorder, *Comprehensive Psychiatry*, 47: 77–87.

Phillips, K.A., Menard, W., Pagano, M.E. et al. (2006b) Delusional versus nondelusional body dysmorphic disorder: clinical features and course of illness, *Journal of Psychiatric Research*, 40: 95–104.

Phillips, K.A., Pinto, A., Hart, A.S. et al. (2012) A comparison of insight in body dysmorphic disorder and obsessive-compulsive disorder, *Journal of Psychiatric Research*, 46: 1293–99.

Phillips, K.A., Quinn, G. and Stout, R.L. (2008) Functional impairment in body dysmorphic disorder: a prospective, follow-up study, *Journal of Psychiatric Research*, 42: 701–7.

Phillips, K.A. and Rasmussen, S.A. (2004) Change in psychosocial functioning and quality of life of patients with body dysmorphic disorder treated with fluoxetine: a placebo-controlled study, *Psychosomatics*, 45: 438–44.

Piccinelli, M. and Wilkinson, G. (2000) Gender differences in depression: critical review, *British Journal of Psychiatry*, 177: 486–92.

Pickering, T.A., Wyman, P.A., Schmeelk-Cone, K. et al. (2018) Diffusion of a peer-led suicide preventive intervention through school-based student peer and adult networks, *Frontiers in Psychiatry*, 9: 598 [https://doi.org/10.3389/fpsyt.2018.00598].

Pigot, M., Loo, C. and Sachdev, P. (2008) Repetitive transcranial magnetic stimulation as treatment for anxiety disorders, *Expert Review of Neurotherapeutics*, 8: 1449–55.

Piper, A. and Merskey, H. (2004) The persistence of folly: a critical examination of dissociative identity disorder. Part I. The excesses of an improbable concept, *Canadian Journal of Psychiatry*, 49: 592–600.

Pirkola, S., Isometsä, E., Aro, H. et al. (2005) Childhood adversities as risk factors for adult mental disorders, *Social Psychiatry and Epidemiology*, 40: 769–77.

Pisani, A.R., Wyman, P.A., Gurditta, K. et al. (2018) Mobile phone intervention to reduce youth suicide in rural communities: field test, *JMIR Mental Health*, 5: e10425 [https://doi.org/10.2196/10425].

Pithers, W.D. (1990) Relapse prevention with sexual aggressors: a method for maintaining therapeutic gain and enhancing external supervision, in W.L. Marshall, D.R. Laws and H.E. Barbaree (eds.) *Handbook of Sexual Assault: Issues, Theories, and Treatment of the Offender*, New York: Plenum Press.

Piwowarczyk, A., Horvath, A., Lukasik, J. et al. (2018) Gluten- and casein-free diet and autism spectrum disorders in children: a systematic review, *European Journal of Nutrition*, 57: 433–40.

Pjerk, E., Winkler, D. and Kasper, S. (2005) Pharmacotherapy of seasonal affective disorder, *CNS Spectrums*, 10: 664–69.

Pjerk, E., Winkler, D., Statsny, J. et al. (2004) Bright light therapy in seasonal affective disorder – does it suffice?, *European Neuropsychopharmacology*, 14: 347–51.

Poli, R. and Agrimi, E. (2012) Internet addiction disorder: prevalence in an Italian student population, *Nordic Journal of Psychiatry*, 66: 55–59.

Pompoli, A., Furukawa, T.A., Efthimiou, O. et al. (2018) Dismantling cognitive-behaviour therapy for panic disorder: a systematic review and component network meta-analysis, *Psychological Medicine*, 48: 1945–53.

Pope, K.S. and Feldman-Summers, S. (1992) National survey of psychologists' sexual and physical abuse history and their evaluation of training and competence in these areas, *Professional Psychology: Research and Practice*, 23: 353–61.

Poulton, R., Caspi, A., Moffitt, T.E. et al. (2000) Children's self-reported psychotic symptoms and adult schizophreniform disorder: a 15-year longitudinal study, *Archives of General Psychiatry*, 57: 1053–58.

Powers, A.R., III, Kelley, M.S. and Corlett, P.R. (2017) Varieties of voice-hearing: psychics and the psychosis continuum, *Schizophrenia Bulletin*, 43: 84–98.

Prescott, C.A. and Kendler, K.S. (1999) Genetic and environmental contributions to alcohol abuse and dependence in a population-based sample of male twins, *American Journal of Psychiatry*, 156: 34–40.

Preti, A., Girolamo, G.D., Vilagut, G. et al. (2009) The epidemiology of eating disorders in six European countries: results of the ESEMeD-WMH project, *Journal of Psychiatric Research*, 43: 1125–32

Project MATCH Research Group (1998) Matching alcoholism treatments to client heterogeneity: project MATCH three-year drinking outcomes, *Alcoholism: Clinical and Experimental Research*, 22: 1300–11.

Pruessner, J.C., Champagne, F., Meaney, M.J. et al. (2004) Dopamine release in response to a psychological stress in humans and its relationship to early life maternal care: a positron emission tomography study using [11C]raclopride, *Journal of Neuroscience*, 24: 2825–31.

Pulikkan, J., Mazumder, A. and Grace, T. (2019) Role of the gut microbiome in autism spectrum disorders, *Advances in Experimental and Medical Biology*, 1118: 253–69.

Putnam, F.W. (1997) *Dissociation in Children and Adolescents*, New York: Guilford Press.

Quirk, S.E., Berk, M., Pasco, J.A. et al. (2017) The prevalence, age distribution and comorbidity of personality disorders in Australian women, *Australian and New Zealand Journal of Psychiatry*, 51: 141–50.

Rachman, S. (2003) *The Treatment of Obsessions*, Oxford: Oxford University Press.

Raine, A., Reynolds, C. and Venables, P.H. (1998) Fearlessness, stimulation seeking, and large body size at 3 years as early predispositions to childhood aggression at age 11 years, *Archives of General Psychiatry*, 55: 745–51.

Rajkumar, R.P. (2015) The impact of disrupted childhood attachment on the presentation of psychogenic erectile dysfunction: an exploratory study, *Journal of Sexual Medicine*, 12: 798–803.

Ralevski, E., Sanislow, C.A. and Grilo, C.M. (2005) Avoidant personality disorder and social phobia: distinct enough to be separate disorders?, *Acta Psychiatrica Scandinavica*, 112: 208–14.

Ramacciotti, C.E., Coli, E., Marazziti, D. et al. (2013) Therapeutic options for binge eating disorder, *Eating and Weight Disorders*, 18: 3–9.

Ramos, V., Canta, G., de Castro, F. et al. (2016) The relation between attachment, personality, internalizing, and externalizing dimensions in adolescents with borderline personality disorder, *Bulletin of the Menninger Clinic*, 80: 213–33.

Rampello, L., Nicoletti, F. and Nicoletti, F. (2000) Dopamine and depression: therapeutic implications, *CNS Drugs*, 13: 35–45.

Ramsay, J.R. (2010) CBT for adult ADHD: adaptations and hypothesized mechanisms of change, *Journal of Cognitive Psychotherapy*, 24: 37–45.

Rapee, R., Mattick, R. and Murrell, E. (1986) Cognitive mediation of anxiety and panic: a cognitive account, *Journal of Behavior Therapy and Experimental Psychiatry*, 17: 245–53.

Rassin, E., Muris, P., Franken, I. et al. (2008) The feature-positive effect and hypochondriacal concerns, *Behaviour Research and Therapy*, 46: 263–69.

Raynsford, J. (2019) Antidepressant discontinuation can be problematic for patients but relapse rates might be reduced with cognitive behavioural therapy or mindfulness-based cognitive therapy, *Evidence-Based Nursing*, 22: 112 [https://doi.org/10.1136/ebnurs-2019-103085].

Razali, M.S. (1995) Psychiatrists and folk healers in Malaysia, *World Health Forum*, 16: 56–58.

Razali, S.M. and Najib, M.A. (2000) Help-seeking pathways among Malay psychiatric patients, *International Journal of Social Psychiatry*, 46: 281–89.

Rea, M., Tompson, M., Miklowitz, D. et al. (2003) Family-focused treatment versus individual treatment for bipolar disorder: results of a randomized clinical trial, *Journal of Consulting and Clinical Psychology*, 71: 482–92.

Read, J., Harrop, C., Geekie, J. et al. (2018) An audit of ECT in England 2011–2015: usage, demographics, and adherence to guidelines and legislation, *Psychology and Psychotherapy*, 91: 263–77.

Rees, S., Steel, Z., Creamer, M. et al. (2014) Onset of common mental disorders and suicidal behavior following women's first exposure to gender based violence: a retrospective, population-based study, *BMC Psychiatry*, 14: 312 [https://doi.org/10.1186/s12888-014-0312-x].

Regier, D.A., Rae, D.S., Narrow, W.E. et al. (1998) Prevalence of anxiety disorders and their comorbidity with mood and addictive disorders, *British Journal of Psychiatry*, 173 (suppl. 34): 24–26.

Reichborn-Kjennerud, T., Czajkowski, N., Neale, M.C. et al. (2007) Genetic and environmental influences on dimensional representations of DSM-IV cluster C personality disorders: a population-based multivariate twin study, *Psychological Medicine*, 37: 645–53.

Reichelt, K.L., Knivsberg, A.M., Lind, G. et al. (1991) Probable etiology and possible treatment of childhood autism, *Brain Dysfunction*, 4: 308–19.

Reid, W.H. and Gacono, C. (2000) Treatment of antisocial personality, psychopathy, and other characterologic antisocial syndromes, *Behavioral Science and Law*, 18: 647–62.

Reine, I., Novo, M. and Hammarström, A. (2008) Does transition from an unstable labour market position to permanent employment protect mental health? Results from a 14-year follow-up of school-leavers, *BMC Public Health*, 8: 159 [https://doi.org/10.1186/1471-2458-8-159].

Research Units on Pediatric Psychopharmacology Autism Network (2005) Risperidone treatment of autistic disorder: longer-term benefits and blinded discontinuation after 6 months, *American Journal of Psychiatry*, 162: 1361–69.

Rey, J.M., Walter, G., Plapp, J.M. et al. (2000) Family environment in attention deficit hyperactivity, oppositional defiant and conduct disorders, *Australia and New Zealand Journal of Psychiatry*, 34: 453–57.

Rho, M.J., Lee, H., Lee, T.H. et al. (2017) Risk factors for internet gaming disorder: psychological factors and internet gaming characteristics, *International Journal of Environmental Research and Public Health*, 15: 40 [https://doi.org/10.3390/ijerph15010040].

Rice, M.E., Harris, G.T. and Cormier, C.A. (1992) An evaluation of a maximum security therapeutic community for psychopaths and other mentally disordered offenders, *Law and Human Behavior*, 16: 399–412.

Rice, M.E., Quinsey, V.L. and Harris, G.T. (1991) Sexual recidivism among child molesters released from a maximum security psychiatric institution, *Journal of Consulting and Clinical Psychology*, 59: 381–86.

Rief, W. and Barsky, A.J. (2005) Psychobiological perspectives on somatoform disorders, *Psychoneuroendocrinology*, 30: 996–1002.

Rief, W., Heitmüller, A.M., Reisberg, K. et al. (2006) Why reassurance fails in patients with unexplained symptoms – an experimental investigation of remembered probabilities, *PLoS Medicine*, 3: e269 [https://doi.org/10.1371/journal.pmed.0030269].

Rief, W., Pilger, F., Ihle, D. et al. (2004) Psychobiological aspects of somatoform disorders: contributions of monoaminergic transmitter systems, *Neuropsychobiology*, 49: 24–29.

Riley, D.E. (2002) Reversible transvestic fetishism in a man with Parkinson's disease treated with selegiline, *Clinical Neuropharmacology*, 25: 234–37.

Rinne, T., Van den Brink, W., Wouters, L. et al. (2002) SSRI treatment of borderline personality disorder: a randomized, placebo-controlled clinical trial for female patients with borderline personality disorder, *American Journal of Psychiatry*, 159: 2048–54.

Ritsher, J.E.B., Warner, V., Johnson, J.G. et al. (2001) Inter-generation longitudinal study of social class and depression: a test of social causation and social selection models, *British Journal of Psychiatry*, 178 (suppl. 40): S84–S90.

Rivera, P., Elliott, T.R., Berry, J.W. et al. (2007) Predictors of caregiver depression among community-residing families living with traumatic brain injury, *NeuroRehabilitation*, 22: 3–8.

Rivera, P.A., Elliott, T.R., Berry, J.W. et al. (2008) Problem-solving training for family caregivers of persons with traumatic brain injuries: a randomized controlled trial, *Archives of Physical Medicine and Rehabilitation*, 89: 931–41.

Rizzo, M.A., Hadjimichael, O.C., Preiningerova, J. et al. (2004) Prevalence and treatment of spasticity reported by multiple sclerosis patients, *Multiple Sclerosis*, 10: 589–95.

Roberts, N.P., Kitchiner, N.J., Kenardy, J. et al. (2019) Early psychological intervention following recent trauma: a systematic review and meta-analysis, *European Journal of Psychotraumatology*, 10: 1695486 [https://doi.org/10.1080/20008198.2019.1695486].

Robins, A.L., Siegel, P.T. and Moye, A. (1995) Family therapy versus individual therapy for anorexia: impact on family conflict, *International Journal of Eating Disorders*, 17: 313–22.

Robinson, D.G., Woerner, M.G., McMeniman, M. et al. (2004) Symptomatic and functional recovery from a first episode of schizophrenia or schizoaffective disorder, *American Journal of Psychiatry*, 161: 473–79.

Robinson, M., Lee, B.Y. and Hane, F.T. (2017) Recent progress in Alzheimer's disease research, part 2: genetics and epidemiology, *Journal of Alzheimer's Disease*, 57: 317–30.

Robinson, T.E. and Berridge, K.C. (2008) The incentive sensitization theory of addiction: some current issues, *Philosophical Transactions of the Royal Society of London B: Biological Sciences*, 363: 3137–46.

Rocca, P., Marchiaro, L., Cocuzza, E. et al. (2002) Treatment of borderline personality disorder with risperidone, *Journal of Clinical Psychiatry*, 63: 241–44.

Rocchi, A., Pellegrini, S. and Siciliano, G. (2003) Causative and susceptibility genes for Alzheimer's disease: a review, *Brain Research Bulletin*, 61: 1–24.

Roecklein, K.A. and Rohan, K.J. (2005) Seasonal affective disorder: an overview and update, *Psychiatry*, 2: 20–26.

Roeleveld, N., Zielhuis, G.A. and Gabreels, F. (1997) The prevalence of mental retardation: a critical review of recent literature, *Developmental Medicine and Child Neurology*, 39: 125–32.

Roelofs, K., Hoogduin, K.A., Keijsers, G.P. et al. (2002) Hypnotic susceptibility in patients with conversion disorder, *Journal of Abnormal Psychology*, 111: 390–95.

Roepke, S., Merkl, A., Dams, A. et al. (2008) Preliminary evidence of improvement of depressive symptoms but not impulsivity in cluster B personality disorder patients treated with quetiapine: an open label trial, *Pharmacopsychiatry*, 41: 176–81.

Roerig, J.L., Steffen, K.J., Mitchell, J.E. et al. (2010) Laxative abuse: epidemiology, diagnosis and management, *Drugs*, 70: 1487–503.

Rogers, C.R. (1961) *On Becoming a Person*, Boston, MA: Houghton Mifflin.

Rogers, S.L., Farrow, M.R., Doody, R.S. et al. (1998) A 24-week, double-blind, placebo-controlled trial of donepezil in patients with Alzheimer' disease, *Neurology*, 50: 136–45.

Rohan, K.J. (2008) *Coping with the Seasons: A Cognitive-behavioral Approach to Seasonal Affective Disorder – Therapist Guide*, New York: Oxford University Press.

Rohan, K.J., Meyerhoff, J., Ho, S.Y. et al. (2016) Outcomes one and two winters following cognitive-behavioral therapy or light therapy for seasonal affective disorder, *American Journal of Psychiatry*, 173: 244–51.

Rohan, K., Roecklein, K. and Haaga, D. (2009) Biological and psychological mechanisms of seasonal affective disorder: a review and integration, *Current Psychiatry Reviews*, 5: 1 [https://doi.org/10.2174/157340009787315299].

Romme, M. and Escher, S. (2000) *Making Sense of Voices*, London: MIND Publications.

Rosati, G. (2001) The prevalence of multiple sclerosis in the world: an update, *Neurological Sciences*, 22: 117–39.

Rose, S., Bisson, J. and Wessely, W. (2002) Psychological debriefing for preventing post-traumatic stress disorder (PTSD), *Cochrane Database of Systematic Reviews*, 2: CD000560 [https://doi.org/10.1002/14651858.CD000560].

Rosen, J.C. (1996) Body dysmorphic disorder: assessment and treatment, in J.K. Thompson (ed.) *Body Image, Eating Disorders, and Obesity*, Washington, DC: American Psychological Association.

Rosenthal, N.E., Sack, D.A., Gillin, J.C. et al. (1984) Seasonal affective disorder: a description of the syndrome and preliminary findings with light therapy, *Archives of General Psychiatry*, 41: 72–80.

Rösler, A. and Witztum, E. (1998) Treatment of men with paraphilia with a long-acting analogue of gonadotropin-releasing hormone, *New England Journal of Medicine*, 338: 416–22.

Ross, J.A., Gliebus, G. and Van Bockstaele, E.J. (2018) Stress induced neural reorganization: a conceptual framework linking depression and Alzheimer's disease, *Progress in Neuropsychopharmacology and Biological Psychiatry*, 85: 136–51.

Rossel, R. (1998) Multiplicity: the challenges of finding place in experience, *Journal of Constructivist Psychology*, 11: 221–40.

Rossell, S.L. and Boundy, C.L. (2005) Are auditory-verbal hallucinations associated with auditory affective processing deficits?, *Schizophrenia Research*, 78: 95–106.

Roth, A. and Fonagy, P. (1998) *What Works for Whom? A Critical Review of Psychotherapy Research*, New York: Guilford Press.

Routsalainen, J., Serra, C., Marine, A. et al. (2008) Systematic review of interventions for reducing occupational stress in health care workers, *Scandinavian Journal of Work, Environment, and Health*, 34: 169–78.

Roy, A., Roy, M., Deb, S. et al. (2015) Are opioid antagonists effective in attenuating the core symptoms of autism spectrum conditions in children: a systematic review, *Journal of Intellectual Disability Research*, 59: 293–306.

Rubinstein, S. and Caballero, B. (2000) Is Miss America an undernourished role model?, *Journal of the American Medical Association*, 283: 1569.

Rudd, M.D. (2000) The suicidal mode: a cognitive-behavioral model of suicidality, *Suicide and Life Threatening Behavior*, 30: 18–33.

Ruffolo, J.S., Phillips, K.A., Menard, W. et al. (2006) Comorbidity of body dysmorphic disorder and eating disorders: severity of psychopathology and body image disturbance, *International Journal of Eating Disorders*, 39: 11–19.

Ruocco, A.C., Amirthavasagam, S., Choi-Kain, L.W. et al. (2013) Neural correlates of negative emotionality in borderline personality disorder: an activation-likelihood-estimation meta-analysis, *Biological Psychiatry*, 73: 153–60.

Rush, A.J., Trivedi, M.H., Ibrahim, H.M. et al. (2003) The 16-item Quick Inventory of Depressive Symptomatology (QIDS) clinical rating (QIDS-C) and self-report (QIDS-SR): a psychometric evaluation in patients with chronic major depression, *Biological Psychiatry*, 54: 573–583.

Russell, D.W., Clavél, F.D., Cutrona, C.E. et al. (2018) Neighborhood racial discrimination and the development of major depression, *Journal of Abnormal Psychology*, 127: 150–59.

Russell, F. (2007) Portage in the UK: recent developments, *Child: Care, Health and Development*, 33: 677–83.

Russell, G.F.M., Szmukler, G.I., Dare, C. et al. (1987) An evaluation of family therapy in anorexia nervosa and bulimia nervosa, *Archives of General Psychiatry*, 44: 1047–56.

Russell, V.A., Sagvolden, T. and Johansen, E.B. (2005) Animal models of attention-deficit hyper-activity disorder, *Behavioral and Brain Functions*, 1: 9 [https://doi.org/10.1186/1744-9081-1-9].

Russon, L. and Alison, D. (1998) Palliative care does not mean giving up, *British Medical Journal*, 317: 195–97.

Ryle, A. and Kerr, I.B. (2002) *Introducing Cognitive Analytic Therapy: Principles and Practice*, Chichester: Wiley-Blackwell.

Sachs-Ericsson, N., Plant, E.A. and Blazer, D.G. (2005) Racial differences in the frequency of depressive symptoms among community dwelling elders: the role of socio-economic factors, *Aging and Mental Health*, 9: 201–9.

Sadeh, N. and Verona, E. (2008) Psychopathic personality traits associated with abnormal selective attention and impaired cognitive control, *Neuropsychology*, 22: 669–80.

Sagvolden, T., Johansen, E.B., Aase, H. et al. (2005) A dynamic developmental theory of attention-deficit/hyperactivity disorder (ADHD) predominantly hyperactive/impulsive and combined subtypes, *Behavioral and Brain Sciences*, 28: 397–419.

Saiz, P.A., Garcia-Portilla, M.P., Florez, G. et al. (2009) Polymorphisms of the IL-1 gene complex are associated with alcohol dependence in Spanish Caucasians: data from an association study, *Alcoholism: Clinical and Experimental Research*, 33: 2147–53.

Sala, M., Caverzasi, E., Marraffini, E. et al. (2008) Cognitive memory control in borderline personality disorder patients, *Psychological Medicine*, 20: 1–9.

Salcedo, S., Gold, A.K., Sheikh, S. et al. (2016) Empirically supported psychosocial interventions for bipolar disorder: current state of the research, *Journal of Affective Disorders*, 201: 203–14.

Salekin, R.T. (2002) Psychopathy and therapeutic pessimism: clinical lore or clinical reality?, *Clinical Psychology Review*, 22: 79–112.

Salerno, L., Rhind, C., Hibbs, R. et al. (2016) An examination of the impact of care giving styles (accommodation and skilful communication and support) on the one year outcome of adolescent anorexia nervosa: testing the assumptions of the cognitive interpersonal model in anorexia nervosa, *Journal of Affective Disorders*, 191: 230–36.

Salkovskis, P. and Kirk, J. (1997) Obsessive-compulsive disorder, in D.M. Clark and C.G. Fairburn (eds.) *Science and Practice of Cognitive Behaviour Therapy*, Oxford: Oxford University Press.

Salokangas, R.K.R., From, T., Luutonen, S. et al. (2018) Adverse childhood experiences leads to perceived negative attitude of others and the effect of adverse childhood experiences on depression in adulthood is mediated via negative attitude of others, *European Psychiatry*, 54: 27–34.

Samuel, D.B. and Widiger, T.A. (2008) A meta-analytic review of the relationships between the five-factor model and DSM-IV-TR personality disorders: a facet level analysis, *Clinical Psychology Review*, 28: 1326–42.

Sandberg, S. (2005) The biopsychosocial context of ADHD, *Behavioral and Brain Sciences*, 28: 441–42.

Sareen, J. (2014) Posttraumatic stress disorder in adults: impact, comorbidity, risk factors, and treatment, *Canadian Journal of Psychiatry*, 59: 460–67.

Sassi, R.B., Stanley, J.A., Axelson, D. et al. (2005) Reduced NAA levels in the dorsolateral prefrontal cortex of young bipolar patients, *American Journal of Psychiatry*, 162: 2109–15.

Sax, W. (2014) Ritual healing and mental health in India, *Transcultural Psychiatry*, 51: 829–49.

Sayal, K., Prasad, V., Daley, D. et al. (2018) ADHD in children and young people: prevalence, care pathways, and service provision, *Lancet Psychiatry*, 5: 175–86.

Scarella, T.M., Boland, R.J. and Barsky, A.J. (2019) Illness anxiety disorder: psychopathology, epidemiology, clinical characteristics, and treatment, *Psychosomatic Medicine*, 81: 398–407.

Scharkow, M., Festl, R. and Quandt, T. (2014) Longitudinal patterns of problematic computer game use among adolescents and adults – a 2-year panel study, *Addiction*, 109: 1910–17.

Schell, T.L., Marshall, G.N. and Jaycox, L.H. (2004) All symptoms are not created equal: the prominent role of hyperarousal in the natural course of posttraumatic psychological distress, *Journal of Abnormal Psychology*, 113: 189–97.

Schenk, D., Barbour, R., Dunn, W. et al. (1999) Immunization with amyloid beta attenuates Alzheimer-disease-like pathology in the PDAPP mouse, *Nature*, 400: 173–77.

Scher, C.D., Ingram, R.E. and Segal, Z.V. (2005) Cognitive reactivity and vulnerability: empirical evaluation of construct activation and cognitive diatheses in unipolar depression, *Clinical Psychology Review*, 25: 487–510.

Scherbaum, N., Kluwig, J., Specka, M. et al. (2005) Group psychotherapy for opiate addicts in methadone maintenance treatment – a controlled trial, *European Addiction Research*, 11: 163–71.

Schiffer, B., Krueger, T., Paul, T. et al. (2008) Brain response to visual sexual stimuli in homosexual pedophiles, *Journal of Psychiatry and Neuroscience*, 33: 23–33.

Schipper, H.M. (2011) Apolipoprotein E: implications for AD neurobiology, epidemiology and risk assessment, *Neurobiology of Aging*, 32: 778–90.

Schmidt, U., Lee, S., Beecham, J. et al. (2007) A randomized controlled trial of family therapy and cognitive behavior therapy guided self-care for adolescents with bulimia nervosa and related disorders, *American Journal of Psychiatry*, 164: 591–98.

Schonert-Reichl, K.A., Oberle, E., Lawlor, M.S. et al. (2015) Enhancing cognitive and social-emotional development through a simple-to-administer mindfulness-based school program for elementary school children: a randomized controlled trial, *Developmental Psychology*, 51: 52–66.

Schooler, C., Caplan, L.J., Revell, A.J. et al. (2008) Brain lesion and memory functioning: short-term memory deficit is independent of lesion location, *Psychonomic Bulletin Review*, 15: 521–27.

Schulze, L., Schmahl, C. and Niedtfeld, I. (2016) Neural correlates of disturbed emotion processing in borderline personality disorder: a multimodal meta-analysis, *Biological Psychiatry*, 79: 97–106.

Schulze, L.N., Stenzel, U., Leipert, J. et al. (2019) Improving medication adherence with telemedicine for adults with severe mental illness, *Psychiatric Services*, 70: 225–28.

Schulze-Rauschenbach, S.C., Harms, U., Schlaepfer, T.E. et al. (2005) Distinctive neurocognitive effects of repetitive transcranial magnetic stimulation and electroconvulsive therapy in major depression, *British Journal of Psychiatry*, 186: 410–16.

Schwartz, C.E., Foley, F.W., Rao, S.M. et al. (1999) Stress and course of disease in multiple sclerosis, *Behavioral Medicine*, 25: 110–16.

Schwarz, A. (2016) *ADHD Nation: Children, Doctors, Big Pharma and the Making of an American Epidemic*, New York: Scribner.

Schwitzer, A.M., Rodriguez, L.E., Thomas, C. et al. (2001) The eating disorders NOS diagnostic profile among college women, *Journal of the American College of Health*, 49: 157–66.

Scocco, P., Barbieri, I. and Frank, E. (2007) Interpersonal problem areas and onset of panic disorder, *Psychopathology*, 40: 8–13.

Scott, J. (2001) Cognitive-behavioral management of patients with bipolar disorder who relapse while on lithium prophylaxis, *Journal of Clinical Psychiatry*, 62: 556–59.

Scott, J., Stanton, B., Garland, A. et al. (2000) Cognitive vulnerability in patients with bipolar disorder, *Psychological Medicine*, 30: 467–72.

Sel, R. (1997) Dissociation as complex adaptation, *Medical Hypothesis*, 48: 2205–8.

Seligman, M.E.P. (1971) Phobias and preparedness, *Behavior Therapy*, 2: 307–20.

Seligman, M.E.P. (1975) *Helplessness*, San Francisco, CA: Freeman.

Sella, F., Re, A.M., Lucangeli, D. et al. (2019) Strategy selection in ADHD characteristics children: a study in arithmetic, *Journal of Attention Disorders*, 23: 87–98.

Semrud-Clikeman, M., Nielsen, K.H., Clinton, A. et al. (1999) An intervention approach for the children with teacher- and parent-identified attentional difficulties, *Journal of Learning Disabilities*, 32: 581–90.

Seto, M.C. and Barbaree, H.E. (1999) Psychopathy, treatment behavior, and sex offender recidivism, *Journal of Interpersonal Violence*, 14: 1235–48.

Shahmanesh, M., Wayal, S., Cowan, F. et al. (2009) Suicidal behavior among female sex workers in Goa, India: the silent epidemic, *American Journal of Public Health*, 99: 1239–46.

Shallice, T. (1988) *From Neuropsychology to Mental Structure*, Cambridge: Cambridge University Press.

Shapiro, D.A. and Shapiro, D. (1983) Comparative therapy outcome research: methodological implications of meta-analysis, *Journal of Consulting and Clinical Psychology*, 45: 543–51.

Shapiro, F. (1995) *Eye Movement Desensitization and Reprocessing: Basic Principles*, New York: Guilford Press.

Sharma, A. and Couture, J. (2014) A review of the pathophysiology, etiology, and treatment of attention-deficit hyperactivity disorder (ADHD), *Annals of Pharmacotherapy*, 48: 209–25.

Sharpe, L. (2002) A reformulated cognitive-behavioral model of problem gambling: a biopsycho-social perspective, *Clinical Psychology Review*, 22: 1–25.

Shaw, M.E., Moores, K.A., Clark, R.C. et al. (2009) Functional connectivity reveals inefficient working memory systems in post-traumatic stress disorder, *Psychiatry Research: Neuroimaging*, 172: 235–41.

Shea, M.T., Edelen, M.O., Pinto, A. et al. (2009) Improvement in borderline personality disorder in relationship to age, *Acta Psychiatrica Scandinavica*, 119: 143–48.

Shea, M.T., Elkin, I., Imber, S.D. et al. (1992) Course of depressive symptoms over follow-up: findings from the National Institute of Mental Health Treatment of Depression Collaborative Research Program, *Archives of General Psychiatry*, 49: 782–87.

Shelton, R.C., Haman, K.L., Rapaport, M.H. et al. (2006) A randomized, double-blind, active-control study of sertraline versus venlafaxine XR in major depressive disorder, *Journal of Clinical Psychiatry*, 67: 1674–81.

Shensa, A., Escobar-Viera, C.G., Sidani, J.E. et al. (2017) Problematic social media use and depressive symptoms among U.S. young adults: a nationally-representative study, *Social Science and Medicine*, 182: 150–57.

Shi, J., Baxter, L.C. and Kuniyoshi, S.M. (2014) Pathologic and imaging correlates of cognitive deficits in multiple sclerosis: changing the paradigm of diagnosis and prognosis, *Cognitive and Behavioral Neurology*, 27: 1–7.

Shum, D., Fleming, J., Gill, H. et al. (2011) A randomized controlled trial of prospective memory rehabilitation in adults with traumatic brain injury, *Journal of Rehabilitation Medicine*, 43: 216–23.

Sibley, M.H., Rohde, L.A., Swanson, J.M. et al. (2018) Late-onset ADHD reconsidered with comprehensive repeated assessments between ages 10 and 25, *American Journal of Psychiatry*, 175: 140–49.

Siegel, J.Z. and Crockett, M.J. (2013) How serotonin shapes moral judgment and behaviour, *Annals of the New York Academy of Sciences*, 1299: 42–51.

Siev, J. and Chambless, D.L. (2007) Specificity of treatment effects: cognitive therapy and relaxation for generalized anxiety and panic disorders, *Journal of Consulting and Clinical Psychology*, 75: 513–22.

Sigitova, E., Fi ar, Z., Hroudová, J. et al. (2017) Biological hypotheses and biomarkers of bipolar disorder, *Psychiatry and Clinical. Neurosciences*, 71: 77–103.

Simeon, D., Greenberg, J., Nelson, D. et al. (2005) Dissociation and posttraumatic stress 1 year after the World Trade Center disaster: follow-up of a longitudinal survey, *Journal of Clinical Psychiatry*, 66: 231–37.

Sinclair, J.D. (2001) Evidence about the use of naltrexone and for different ways of using it in the treatment of alcoholism, *Alcohol and Alcoholism*, 36: 2–10.

Sinha, S., Anderson, J., John, V. et al. (2000) Recent advances in the understanding of the processing of APP to beta amyloid peptide, *Annals of the New York Academy of Sciences*, 920: 206–8.

Sinnakaruppan, I. and Williams, D.M. (2001) Head injury and family carers: a critical appraisal of case management programmes in the community, *Brain Injury*, 15: 653–72.

Sirey, J.A., Bruce, M.L., Alexopoulos, G.S. et al. (2001) Stigma as a barrier to recovery: perceived stigma and patient-rated severity of illness as predictors of antidepressant drug adherence, *Psychiatric Services*, 52: 1615–20.

Skinner, B.F. (1953) *Science and Human Behavior*, New York: Macmillan.

Skokauskas, N. and Satkeviciute, R. (2007) Adolescent pathological gambling in Kaunas, Lithuania, *Nordic Journal of Psychiatry*, 61: 86–91.

Skre, I., Onstad., S., Torgersen, S. et al. (2000) The heritability of common phobic fear: a twin study of a clinical sample, *Journal of Anxiety Disorders*, 14: 549–62.

Skrzypek, S., Wehmeier, P.M. and Remschmidt, H. (2001) Body image assessment using body size estimation in recent studies on anorexia nervosa: a brief review, *European Child and Adolescent Psychiatry*, 10: 215–21.

Slutske, W.S., Meier, M.H., Zhu, G. et al. (2009) The Australian Twin Study of Gambling (OZ-GAM): rationale, sample description, predictors of participation, and a first look at sources of individual differences in gambling involvement, *Twin Research and Human Genetics*, 12: 63–78.

Smink, F.R., van Hoeken, D. and Hoek, H.W. (2012) Epidemiology of eating disorders: incidence, prevalence and mortality rates, *Current Psychiatry Reports*, 14: 406–14.

Smith, D.P., Fairweather-Schmidt, A.K., Harvey, P.W. et al. (2018) How does routinely delivered cognitive-behavioural therapy for gambling disorder compare to 'gold standard' clinical trial?, *Clinical Psychology and Psychotherapy*, 25: 302–10.

Smyth, B.P., O'Brien, M. and Barry, J. (2000) Trends in treated opiate misuse in Dublin: the emergence of chasing the dragon, *Addiction*, 95: 1217–23.

Sobanski, E. and Schmidt, M.H. (2000) 'Everybody looks at my pubic bone': a case report of an adolescent patient with body dysmorphic disorder, *Acta Psychiatrica Scandinavica*, 101: 80–82.

Sobczak, S., Riedel, W.J., Booij, I. et al. (2002) Cognition following acute tryptophan depletion: difference between first-degree relatives of bipolar disorder patients and matched healthy control volunteers, *Psychological Medicine*, 32: 503–15.

Södersten, P., Bergh, C., Leon, M. et al. (2017) Cognitive behavior therapy for eating disorders versus normalization of eating behaviour, *Physiology and Behavior*, 174: 178–90.

Sohlberg, M.M., Johnson, L., Paule, L. et al. (2001) *Attention Process Training-II: A Program to Address Attentional Deficits for Persons with Mild Cognitive Dysfunction*, 2nd edition, Wake Forest, NC: Lash & Associates.

Sohlberg, M.M. and Mateer, C.A. (2001) Improving attention and managing attentional problems: adapting rehabilitation techniques to adults with ADD, *Annals of the New York Academy of Sciences*, 931: 359–75.

Soo, C. and Tate, R. (2007) Psychological treatment for anxiety in people with traumatic brain injury, *Cochrane Database of Systematic Reviews*, 3: CD005239 [https://doi.org/10.1002/14651858.CD005239.pub2].

Sorenson, M., Janusek, L. and Mathews, H. (2013) Psychological stress and cytokine production in multiple sclerosis: correlation with disease symptomatology, *Biological Research for Nursing*, 15: 226–33.

Spada, M.M., Giustina, L., Rolandi, S. et al. (2015) Profiling metacognition in gambling disorder, *Behavioural and Cognitive Psychotherapy*, 43: 614–22.

Spanos, N.P. (1994) Multiple identity enactments and multiple personality disorder: a sociocognitive perspective, *Psychological Bulletin*, 116: 143–65.

Sparks, D.L., Sabbagh, M.N., Connor, D.J. et al. (2005) Atorvastatin for the treatment of mild to moderate Alzheimer disease: preliminary results, *Archives of Neurology*, 62: 753–57.

Spiegel, D.A. and Barlow, D.H. (2000) Generalized anxiety disorders, in M.G. Gelder, J.J. Lopez-Ibor, Jr. and N.C. Andreasen (eds.) *New Oxford Textbook of Psychiatry*, Oxford: Oxford University Press.

Spielberger, C.D., Gorsuch, R.L., Lushene, R. et al. (1983) *Manual for the State-Trait Anxiety Inventory (STAI)*, Palo Alto, CA: Consulting Psychologists Press.

Starcevic, V. and Janca, A. (2018) Pharmacotherapy of borderline personality disorder: replacing confusion with prudent pragmatism, *Current Opinion in Psychiatry*, 31: 69–73.

Steege, M.W., Wacker, D.P., Cigrand, K.C. et al. (1990) Use of negative reinforcement in the treatment of self-injurious behavior, *Journal of Applied Behavior Analysis*, 23: 459–67.

Stefanopoulou, E., Hogarth, H., Taylor, M. et al. (2020) Are digital interventions effective in reducing suicidal ideation and self-harm? A systematic review, *Journal of Mental Health*, 29: 207–16.

Steiger, H., Gauvin, L., Engelberg, M.J. et al. (2005) Mood- and restraint-based antecedents to binge episodes in bulimia nervosa: possible influences of the serotonin system, *Psychological Medicine*, 35: 1553–62.

Stein, K.F. and Corte, C. (2003) Reconceptualizing causative factors and intervention strategies in the eating disorders: a shift from body image to self-concept impairments, *Archives of Psychiatric Nursing*, 17: 57–66.

Steiner, H., Smith, C., Rosenkranz, R.T. et al. (1991) The early care and feeding of anorexics, *Child Psychiatry and Human Development*, 21: 163–67.

Stella, L., D'Ambra, C., Mazzeo, F. et al. (2005) Naltrexone plus benzodiazepine aids abstinence in opioid-dependent patients, *Life Sciences*, 77: 2717–22.

Stephens, D.L., Collins, M.D. and Dodder, R.A. (2005) A longitudinal study of employment and skill acquisition among individuals with developmental disabilities, *Research in Developmental Disabilities*, 26: 469–86.

Steward, K.A., Kennedy, R., Novack, T.A. et al. (2018) The role of cognitive reserve in recovery from traumatic brain injury, *Journal of Head Trauma Rehabilitation*, 33: E18–E27.

Stewart, R.M. and Brown, R.I. (1988) An outcome study of Gamblers Anonymous, *British Journal of Psychiatry*, 152: 284–88.

Stewart, S.M., Kennard, B.D., Lee, P.W. et al. (2005) Hopelessness and suicidal ideation among adolescents in two cultures, *Journal of Child Psychology and Psychiatry*, 46: 364–72.

Stitzer, M. and Petry, N. (2006) Contingency management for treatment of substance abuse, *Annual Review of Clinical Psychology*, 2: 411–34.

Stoffers-Winterling, J.M., Völlm, B.A., Rücker, G. et al. (2012) Psychological therapies for people with borderline personality disorder, *Cochrane Database of Systematic Reviews*, 8: CD005652 [https://doi.org/10.1002/14651858.CD005652.pub2].

Stone, J., Carson, A., Duncan, R. et al. (2010) Who is referred to neurology clinics? The diagnoses made in 3781 new patients, *Clinical Neurology and Neurosurgery*, 112: 747–51.

Storebø, O.J., Krogh, H.B., Ramstad, E. et al. (2015) Methylphenidate for attention-deficit/hyperactivity disorder in children and adolescents: Cochrane systematic review with meta-analyses and trial sequential analyses of randomised clinical trials, *British Medical Journal*, 351: h5203 [https://doi.org/10.1136/bmj.h5203].

Story, T.J. and Craske, M.G. (2008) Responses to false physiological feedback in individuals with panic attacks and elevated anxiety sensitivity, *Behaviour Research and Therapy*, 46: 1001–8.

Strang, J., Sheridan, J., Hunt, C. et al. (2005) The prescribing of methadone and other opioids to addicts: national survey of GPs in England and Wales, *British Journal of General Practice*, 55: 444–51.

Strange, P.G. (1992) *Brain Biochemistry and Brain Disorders*, New York: Oxford University Press.

Striegel-Moore, R.H., Franko, D.L., Thompson, D. et al. (2004) Changes in weight and body image over time in women with eating disorders, *International Journal of Eating Disorders*, 36: 315–27.

Striegel-Moore, R.H. and Smolak, L. (2000) The influence of ethnicity on eating disorders in women, in R.M. Esler and M. Hersen (eds.) *Handbook of Gender, Culture, and Health*, Mahwah, NJ: Erlbaum.

Strong, R.E., Marchant, B.K., Reimherr, F.W. et al. (2009) Narrow-band blue-light treatment of seasonal affective disorder in adults and the influence of additional nonseasonal symptoms, *Depression and Anxiety*, 26: 273–78.

Strosahl, K.D., Hayes, S.C., Wilson, K.G. et al. (2004) An ACT primer: core therapy processes, intervention strategies, and therapist competencies, in S.C. Hayes and K.D. Strosahl (eds.) *A Practical Guide to Acceptance and Commitment Therapy*, New York: Springer.

Struewing, J.P. and Gray, G.C. (1990) An epidemic of respiratory complaints exacerbated by mass psychogenic illness in a military recruit population, *American Journal of Epidemiology*, 132: 1120–29.

Suchy, Y., Eastvold, A.D., Strassberg, D.S. et al. (2014) Understanding processing speed weaknesses among pedophilic child molesters: response style vs. neuropathology, *Journal of Abnormal Psychology*, 123: 273–85.

Sukhodolsky, D.G. and Ruchkin, V.V. (2004) Association of normative beliefs and anger with aggression and antisocial behavior in Russian male juvenile offenders and high school students, *Journal of Abnormal Child Psychology*, 32: 225–36.

Sullivan, G.M. and Neria, Y. (2009) Pharmacotherapy in post-traumatic stress disorder: evidence from randomized controlled trials, *Current Opinion in Investigational Drugs*, 10: 35–45.

Sullivan, H.S. (1953) *The Interpersonal Theory of Psychiatry*, New York: Norton.

Sumaya, I., Rienzi, B.M., Deegan, J.F., II et al. (2001) Bright light treatment decreases depression in institutionalized older adults: a placebo-controlled crossover study, *Journals of Gerontology A: Medical Sciences*, 56: M356–M360.

Suppes, T., Baldessarini, R.J., Faedda, G.L. et al. (1991) Risk of recurrence following discontinuation of lithium treatment in bipolar disorder, *Archives of General Psychiatry*, 48: 1082–88.

Surtees, P.G., Wainwright, N.W., Willis-Owen, S.A. et al. (2006) Social adversity, the serotonin transporter (5-HTTLPR) polymorphism and major depressive disorder, *Biological Psychiatry*, 58: 451–56.

Svartberg, M., Stiles, T.C. and Seltzer, M.H. (2004) Randomized, controlled trial of the effectiveness of short-term dynamic psychotherapy and cognitive therapy for cluster C personality disorders, *American Journal of Psychiatry*, 161: 810–17.

Sveen, U., Røe, C., Sigurdardottir, S. et al. (2016) Rehabilitation pathways and functional independence one year after severe traumatic brain injury, *European Journal of Physical and Rehabilitation Medicine*, 52: 650–61.

Swannell, S., Martin, G., Page, A. et al. (2012) Child maltreatment, subsequent non-suicidal self-injury and the mediating roles of dissociation, alexithymia and self-blame, *Child Abuse and Neglect*, 36: 572–84.

Swift, W., Maher, L. and Sunjic, S. (1999) Transitions between routes of heroin administration: a study of Caucasian and Indochinese heroin users in south-western Sydney, Australia, *Addiction*, 94: 71–82.

Swinson, R. and McCabe, R.E. (2019) Pharmacotherapy for specific phobia in adults, *UpToDate.com* [https://www.uptodate.com/contents/pharmacotherapy-for-specific-phobia-in-adults].

Tarrier, N., Kinney, C., McCarthy, E. et al. (2000) Two-year follow-up of cognitive-behavioural therapy and supportive counselling in the treatment of persistent symptoms in chronic schizophrenia, *Journal of Consulting and Clinical Psychology*, 68: 917–22.

Tasca, G.A. and Balfour, L. (2014) Attachment and eating disorders: a review of current research, *International Journal of Eating Disorders*, 47: 710–17.

Tatangelo, G., McCabe, M., Mellor, D. et al. (2016) A systematic review of body dissatisfaction and sociocultural messages related to the body among preschool children, *Body Image*, 18: 86–95.

Taylor, B., Miller, E., Farringdon, C.P. et al. (1999) MMR vaccine and autism: no epidemiological evidence of a causal association, *Lancet*, 353: 2026–29.

Tcheremissine, O.V. and Lieving, L.M. (2006) Pharmacological aspects of the treatment of conduct disorder in children and adolescents, *CNS Drugs*, 20: 549–65.

Teasdale, J.D. (1993) Emotion and two kinds of meaning: cognitive therapy and applied cognitive science, *Behaviour Research and Therapy*, 31: 339–54.

Teasdale, J.D., Segal, Z. and Williams, J.M.G. (1995) How does cognitive therapy prevent depressive relapse and why should attentional control (mindfulness) training help?, *Behaviour Research and Therapy*, 33: 25–39.

Teasdale, J.D., Segal, Z.V., Williams, J.M.G. et al. (2000) Prevention of relapse/recurrence in major depression by mindfulness-based cognitive therapy, *Journal of Consulting and Clinical Psychology*, 68: 615–23.

Tee, S.F., Chow, T.J., Tang, P.Y. et al. (2010) Linkage of schizophrenia with TPH2 and 5-HTR2A gene polymorphisms in the Malay population, *Genetics and Molecular Research*, 9: 1274–78.

Terman, M. (1988) On the question of mechanism in phototherapy for seasonal affective disorder: considerations of clinical efficacy and epidemiology, *Journal of Biological Rhythms*, 3: 155–72.

Terman, M.A., Terman, J.S., Quitkin, F.M. et al. (1989) Light therapy for seasonal affective disorder: a review of efficacy, *Neuropsychopharmacology*, 2: 1–22.

Thaler, K., Delivuk, M., Chapman, A. et al. (2011) Second-generation antidepressants for seasonal affective disorder, *Cochrane Database of Systematic Reviews*, 12: CD008591 [https://doi.org/10.1002/14651858.CD008591.pub2].

Thapar, A., O'Donovan, M. and Owen, M.J. (2005) The genetics of attention deficit hyperactivity disorder, *Human Molecular Genetics*, 14 (suppl. 2): R275–R282.

Tharyan, P. and Adams, C.E. (2005) Electroconvulsive therapy for schizophrenia, *Cochrane Database of Systematic Reviews*, 2: CD000076 [https://doi.org/10.1002/14651858.CD000076.pub2].

Thaut, M.H., Peterson, D.A., McIntosh, G.C. et al. (2014) Music mnemonics aid verbal memory and induce learning-related brain plasticity in multiple sclerosis, *Frontiers in Human Neuroscience*, 8: 395 [https://doi.org/10.3389/fnhum.2014.00395].

Thomas, J.J., Vartanian, L.R. and Brownell, K.D. (2009) The relationship between eating disorder not otherwise specified (EDNOS) and officially recognized eating disorders: meta-analysis and implications for DSM, *Psychological Bulletin*, 135: 407–33.

Thompson, C. and Briggs, M. (2000) Support for carers of people with Alzheimer's type dementia, *Cochrane Database of Systematic Reviews*, 2: CD000454 [https://doi.org/10.1002/14651858.CD000454].

Thompson, C., Raheja, S.K. and King, E.A. (1995) A follow-up study of seasonal affective disorder, *British Journal of Psychiatry*, 167: 380–84.

Thompson-Brenner, H. (2016) Improving psychotherapy for anorexia nervosa: introduction to the special section on innovative treatment approaches, *Psychotherapy*, 53: 220–22.

Thorgaard, M.V., Frostholm, L., Walker, L.S. et al. (2017) Effects of maternal health anxiety on children's health complaints, emotional symptoms, and quality of life, *European Child and Adolescent Psychiatry*, 26: 591–60.

Tienari, P., Wynne, L.C., Moring, J. et al. (2000) Finnish adoptive family study: sample selection and adoptee DSM-III-R diagnoses, *Acta Psychiatrica Scandinavica*, 101: 433–43.

Timko, C., Moos, R.H., Finney, J.W. et al. (2000) Long-term outcomes of alcohol use disorders: comparing untreated individuals with those in Alcoholics Anonymous and formal treatment, *Journal of Studies in Alcohol*, 61: 529–40.

Tizaoui, K. (2018) Multiple sclerosis genetics: results from meta-analyses of candidate-gene association studies, *Cytokine*, 106: 154–64.

Togher, L., McDonald, S., Tate, R. et al. (2013) Training communication partners of people with severe traumatic brain injury improves everyday conversations: a multicenter single blind clinical trial, *Journal of Rehabilitation Medicine*, 45: 637–45.

Toh, W.L., Grace, S.A., Rossell, S.L. et al. (2020) Body parts of clinical concern in anorexia nervosa versus body dysmorphic disorder: a cross-diagnostic comparison, *Australasian Psychiatry*, 28: 134–39.

Tolin, D.F., Maltby, N., Diefenbach, G.J. et al. (2004) Cognitive-behavioral therapy for medication nonresponders with obsessive-compulsive disorder: a wait-list-controlled open trial, *Journal of Clinical Psychiatry*, 65: 922–31.

Tondi, L., Ribani, L., Bottazzi, M. et al. (2007) Validation therapy (VT) in nursing home: a case-control study, *Archives of Gerontology and Geriatrics*, 44 (suppl. 1): 407–11.

Tondo, L., Vázquez, G.H. and Baldessarini, R.J. (2017) Depression and mania in bipolar disorder, *Current Neuropharmacology*, 15: 353–58.

Torgersen, S., Kringlen, E. and Cramer, V. (2001) The prevalence of personality disorders in a community sample, *Archives of General Psychiatry*, 58: 590–96.

Torgersen, S., Lygren, S., Oien, P.A. et al. (2000) A twin study of personality disorders, *Comprehensive Psychiatry*, 41: 416–25.

Touchette, P.E., McDonald, R.F. and Langer, S.N. (1985) A scatter plot for identifying stimulus control of problem behavior, *Journal of Applied Behavior Analysis*, 18: 343–51.

Treasure, T. (2001) *The Mental Health Act and Eating Disorders*, London: Institute of Psychiatry, Division of Psychological Medicine, Eating Disorders Research Unit.

Tremlett, H.L., Luscombe, D.K. and Wiles, C.M. et al. (2001) Prescribing for multiple sclerosis patients in general practice: a case-control study, *Journal of Clinical Pharmacy and Therapeutics*, 26: 437–44.

Troisi, A., Massaroni, P. and Cuzzolaro, M. (2005) Early separation anxiety and adult attachment style in women with eating disorders, *British Journal of Clinical Psychology*, 44: 89–97.

Tripp, G. and Wickens, J.R. (2009) Neurobiology of ADHD, *Neuropharmacology*, 57: 579–89.

Truax, C.B. (1966) Reinforcement and nonreinforcement in Rogerian psychotherapy, *Journal of Abnormal Psychology*, 71: 1–9.

Tsai, S.J., Hong, C.J., Liou, Y.J. et al. (2009) Tryptophan hydroxylase 2 gene is associated with major depression and antidepressant treatment response, *Progress in Neuropsychopharmacology and Biological Psychiatry*, 33: 637–41.

Tsai, Y.F., Yeh, S.H. and Tsai, H.H. (2005) Prevalence and risk factors for depressive symptoms among community-dwelling elders in Taiwan, *International Journal of Geriatric Psychiatry*, 20: 1097–102.

Tsao, J.C.I., Mystkowski, J.L., Zucker, B.G. et al. (2002) Effects of cognitive behaviour therapy for panic disorder on comorbid conditions: replication and extension, *Behaviour Therapy*, 33: 493–509.

Tucker, T.K. and Ritter, A.J. (2000) Naltrexone in the treatment of heroin dependence: a literature review, *Drug and Alcohol Review*, 19: 73–82.

Tulloch, H., Greenman, P.S. and Tassé, V. (2015) Post-traumatic stress disorder among cardiac patients: prevalence, risk factors, and considerations for assessment and treatment, *Behavioral Sciences*, 5: 27–40.

Turner, D. and Briken, P. (2017) Treatment of paraphilic disorders in sexual offenders or men with risk of sexual offending with luteinizing hormone-releasing hormone agonists: an updated systematic review, *Journal of Sexual Medicine*, 15: 77–93.

Turner, N.E., Preston, D.L., Saunders, C. et al. (2009) The relationship of problem gambling to criminal behavior in a sample of Canadian male federal offenders, *Journal of Gambling Studies*, 25: 153–69.

Tyrer, P., Reed, G.M. and Crawford, M.J. (2015) Classification, assessment, prevalence, and effect of personality disorder, *Lancet*, 385: 717–26.

Tyrer, P., Seivewright, N., Ferguson, B. et al. (1993) The Nottingham study of neurotic disorder: effect of personality status on response to drug treatment, cognitive therapy and self-help over two years, *British Journal of Psychiatry*, 162: 219–26.

Úbeda-Gómez, J., León-Palacios, M.G., Escudero-Pérez, S. et al. (2015) Relationship between self-focused attention, mindfulness and distress in individuals with auditory verbal hallucinations, *Cognitive Neuropsychiatry*, 20: 482–88.

Ulfvebrand, S., Birgegard, A., Norring, C. et al. (2015) Psychiatric comorbidity in women and men with eating disorders: results from a large clinical database, *Psychiatry Research*, 230: 294–99.

Ullrich, S., Borkenau, P. and Marneros, A. (2001) Personality disorders in offenders: categorical versus dimensional approaches, *Journal of Personality Disorders*, 15: 442–49.

Ulvik, A., Kvale, R., Wentzel-Larsen, T. et al. (2008) Quality of life 2–7 years after major trauma, *Acta Anaesthesiologica Scandinavica*, 52: 195–201.

US Department of Education (2006) *Teaching Children with Attention Deficit Hyperactivity Disorder: Instructional strategies and practices*, Washington, DC: US Department of Education, Office of Special Education and Rehabilitative Services, Office of Special Education Programs [https://files.eric.ed.gov/fulltext/ED495483.pdf].

Van Apeldoorn, F.J., Timmerman, M.E., Mersch, P.P. et al. (2010) A randomized trial of cognitive-behavioral therapy or selective serotonin reuptake inhibitor or both combined for panic disorder with or without agoraphobia: treatment results through 1-year follow-up, *Journal of Clinical Psychiatry*, 71: 574–86.

Van Assche, L., Van de Ven, L., Vandenbulcke, M. et al. (2020) Ghosts from the past? The association between childhood interpersonal trauma, attachment and anxiety and depression in late life, *Aging and Mental Health*, 24: 898–905.

Van den Akker, L.E., Beckerman, H., Collette, E.H. et al. (2016) Effectiveness of cognitive behavioral therapy for the treatment of fatigue in patients with multiple sclerosis: a systematic review and meta-analysis, *Journal of Psychosomatic Research*, 90: 33–42.

Van den Bosch, L.M., Koeter, M.W., Stijnen, T. et al. (2005) Sustained efficacy of dialectical behaviour therapy for borderline personality disorder, *Behaviour Research and Therapy*, 43: 1231–41.

Van der Naalt, J., Timmerman, M.E., de Koning, M.E. et al. (2017) Early predictors of outcome after mild traumatic brain injury (UPFRONT): an observational cohort study, *Lancet Neurology*, 16: 532–40.

Van der Sande, R., Buskens, E., Hart, E. et al. (1997) Psychosocial intervention following suicide attempt: a systematic review of treatment interventions, *Acta Psychiatrica Scandinavica*, 96: 43–50.

Van der Watt, A.S.J., Nortje, G., Kola, L. et al. (2017) Collaboration between biomedical and complementary and alternative care providers: barriers and pathways, *Qualitative Health Research*, 27: 2177–88.

Van Dessel, N., den Boeft, M., van der Wouden, J.C. et al. (2014) Non-pharmacological interventions for somatoform disorders and medically unexplained physical symptoms (MUPS) in adults, *Cochrane Database of Systematic Reviews*, 11: CD011142 [https://doi.org/10.1002/14651858.CD011142.pub2].

Vandiver, D.M. (2006) Female sex offenders: a comparison of solo offenders and co-offenders, *Violence and Victims*, 21: 339–54.

Van Grootheest, D., Cath, D., Beekman, A. et al. (2005) Twin studies on obsessive–compulsive disorder: a review, *Twin Research and Human Genetics*, 8: 450–58.

Vanheule, S., Desmet, M., Meganck, R. et al. (2014) Reliability in psychiatric diagnosis with the DSM: old wine in new barrels, *Psychotherapy and Psychosomatics*, 83: 313–14.

Van Lankveld, J.J., ter Kuile, M.M., de Groot, H.E. et al. (2006) Cognitive-behavioral therapy for women with lifelong vaginismus: a randomized waiting-list controlled trial of efficacy, *Journal of Consulting and Clinical Psychology*, 74: 168–78.

Van Trotsenburg, A.S., Vulsma, T., Rutgers van Rozenburg-Marres, S.L. et al. (2005) The effect of thyroxine treatment started in the neonatal period on development and growth of two-year-old Down syndrome children: a randomized clinical trial, *Journal of Clinical Endocrinology and Metabolism*, 90: 3304–11.

Varela, R.E. and Hensley-Maloney, L. (2009) The influence of culture on anxiety in Latino youth: a review, *Clinical Child and Family Psychology Review*, 12: 217–33.

Varese, F., Smeets, F., Drukker, M. et al. (2012) Childhood adversities increase the risk of psychosis: a meta-analysis of patient-control, prospective- and cross-sectional cohort studies, *Schizophrenia Bulletin*, 38: 661–71.

Vaughn, C.E. and Leff, J.P. (1976) The influence of family and social factors on the course of psychiatric patients, *British Journal of Psychiatry*, 129: 125–37.

Veale, D. (2004) Advances in a cognitive behavioural model of body dysmorphic disorder, *Body Image*, 1: 113–25.

Veling, W., Hoek, H.W., Wiersma, D. et al. (2010) Ethnic identity and the risk of schizophrenia in ethnic minorities: a case-control study, *Schizophrenia Bulletin*, 36: 1149–56.

Vickers, K., Jafarpour, S., Mofidibi, A. et al. (2012) The 35% carbon dioxide test in stress and panic research: overview of effects and integration of findings, *Clinical Psychology Review*, 32: 153–64.

Viding, E., Larsson, H. and Jones, A.P. (2008) Quantitative genetic studies of antisocial behaviour, *Philosophical Transactions of the Royal Society of London B: Biological Sciences*, 363: 2519–27.

Viinamäki, H., Tanskanen, A., Koivumaa-Honkanen, H. et al. (2003) Cluster C personality disorder and recovery from major depression: 24-month prospective follow-up, *Journal of Personality Disorders*, 17: 341–50.

Vitaro, F., Arseneault, L. and Tremblay, R.E. (1999) Impulsivity predicts problem gambling in low SES adolescent males, *Addiction*, 94: 565–75.

Vuilleumier, P. (2014) Brain circuits implicated in psychogenic paralysis in conversion disorders and hypnosis, *Neurophysiologie Clinique*, 44: 323–37.

Wagner, A., Aizenstein, H., Venkatraman, V.K. et al. (2006) Altered reward processing in women recovered from anorexia nervosa, *American Journal of Psychiatry*, 164: 1842–49.

Wahlberg, K.-E., Jackson, D., Haley, H. et al. (2000) Gene-environment interaction in vulnerability to schizophrenia: findings from the Finnish Adoptive Family Study of Schizophrenia, *American Journal of Psychiatry*, 154: 355–62.

Wakefield, A.J., Murch, S.H., Anthony, A. et al. (1998) Ileal-lymphoid-nodular hyperplasia, non-specific colitis, and pervasive developmental disorder in children, *Lancet*, 351: 637–41.

Wallien, M.S. and Cohen-Kettenis, P.T. (2008) Psychosexual outcome of gender-dysphoric children, *Journal of the American Academy of Child and Adolescent Psychiatry*, 47: 1413–23.

Walsh, B.T., Agras, W.S., Devlin, M.J. et al. (2000) Fluoxetine for bulimia nervosa following poor response to psychotherapy, *American Journal of Psychiatry*, 157: 1332–34.

Walshe, D.G., Lewis, E.J., Kim, S.I. et al. (2003) Exploring the use of computer games and virtual reality in exposure therapy for fear of driving following a motor vehicle accident, *Cyberpsychology and Behavior*, 6: 329–34.

Wampold, B.E. (2015) How important are the common factors in psychotherapy? An update, *World Psychiatry*, 14: 270–77.

Wang, J., Guo, W.-J., Mo, L.-L. et al. (2017) Prevalence and strong association of high somatic symptom severity with depression and anxiety in a Chinese inpatient population, *Asia Pacific Psychiatry*, 9: e12282 [https://doi.org/10.1111/appy.12282].

Wang, J.J. (2007) Group reminiscence therapy for cognitive and affective function of demented elderly in Taiwan, *International Journal of Geriatric Psychiatry*, 22: 1235–40.

Wang, S.M., Han, C., Lee, S.J. et al. (2017) Modafinil for the treatment of attention-deficit/hyperactivity disorder: a meta-analysis, *Journal of Psychiatric Research*, 84: 292–300.

Ward, A., Ramsay, R., Turnbull, S. et al. (2001) Attachment in anorexia nervosa: a transgenerational perspective, *British Journal of Medical Psychology*, 74: 497–505.

Ward, T. and Siegert, R.J. (2002) Toward a comprehensive theory of child sexual abuse: a theory knitting perspective, *Psychology, Crime, and Law*, 9: 319–51.

Wardenaar, K.J., Lim, C., Al-Hamzawi, A. et al. (2017) The cross-national epidemiology of specific phobia in the World Mental Health Surveys, *Psychological Medicine*, 47: 1744–60.

Warwick, H.M. and Salkovskis, P.M. (1990) Hypochondriasis, *Behaviour Research and Therapy*, 28: 105–17.

Watanabe, Y., Someya, T. and Nawa, H. (2010) Cytokine hypothesis of schizophrenia pathogenesis: evidence from human studies and animal models, *Psychiatry and Clinical Neurosciences*, 64: 217–30.

Watson, J.B. and Rayner, R. (1920) Conditioned emotional reaction, *Journal of Experimental Psychology*, 3: 1–14.

Watzlawick, P., Weakland, J.H. and Fisch, R. (1974) *Change: Principles of Problem Formulation and Problem Resolution*, New York: Norton.

Webb, J. and Whitaker, S. (2012) Defining learning disability, *The Psychologist*, 25: 440–43.

Wechsler, T.F., Kümpers. F. and Mühlberger, A. (2019) Inferiority or even superiority of virtual reality exposure therapy in phobias? A systematic review and quantitative meta-analysis on randomized controlled trials specifically comparing the efficacy of virtual reality exposure to gold standard in vivo exposure in agoraphobia, specific phobia, and social phobia, *Frontiers in Psychology*, 10: 1758 [https://doi.org/10.3389/fpsyg.2019.01758].

Weich, S., Sloggett, A. and Lewis, G. (1998) Social roles and gender difference in the prevalence of common mental disorders, *British Journal of Psychiatry*, 173: 489–93.

Weiner, H.L., Lemere, C.A., Maron, R. et al. (2000) Nasal administration of amyloid-beta peptide decreases cerebral amyloid burden in a mouse model of Alzheimer's disease, *Annals of Neurology*, 48: 567–79.

Weiner, L. and Avery-Clark, C. (2014) Sensate Focus: clarifying the Masters and Johnson's model, *Sexual and Relationship Therapy*, 29: 307–19.

Weinmeyer, R. (2016) Needle exchange programs' status in US politics, *American Medical Association Journal of Ethics*, 18: 252–57.

Weinstein, A. and Lejoyeux, M. (2010) Internet addiction or excessive internet use, *American Journal of Drug and Alcohol Abuse*, 36: 277–83.

Weintraub, M.J., Hall, D.L., Carbonella, J.Y. et al. (2017) Integrity of literature on expressed emotion and relapse in patients with schizophrenia verified by a p-curve analysis, *Family Process*, 56: 436–44.

Wells, A. (1995) Meta-cognition and worry: a cognitive model of generalized anxiety disorder, *Behavioural and Cognitive Psychotherapy*, 23: 301–20.

Wells, A. (2000) *Emotional Disorders and Metacognition: Innovative Cognitive Therapy*, Chichester: Wiley.

Wells, A. and Sembi, S. (2004) Metacognitive therapy for PTSD: a preliminary investigation of a new brief treatment, *Journal of Behavior Therapy*, 35: 307–18.

Wender, P.H., Wolf, L.E. and Wasserstein, J. (2001) Adults with ADHD: an overview, *Annals of the New York Academy of Sciences*, 931: 1–16.

Wenzel, A. and Beck, A.T. (2008) A cognitive model of suicidal behavior: theory and treatment, *Applied and Preventive Psychology*, 12: 189–201.

Wenzel, A., Brendle, J.R., Kerr, P.L. et al. (2007) A quantitative estimate of schema abnormality in socially anxious and non-anxious individuals, *Cognitive Behaviour Therapy*, 36: 220–29.

Werner, S., Malaspina, D. and Rabinowitz, J. (2007) Socioeconomic status at birth is associated with risk of schizophrenia: population-based multilevel study, *Schizophrenia Bulletin*, 33: 1373–78.

Werner-Seidler, A., Afzali, M.H., Chapman, C. et al. (2017) The relationship between social support networks and depression in the 2007 National Survey of Mental Health and Well-being, *Social Psychiatry and Psychiatric Epidemiology*, 52: 1463–73.

Weyers, S., Elaut, E., De Sutter, P. et al. (2009) Long-term assessment of the physical, mental, and sexual health among transsexual women, *Journal of Sexual Medicine*, 6: 752–60.

Whitaker-Azmitia, P.M. (2005) Behavioral and cellular consequences of increasing serotonergic activity during brain development: a role in autism?, *International Journal of Developmental Neuroscience*, 23: 75–83.

White, J., Greene, G., Farewell, D. et al. (2017) Improving mental health through the regeneration of deprived neighborhoods: a natural experiment, *American Journal of Epidemiology*, 186: 473–80.

Whitehouse, P.J., Struble, R.G., Clark, A.W. et al. (1982) Alzheimer disease: plagues, tangles, and the basal forebrain, *Annals of Neurology*, 12: 494.

Whittal, M.L. and Zaretsky, A. (1996) Cognitive-behavioral strategies for the treatment of eating disorders, in M.H. Pollack, M.W. Otto and J.F. Rosenbaum (eds.) *Challenges in Clinical Practice: Pharmacologic and Psychosocial Strategies*, New York: Guilford Press.

Widiger, T.A. (2011) The DSM-5 dimensional model of personality disorder: rationale and empirical support, *Journal of Personality Disorders*, 25: 222–34.

Widiger, T.A., Livesley, W.J. and Clark, L.A. (2009) An integrative dimensional classification of personality disorder, *Psychological Assessment*, 21: 243–55.

Widom, C.S., Czaja, S.J., Kozakowski, S.S. et al. (2018) Does adult attachment style mediate the relationship between childhood maltreatment and mental and physical health outcomes?, *Child Abuse and Neglect*, 76: 533–45.

Wiers, R.W. and Stacy, A.W. (eds.) (2006) *Handbook of Implicit Cognition and Addiction*, London: Sage.

Wileman, S.M., Eagles, J.M., Andrew, J.E. et al. (2001) Light therapy for seasonal affective disorder in primary care, *British Journal of Psychiatry*, 178: 311–16.

Wilkinson, R. and Pickett, K. (2018) *The Inner Level: How More Equal Societies Reduce Stress, Restore Sanity and Improve Everyone's Well-being*, London: Penguin.

Willemse-van Son, A.H., Ribbers, G.M., Verhagen, A.P. et al. (2007) Prognostic factors of long-term functioning and productivity after traumatic brain injury: a systematic review of prospective cohort studies, *Clinical Rehabilitation*, 21: 1024–37.

Willemsen-Swinkels, S.H., Buitlaar, J.K., Nijhof, G.J. et al. (1995) Failure of naltrexone hydrochloride to reduce self-injurious and autistic behavior in mentally retarded adults: double-blind placebo-controlled studies, *Archives of General Psychiatry*, 52: 766–73.

Willner, P., Rose, J., Jahoda, A. et al. (2013) Group-based cognitive-behavioural anger management for people with mild to moderate intellectual disabilities: cluster randomised controlled trial, *British Journal of Psychiatry*, 203: 288–96.

Wilson, B. (1989) Models of cognitive rehabilitation, in R.L. Wood and P.G. Eames (eds.) *Models of Brain Injury Rehabilitation*, Baltimore, MD: Johns Hopkins University Press.

Wilson, B.A. (2001) Assessment and management of people with severe brain injury and reduced states of awareness, *Brain Impairment*, 2: 52.

Wilson, B.A. (2005) The effective rehabilitation of memory-related disabilities, in P.W. Halligan and D.T. Wade (eds.) *Effectiveness of Rehabilitation for Cognitive Deficits*, New York: Oxford University Press.

Wilson, B.A., Emslie, H., Quirk, K. et al. (2005) A randomized control trial to evaluate a paging system for people with traumatic brain injury (abstract), *Brain Injury*, 19: 891–94.

Winters, K.C. and Neale, J.M. (1985) Mania and low self-esteem, *Journal of Abnormal Psychology*, 94: 282–90.

Wolfensberger, W. (1972) *The Principle of Normalization in Human Services*, Toronto: National Institutes of Mental Retardation.

Wolfensberger, W. (1983) Social role valorization: a proposed new term for the principle of normalization, *Mental Retardation*, 21: 234–39.

Wolitzky-Taylor, K.B., Horowitz, J.D., Powers, M.B. et al. (2008) Psychological approaches in the treatment of specific phobias: a meta-analysis, *Clinical Psychology Review*, 28: 1021–37.

Wolke, D., Schreier, A., Zanarini, M.C. et al. (2012) Bullied by peers in childhood and borderline personality symptoms at 11 years of age: a prospective study, *Journal of Child Psychology and Psychiatry, and Allied Disciplines*, 53: 846–55.

Wolpe, J. (1982) *The Practice of Behavior Therapy*, 3rd edition, New York: Pergamon Press.

Wong, S. and Hare, R.D. (2002) *Program Guidelines for the Institutional Treatment of Violent Psychopathic Offenders*, Toronto: Multi-Health Systems.

Wong, S., Yip, B., Mak, W. et al. (2016) Mindfulness-based cognitive therapy *v.* group psychoeducation for people with generalised anxiety disorder: randomised controlled trial, *British Journal of Psychiatry*, 209: 68–75.

Wood, S.J., Yucel, M., Velakoulis, D. et al. (2005) Hippocampal and anterior cingulate morphology in subjects at ultra-high-risk for psychosis: the role of family history of psychotic illness, *Schizophrenia Research*, 75: 295–301.

Woods, B., O'Philbin, L., Farrell, E.M. et al. (2018) Reminiscence therapy for dementia (review), *Cochrane Database of Systematic Reviews*, 3: CD001120 [https://doi.org/10.1002/14651858. CD001120.pub3].

Woods, R. and Bird, M. (1999) Non-pharmacological approaches to treatment, in G.K. Wilcock, R.S. Bucks and K. Rockwood (eds.) *Diagnosis and Management of Dementia: A Manual for Memory Disorders Teams*, Oxford: Oxford University Press.

Woods, R. and Roth, A. (1996) Effectiveness of psychological therapy with older people, in A. Roth and P. Fonagy (eds.) *What Works for Whom? A Critical Review of Psychotherapy Research*, New York: Guilford Press.

World Health Organization (WHO) (2004) *Promoting Mental Health. Concepts. Emerging evidence. Practice*, Summary Report. Geneva: WHO [https://www.who.int/mental_health/evidence/en/promoting_mhh.pdf].

World Health Organization (WHO) (2012) *Public Health Action for the Prevention of Suicide: A framework*, Geneva: WHO [https://www.who.int/mental_health/publications/prevention_suicide_2012/en/].

World Health Organization (WHO) (2017) *Suicide Rate Estimates, Age-standardized: Estimates by country*, Geneva: WHO [https://apps.who.int/gho/data/node.main.MHSUICIDEASDR?lang=en].

World Health Organization (WHO) (2018a) *International Classification of Diseases, 11th revision* (ICD-11), Geneva: WHO [https://www.who.int/classifications/icd/en/].

World Health Organization (2018b) *World Drug Report*, Geneva: WHO [https://www.unodc.org/wdr2018/].

World Health Organization (WHO) (2019) *Duration of Antidepressant Treatment*, Geneva: WHO [https://www.who.int/mental_health/mhgap/evidence/depression/q2/en/].

World Health Organization and Calouste Gulbenkian Foundation (WHO/CGF) (2014) *Social Determinants of Mental Health*, Geneva: WHO [https://www.who.int/mental_health/publications/gulbenkian_paper_social_determinants_of_mental_health/en/].

Wupperman, P., Neumann, C.S. and Axelrod, S.R. (2008) Do deficits in mindfulness underlie borderline personality features and core difficulties?, *Journal of Personality Disorder*, 22: 466–82.

Wyatt, R.B., de Jong, D.C. and Holden, C.J. (2019) Spectatoring mediates the association between penis appearance concerns and sexual dysfunction, *Journal of Sex and Marital Therapy*, 45: 328–38.

Xu, K., Lichtermann, D., Lipsky, R.H. et al. (2004) Association of specific haplotypes of D2 dopamine receptor gene with vulnerability to heroin dependence in 2 distinct populations, *Archives of General Psychiatry*, 61: 597–606.

Yale, R. (1995) *Developing Support Groups for Individuals with Early Stage Alzheimer's Disease: Planning, Implementation and Evaluation*, Baltimore, MD: Health Profession Press.

Yalom, I.D., Green, R. and Fisk, N. (1973) Prenatal exposure to female hormones: effect on psychosocial development in boys, *Archives of General Psychiatry*, 28: 554–61.

Yang, L.H., Phillips, M.R., Licht, D.M. et al. (2004) Causal attributions about schizophrenia in families in China: expressed emotion and patient relapse, *Journal of Abnormal Psychology*, 113: 592–602.

Yang, Y., Wang, C., Li, X. et al. (2019) The 5-HTTLPR polymorphism impacts moral permissibility of impersonal harmful behaviors, *Social Cognitive and Affective Neuroscience*, 14: 911–18.

Yatham, L.N., Kauer-Sant'Anna, M., Bond, D.J. et al. (2009) Course and outcome after the first manic episode in patients with bipolar disorder: prospective 12-month data from the Systematic Treatment Optimization Program for Early Mania Project, *Canadian Journal of Psychiatry*, 54: 105–12.

Yerevanian, B.I., Koek, R.J., Feusner, J.D. et al. (2004) Antidepressants and suicidal behaviour in unipolar depression, *Acta Psychiatrica Scandinavica*, 110: 452–58.

Yoon, S., Kleinman, M., Mertz, J. et al. (2019) Is social network site usage related to depression? A meta-analysis of Facebook–depression relations, *Journal of Affective Disorders*, 248: 65–72.

Young, J.E. (1999) *Cognitive Therapy for Personality Disorders: A Schema-Focused Approach*, Sarasota, FL: Professional Resource Exchange Inc.

Young, J.E., Klosko, J.S. and Weishaar, M.E. (2003) *Schema Therapy: A Practitioner's Guide*, New York: Guilford Press.

Young, J.E. and Lindemann, M.D. (1992) An integrative schema-focused model for personality disorders, *Journal of Cognitive Psychotherapy*, 6: 11–23.

Young, M.A. and Azam, O.A. (2003) Ruminative response style and the severity of seasonal affective disorder, *Cognitive Therapy and Research*, 27: 223–32.

Zablotsky, B., Black, L.I. and Blumberg, S.J. (2017) Estimated prevalence of children with diagnosed developmental disabilities in the United States, 2014–2016, *NCHS Data Brief*, 291: 1–8.

Zack, M. and Poulos, C.X. (2009) Parallel roles for dopamine in pathological gambling and psychostimulant addiction, *Current Drug Abuse Reviews*, 2: 11–25.

Zahavi, A.Y., Sabbagh, M.A., Washburn, D. et al. (2016) Serotonin and dopamine gene variation and theory of mind decoding accuracy in major depression: a preliminary investigation, *PloS One*, 11: e0150872 [https://doi.org/10.1371/journal.pone.0150872].

Zanarini, M.C., Frankenburg, F.R., Hennen, J. et al. (2005) The McLean Study of Adult Development (MSAD): overview and implications of the first six years of prospective follow-up, *Journal of Personality Disorders*, 19: 505–23.

Zanarini, M.C., Frankenburg, F.R. and Vujanovic, A.A. (2002) Inter-rater and test-retest reliability of the Revised Diagnostic Interview for Borderlines, *Journal of Personality Disorders*, 16: 270–76.

Zarros, A.C., Kalopita, K.S. and Tsakiris, S.T. (2005) Serotoninergic impairment and aggressive behavior in Alzheimer's disease, *Acta Neurobiologiae Experimentalis*, 65: 277–86.

Zerbe, K.J. (2001) The crucial role of psychodynamic understanding in the treatment of eating disorders, *Psychiatric Clinics of North America*, 24: 305–13.

Zhou, J.-N., Hofman, M.A. and Black, K. (1995) A sex difference in the human brain and its relation to transsexuality, *Nature*, 378: 68–70.

Zilbergeld, B. (1992) *The New Male Sexuality*, New York: Bantam.

Zimmerman, J. and Grosz, H.J. (1966) 'Visual' performance of a functionally blind person, *Behaviour Research and Therapy*, 4: 119–34.

Zipfel, S., Wild, B., Gross, G. et al. (2014) Focal psychodynamic therapy, cognitive behaviour therapy, and optimised treatment as usual in outpatients with anorexia nervosa (ANTOP study): randomised controlled trial, *Lancet*, 383: 127–37.

Zola, S.M. (1998) Memory, amnesia, and the issue of recovered memory: neurobiological aspects, *Clinical Psychology Review*, 18: 915–32.

Zucker, K.J. (2017) Epidemiology of gender dysphoria and transgender identity, *Sexual Health*, 14: 404–11.

Zucker, K.J. and Bradley, S.J. (1995) *Gender Identity Disorder and Psychosexual Problems in Children and Adolescents*, New York: Guilford Press.

Zucker, K.J., Green, R., Garofano, C. et al. (1994) Prenatal gender preference of mothers of feminine and masculine boys: relation to sibling sex composition and birth order, *Journal of Abnormal Child Psychology*, 22: 1–13.

Zweig-Frank, H. and Paris, J. (2002) Predictors of outcome in a 27-year follow-up of patients with borderline personality disorder, *Comprehensive Psychiatry*, 43: 103–7.

Index